TAYLOR'S CLINICAL
NURSING SKILLS

A Nursing Process Approach

TAYLOR'S CLINICAL NURSING SKILLS

A Nursing Process Approach

Pamela Evans-Smith, MSN, FNP

Clinical Nursing Instructor

University of Missouri

Columbia, Missouri

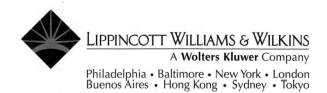

LIPPINCOTT WILLIAMS & WILKINS
A **Wolters Kluwer** Company

Philadelphia • Baltimore • New York • London
Buenos Aires • Hong Kong • Sydney • Tokyo

Senior Acquisitions Editor: Elizabeth Nieginski	*Art Director:* Carolyn O'Brien
Senior Developmental Editor: Danielle DiPalma	*Illustration Coordinator:* Brett MacNaughton
Editorial Assistant: Josh Levandowski	*Cover Designer:* Anthony Grover
Senior Production Editor: Rosanne Hallowell	*Senior Manufacturing Manager:* William Alberti
Copy-editor: Wendy Walker	*Indexer:* Michael Ferreira
Director of Nursing Production: Helen Ewan	*Compositor:* Circle Graphics
Managing Editor / Production: Erika Kors	*Printer:* R. R. Donnelley / Willard

9 8 7 6 5 4 3 2 1

Library of Congress Cataloging-in-Publication Data

Taylor's clinical nursing skills : a nursing process approach / [edited by] Pamela Evans-Smith.
   p. ; cm.
  Includes index.
  To accompany: Fundamentals of nursing / Carol Taylor, Carol Lillis, Priscilla LeMone. 5th ed. c2005.
  ISBN 0-7817-5138-1 (pbk.)
  1. Nursing. I. Title: Clinical nursing skills. II. Taylor, Carol, CSFN. III. Evans-Smith, Pamela. IV. Taylor, Carol, CSFN. Fundamentals of nursing.
  [DNLM: 1. Nursing Process. 2. Nursing Care--methods. WY 100 T247 2005]
RT41.T398 2005
610.73--dc22

To my children, husband, parents, and friends, thank you for your support during this endeavor.

To Mr. Graham, thank you for always seeing my true potential.

Contributors

Pamela B. Lynn, RN, MSN
Lecturer
School of Nursing
Gwynedd-Mercy College
Gwynedd Valley, Pennsylvania
   Chapter 8: Skin Integrity and Wound Care
   Chapter 9: Activity

Sheryl Kathleen Buckner, RN, MS
Clinical Instructor and Professional Practice Lab Coordinator
University of Oklahoma, College of Nursing
Oklahoma City, Oklahoma
   Unit III: Integrated Case Studies

Connie J. Hollen, RN, MS
Adjunct Instructor
University of Oklahoma, College of Allied Health
Oklahoma City, Oklahoma
   Unit III: Integrated Case Studies

Loren Nell Melton Stein, RNC, MSN
Adjunct Instructor
University of Oklahoma, College of Allied Health
Oklahoma City, Oklahoma
   Unit III: Integrated Case Studies

Clinical Consultants

Sheryl Kathleen Buckner, RN, MS
Clinical Instructor and Professional Practice Lab Coordinator
University of Oklahoma, College of Nursing
Oklahoma City, Oklahoma
   Chapters 1–17

Maryann Foley, RN, BSN
Flourtown, Pennsylvania
   Chapters 1–17; Unit III: Integrated Case Studies

Suzy Harrington, MS, RN, CHES
Director of Education
Central Colorado Area Health Education Center (AHEC)
Denver, Colorado
   Chapter 16: Cardiovascular Care

Connie J. Hollen, RN, MS
Adjunct Instructor
University of Oklahoma, College of Allied Health
Oklahoma City, Oklahoma
   Chapters 1–17

Loren Nell Melton Stein, RNC, MSN
Adjunct Instructor
University of Oklahoma, College of Allied Health
Oklahoma City, Oklahoma
   Chapters 1–17

Reviewers

Harrison Applin, RN, BScN, Med
Nursing Instructor
Grant MacEwan College
City Centre Campus
Edmonton, Alberta
Canada

Madeleine Buck, BScN, MSc(A)
School of Nursing
McGill University
Montreal, Quebec
Canada

Martha A. Conrad, RN, MSN, CNS, C
Coordinator, Learning Resources Center
College of Nursing
University of Akron
Akron, Ohio

Karen D. Danielson, RN, MSN
Associate Professor
North Central State College
Mansfield, Ohio

Joseph A. Foley, RN, MSN, CPNP, CNS
Instructor, Pediatric Nursing
College of Nursing
The University of Akron
Akron, Ohio

Judy L. Goodhart, MSN, RN
Professor of Nursing
Department of Nursing
Mesa State College
Grand Junction, Colorado

Pamela Gwin, RNC
Director, Vocational Program
Brazosport College
Lake Jackson, Texas

Lynda Johnston, RN, BSN, IBCLC
Nursing Instructor
Douglas College
New Westminster, British Columbia
Canada

Virginia Lester, RN, BSN, MSN, CNS
Assistant Professor
Angelo State University
San Angelo, Texas

Maureen Marthaler
Assistant Professor
School of Nursing
Purdue University Calumet
Hammond, Indiana

Patti Simmons, RN, MN
Assistant Professor of Nursing
North Georgia College and State University
Dahlonega, Georgia

Preface

Taylor's Clinical Nursing Skills: A Nursing Process Approach aims to help nursing students or graduate nurses incorporate cognitive, technical, interpersonal, and ethical/legal skills into safe and effective patient care. This book is written to meet the needs of novice to advanced nurses. Many of the skills shown in this book may not be encountered in nursing school but may be encountered once the graduate nurse has entered the workforce.

Because it emphasizes the basic principles of patient care, we believe this book can easily be used with any Fundamentals text. However, this Skills book was specifically designed to accompany *Fundamentals of Nursing: The Art and Science of Nursing Care,* fifth edition, by Taylor, Lillis, and LeMone, to provide a seamless learning experience. Some of the Skills and Guidelines for Nursing Care from the Taylor Fundamentals book may also be found in this book, but the content has been embellished here to:
- Highlight the nursing process
- Emphasize unexpected situations that the nurse may encounter, along with related interventions for how to respond to these unexpected situations
- Draw attention to critical actions within skills
- Illustrate specific actions within a skill through the use of over 1,000 four-color photographs and illustrations

Additionally, this book contains numerous higher-level skills that are not addressed in the Taylor Fundamentals book.

ORGANIZATION

Taylor's Clinical Nursing Skills is organized into three units. Ideally, the text will be followed sequentially, but every effort has been made to respect the differing needs of diverse curricula and students. Thus, each chapter stands on its own merit and may be read independently of others.

Unit I, Actions Basic to Nursing Care

This unit introduces the foundational skills used by nurses: measuring vital signs, assessing health, promoting safety, maintaining asepsis, administering medication, and caring for surgical patients.

Unit II, Promoting Healthy Physiologic Responses

This unit focuses on the physiologic needs of patients: hygiene; skin integrity and wound care; activity; comfort; nutrition; urinary elimination; bowel elimination; oxygenation; fluid, electrolyte, and acid–base balance; neurological care; and cardiovascular care.

Unit III, Integrated Case Studies

Although nursing skills textbooks generally present content in a linear fashion for ease of understanding, in reality many nursing skills are performed in combination for patients with complicated health needs. The integrated case studies in this unit are designed to challenge the reader to think critically, think outside the norm, consider the multiple needs of patients, and prioritize care appropriately—ultimately preparing the student and graduate nurse for complex situations that may arise in everyday practice.

FEATURES

Focusing on Patient Care

Each chapter in Units I and II begins with a description of three real-world case scenarios that put the skills into context. These scenarios provide a framework for the chapter content to be covered.

Review Material

Because of the breadth and depth of nursing knowledge that must be absorbed, nursing students and graduate nurses can easily become overwhelmed. Thus, this book is designed to eliminate excessive content and redundancy and to better focus the reader's attention. To this end, each chapter in Units I and II opens with several boxes, tables, or figures that summarize important theoretical concepts that should be understood prior to performing a skill. For a more in-depth study of these concepts, readers are encouraged to refer to their Fundamentals textbook.

Step-by-Step Skills

Each chapter presents a host of related step-by step skills. The skills are presented in a concise, straightforward, and simplified two-column format to facilitate competent performance of nursing skills.
- **Scientific rationales** accompany each nursing action to promote a deeper understanding of the basic principles supporting nursing care.

- The **nursing process** framework is used to integrate related nursing responsibilities for each of the five steps.
- **Nursing Alerts** (in red type) draw attention to crucial information.
- **Sample Documentation** figures are unique "handwritten" notes found within the intervention section of the nursing process. These figures show students and graduate nurses how to properly document the skill and their findings.
- **Infant, Child and Older Adult Considerations** as well as **Home Health** and **Special Considerations** (eg, modifications and home care) appear throughout to explain the varying needs of patients across the lifespan and in various settings.
- **Unexpected Situations** are provided after the explanation of normal outcomes. Each situation is followed by an explanation of how best to react, with rationales. This feature serves as a starting point for group discussion.

Photo Atlas Approach

When learning a new skill, it is often overwhelming to just read how to perform a skill. With over 1,000 *NEW* photographs, this book offers a pictorial guide to performing each skill. The skill will not only be learned but also remembered through the use of text with pictures.

Developing Critical Thinking Skills

Critical thinking questions at the end of the chapter reflect back to the opening scenarios for added cohesion throughout the chapters. Readers are challenged to apply the skills and use the new knowledge they have gained to "think through" learning exercises designed to show how critical thinking can impact patient care and possibly change outcomes.

TEACHING/LEARNING PACKAGE

To facilitate mastery of this text's content, a comprehensive teaching/learning package has been developed to assist faculty and students.

Instructor's Resource CD-ROM

This all-in-one resource features an Instructor's Manual and Image Bank.
- The Instructor's Manual contains a detailed step-by-step plan for setting up a skills course and provides answers to Developing Critical Thinking Skills questions found within the text. The unique "Build-a-Skill" feature allows instructors to customize nursing skills.

- The Image Bank provides free access to all of the textbook's illustrations and photos for use in Powerpoint, handouts, and so forth.

Student Resources

Students resources include a free back-of-book CD-ROM, Skill Checklists, and an Interactive CD-ROM:
- FREE Back of Book CD-ROM features a PDA download of selected skills for use with handheld devices
- *Skill Checklists to Accompany Taylor's Clinical Nursing Skills* by Pamela Evans-Smith and Marilee LeBon was designed to accompany the skills textbook and promote proper technique while increasing confidence.

TAYLOR SUITE OF PRODUCTS

From traditional texts to video and interactive products, the Taylor Fundamentals/Skills suite is tailored to fit every learning style. This integrated suite of products offers students a seamless learning experience you won't find anywhere else. The following products accompany *Taylor's Clinical Nursing Skills:*
- *Fundamentals of Nursing: The Art and Science of Nursing Care,* fifth edition, by Carol Taylor, Carol Lillis, and Priscilla LeMone. This traditional Fundamentals text promotes nursing as an evolving art and science, directed to human health and well-being. It challenges students to focus on the four blended skills of nursing care, which prepare students to combine the highest level of scientific knowledge and technologic skill with responsible, caring practice. The text includes engaging features to promote critical thinking and comprehension.
- *Taylor's Video Guide to Clinical Nursing Skills.* Hosted by a nurse expert, this video series offers engaging reality-based footage, interviews with patients, caregivers, and nurses, and detailed step-by-step demonstration of skills. Each of the 17 modules corresponds with a unit of the parent text so students can refer to the fifth edition as they follow along with the video.
- *Taylor's Interactive Nursing Skills (CD-ROM).* This high-quality interactive electronic product provides a consistent learning structure for both Skills and Fundamentals. The two parts to *Taylor's Interactive Nursing Skills CD-ROM* are
  - *Interactive Skills:* Students develop skills by answering critical thinking questions, as well as NCLEX-type questions.
  - *Interactive Tutorials:* Students engage in tutorials covering fundamentals concepts.

Pamela Evans-Smith, MSN, FNP

Acknowledgments

I could not have written this book without the help of many people. Thanks to Priscilla LeMone for introducing me to Lippincott Williams & Wilkins. Thanks to Carol Lillis for offering many encouraging words. Thanks to Elizabeth Nieginski for inviting me to write this book. Thanks to Maryann Foley, Sarah Kyle, and Kelly Trakalo for putting so much time and effort into helping this dream become a reality. A special thanks to Danielle DiPalma, Senior Developmental Editor, for all of her encouragement, guidance, and understanding. Thanks to Rosanne Hallowell, Senior Production Editor, Carolyn O'Brien, Art Director, and Brett MacNaughton, Illustration Coordinator, for patiently pulling all of the pieces together during production. Thanks to the contributors, clinical consultants, and reviewers who generously gave their wisdom, ideas, and time. I'd like to thank Joan Robinson and Judy McCann for their understanding, assistance, and provision of content from *Nursing Procedures,* fourth edition, and *Nursing Procedures Made Incredibly Easy* for Chapters 2, 10, and 16.

I would also like to thank all of the faculty at the University of Missouri-Columbia for sharing their insights into the world of nursing. A special thanks to Cheryl Bausler for being an exceptional mentor and never tiring of my questions.

A special thanks to all of my nursing students for never letting me become complacent with my job, keeping me on my toes through your interesting questions, and reinforcing to me my love of nursing.

Pamela Evans-Smith, MSN, FNP

Contents

TAYLOR'S CLINICAL NURSING SKILLS
A Nursing Process Approach

Actions Basic to Nursing Care

Vital Signs

This chapter will explain some of the skills needed to care for the following patients:

Tyrone Jeffries, age 5, is in the emergency department with a temperature of 38.9°C.

Toby White, age 26, has a history of asthma and is now breathing 32 times per minute.

Carl Glatz, age 58, has recently started taking medications to control his hypertension.

Learning Outcomes

After studying this chapter the reader should be able to:

1. Assess temperature via the oral, rectal, tympanic, and axillary routes.
2. Assess the respiratory rate.
3. Assess the pulse via the radial and apical routes.
4. Assess blood pressure with auscultation, using an ultrasound Doppler, or using a machine.
5. Weigh a patient using a bed scale.
6. Monitor a newborn's temperature while using a radiant overhead warmer.

Key Terms

afebrile: a condition in which the body temperature is not elevated

apnea: absence of breathing

bell: (of stethoscope) hollowed, upright, curved portion used to auscultate low-pitched sounds such as murmurs

blood pressure: force of blood against arterial walls

bradycardia: slow heart rate

bradypnea: abnormally slow rate of breathing

diaphragm: (of stethoscope) large, flat disk on the stethoscope used to auscultate high-pitched sounds such as respiratory sounds

diastolic pressure: least amount of pressure exerted on arterial walls, which occurs when the heart is at rest between ventricular contractions

dyspnea: difficult or labored breathing

dysrhythmia: an abnormal cardiac rhythm; synonym is arrhythmia

eupnea: normal respirations

expiration: act of breathing out; synonym is exhalation

febrile: a condition in which the body temperature is elevated

hyperpyrexia: high fever, above 41°C

hypertension: blood pressure elevated above the upper limit of normal

hypotension: blood pressure below the lower limit of normal

hypothermia: body temperature below the lower limit of normal

inspiration: act of breathing in; synonym is inhalation

Korotkoff sounds: series of sounds that correspond to changes in blood flow through an artery as pressure is released

orthopnea: type of dyspnea in which breathing is easier when the patient sits or stands

orthostatic hypotension: temporary fall in blood pressure associated with assuming an upright position; synonym for postural hypotension

pulse deficit: difference between the apical and radial pulse rates

pulse pressure: difference between systolic and diastolic pressures

continues

Key Terms (continued)

pyrexia: elevation above the upper limit of normal body temperature; synonym for fever

respiration: act of breathing and using oxygen in body cells

systolic pressure: highest point of pressure on arterial walls when the ventricles contract

tachycardia: rapid heart rate

tachypnea: abnormally rapid rate of breathing

vital signs: body temperature, pulse, and respiratory rates, and blood pressure; synonym for cardinal signs

Vital signs are a person's temperature, pulse, respiration, and blood pressure. (Pain, often called the fifth vital sign, is discussed in Chapter 10). A person's physiologic status is reflected by these indicators of body function, which are normally regulated through homeostatic mechanisms and fall within certain normal ranges. A change in vital signs may indicate a change in health.

Vital signs are taken and compared with accepted normal values and the patient's usual patterns in a wide variety of instances, including screenings at health fairs and clinics, in the home, upon admission to a healthcare setting, when certain medications are given, before and after diagnostic and surgical procedures, before and after certain nursing interventions, and in emergency situations. Nurses take vital signs as often as the condition of a patient requires such assessment.

Careful attention to the details of vital sign procedures and accuracy in the interpretation of the findings are extremely important. It is the nurse's role to interpret vital sign findings. How to assess each of the vital signs is presented in this chapter. Please look over the summary table and boxes at the beginning of this chapter for a quick review of critical knowledge to assist you in understanding the skills related to measuring vital signs.

TABLE 1-1 Age-Related Variations in Normal Vital Signs

Age	Temperature (°C)	Pulse (beats/min)	Respirations (breaths/min)	Blood Pressure (mm Hg)
Newborn	36.8 (Axillary)	80–180	30–60	73/55
1–3 yr	37.7 (Rectal)	80–140	20–40	90/55
6–8 yr	37 (Oral)	75–120	15–25	95/75
10 yr	37 (Oral)	75–110	15–25	102/62
Teens	37 (Oral)	60–100	15–20	102/80
Adults	37 (Oral)	60–100	12–20	120/80
>70 yr	36 (Oral)	60–100	15–20	120/80 (May normally be up to 160/95)

BOX 1-1 Infant and Child Vital Sign Techniques

- Due to the "fear factor" of blood pressure measurement, save the blood pressure for last. Children and infants often begin to cry during blood pressure assessment, and this may affect the respiration and pulse rate assessment.
- Perform as many tasks as possible while the child is sitting on the parent's lap or in a chair next to the parent.
- Let the child see and touch the equipment before you begin to use it.
- Make measuring vital signs a game. For instance, if you are using a tympanic thermometer that makes a chirping sound, tell the child you are looking for "birdies" in the ear. While auscultating the pulse, tell the child you are listening for another type of animal.
- If the child has a doll or stuffed animal, pretend to take the doll's vital signs first.

TABLE 1-2 Equivalent Centigrade and Fahrenheit Temperatures*

Centigrade	Fahrenheit	Centigrade	Fahrenheit
34.0	93.2	38.5	101.3
35.0	95.0	39.0	102.2
36.0	96.8	40.0	104.0
36.5	97.7	41.0	105.8
37.0	98.6	42.0	107.6
37.5	99.5	43.0	109.4
38.0	100.4	44.0	111.2

* To convert centigrade to Fahrenheit, multiply by $^9/_5$ and add 32. To change Fahrenheit to centigrade, subtract 32 and multiply by $^5/_9$.

BOX 1-2 Pulse Sites and Pulse Amplitude

Pulse Sites

Arteries commonly used for assessing the pulse include the temporal, carotid, brachial, radial, femoral, popliteal, posterior tibial, and dorsalis pedis.

Pulse Amplitude

Pulse amplitude typically is graded as 0 to 4:

0 (absent pulse): pulse cannot be felt, even with the application of extreme pressure

1+ (thready pulse): pulse is very difficult to feel, and applying slight pressure causes pulse to disappear

2+ (weak pulse): pulse is stronger than a thready pulse, but applying light pressure causes pulse to disappear

3+ (normal pulse): pulse is easily felt and requires moderate pressure to make it disappear

4+ (bounding pulse): pulse is strong and does not disappear with moderate pressure

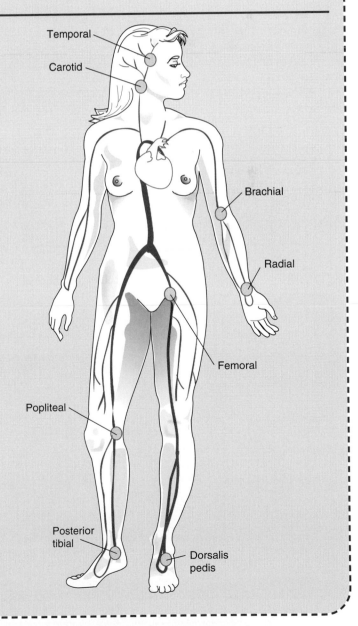

TABLE 1-3 Categories for Blood Pressure Levels in Adults (Ages 18 and Older)

Category	Blood Pressure Level (mm Hg)	
	Systolic	Diastolic
Normal	<120	<80
Prehypertension	120–139	80–89
High Blood Pressure		
Stage 1	140–159	90–99
Stage 2	≥160	≥100

These categories are from the National High Blood Pressure Education Program, National Heart, Lung, and Blood Institute, National Institutes of Health, and are available from www.nhlbi.nih.gov/hbp/detect/categ.htm.

TABLE 1-4 Blood Pressure Assessment Errors and Contributing Causes

Error	Contributing Causes	Error	Contributing Causes
Falsely low assessments	• Hearing deficit • Noise in the environment • Viewing the meniscus from above eye level • Applying too wide a cuff • Inserting eartips of stethoscope incorrectly • Using cracked or kinked tubing • Releasing the valve rapidly • Misplacing the bell beyond the direct area of the artery • Failing to pump the cuff 20 to 30 mm Hg above the disappearance of the pulse	Falsely high assessments	• Using a manometer not calibrated at the zero mark • Assessing the blood pressure immediately after exercise • Viewing the meniscus from below eye level • Applying a cuff that is too narrow • Releasing the valve too slowly • Reinflating the bladder during auscultation

TABLE 1-5 Acceptable Bladder Dimensions (in cm) for Arms of Different Sizes*

Cuff	Bladder Width (cm)	Bladder Length (cm)	Arm Circumference Range at Midpoint (cm)
Newborn	3	6	<6
Infant	5	15	6–15†
Child	8	21	16–21†
Small adult	10	24	22–26
Adult	13	30	27–34
Large adult	16	38	35–44
Adult thigh	20	42	45–52

*There is some overlapping of the recommended range for arm circumferences in order to limit the number of cuffs; it is recommended that the larger cuff be used when available.
†To approximate the bladder width: arm circumference ratio of 0.40 more closely in infants and children, additional cuffs are available.
Requests for reprints should be sent to the Office of Scientific Affairs, American Heart Association, 7272 Greenville Avenue, Dallas, TX 75231-4596.
(From *Circulation, 88*, 2460–2467, 1993.)

TABLE 1-6 **Korotkoff Sounds**

Phase	Description	Illustration
Phase I	Characterized by the first appearance of faint but clear tapping sounds that gradually increase in intensity; the first tapping sound is the systolic pressure	
Phase II	Characterized by muffled or swishing sounds; these sounds may temporarily disappear, especially in hypertensive people; the disappearance of the sound during the latter part of phase I and during phase II is called the *auscultatory gap* and may cover a range of as much as 40 mm Hg; failing to recognize this gap may cause serious errors of underestimating systolic pressure or overestimating diastolic pressure.	
Phase III	Characterized by distinct, loud sounds as the blood flows relatively freely through an increasingly open artery	
Phase IV	Characterized by a distinct, abrupt, muffling sound with a soft, blowing quality; in adults, the onset of this phase is considered to be the first diastolic figure	
Phase V	The last sound heard before a period of continuous silence; the pressure at which the last sound is heard is the second diastolic measurement	

SKILL 1-1   Assessing a Temperature

Body temperature is the heat of the body measured in degrees. Body temperature indicates the difference between production of heat and loss of heat. Heat is generated by metabolic processes in the core tissues of the body, transferred to the skin surface by the circulating blood, and then dissipated to the environment. Core body temperature is normally maintained within a range of 36.0°C (97.0°F) to 37.5°C (99.5°F). There are individual variations of these temperatures as well as normal changes during the day, with core body temperatures being lowest in the early morning and highest in the late afternoon (Porth, 2002).

Temperatures differ in various parts of the body, with core body temperatures being higher than surface body temperatures. Core temperatures are measured at tympanic or rectal sites, but they may also be measured in the esophagus, pulmonary artery, or bladder by invasive monitoring devices. Surface body temperatures are measured at oral (sublingual) and axillary sites.

Several types of equipment and different procedures might be used to measure body temperature. To obtain an accurate measurement, you must choose the correct equipment, the best site, and the appropriate tool based on the patient's condition. If a temperature reading is obtained from a site other than the oral route, document the site used along with the measurement. If no site is listed, it is generally assumed to be the oral route.

Equipment

- Digital, electronic, or glass thermometer
- Probe covers for electronic thermometer
- Pencil or pen, paper or flow sheet

ASSESSMENT

Assess the patient to ensure that his or her cognitive functioning is intact. If not, an oral temperature is to be taken, the patient could harm himself or herself by biting down on the thermometer. Also assess whether the patient can close his or her lips around the thermometer; if the patient cannot, select a different method. Assess the oral cavity for any sores, diseases of the oral cavity, or previous surgery of the nose or mouth. Avoid taking an oral temperature if the patient has any of these conditions. Ask the patient if he or she has recently smoked, has been chewing gum, or was eating and drinking immediately before assessing temperature. If the patient has done any of these things, wait 15 to 30 minutes before taking an oral temperature because of the possible direct influence on the patient's temperature.

If you are taking a rectal temperature, review the patient's platelet level (if ordered). Do not insert a rectal thermometer into a patient who has a low platelet count. The rectum is very vascular and a thermometer could cause rectal bleeding. With a low platelet count, the patient could lose a large amount of blood. Taking a rectal temperature is contraindicated in a patient who is immunosuppressed because of the risk of rectal abscess. Before assessing a rectal temperature, look at the patient's diagnosis. Many institutions will not allow a rectal temperature to be taken on patients with heart disease or those who have recently undergone thoracic surgery due to chance of stimulating the vagus nerve and causing bradycardia.

If patient has an earache, do not use the affected ear to take a tympanic temperature. The movement of the tragus may cause severe discomfort. Assess the patient for significant ear drainage or a scarred tympanic membrane. These conditions can provide inaccurate results and could cause problems for the patient. However, an ear infection or the presence of earwax in the canal will not significantly affect a tympanic thermometer reading. If the patient has been sleeping with the head turned to one side, take a tympanic temperature in the other ear. Heat may be increased on the side that was against the pillow, especially if it is a plastic-covered pillow.

continues

Assessing a Temperature (continued)

**NURSING
DIAGNOSIS**

Determine the related factors for the nursing diagnoses based on the patient's current status. Appropriate nursing diagnoses may include:

- Risk for Trauma
- Hyperthermia
- Hypothermia
- Risk for Imbalanced Body Temperature
- Ineffective Thermoregulation

**OUTCOME
IDENTIFICATION
AND PLANNING**

The expected outcomes to achieve when performing temperature assessment are that an accurate temperature is assessed and that the patient experiences no trauma. Other outcomes may be appropriate depending on the patient's nursing diagnosis.

IMPLEMENTATION

ACTION	RATIONALE
Measuring Temperature Regardless of Route	
1. Check physician's order or nursing care plan for frequency and route.	This provides for patient safety.
2. Identify the patient.	This provides for patient safety.
3. Explain the procedure to the patient.	Explanation reduces apprehension and encourages cooperation.
4. Ensure that the electronic or digital thermometer is in operating condition.	An improperly functioning thermometer may not give an accurate reading.
5. Perform hand hygiene and don gloves if appropriate or indicated.	Hand hygiene deters the spread of microorganisms.
6. Select the appropriate site.	Assess the patient's age and mental and physical condition to ensure safety and accuracy of measurement.
7. Follow the steps as outlined below for the appropriate type of thermometer.	
8. Perform hand hygiene. If gloves are worn, discard them in the proper receptacle.	Hand hygiene deters the spread of microorganisms.
9. Record temperature on paper, flow sheet, or computerized record. Report abnormal findings to the appropriate person. Identify the site of assessment if other than oral.	Recording and reporting ensure accurate documentation and communication.

10/29/06 0800   Tympanic temperature assessed. Temperature 38.7°C. Physician notified. Ordered to give 650 mg PO acetaminophen. Incentive spirometer × 10 Q 1 hours until temperature less than 38.0°C.—M. Evans, RN

Action 9: Documentation.

Measuring Tympanic Membrane Temperature	
1. If necessary, push the "on" button and wait for the "ready" signal on the unit.	For proper function, thermometer must be turned on and warmed up.
2. Attach tympanic probe covering.	Use of the covering deters the spread of microorganisms.
3. **Insert the probe snugly into the external ear, using gentle but firm pressure, angling the thermometer toward the patient's jaw line. Pull pinna up and back to straighten the ear canal in an adult.**	If the probe is not inserted correctly, the patient's temperature will be noted as lower than normal.

continues

Assessing a Temperature (continued)

ACTION

RATIONALE

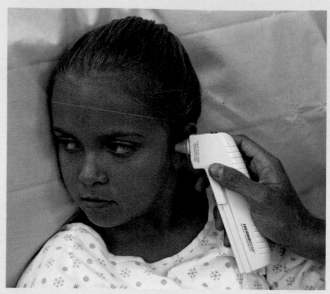

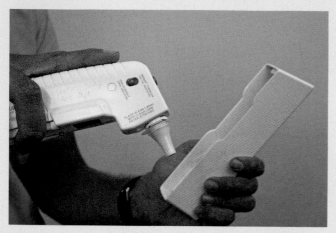

Action 1: Turn unit on and await the ready signal.

Action 3: Insert tympanic thermometer into the patient's ear.

4. Activate the unit by pushing the trigger button. The reading is immediate (usually within 2 seconds). Note the reading.

5. Discard the probe cover in an appropriate receptacle by pushing the probe release button, and replace the thermometer in its charger.

The digital thermometer must be activated to record the temperature.

Discarding the probe cover ensures that it will not be reused accidentally on another patient. The thermometer must stay on the charger so that it is ready to use at all times.

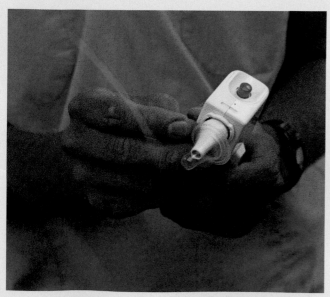

Action 5: Dispose of probe cover.

continues

SKILL
1-1

Assessing a Temperature (continued)

ACTION

RATIONALE

Assessing Oral Temperature With an Electronic or Digital Thermometer

1. Remove the electronic unit from the charging unit, and remove the probe from within the recording unit.

2. Cover thermometer probe with disposable probe cover and slide it into place until it snaps into place.

3. **Place the probe beneath the patient's tongue in the posterior sublingual pocket. Ask the patient to close his or her lips around the probe.**

Electronic unit must be taken into the patient's room to assess the patient's temperature. On some models, by removing the probe the machine is already turned on.

Using a cover prevents contamination of the thermometer probe.

When the probe rests deep in the posterior sublingual pocket, it is in contact with blood vessels lying close to the surface.

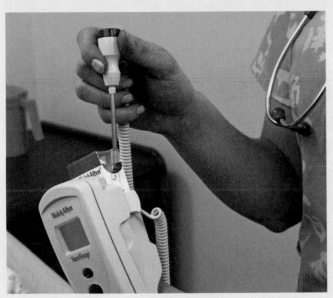

Action 2: Put probe cover on the thermometer.

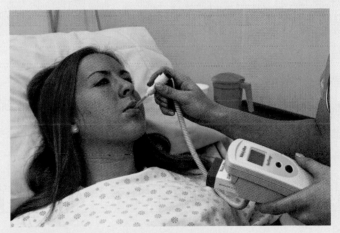

Action 3: Insert thermometer under the tongue.

4. **Continue to hold the probe until you hear a beep.** Note the temperature reading.

5. Remove the probe from the patient's mouth and dispose of the probe cover by holding the probe over an appropriate receptacle and pressing the probe release button.

6. Return the thermometer probe to the storage place within the unit and return the electronic unit to the charging unit to make sure it is fully charged.

If left unsupported, the weight of the probe tends to pull it away from the correct location. The signal indicates the measurement is completed. The electronic thermometer provides a digital display of the measured temperature.

Disposing of the probe cover ensures that it will not be reused accidentally on another patient.

The thermometer needs to be recharged for future use.

continues

Assessing a Temperature (continued)

ACTION   **RATIONALE**

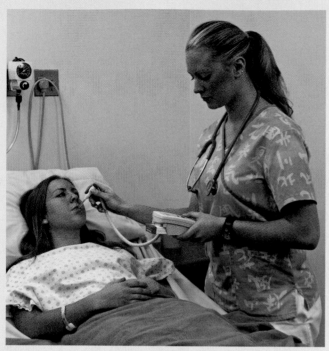

Action 4: Hold probe in the patient's mouth.

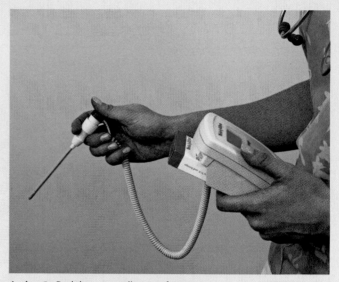

Action 5: Push button to dispose of cover.

Assessing Rectal Temperature With an Electronic or Digital Thermometer

1. Put on gloves.

2. Provide privacy by closing the door or curtain.

3. Place the bed at an appropriate working height.

4. Assist the patient to a side-lying position. Pull back the covers enough to expose only the buttocks.

5. Remove the probe from within the recording unit of the electronic thermometer. Cover the probe with a disposable probe cover and slide it into place until it snaps in place.

6. **Lubricate about 1″ of the probe with a water-soluble lubricant.**

7. Reassure the patient. Separate the buttocks until the anal sphincter is clearly visible.

8. **Insert the thermometer probe into the anus about 1.5″ in an adult or 1″ in a child.**

Gloves protect nurse from microorganisms in the feces.

Privacy preserves the patient's dignity.

Having the bed at the right height reduces strain on the nurse's back.

The side-lying position allows the nurse to visualize the buttocks. Exposing only the buttocks keeps the patient warm and maintains his or her dignity.

Using a cover prevents contamination of the thermometer.

Lubrication reduces friction and facilitates insertion, minimizing the risk of irritation or injury to the rectal mucous membranes.

If not placed directly into the anal opening, the thermometer probe may injure adjacent tissue or cause discomfort.

Depth of insertion must be adjusted based on the patient's age. Rectal temperatures are not normally taken in an infant.

continues

Assessing a Temperature (continued)

ACTION   **RATIONALE**

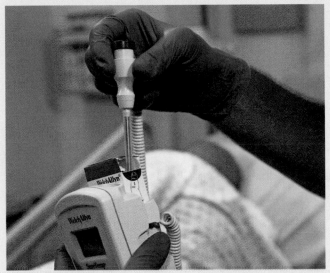

Action 5: Remove appropriate probe and attach disposable probe cover.

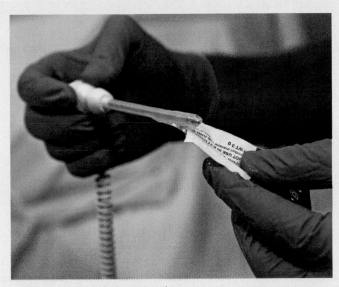

Action 6: Lubricate thermometer tip.

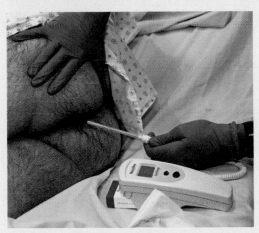

Action 8: Insert thermometer into the anus.

9. Hold the probe in place until you hear a beep, then carefully remove the probe. Note the temperature reading on the display.

10. Dispose of the probe cover by holding the probe over an appropriate waste receptacle and pressing the release button.

11. Using toilet tissue, wipe the anus of any feces or excess lubricant. Dispose of the toilet tissue.

12. Remove gloves and discard them. Perform hand hygiene.

13. Cover the patient and help him or her to a position of comfort. Place the bed in the lowest position; elevate rails as needed.

14. Return the thermometer to the charging unit.

If left unsupported, the weight of the probe tends to pull it away from the correct location. The signal indicates the measurement is completed. The electronic thermometer provides a digital display of the measured temperature.

Proper probe cover disposal reduces risk of microorganism transmission.

Wiping promotes cleanliness. Disposing of the toilet tissue avoids transmission of microorganisms.

Hand hygiene avoids transmission of microorganisms.

These actions provide for the patient's comfort and safety.

The thermometer needs to be recharged for future use.

continues

SKILL 1-1   Assessing a Temperature (continued)

ACTION	RATIONALE

Assessing Axillary Temperature With an Electronic or Digital Thermometer

1. Ensure privacy by closing the door or curtain.

   Privacy protects the patient's dignity.

2. Place the bed at an appropriate working height.

   Having the bed at the right height reduces strain on the nurse's back.

3. Move the patient's clothing to expose only the axilla.

   The axilla must be exposed for placement of the thermometer.

4. Remove the probe from the recording unit of the electronic thermometer. Place a disposable probe cover on by sliding it on and snapping it securely.

   Using a cover prevents contamination of the thermometer probe.

5. **Place the end of the probe in the center of the axilla. Have the patient bring the arm down and close to the body.**

   The deepest area of the axilla provides the most accurate measurement; surrounding the bulb with skin surface provides a more reliable measurement.

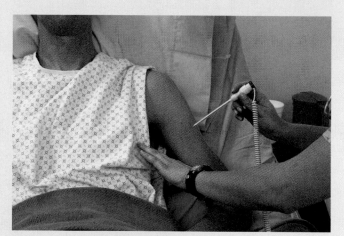

Action 3: Expose axilla to assess temperature.

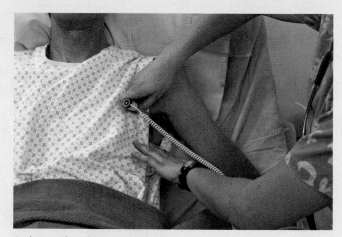

Action 5: Place thermometer in center of axilla.

6. Hold the probe in place until you hear a beep, and then carefully remove the probe. Note the temperature reading.

   Axillary thermometers must be held in place to obtain an accurate temperature.

7. Dispose of the probe cover by holding the probe over an appropriate waste receptacle and pushing the release button.

   Discarding the probe cover ensures that it will not be reused accidentally on another patient.

8. Place the bed in the lowest position and elevate rails as needed. Leave the patient clean and comfortable.

   Low bed position and elevated side rails provide for patient safety.

9. Return the electronic thermometer to the charging unit.

   Thermometer needs to be recharged for future use.

Assessing Temperature With a Glass Thermometer

1. If it is stored in a chemical solution, wipe the thermometer dry with a soft tissue, using a firm twisting motion. Wipe from the bulb toward the fingers.

   Chemical solutions may irritate mucous membranes and have an objectionable taste. Twisting helps cover the entire surface. Wiping from an area of few or no organisms to an area where organisms might be present minimizes spread to a cleaner area.

2. Grasp the thermometer firmly with the thumb and the forefinger and, using strong wrist movements, shake it until the chemical line reaches at least 36°C.

   Moves the chemical back into the bulb below the previous measurement.

continues

Assessing a Temperature (continued)

ACTION	RATIONALE

ACTION

3. **Read the thermometer by holding it horizontally at eye level, and rotate it between your fingers until you can see the chemical line.**

4. **For oral use, place the bulb of the thermometer within the back of the right or left pocket under the patient's tongue and tell the patient to close the lips around the thermometer. For rectal use, place the thermometer bulb in the rectum as described when using an electronic thermometer. For axillary use, place the thermometer bulb in the center of the axilla with the patient's arm against the chest wall.**

5. **Leave the thermometer in place for 3 minutes or according to agency protocol (for oral use); 2 to 3 minutes (for rectal use); and 10 minutes (for axillary use).**

RATIONALE

This position makes it easier to see the chemical line.

The probe must be inserted correctly to obtain an accurate reading.

Time is needed for the chemical in the thermometer to expand and accurately measure temperature. Axillary measurement takes a longer time for the chemical to expand. Staying with the patient ensures that the thermometer remains in the correct position and is not broken.

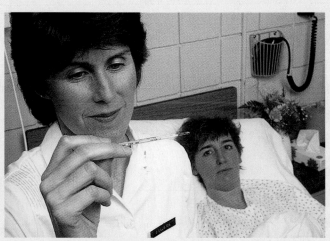

Action 3: Read thermometer.

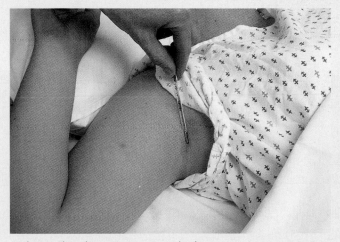

Action 4: Place thermometer appropriately.

6. Remove the thermometer, and wipe it once from the fingers down to the bulb, using a firm, twisting motion.

Wiping the thermometer minimizes the spread of organisms from an area of higher concentration to a cleaner area; friction helps loosen material from the thermometer surface.

7. Dispose of the tissues in a receptacle for contaminated items.

Confining contaminated articles helps reduce the spread of pathogens.

8. Read the thermometer to the nearest tenth of a degree.

The chemical may rise a bit above or below the calibration lines.

9. Wash thermometer in lukewarm, soapy water. Rinse it in cool water. Dry and replace the thermometer in its container.

Washing removes organic material and organisms.

continues

SKILL 1-1   Assessing a Temperature (continued)

EVALUATION

The expected outcomes are met when the patient's temperature is assessed accurately and the patient experiences no trauma.

Unexpected Situations and Associated Interventions

- *Temperature reading is higher or lower than expected based on how the patient's skin feels:* Reassess temperature with a different thermometer. The thermometer may not be calibrated correctly. If using a tympanic thermometer, you will get lower readings if the probe is not inserted far enough into the ear.
- *During rectal temperature assessment, the patient reports feeling lightheaded or passes out:* Remove the thermometer immediately. Quickly assess the patient's blood pressure and heart rate. Notify the physician. Do not attempt to take another rectal temperature on this patient.

Infant and Child Considerations

Small children have a limited attention span and have difficulty keeping their lips closed long enough to obtain an accurate oral temperature reading. For children younger than 6 years, use the axillary or tympanic site or use a temperature-sensitive tape (although research is ongoing to determine the accuracy of the measurements).

Home Care Considerations

Use the axillary or tympanic site for a confused, disoriented, or comatose adult. Axillary temperatures are generally about one degree less than oral temperatures; rectal temperatures are generally about one degree higher.

SKILL 1-2   Assessing a Pulse

The pulse is a throbbing sensation that can be palpated over a peripheral artery or auscultated (listened to) over the apex of the heart. It results from a wave of blood being pumped into the arterial circulation by the contraction of the left ventricle. Each time the left ventricle contracts to eject blood into an already full aorta, the arterial walls in the cardiovascular system expand to compensate for the increase in pressure of the blood. Characteristics of the pulse, including rate, quality, rhythm, and volume, provide information about the effectiveness of the heart as a pump and the adequacy of peripheral blood flow.

The pulse may be assessed by palpating peripheral arteries or the carotid artery, by auscultating the apical pulse with a stethoscope, or by using a Doppler ultrasound. To assess the pulse accurately, you need to know which site to choose and what method is most appropriate for the patient. When palpating pulses, place your fingers over the artery so that the ends of your fingers are flat against the patient's skin. Do not press with the tip of the fingers only. Pulse rates are measured in beats per minute.

Equipment

- Watch with second hand or digital readout
- Stethoscope (for apical pulse)
- Alcohol swab (for stethoscope)
- Gel (for Doppler)
- Pencil or pen, paper or flow sheet
- Indelible marker (for Doppler)
- Tissue (for Doppler)

continues

SKILL 1-2   Assessing a Pulse (continued)

ASSESSMENT

Choose a site to assess the pulse. For an adult patient the most common site is the radial or apical pulse. For a child older than 2 years the radial pulse may be palpated. In infants and young children the brachial pulse may be palpated or the apical pulse may be auscultated.

NURSING DIAGNOSIS

Determine the related factors for the nursing diagnoses based on the patient's current status. Appropriate nursing diagnoses may include:

- Decreased Cardiac Output
- Ineffective Tissue Perfusion
- Deficient Fluid Volume
- Acute Pain

OUTCOME IDENTIFICATION AND PLANNING

The expected outcomes to achieve when taking a pulse rate are that the patient's pulse is palpated or auscultated and the patient experiences no trauma. Other outcomes may be appropriate depending on the patient's nursing diagnosis.

IMPLEMENTATION

ACTION	RATIONALE
For All Sites and Methods	
1. Identify the patient.	Identifying the patient ensure patient safety.
2. Explain the procedure to the patient.	Explanation reduces apprehension and encourages cooperation.
3. Gather equipment.	Having all equipment on hand provides for an organized approach to the task.
4. Perform hand hygiene and don gloves as appropriate.	Gloves and hand hygiene deter the spread of microorganisms.
5. Select the appropriate site.	Different arteries may be used to assess the pulse; apical pulses are assessed if the peripheral pulse is rapid, irregular, or nonpalpable.
6. Follow the steps as outlined below for the appropriate pulse assessment.	
7. Perform hand hygiene.	Hand hygiene deters the spread of microorganisms.
8. Record pulse rate and site on paper, flow sheet, or computerized record. Report abnormal findings to the appropriate person. Identify site of assessment if other than apical.	These actions provide accurate documentation and reporting.

> 10/15/06   0745   Pulse is regular, 2+ and equal in radial, popliteal, and dorsalis pedal.
> —M. Evans, RN

Action 8: Documentation.

Palpating the Radial Pulse	
1. The patient may either be supine with the arm alongside the body, wrist extended, and palms of the hand lateral or facing down or sitting with the forearm at a 90-degree angle to the body resting on a support with the wrist extended and the palm downward or facing laterally.	These positions are comfortable for the patient and convenient for the nurse.
2. **Place your first, second, and third fingers along the patient's radial artery, and press gently against the radius.** Rest your thumb on the back of the patient's wrist.	The sensitive fingertips can feel the pulsation of the artery.

continues

Assessing a Pulse (continued)

ACTION	RATIONALE

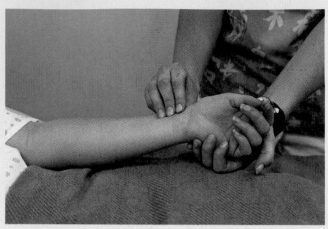

Action 2: Palpate the radial pulse.

3. Apply only enough pressure so that the artery can be felt distinctly.

   Moderate pressure facilitates palpation of the pulsations. Too much pressure obliterates the pulse; with too little pressure, the pulse is imperceptible.

4. Using a watch with a second hand, count the number of pulsations felt for 30 seconds. Multiply this number by 2 to calculate the rate for 1 minute. If the rate, rhythm, or amplitude of the pulse is abnormal in any way, palpate and count the pulse for 1 minute or longer.

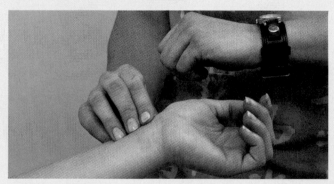

Action 4: Count the pulse.

Auscultating the Apical Pulse Rate

1. Use alcohol swab to clean earpieces and diaphragm of the stethoscope.

   Cleaning with alcohol deters transmission of microorganisms.

2. Assist patient in sitting in a chair or in bed, and expose chest area.

   This position facilitates identification of site for stethoscope placement.

3. Hold the stethoscope diaphragm against the palm of your hand for a few seconds.

   Warming the diaphragm promotes patient comfort.

4. **Palpate the fifth intercostal space, and move to the left midclavicular line.** Place the diaphragm over the apex of the heart (see illustration, p. 19).

   This is the point of maximum impulse, where the heartbeat is best heard.

5. Listen for heart sounds ("lub-dub").

   These sounds occur as the heart valves close. Each "lub-dub" counts as one beat.

6. **Using a watch with a second hand, count the heartbeat for 1 minute.**

   Counting for a full minute increases the accuracy of assessment.

continues

Assessing a Pulse (continued)

ACTION	RATIONALE

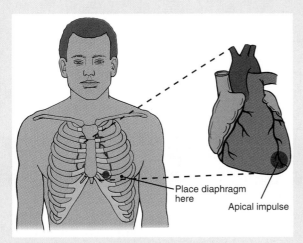

Action 4: Auscultating the apical pulse: apex area.

Place diaphragm here

Apical impulse

Using a Doppler to Assess the Pulse Rate

ACTION	RATIONALE
1. Remove Doppler from charger and turn it on. Make sure that volume is set at low.	Doppler needs to be charged and ready for use at all times. If the volume is turned up high, it may alarm the patient.
2. **Apply Doppler gel to the site where you are auscultating the pulse.**	For the Doppler to pick up the sound waves, a medium such as gel is needed.
3. Hold the Doppler in your nondominant hand. With your dominant hand place the Doppler tip in the gel. Adjust the volume as needed. Move the Doppler tip around until the pulse is heard.	Anatomic locations may vary slightly from person to person. The Doppler may need to be moved to locate the appropriate site.
4. **Using a watch with a second hand, count the heartbeat for 1 minute.**	Measuring for a full minute increases the accuracy of assessment.
5. Remove the Doppler tip and turn the Doppler off. Wipe the gel off of the patient's extremity with tissue.	If the Doppler is left on, the battery will wear down. Removing gel ensures the patient's comfort.
6. Return the Doppler to the charge base.	The Doppler needs to be recharged for future use.

EVALUATION   The expected outcomes are met when the patient's pulse is palpated or auscultated and the patient experiences no trauma.

Unexpected Situations and Associated Interventions

- *The pulse is irregular:* Monitor the pulse for a full minute. If this is a change for the patient, notify the physician.
- *The pulse is palpated easily but then disappears:* Apply only moderate pressure to the pulse. Applying too much pressure may obliterate the pulse.
- *You cannot palpate a pulse:* Use an ultrasound Doppler to assess the pulse. If this is a change in assessment, notify the physician. If you cannot find the pulse using an ultrasound Doppler, notify the physician. If you can find the pulse using an ultrasound Doppler, place a small X over the spot where the pulse is located. This can make palpating the pulse easier since the exact location of the pulse is known.

Infant and Child Considerations

- The apical pulse is the most reliable for infants and small children.

continues

SKILL 1-2   Assessing a Pulse (continued)

Home Care Considerations
- Teach the patient and family members how to take the patient's pulse.
- Inform the patient and family about digital pulse monitoring devices.
- Teach family members how to locate and monitor peripheral pulse sites.

Special Considerations
- The normal heart rate varies by age.
- When palpating a carotid pulse, lightly press only one side of the neck at a time. Never attempt to palpate both carotid arteries at the same time.

SKILL 1-3   Assessing Respiration

Respiration involves several physiologic events. Pulmonary ventilation (or breathing) is movement of air in and out of the lungs; inspiration (or inhalation) is the act of breathing in, and expiration (or exhalation) is the act of breathing out. External respiration is the exchange of oxygen and carbon dioxide between the alveoli of the lungs and the circulating blood through diffusion. Internal respiration is the exchange of oxygen and carbon dioxide between the circulating blood and tissue cells. Although nurses assess the manifestations of changes in all of these respiratory events, the part that is measured as a vital sign is pulmonary ventilation, called respirations.

The nurse assesses respiratory rate, depth, and rhythm by inspection (observing and listening) or by listening with the stethoscope. The nurse determines the rate by counting the number of breaths per minute. If respirations are very shallow and difficult to visually detect, observe the sternal notch, where respiration is more apparent. With an infant or young child, assess respirations before taking the temperature so the child is not crying, which would alter the respiratory status.

Move right from the pulse assessment to counting the respiratory rate to avoid letting the patient know you are counting respirations. Patients should be unaware of the respiratory assessment because if they are conscious of the procedure, they might alter their breathing patterns or rate.

Equipment
- Watch with second hand or digital readout
- Pencil or pen, paper, or flow sheet

ASSESSMENT

Assess patient for any signs of respiratory distress, which include retractions, nasal flaring, grunting, orthopnea, or tachypnea.

NURSING DIAGNOSIS

Determine the related factors for the nursing diagnoses based on the patient's current status. Appropriate nursing diagnoses may include:
- Ineffective Breathing Pattern
- Impaired Gas Exchange
- Risk for Activity Intolerance

OUTCOME IDENTIFICATION AND PLANNING

The expected outcomes to achieve when measuring respirations are that the patient's respiratory rate is counted successfully; the patient's respiratory rhythm and depth are observed accurately; and the patient experiences no trauma. Other outcomes may be appropriate depending on the patient's nursing diagnosis.

continues

Assessing Respiration (continued)

IMPLEMENTATION
ACTION

RATIONALE

1. **While your fingers are still in place after counting the pulse rate, observe the patient's respirations.**

The patient may alter the rate of respirations if he or she is aware they are being counted.

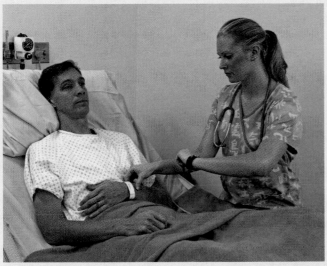

Action 1: Assess respirations.

2. Note the rise and fall of the patient's chest.

A complete cycle of an inspiration and an expiration composes one respiration.

3. Using a watch with a second hand, count the number of respirations for at least 30 seconds. Multiply this number by 2 to calculate the respiratory rate per minute.

Sufficient time is necessary to observe the rate, depth, and other characteristics.

4. If respirations are abnormal in any way, count the respirations for at least 1 full minute.

Increased time allows the detection of unequal timing between respirations.

5. Perform hand hygiene.

Hand hygiene deters the spread of microorganisms.

6. Document respiratory rate on paper, flow sheet, or computerized record. Report any abnormal findings to the appropriate person.

These actions provide for accurate documentation and reporting.

10/23/06   0830   Respirations 16/min.
Regular and unlabored—M. Evans, RN

Action 6: Documentation.

EVALUATION

The expected outcome is met when the patient's respirations are assessed without the patient altering the rate, rhythm, or depth.

Unexpected Situations and Associated Interventions

- *The patient is breathing with such shallow respirations that you cannot count the rate:* Sometimes it is easier to count respirations by auscultating the lung sounds. Notify the physician of respiratory rate and the shallowness of the respirations.

Infant and Child Considerations

- In infants, count respirations for 1 full minute due to a normally irregular rhythm.

Assessing Blood Pressure

Blood pressure refers to the force of the blood against the arterial walls. Maximum blood pressure is exerted on the walls of arteries when the left ventricle of the heart pushes blood through the aortic valve into the aorta at the beginning of systole. The pressure rises as the ventricle contracts and falls as the heart relaxes. This continuous contraction and relaxation of the left ventricle creates a pressure wave that is transmitted through the arterial system (Porth, 2002). The highest pressure is the systolic pressure. When the heart rests between beats during diastole, the pressure drops. The lowest pressure present on arterial walls at this time is the diastolic pressure. The difference between the two is called the pulse pressure.

Blood pressure is measured in millimeters of mercury (mm Hg) and is recorded as a fraction. The numerator is the systolic pressure; the denominator is the diastolic pressure. For example, if the blood pressure is 120/80 mm Hg, 120 is the systolic pressure and 80 is the diastolic pressure. The pulse pressure, in this case, is 40.

To get an accurate assessment of blood pressure, you should know what equipment to use, which site to choose, and how to identify the sounds you hear. Routine measurement should be taken after the patient has rested for a minimum of 5 minutes. In addition, the patient should not have any caffeine or nicotine 30 minutes before the blood pressure is measured.

Automatic, electronic equipment is often used to monitor blood pressure in acute care settings, during anesthesia, postoperatively, or any time frequent assessments are necessary. This unit determines blood pressure by analyzing the sounds of blood flow or measuring oscillations. The machine can be set to take and record blood pressure readings at preset intervals. Irregular heart rates, excessive patient movement, and environmental noise can interfere with the readings. Because electronic equipment is more sensitive to outside interference, these readings are susceptible to error. The cuff is applied in the same manner as the auscultatory method, with the microphone or pressure sensor positioned directly over the artery. When using an automatic blood pressure device for serial readings, check the cuffed limb frequently. Incomplete deflation of the cuff between measurements can lead to inadequate arterial perfusion and venous drainage, compromising the circulation in the limb.

Equipment

- Stethoscope
- Sphygmomanometer
- Blood pressure cuff of appropriate size
- Pencil or pen, paper or flow sheet
- Alcohol swab
- Blood pressure machine (if using electronic)
- Doppler (if needed)
- Gel (for Doppler)

ASSESSMENT

Palpate the brachial artery. Assess for an intravenous infusion, breast or axilla surgery on that side, cast, arteriovenous shunt, or injured or diseased limb. If any of these conditions are present, do not use the affected arm to monitor blood pressure. Assess the size of the arm so that the appropriate-sized blood pressure cuff can be used. Assess the patient for pain. If the patient reports pain, give pain medication as ordered before assessing blood pressure. If the blood pressure is taken while the patient is in pain, make a notation concerning the pain if the blood pressure is elevated.

**NURSING
DIAGNOSIS**

Determine the related factors for the nursing diagnoses based on the patient's current status. Appropriate nursing diagnoses may include:

- Decreased Cardiac Output
- Ineffective Health Maintenance
- Effective Therapeutic Regimen Management
- Risk for Falls

continues

Assessing Blood Pressure (continued)

| OUTCOME IDENTIFICATION AND PLANNING | The expected outcomes to achieve when measuring blood pressure are that the patient's blood pressure is measured accurately and the patient experiences no trauma. Other outcomes may be appropriate depending on the patient's nursing diagnosis. |

IMPLEMENTATION

ACTION	RATIONALE
Taking Blood Pressure Using a Blood Pressure Cuff and Stethoscope	
1. Identify the patient.	Identifying the patient provides patient safety.
2. Explain the procedure to the patient.	Explanation reduces apprehension and encourages cooperation.
3. Gather equipment.	Having all equipment on hand provides for an organized approach to the task.
4. Perform hand hygiene.	Hand hygiene deters the spread of microorganisms.
5. Delay obtaining the blood pressure if the patient is emotionally upset, is in pain, or has just exercised (unless measurement is urgent).	Factors such as emotional upset, exercise, and pain alter blood pressure.
6. **Select the appropriate arm for application of cuff (no intravenous infusion, breast or axilla surgery on that side, cast, arteriovenous shunt, or injured or diseased limb).**	Measurement of blood pressure may temporarily impede circulation to the extremity.
7. Have the patient assume a comfortable lying or sitting position with the forearm supported at the level of the heart and the palm of the hand upward.	This position places the brachial artery on the inner aspect of the elbow so that the bell or diaphragm of the stethoscope can rest on it easily.

Action 7: Proper position for blood pressure assessment.

| 8. Expose the brachial artery by removing garments, or move a sleeve, if it is not too tight, above the area where the cuff will be placed. | Clothing over the artery interferes with the ability to hear sounds and may cause inaccurate blood pressure readings. A tight sleeve would cause congestion of blood and possibly inaccurate readings. |

continues

SKILL
1-4   **Assessing Blood Pressure** (continued)

ACTION

RATIONALE

9. **Center the bladder of the cuff over the brachial artery, about midway on the arm, so that the lower edge of the cuff is about 2.5 to 5 cm (1" to 2") above the inner aspect of the elbow. The tubing should extend from the edge of the cuff nearer the patient's elbow.**

Pressure in the cuff applied directly to the artery provides the most accurate readings. If the cuff gets in the way of the stethoscope, readings are likely to be inaccurate. A cuff placed upside-down with the tubing toward the patient's head may give a false reading.

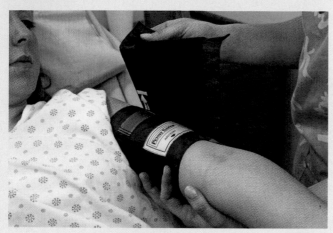

Action 9: Place the blood pressure cuff.

10. Wrap the cuff around the arm smoothly and snugly, and fasten it securely or tuck the end of the cuff well under the preceding wrapping. Do not allow any clothing to interfere with the proper placement of the cuff.

A smooth cuff and snug wrapping produce equal pressure and help promote an accurate measurement. A cuff too loosely wrapped results in an inaccurate reading.

11. Check that the needle on the aneroid gauge is within the zero mark. If using a mercury manometer, check to see that the manometer is in the vertical position and that the mercury is within the zero level with the gauge at eye level.

If the needle is not in the zero area, the blood pressure may not be accurate. Tilting a mercury manometer, inaccurate calibration, or improper height for reading the gauge can lead to errors in determining the pressure measurements.

12. **Palpate the pulse at the brachial or radial artery by pressing gently with the fingertips.**

Palpation allows for measurement of the approximate systolic reading.

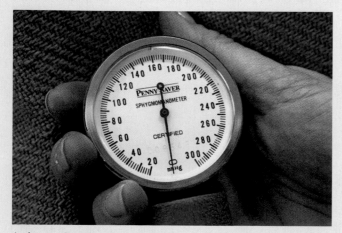

Action 11: Ensure gauge starts at zero.

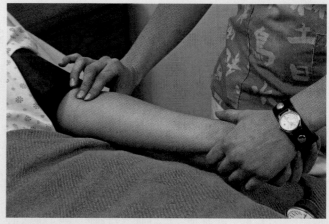

Action 12: Palpate the brachial pulse.

continues

Assessing Blood Pressure (continued)

ACTION	RATIONALE
13. Tighten the screw valve on the air pump.	The bladder within the cuff will not inflate with the valve open.
14. **Inflate the cuff while continuing to palpate the artery. Note the point on the gauge where the pulse disappears.**	The point where the pulse disappears provides an estimate of the systolic pressure. To identify the first Korotkoff sound accurately, the cuff must be inflated to a pressure above the point at which the pulse can no longer be felt.
15. Deflate the cuff and wait 15 seconds.	Allowing a brief pause before continuing permits the blood to refill and circulate through the arm.
16. **Assume a position that is no more than 3 feet away from the gauge.**	A distance of more than about 3 feet can interfere with accurate readings of the numbers on the gauge.
17. Place the stethoscope earpieces in your ears. Direct the earpieces forward into the canal and not against the ear itself.	Proper placement blocks extraneous noise and allows sound to travel more clearly.
18. **Place the bell or diaphragm of the stethoscope firmly but with as little pressure as possible over the brachial artery. Do not allow the stethoscope to touch clothing or the cuff.**	Having the bell or diaphragm directly over the artery allows more accurate readings. Heavy pressure on the brachial artery distorts the shape of the artery and the sound. Placing the bell or diaphragm away from clothing and the cuff prevents noise, which would distract from the sounds made by blood flowing through the artery.
19. Pump the pressure 30 mm Hg above the point at which the systolic pressure was palpated and estimated. Open the valve on the manometer and allow air to escape slowly (allowing the gauge to drop 2 to 3 mm per heartbeat).	Increasing the pressure above the point where the pulse disappeared ensures a period before hearing the first sound that corresponds with the systolic pressure. It prevents misinterpreting phase II sounds as phase I.
20. **Note the point on the gauge at which the first faint, but clear, sound appears that slowly increases in intensity. Note this number as the systolic pressure.**	Systolic pressure is the point at which the blood in the artery is first able to force its way through the vessel at a similar pressure exerted by the air bladder in the cuff. The first sound is phase I of Korotkoff sounds.

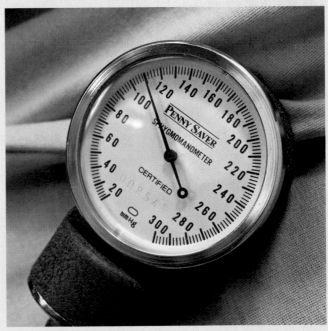

Action 18: Proper placement of diaphragm of stethoscope.

Action 19: Measure systolic blood pressure.

continues

SKILL 1-4 Assessing Blood Pressure (continued)

ACTION	RATIONALE
21. Read the pressure to the closest even number.	It is common practice to read blood pressure to the closest even number.
22. Do not reinflate the cuff once the air is being released to recheck the systolic pressure reading.	Reinflating the cuff while obtaining the blood pressure is uncomfortable for the patient and may cause an inaccurate reading. Reinflating the cuff causes congestion of blood in the lower arm, which lessens the loudness of Korotkoff sounds.
23. **Note the pressure at which the sound first becomes muffled. Also observe the point at which the sound completely disappears. These may occur separately or at the same point.**	The point at which the sound changes corresponds to phase IV Korotkoff sounds and is considered the first diastolic pressure reading. According to the American Heart Association, this is used as the diastolic pressure recording in children. The last sound heard is the beginning of phase V and is the second diastolic measurement.

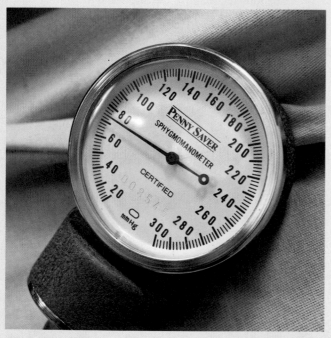

Action 23: Measure diastolic blood pressure.

24. Allow the remaining air to escape quickly. Repeat any suspicious reading, but wait 30 to 60 seconds between readings to allow normal circulation to return in the limb. Deflate the cuff completely between attempts to check the blood pressure.	False readings are likely to occur if there is congestion of blood in the limb while obtaining repeated readings.
25. Remove the cuff, and clean and store the equipment.	Equipment should be left ready for use.
26. Perform hand hygiene. If gloves were worn, discard them in the proper receptacle.	Hand hygiene deters the spread of microorganisms.

continues

SKILL 1-4   **Assessing Blood Pressure** (continued)

ACTION

27. Record the findings on paper, flow sheet, or computerized record. Report abnormal findings to the appropriate person. Identify arm used and site of assessment if other than brachial.

RATIONALE

Reporting and recording ensure accurate documentation and communication.

> 10/18/06   0945   Blood pressure taken in right arm 180/100/88. Physician notified. Ordered Captopril 25 PO mg BID. Blood pressure to be repeated 30 minutes after administering medication.—M. Evans, RN

Action 27: Documentation.

Assessing Blood Pressure With An Electronic Device

To assess a blood pressure with an electronic machine, follow steps 1 to 10 above, then:

11. Turn the machine on. **If the machine has different settings for infants, children, and adults, select the appropriate setting.** Push the start button. **Instruct the patient to hold the arm still.**

The machine is preprogrammed to inflate to a certain systolic pressure. If the machine is set for an infant, it will not inflate as high. The machine will continue to inflate if the patient is moving the arm, which becomes painful for the patient.

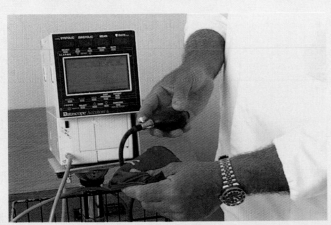

Action 11: Electronic blood pressure machine.

12. Wait until the machine beeps and the blood pressure reading appears. Remove the cuff from the patient's arm and clean and store the equipment.

Equipment should be left ready for use.

13. Perform hand hygiene. If gloves are worn, discard them in the proper receptacle.

Hand hygiene deters the spread of microorganisms.

14. Record the findings on paper, flow sheet, or computerized record. Report abnormal findings to the appropriate person. Identify arm used and site of assessment if other than brachial.

Reporting and recording ensure accurate documentation and communication.

continues

ACTION	RATIONALE

Using a Doppler Ultrasound to Measure Blood Pressure

If the blood pressure is low and you cannot auscultate a blood pressure, you may be able to measure blood pressure using Doppler ultrasound. Follow actions 1 to 11 above, then:

12. Place a small amount of gel over the brachial artery.

> For the Doppler to pick up the sound waves, a medium such as gel or lubricant is needed.

13. Hold the Doppler in your nondominant hand. Using your dominant hand place the Doppler tip in the gel. Adjust the volume as needed. Move the Doppler tip around until you hear the pulse.

> Anatomic locations may vary slightly from person to person. The Doppler may need to be moved to locate the appropriate site.

14. Once the pulse is found using the Doppler, close the valve to the sphygmomanometer. Tighten the screw valve on the air pump.

> The bladder within the cuff will not inflate with the valve open.

15. **Inflate the cuff while continuing to use the Doppler on the artery. Note the point on the gauge where the pulse disappears.**

> The point where the pulse disappears provides an estimate of the systolic pressure.

16. Allow the remaining air to escape quickly. Repeat any suspicious reading, but wait 30 to 60 seconds between readings to allow normal circulation to return in the limb. Deflate the cuff completely between attempts to check the blood pressure.

> False readings are likely to occur if there is congestion of blood in the limb while obtaining repeated readings.

17. Remove the cuff, and clean and store the equipment.

> Equipment should be left ready for use.

18. Perform hand hygiene. If gloves are worn, discard them in the proper receptacle.

> Hand hygiene deters the spread of microorganisms.

19. Record the findings on paper, flow sheet, or computerized record. Report abnormal findings to the appropriate person. Identify arm used and site of assessment if other than brachial.

> Reporting and recording ensure accurate documentation and communication.

> 10/23/06   Doppler blood pressure in right arm 86. Physician notified and at bedside. —M. Evans, RN

Action 19: Documentation.

EVALUATION

The expected outcomes are met when the blood pressure is measured accurately and the patient experiences no trauma.

Infant and Child Considerations

- In infants and small children, the lower extremities are commonly used for blood pressure monitoring. The more common sites are the popliteal, dorsalis pedis, and posterior tibial. Blood pressures obtained in the lower extremities are generally higher than if taken in the upper extremities.
- In newborns, take blood pressure in all four extremities and document. Large differences among blood pressure readings can indicate heart defects.

continues

Assessing Blood Pressure (continued)

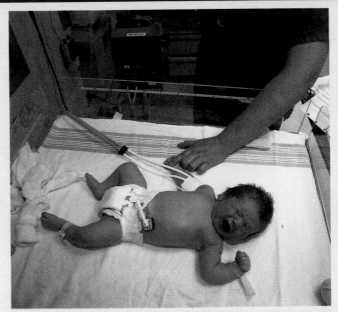

Measuring blood pressure of a newborn using an electronic blood pressure machine and properly sized cuff.   (Photo by Joe Mitchell)

Home Care Considerations

- Use a cuff size appropriate for limb circumference. Inform the patient that cuff sizes range from a pediatric cuff to a large thigh cuff and that a poorly fitting cuff may result in an inaccurate measurement.
- Inform patient about digital blood pressure monitoring equipment. Though costly, most provide an easy-to-read recording of systolic and diastolic measurements.

Special Considerations

- If this is the initial nursing assessment of a patient, take the blood pressure on both arms. It is normal to have a 5- to 10-mm Hg difference in the systolic reading between arms. Use the arm with the higher reading for subsequent pressures.
- If you have difficulty hearing the blood pressure sounds, raise the patient's arm, with cuff in place, over his or her head for 15 seconds before rechecking the blood pressure. Inflate the cuff while the arm is elevated, and then gently lower the arm while continuing to support it. Position the stethoscope and deflate the cuff at the usual rate while listening for Korotkoff sounds. Raising the arm over the head helps relieve congestion of blood in the limb, increases pressure differences, and makes the sounds louder and more distinct when blood enters the lower arm.
- Many electronic devices are not recommended for patients with irregular heart rates, tremors, or the inability to hold the extremity still. The machine will continue to inflate, causing pain for the patient.

Using a Bed Scale

Obtaining a patient's weight is an important component of assessment. In addition to providing baseline information of the patient's overall status, weight is a valuable indicator of nutritional status and fluid balance. Changes in a patient's weight can provide clues to underlying problems such as nutritional deficiencies or fluid excess or deficiency or indicate the development of new problems, such as fluid overload. Weight also can be used to evaluate a patient's response to treatment. For example, if a patient was receiving nutritional supplementation, obtaining daily or biweekly weights would be used to determine achievement of the expected outcome (that is, weight gain).

Typically, weight is measured by having the patient stand on an upright scale. However, doing so requires that the patient is mobile and can maintain his or her balance. For patients who are confined to the bed, have limited mobility, or cannot maintain a balanced standing position for a short period of time, a bed scale can be used. With a bed scale, the patient is placed in a sling and raised above the bed, if the scale is not built into the bed. To ensure safety, a second nurse should be on hand to assist you with weighing the patient.

Equipment	• Bed scale with sling • Cover for sling
ASSESSMENT	Assess the patient's ability to stand for a weight measurement. If patient cannot stand, assess the patient's ability to lie still for a weight measurement. Assess the patient for pain; medication may be given for pain or sedation before placing the patient on a bed scale.
NURSING DIAGNOSIS	Determine the related factors for the nursing diagnosis based on the patient's current status. An appropriate nursing diagnosis is Risk for Injury.
OUTCOME IDENTIFICATION AND PLANNING	The expected outcomes to achieve when weighing the patient are that an accurate weight is measured using the bed scale and the patient experiences no injury.

IMPLEMENTATION

ACTION	RATIONALE
1. Identify the patient.	Identifying the patient provides patient safety.
2. Explain the procedure to the patient.	Explanation reduces apprehension and encourages cooperation.
3. Gather equipment.	Having all equipment on hand provides for an organized approach to the task.
4. Perform hand hygiene.	Hand hygiene deters the spread of microorganisms.
5. Unplug the bed scale from the electrical outlet. Slide the disposable plastic cover over the sling of the bed scale.	Using a cover deters the spread of microorganisms.
6. Attach the sling to the bed scale. Turn the scale on. **Adjust the dial so that weight reads 0.0.**	Scale will add the sling into the weight unless it is zeroed with the sling and cover.
7. Remove the sling from the scale. Raise bed to a comfortable working level. Roll sling long ways. Raise side rail. Turn patient onto side facing side rail. Place rolled sling under patient.	Raising the bed to the appropriate height prevents strain to the nurse's back. This position facilitates placing the patient onto the sling.
8. Roll patient back over sling and up on other side. Pull sling through (as if placing sheet under patient).	This facilitates placing patient onto sling.

continues

SKILL 1-5

Using a Bed Scale (continued)

ACTION	RATIONALE
9. Roll scale so that arms of scale are directly over patient. **Spread the base of the scale.** Remove pillow and blankets. Lower arms of the scale and place hooks into holes on the sling.	By spreading the base, you are giving the scale a wider base, thus preventing the scale from toppling over with the patient.
10. Once scale arms are hooked onto the sling, begin to crank scale so that patient is lifted up off of the bed. **Assess all tubes and drains, making sure that none have tension placed on them as the scale is lifted. Once the sling is no longer touching the bed, ensure that nothing else is hanging onto the sling (e.g., ventilator tubing, intravenous tubing). If any tubing is connected to the patient, raise it up so that it is not adding any weight to the patient.**	Scale must be hanging free to obtain an accurate weight. Any tubing that is hanging off the scale will add weight to the patient.
11. Note weight on the scale. Slowly and gently, lower patient back onto the bed. Disconnect scale arms from sling. Close base of scale and remove from room.	Lowering patient slowly does not alarm patient. Closing the base of the scale facilitates removing from the room.
12. Raise side rail. Turn patient to side rail. Roll the sling up against the patient's backside.	Raising the side rail is a safety measure.
13. Raise the other side rail. Roll patient back over the sling and up facing the other side rail. Remove sling from bed.	Patient needs to be removed from sling before it can be removed from the bed.
14. Place patient in comfortable position. **Lower the bed.**	These actions promote patient comfort and safety.
15. Remove disposable cover from sling and discard in appropriate receptacle. Replace scale and sling in appropriate spot. Plug scale into electrical outlet.	Using a cover deters spread of microorganisms. Scale should be ready for use at any time.
16. Document weight and scale used.	Reporting and recording ensure accurate documentation and communication.

10/15/06 0230   *Patient weighed using bed scale. 75.2 kg. Pt. premedicated with 5 mg Versed prior to weighing.—M. Evans, RN*

Action 16: Documentation.

EVALUATION   The expected outcome is met when the patient is weighed without injury using the bed scale.

Unexpected Situations and Associated Interventions

- *As the patient is being lifted, the scale begins to tip over:* Stop lifting the patient. Slowly lower the patient back to the bed. Ensure that the base of the scale is spread before attempting to weigh the patient.
- *Weight differs from the previous day's weight by more than 1 kg:* Weigh the patient using the same scale at the same time each day. Check calibration of the scale. Make sure that the patient is wearing the same clothing. Make sure that no tubes or containers are hanging on the scale. If the patient is incontinent, make sure undergarments are clean and dry.
- *Patient becomes agitated as the sling is raised into the air:* Stop lifting the patient and reassure him or her. If the patient continues to be agitated, lower him or her back to the bed and obtain an order for sedation before attempting to take another weight.

SKILL 1-6   Monitoring Temperature Using an Overhead Radiant Warmer

Maintaining body temperature is important for overall body function. This is especially true in neonates and infants who are making the transition to extrauterine life and are exposed to stressors or chilling (e.g., from undergoing numerous procedures), or who have an underlying condition that interferes with thermoregulation (e.g., prematurity). This group is highly susceptible to heat loss.

An overhead radiant warmer warms the air to provide a neutral thermal environment, one that is neither too warm nor too cool for the patient. Typically radiant warmers are used for infants who have trouble maintaining body temperature. In addition, use of a radiant warmer minimizes the oxygen and calories that the infant would expend to maintain body temperature, thereby minimizing the effects of body temperature changes on metabolic activity.

Equipment

- Overhead warmer
- Temperature probe
- Aluminum foil probe cover

ASSESSMENT

Assess the patient's temperature using the axillary route and assess the patient's fluid intake and output.

NURSING DIAGNOSIS

Determine the related factors for the nursing diagnoses based on the patient's current status. Appropriate nursing diagnoses may include:

- Hyperthermia
- Hypothermia
- Risk for Imbalanced Body Temperature
- Ineffective Thermoregulation

OUTCOME IDENTIFICATION AND PLANNING

The expected outcomes to achieve when using an overhead warmer are that the infant is placed under the warmer; the temperature is well controlled; and the infant experiences no injury.

IMPLEMENTATION

ACTION	RATIONALE
1. Identify the patient.	Identifying the patient provides for patient safety.
2. Explain the procedure to the family.	Explanation reduces the family's apprehension and encourages family cooperation.
3. Gather equipment.	Having all equipment on hand provides for an organized approach to the task.
4. Perform hand hygiene.	Hand hygiene deters the spread of microorganisms.
5. Plug the warmer in. Turn the warmer to the manual setting. Allow the blankets to warm before placing the infant under the warmer.	By allowing the blankets to warm before placing the infant under the warmer, you are preventing heat loss through conduction. By placing the warmer on the manual setting, you are keeping the warmer at a set temperature no matter how warm the blankets become.
6. **Switch the warmer setting to automatic.** Place the infant under the warmer. Attach probe to the infant so that the probe is directly under the radiant heater but not on a bony area. Cover with a foil patch.	The automatic setting ensures that the warmer will regulate the amount of radiant heat depending on the temperature of the infant's skin. The foil patch prevents direct warming of the probe, allowing the probe to read only the infant's temperature.

continues

Monitoring Temperature Using an Overhead Radiant Warmer (continued)

ACTION   **RATIONALE**

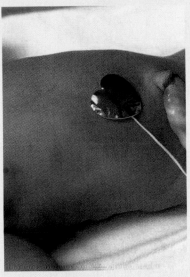

Action 6: Probe in place with foil cover.
(Photo by Joe Mitchell)

7. **Adjust the temperature as ordered.**

The temperature should be adjusted so that the infant does not become too warm or too cold.

8. **Continue to monitor the axillary temperature as ordered.** The temperature may need to be monitored more frequently in the beginning.

By monitoring the infant's axillary temperature, you are watching for signs of fever or hypothermia.

9. Adjust the warmer's temperature as needed according to the axillary temperatures.

This prevents the infant from becoming too warm or too cool.

10. Document the placement of the infant under the radiant warmer and the settings of the radiant warmer.

Documentation promotes communication and continuity of care.

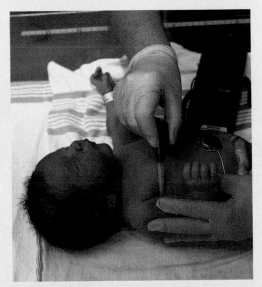

Action 8: Taking infant's axillary temperature.
(Photo by Joe Mitchell)

10/13/06 1110   *Infant placed under radiant warmer. Warmer on automatic setting 36.7, baby's skin temperature 36.8.*
—M. Evans, RN

Action 10: Documentation

continues

EVALUATION	The expected outcomes are met when the infant is placed under a radiant warmer; the temperature is well controlled; and the infant experiences no injury.
Unexpected Situations and Associated Interventions	• *The infant become febrile under the radiant warmer:* Do not turn the warmer off and leave the infant naked. This could cause cold stress and even death. Leave the warmer on automatic and dial the set temperature. Notify the physician. • *The warmer's temperature is fluctuating constantly or is inaccurate:* Change the probe cover. If this does not improve the temperature variations, change the probe as well.
Special Considerations	• Many times, plastic surgeons order overhead radiant warmers to be used for patients who have undergone extremity or digit reattachment surgery. In this case, judge the heat by the probe's reading of the skin temperature.

■ Developing Critical Thinking Skills

1. Tyrone Jeffries, the 5-year-old with a fever of 38.9°C, is suspected of having a middle ear infection. You need to obtain another set of vital signs for him. As you approach with the electronic thermometer, Tyrone begins to scream, saying, "Get away from me with that thing. You're not going to put that thing in me!" How would you respond?
2. Toby White, who is 26 years old with a history of asthma, has a respiratory rate of 32 breaths per minute. What other assessments would be most important to make?
3. Carl Glatz, the 58-year-old man receiving medications for hypertension, asks you about how he should monitor his blood pressure at home. What information would you suggest?

Bibliography

Baue, W. (2003). Phase-out of mercury thermometers continues to rise. SocialFunds.com. Available *www.socialfunds.com/news/article.cgi?sfArticleId=752*.

Bauer, J. (2002). Blood pressure cuffs. *RN, 65*(8), 61–62.

Bauer, J. (2002). Vital signs monitors. *RN, 65*(7), 61–62.

Bauer, J. (2003). Thermometers. *RN, 66*(3), 63–54.

Faria, S. (1999). Assessment of peripheral arterial pulses. *Home Care Provider, 4*(4), 140–141.

Gall, G. (2002). A useful screening tool. *RN, 65*(9), 41–43.

Holtzclaw, B. (2001). Circadian rhythmicity and homeostatic stability in thermoregulation. *Biological Research for Nursing, 2*(4), 221–235.

Lanham, D., Walker, B., Klocke, E., & Jennings, M. (1999). Accuracy of tympanic temperature readings in children under 6 years of age. *Pediatric Nursing, 25*(1), 39–42.

NANDA International. (2003). *Nursing diagnoses: Definitions & classification.* Philadelphia: NANDA.

Porth, C. (2002). *Pathophysiology: Concepts of altered health states* (6th ed.). Philadelphia: Lippincott.

U.S. Department of Health and Human Services. (2003, May). *The seventh report of the joint national committee on prevention, detection, evaluation, and treatment of high blood pressure* (NIH Publication 03-5233). National Institutes of Health, National Heart, Lung, and Blood Institute.

Weber, J., & Kelley, J. (2003). *Health assessment in nursing* (2nd ed.). Philadelphia: Lippincott Williams & Wilkins.

Assessment

This chapter will help you develop some of the skills related to assessment necessary to care for the following patients:

William Lincoln comes to the clinic complaining of cold and flulike symptoms.

Lois Felker, age 30, has a history of type 1 diabetes. She comes to the physician's office for a routine checkup.

Bobby Williams, a teenager brought to the emergency department by his parents, is suspected of having appendicitis.

Learning Outcomes

After studying this chapter, the reader should be able to:

1. Perform a head-to-toe-physical assessment.
2. Collect a venous blood sample via venipuncture.
3. Obtain a blood specimen for culture and sensitivity.

Key Terms

adventitious breath sounds: sounds that are not normally heard in the lungs on auscultation

auscultation: act of listening with a stethoscope to sounds produced within the body

bruits: abnormal "swooshing" sounds heard on auscultation indicating turbulent blood flow

cyanosis: bluish or grayish discoloration of the skin in response to inadequate oxygenation

ecchymosis: a collection of blood in the subcutaneous tissues, causing purplish discoloration

edema: excess fluid in the tissues, characterized by swelling

erythema: redness of the skin

inspection: process of performing deliberate, purposeful observations in a systematic manner

jaundice: yellow color of the skin resulting from liver and gall-bladder diseases, some types of anemia, and hemolysis

pallor: paleness of the skin

palpation: an assessment technique that uses the sense of touch

percussion: the act of striking one object against another to produce sound

petechiae: small hemorrhagic spots caused by capillary bleeding

precordium: the area on the anterior chest corresponding to the aortic, pulmonic, tricuspid, and apical areas and Erb's point

turgor: fullness or elasticity of the skin

Health assessment is an integral component of nursing care and is the basis of

the nursing process. Assessments are used to plan, implement, and evaluate teaching and care in order to promote an optimal level of health through interventions to prevent illness, restore health, and facilitate coping with disabilities or death. Health assessments are a part of nursing care for patients across the lifespan and may be conducted in any setting.

The scope and type of assessment conducted varies based on the setting, the patient's health-care needs, and the acuity of the health problem. A health assessment may be comprehensive, ongoing partial, focused, or emergency. A comprehensive assessment with a health history and complete physical examination is usually conducted when a patient enters a healthcare setting; information is used as a baseline for comparing later assessment. An ongoing partial assessment is one that is conducted at regular intervals (such as at the beginning of each home health visit or each hospital shift) during patient care. This type of assessment focuses on identified health problems to monitor positive or negative changes and evaluate the effectiveness of interventions. A focused assessment is conducted to assess a specific problem. An emergency assessment is a type of rapid focused assessment conducted to determine potentially fatal situations.

A health history is a collection of subjective data that provides a detailed profile of the patient's health status. Nurses use therapeutic communication skills and interviewing techniques during the health history to establish an effective nurse–patient relationship and to gather data to identify actual and potential health problems as well as sources of strength. A physical assessment is the systematic collection of objective data that is directly observed or is elicited through examination techniques. Performing a physical assessment requires knowledge about the equipment being used, proper patient positioning and draping, and the techniques of inspection, palpation, percussion, and auscultation. In addition, laboratory and diagnostic tests provide crucial information about a patient's health. These results become a part of the total health assessment.

This chapter will cover skills to assist the nurse in performing an assessment. Please look over the summary boxes and tables at the beginning of this chapter for a quick review of critical knowledge to assist you in understanding the skills related to assessment.

BOX 2-1 Symptom Analysis

The mnemonic "PQRST" is a helpful guide to analyze a patient's symptoms:

Provocative or palliative: What causes the symptom? What makes it better or worse?

- What were you doing when you first noticed it?
- What seems to trigger it? Stress? Position? Certain activities? An argument? (For a sign such as an eye discharge: What seems to cause it or make it worse? For a psychological symptom such as depression: Does the depression occur after specific events?)
- What relieves the symptom? Changing diet? Changing position? Taking medication? Being active?
- What makes the symptom worse?

Quality or quantity: How does the symptom feel, look, or sound? How much of it are you experiencing now?

- How would you describe the symptom—how it feels, looks, or sounds?
- How much are you experiencing now? Is it so much that it prevents you from performing any activities? Is it more or less than you experienced at any other time?

Region or radiation: Where is the symptom located? Does it spread?

- Where does the symptom occur?
- In the case of pain, does it travel down your back or arms, up your neck, or down your legs?

Severity: How does the symptom rate on a scale of 1 to 10, with 10 being the most severe?

- How bad is the symptom at its worst? Does it force you to lie down, sit down, or slow down?
- Does the symptom seem to be getting better, getting worse, or staying about the same?

Timing: When did the symptom begin? Did it occur suddenly or gradually? How often does it occur?

- On what date and time did the symptom first occur?
- How did the symptom start? Suddenly? Gradually?
- How often do you experience the symptom? Hourly? Daily? Weekly? Monthly?
- When do you usually experience the symptom? During the day? At night? In the early morning? Does it awaken you? Does it occur before, during, or after meals? Does it occur seasonally?
- How long does an episode of the symptom last?

BOX 2-2 Assessment Techniques

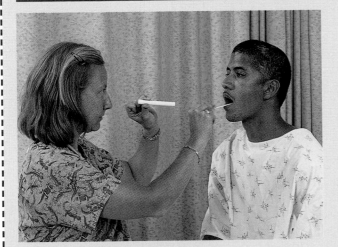

Inspection

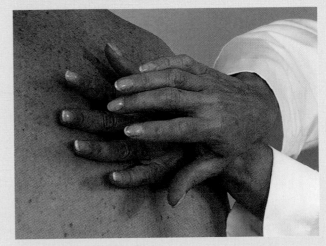

Percussion

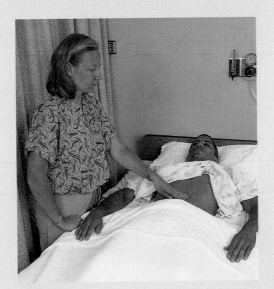

Light palpation

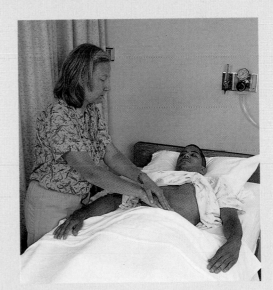

Deep palpation

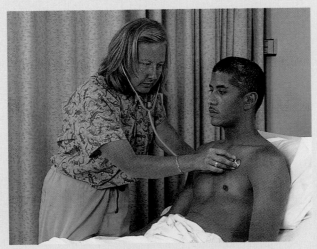

Auscultation

(Photos © B. Proud.)

BOX 2-3 Outline of a Head-to-Toe Physical Assessment

- General survey
- Height and weight
- Vital signs
- Head
    - Skin
    - Face, skull and scalp, hair
    - Eyes
    - Ears
    - Nose and sinuses
    - Mouth and oropharynx
    - Cranial nerves
- Neck
    - Skin
    - Lymph nodes
    - Muscles
    - Thyroid
    - Trachea
    - Carotid arteries
    - Neck veins
- Chest and back
    - Skin
    - Chest size and shape
    - Heart
    - Lungs
    - Breasts and axilla
    - Spine

- Upper extremities
    - Skin, hair, and fingernails
    - Sensation
    - Muscle size, strength, and tone
    - Joint range of motion
    - Radial and brachial pulses
    - Tendon reflexes
- Abdomen
    - Skin
    - Bowel sounds
    - Vascular sounds
    - Abdominal contents
    - Specific organs, such as the liver and bladder
- Genitalia
    - Skin and hair
    - Urethra
    - Males: penis and testes
    - Females: vagina
- Anus and rectum
- Lower extremities
    - Skin, hair, and toenails
    - Gait and balance
    - Muscle size, strength, and tone
    - Joint range of motion
    - Popliteal, posterior tibial, and pedal pulses
    - Tendon and plantar reflexes

BOX 2-4 Normal Breath Sounds

Bronchial Breath Sounds

Pitch: High
Quality: Harsh or hollow
Amplitude: Loud
Duration: Short during inspiration, long in expiration
Location: Trachea and larynx

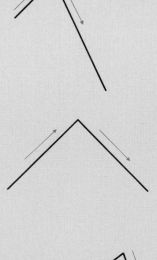

Bronchovesicular Breath Sounds

Pitch: Moderate
Quality: Mixed
Amplitude: Moderate
Duration: Same in inspiration and expiration
Location: Over the major bronchi—posterior: between the scapulae; anterior: around the upper sternum in the first and second intercostal spaces

Vesicular Breath Sounds

Pitch: Low
Quality: Breezy
Amplitude: Soft
Duration: Long in inspiration, short in expiration
Location: Peripheral lung fields

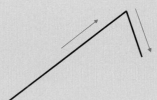

(From Weber, J., & Kelley, J. [2003]. *Health assessment on nursing* [2nd ed.]. Philadelphia: Lippincott Williams & Wilkins.)

TABLE 2-1 **Positions Used in Physical Assessment**

Position	Description
Standing 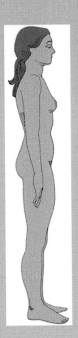	The patient stands erect. This position should not be used for patients who are weak, dizzy, or prone to fall. It is used to assess posture, balance, and gait (while walking upright).
Sitting 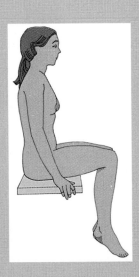	The patient may sit in a chair or on the side of the bed or examining table, or may remain in bed with the head elevated. It allows visualization of the upper body and facilitates full lung expansion and is used to assess vital signs and the head, neck, anterior and posterior thorax and lungs, heart, breasts, and upper extremities.
Supine 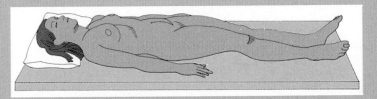	The patient lies flat on the back with legs extended and knees slightly flexed. It facilitates abdominal muscle relaxation and is used to assess vital signs and the head, neck, anterior thorax and lungs, heart, breasts, abdomen, extremities, and peripheral pulses.

continues

TABLE 2-1 continued

Position	Description

Dorsal recumbent

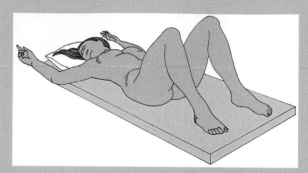

The patient lies on the back with legs separated, knees flexed, and soles of the feet on the bed. It should not be used for abdominal assessment as it causes contraction of abdominal muscles. It is used to assess the head, neck, anterior thorax and lungs, heart, breasts, extremities, and peripheral pulses.

Sims'

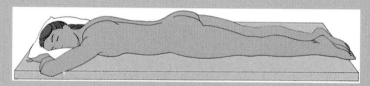

The patient lies on either side with the lower arm below the body and the upper arm flexed at the shoulder and elbow. Both knees are flexed, with the upper leg more acutely flexed. It is used to assess the rectum or vagina.

Prone

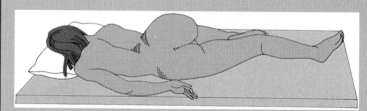

The patient lies flat on the bed on the abdomen with the head turned to one side. It is used to assess the hip joint and the posterior thorax.

Lithotomy

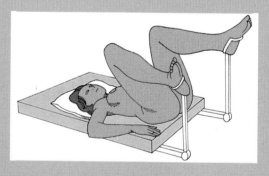

The patient is in the dorsal recumbent position with the buttocks at the edge of the examining table and the heels in stirrups. It is used to assess the female genitalia and rectum.

Knee–chest

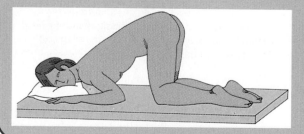

The patient kneels, with the body at a 90-degree angle to the hips, back straight, arms above the head. It is used to assess the anus and rectum.

TABLE 2-2 Percussion Tones

Tone	Relative Intensity	Sample Location
Flat	Soft	Thigh
Dull	Medium	Liver
Resonance	Loud	Normal lung
Hyperresonance	Very loud	Emphysematous lung
Tympany	Loud	Gastric air bubble or puffed-out cheek

TABLE 2-3 Adventitious Breath Sounds

Abnormal Sound	Characteristics	Source	Conditions
Discontinuous Sounds Crackles (fine) 	High-pitched, short, popping sounds heard during inspiration and not cleared with coughing; sounds are discontinuous and can be simulated by rolling a strand of hair between your fingers near your ear.	Inhaled air suddenly opens the small deflated air passages that are coated and sticky with exudate.	Crackles occurring late in inspiration are associated with restrictive diseases such as pneumonia and congestive heart failure. Crackles occurring early in inspiration are associated with obstructive disorders such as bronchitis, asthma, or emphysema.
Crackles (coarse) 	Low-pitched, bubbling, moist sounds that may persist from early inspiration to early expiration; also described as softly separating Velcro.	Inhaled air comes into contact with secretions in the large bronchi and trachea.	Can indicate such things as pneumonia, pulmonary edema, and pulmonary fibrosis. "Velcro rales" of pulmonary fibrosis are heard louder and closer to stethoscope, usually do not change location, and are more common in clients with long-term COPD.
Continuous Sounds Pleural friction rub 	Low-pitched, dry, grating sound. Sound is much like crackles, only more superficial and occurs during both inspiration and expiration.	Sound is the result of rubbing of two inflamed pleural surfaces.	Pleuritis
Wheeze (sibilant) 	High-pitched, musical sounds heard primarily during expiration but may also be heard on inspiration.	Air passing through constricted passages caused by swelling, secretions, or tumor.	Sibilant wheezes are often heard in cases of acute asthma or chronic emphysema.
Wheeze (sonorous) 	Low-pitched snoring or moaning sounds heard primarily during expiration but may be heard throughout the respiratory cycle. These wheezes may clear with coughing.	Same as sibilant wheeze. The pitch of the wheeze cannot be correlated to the size of the passageway that generates it.	Sonorous wheezes are often heard in cases of bronchitis or single obstructions and snoring before an episode of sleep apnea. *Stridor* is a harsh honking wheeze with severe broncholaryngospasm, such as occurs with croup.

Performing a Head-to-Toe Physical Assessment

Nurses perform a complete physical assessment when the patient is admitted to the facility and partial reassessments as the patient's condition warrants. A complete assessment includes a thorough health history and physical examination. The health history includes the chief complaint, a history of the current illness, general medical and surgical histories, a family history, a social history, and a review of systems.

Typically, the physical examination follows a methodical, head-to-toe format. Patient preparation includes providing a clear explanation of the examination as well as proper positioning and draping before and during the examination. The nurse must make every effort to recognize and respect the patient's feelings (particularly embarrassment and anxiety) as well as to provide comfort measures and to take appropriate safety precautions.

Equipment

- Scale with height measurement bar
- Sphygmomanometer
- Watch with second hand
- Stethoscope
- Thermometer
- Patient gown
- Examining table if necessary
- Gloves
- Sheet, bath blanket, or towel, as needed for draping
- Tape
- Lighting, including a flashlight
- Laryngeal mirror
- Tongue blades
- Percussion (reflex) hammer
- Otoscope
- Tuning fork
- Tape measure
- Visual acuity chart
- Ophthalmoscope
- Test tubes of hot and cold water
- Containers of odorous materials (e.g., coffee or chocolate) and substances for taste assessment (sugar, salt, vinegar)
- Miscellaneous items such as coin, pin, cotton, or paper clip
- Waterproof pads
- Water-soluble lubricant
- Facial tissues
- Cotton-tipped applicators

ASSESSMENT

Complete a health history. Obtain biographical data, including the patient's name, address, telephone number, contact person, gender, age and birthdate, birthplace, Social Security number, marital status, education, religion, occupation, race, nationality, and cultural background as well as the names of persons living with the patient. Question the patient about his or her health and illness patterns, the chief complaint, current and past health status, family health status, and condition of body systems. Inquire about health promotion and protection patterns, including health beliefs, personal habits, sleep and wake cycles, exercise, recreation, nutrition, stress level and coping skills, socioeconomic status, environmental health conditions, and occupational health hazards. Explore the patient's role and relationship patterns, including self-concept, cultural and religious influences, family roles and relationships, sexuality and reproductive patterns, social support systems, and any other psychosocial considerations. Finally, review the patient's health history to obtain subjective data about the patient and insight into problem areas and subtle physical changes. Investigate the patient's chief complaint.

continues

NURSING DIAGNOSIS

Determine the related factors for the nursing diagnoses based on the patient's current status. An appropriate nursing diagnosis may be Anxiety. Other appropriate nursing diagnoses may include:

- Fear
- Ineffective Health Maintenance
- Health-Seeking Behaviors
- Deficient Knowledge

Many other nursing diagnoses also may require the use of this skill.

OUTCOME IDENTIFICATION AND PLANNING

The expected outcome to achieve when performing a physical assessment is that the patient participates in the assessment and demonstrates a decrease in anxiety related to assessment and possible findings. Other outcomes may be appropriate depending on the patient's nursing diagnosis.

IMPLEMENTATION

ACTION	RATIONALE
1. Explain the physical examination and answer questions.	Explanation helps to alleviate anxiety, promotes cooperation, and facilitates the examination.
2. Instruct the patient to void if possible. Collect a urine specimen if ordered.	Emptying the bladder increases patient comfort during the examination.
3. Perform hand hygiene.	Hand hygiene deters the risk of microorganism transmission.
4. Help the patient undress, and provide a gown.	Having the patient wear a gown facilitates examination of the various body areas.
5. Measure and record height, weight, and vital signs.	These measurements provide a baseline for future comparisons and provide clues to problems.
6. Assist the patient onto the examination table, stretcher, or bed; position and drape the patient according to the body area to be assessed.	Proper positioning facilitates the examination; draping provides for warmth and maintains privacy. Requirements for positioning and draping vary with the body system and region being assessed. To examine the head, neck, and anterior and posterior thorax, the patient sits on the edge of the examination table or bed. For the abdomen and cardiovascular system, the supine and standing positions are used. For an abdominal assessment in the female patient, a towel is placed over her breasts and upper thorax and the sheet is pulled down as far as her symphysis pubis.

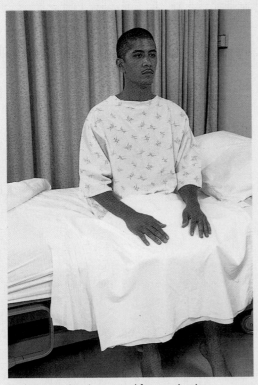

Action 6: Patient is prepared for examination.
(Photo © B. Proud.)

continues

Performing a Head-to-Toe Physical Assessment (continued)

ACTION

7. Perform a physical examination, starting at the head and working in a systematic fashion. Don gloves when indicated.

8. Inspect the head, noting hair color, texture, and distribution. Palpate from the forehead to the posterior triangle of the neck for the posterior cervical lymph nodes.

9. Palpate in front of and behind the ears, under the chin, and in the anterior triangle for the anterior cervical lymph nodes.

10. Palpate the left and then the right carotid arteries and auscultate the arteries.

11. Palpate the trachea and then the suprasternal notch.

RATIONALE

Proceeding in a systematic fashion promotes organization and efficiency, ensuring that all body areas are addressed. Gloves reduce the risk of infection transmission.

This technique can detect asymmetry, size changes, enlarged lymph nodes, and tenderness.

This technique can detect enlarged lymph nodes.

Palpation of this area evaluates circulation through the arteries; auscultation can detect a bruit.

Tracheal palpation evaluates its position; palpation of the suprasternal notch allows evaluation of aortic arch pulsations.

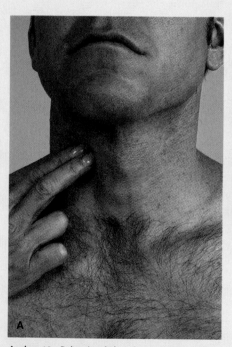
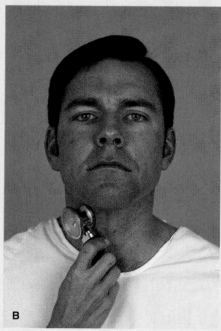
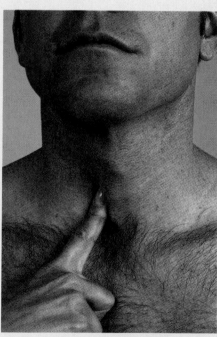
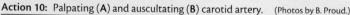

Action 10: Palpating **(A)** and auscultating **(B)** carotid artery.   (Photos by B. Proud.)

Action 11: Palpating to determine position of trachea.   (Photo by B. Proud.)

12. Palpate the supraclavicular area.

13. Palpate and then auscultate the thyroid gland.

14. Have the patient touch his or her chin to chest and to each shoulder, each ear to the corresponding shoulder, and then tip head back as far as possible.

This technique can detect enlarged lymph nodes.

Palpation reveals thyroid enlargement, tenderness, or nodules; auscultation identifies bruits.

These actions evaluate neck range of motion.

continues

Performing a Head-to-Toe Physical Assessment (continued)

ACTION | **RATIONALE**

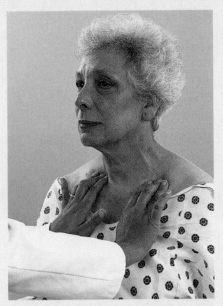

Action 12: Palpating the supraclavicular nodes.
(Photo © B. Proud.)

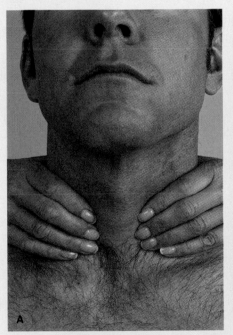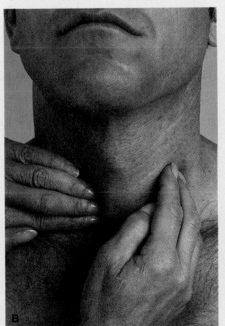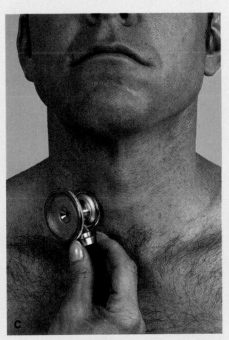

Action 13: (**A**) Palpating the thyroid using a posterior approach. (**B**) Palpating he thyroid using an anterior approach. (**C**) Auscultating the thyroid. (Photos by B. Proud.)

15. Place your hands on the patient's shoulders while he or she shrugs against resistance. Then place your hand on the patient's left cheek, then the right cheek, and have the patient push against it.

These actions check cranial nerve XI (accessory nerve) function and trapezius and sternocleidomastoid muscle strength.

continues

Performing a Head-to-Toe Physical Assessment (continued)

ACTION	**RATIONALE**

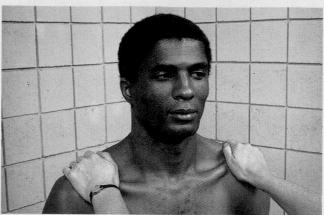

Action 15: Testing accessory nerve. The patient shrugs his shoulders against the resistance of the nurse's hands.   (Photo © Ken Kasper.)

16. Have the patient smile, frown, wrinkle forehead, and puff out cheeks.	This maneuver evaluates the motor function of cranial nerve VII (facial nerve).
17. Occlude one nostril externally with a finger while patient breathes through the other; repeat for the other side.	This technique checks the patency of the nasal passages.
18. Inspect the internal nostrils using an otoscope with a nasal speculum attachment or an ophthalmoscope handle with a nasal attachment.	This technique can detect edema, inflammation, and excessive drainage.

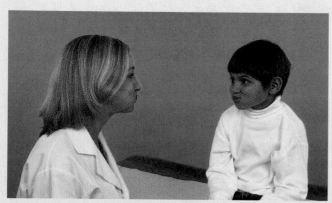

Action 16: Evaluating motor function of facial nerve. The patient puffs out cheeks as instructed.   (Photo by B. Proud.)

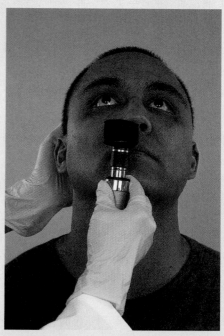

Action 18: Inspecting the internal nostrils. (Photo © B. Proud.)

continues

SKILL 2-1   Performing a Head-to-Toe Physical Assessment (continued)

ACTION	RATIONALE
19. Palpate the nose and then palpate and percuss the frontal and maxillary sinuses. Transilluminate the sinuses if the patient reports tenderness.	Palpation of the nose helps to detect structural abnormalities. Sinus palpation and percussion are used to elicit tenderness, which may indicate sinus congestion or infection.

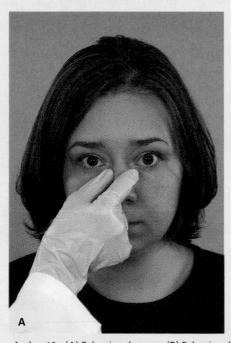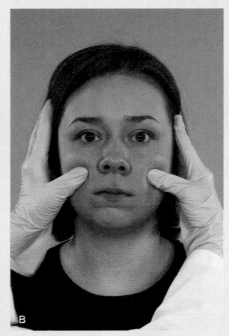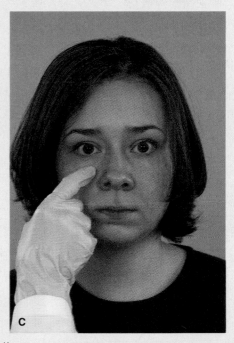

Action 19: (A) Palpating the nose. (B) Palpating the sinuses. (C) Percussing the sinuses.   (Photos © B. Proud.)

20. Palpate the temporomandibular joint as the patient opens and closes the jaw.	The action evaluates the temporomandibular joints and the motor portion of cranial nerve V (trigeminal nerve).
21. Inspect the oral mucosa, gingivae, teeth, and salivary gland openings using a tongue blade and penlight.	This technique evaluates the condition of the oral structures.

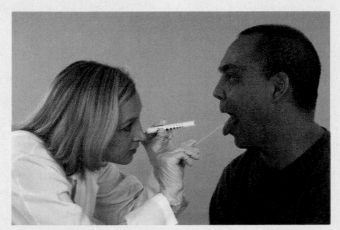

Action 21: Inspecting the mouth using a tongue blade and penlight.
(Photo by B. Proud.)

continues

ACTION

RATIONALE

22. Observe the tongue and hard and soft palates; ask the patient to stick out the tongue; **ask the patient to say "ahh" while sticking out the tongue.** Inspect the visible oral structures.

Observation provides information about the hydration and condition of oral structures. Sticking out the tongue evaluates the function of cranial nerve XII (hypoglossal nerve). Saying "ahh" checks portions of cranial nerve IX and X (glossopharyngeal and vagus nerves).

23. **Test the gag reflex.**

Gagging indicates intact cranial nerves IX and X.

24. Place a tongue blade at the side of the tongue while patient pushes it to the left and right with the tongue.

This action tests cranial nerve XII.

25. Ask the patient to close the eyes and identify the smell of different substances, such as coffee, chocolate, or alcohol.

This action tests the function of cranial nerve I (olfactory nerve).

26. Test the patient's visual acuity with a Snellen chart or another chart; have the patient identify the pattern in a specially prepared page of color dots or plates.

This testing evaluates the patient's distance vision (central vision) and function of cranial nerve II (optic nerve); testing with color dots or plates evaluates color perception.

27. Move the patient's eyes through the six cardinal positions of gaze.

This testing evaluates the function of each of the six extraocular eye muscles and tests cranial nerves III, IV, and VI (oculomotor, trochlear, and abducens nerves).

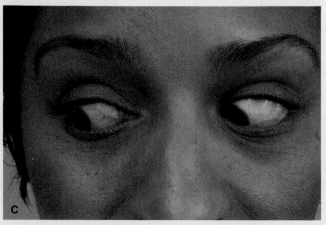

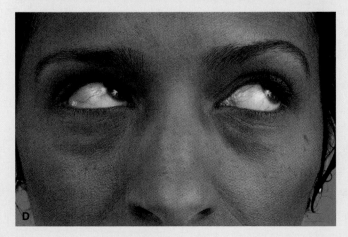

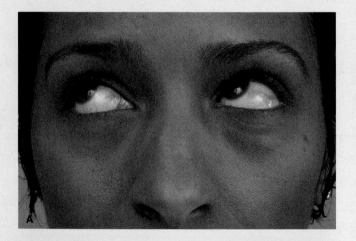

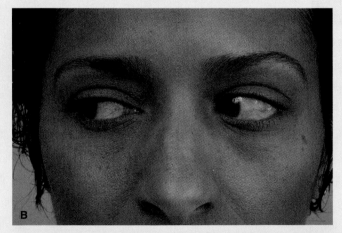

Action 27: Six cardinal positions of gaze.   (Photos by B. Proud.)

continues

Performing a Head-to-Toe Physical Assessment (continued)

ACTION	RATIONALE

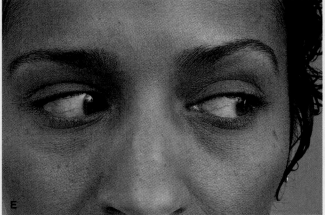

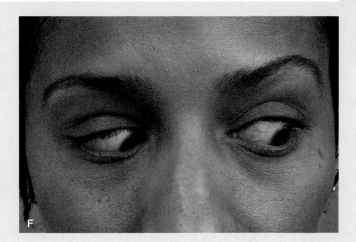

Action 27: (*Continued*)

28. Inspect the external eye structures, conjunctiva, and sclera.

Inspection detects abnormalities such as ptosis, styes, conjunctivitis, or scleral color changes associated with systemic disorders.

29. Inspect the cornea, iris, and anterior chamber by shining a penlight tangentially across the eye.

This technique assesses anterior chamber depth and condition of the iris and cornea.

30. **Examine the pupils for equality of size, shape, reaction to light, and accommodation.**

Testing pupillary response to light and accommodation assesses cranial nerves III, IV, and VI.

31. Using an ophthalmoscope, check the red reflex.

Presence of the red reflex indicates that the cornea, anterior chamber, and lens are free of opacity and clouding.

32. Inspect the ear and perform an otoscopic examination; palpate the ear and mastoid process.

These techniques evaluate the structures of external and middle ear; palpation reveals inflammation or infection, nodules, or lesions.

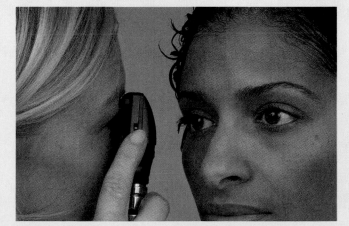

Action 31: Checking red reflex using an ophthalmoscope. (Photo by B. Proud.)

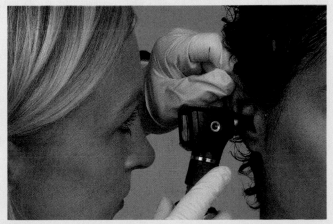

Action 32: Performing an otoscopic examination to evaluate structures of the external and middle ear. For an adult, the pinna is pulled up and back. (Photo by B. Proud.)

continues

Performing a Head-to-Toe Physical Assessment (continued)

ACTION	RATIONALE

33. Use a whispered voice or ticking of a watch to test hearing, one ear at a time.

This testing provides a gross assessment of cranial nerve VII (acoustic nerve).

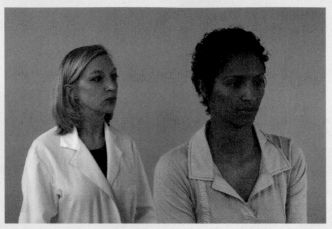

Action 33: Performing the whispered voice test to check hearing.
(Photo by B. Proud.)

34. Use a tuning fork to perform Weber's test and Rinne's test.

These tests help to differentiate conductive from sensorineural hearing loss.

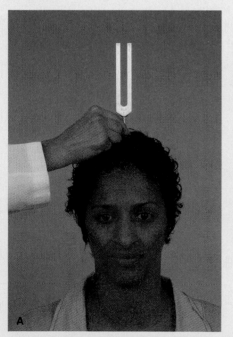
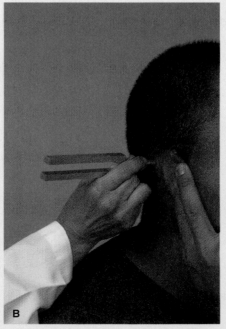
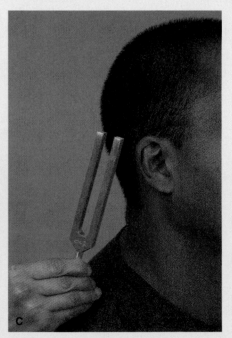

Action 34: (A) Performing a Weber's test. (B and C) Performing the Rinne test. First, the tuning fork base is placed on the mastoid process (B), after which the prongs are moved to the front of the external auditory canal (C). (Photos by B. Proud.)

continues

Performing a Head-to-Toe Physical Assessment (continued)

ACTION	RATIONALE
35. Inspect the posterior thorax. Observe the skin, bones, and muscles of the spine, shoulder blades, and back as well as symmetry of expansion and accessory muscle use.	Observation provides information about lung expansion and accessory muscle use during respirations; it also provides information about deformities that could alter ventilation. Inspection of skin helps identify lesions, abnormalities, or variations such as moles.
36. Assess the anteroposterior and lateral diameters of the thorax.	This assessment helps to detect deformities such as barrel chest.
37. Palpate over the spine and posterior thorax.	Palpation detects pain in the spine and paraspinous muscles, evaluates muscle consistency, and helps detect musculoskeletal inflammation.

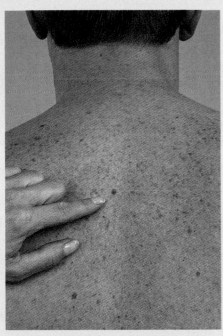

Action 35: Inspecting the skin for abnormalities and variations. Any lesion or mole noted during inspection of the patient's back should be documented in the patient's medical record for follow-up evaluation.   (Photo by B. Proud.)

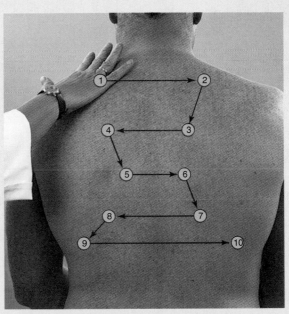

Action 37: Sequence for palpating posterior thorax.

38. Assess respiratory excursion and tactile fremitus (as the patient repeats "ninety-nine").	Respiratory excursion indicates lung expansion; assessing tactile fremitus provides information about content of lungs (vibrations increase over consolidated or fluid-filled areas).
39. Percuss over the posterior and lateral lung fields and for diaphragmatic excursion on each side of the thorax.	Percussion over the lung fields helps identify the density and location of the lungs, diaphragm, and other anatomic structures; diaphragmatic excursion provides information about diaphragm movement during respiration.

continues

Performing a Head-to-Toe Physical Assessment (continued)

ACTION	RATIONALE

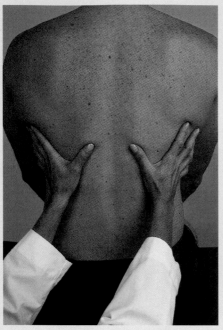

Action 38: Assessing respiratory excursion.
(Photo by B. Proud.)

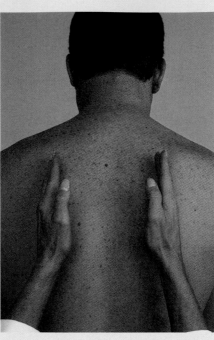

Action 38: Assessing for tactile fremitus.
(Photo by B. Proud.)

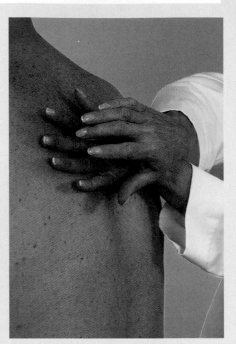

Action 39: Percussing posterior thorax.
(Photo by B. Proud.)

40. **Auscultate the lungs through the posterior thorax as the patient breathes slowly and deeply through the mouth.**

Lung auscultation helps to detect abnormal fluid or mucus accumulation as well as obstructed passageways.

41. Examine the anterior thorax. Observe the skin, bones, and muscles as well as symmetry of expansion and accessory muscle use.

Observation provides information about lung expansion and accessory muscle use during respirations; it also provides information about deformities that could alter ventilation.

42. Inspect the anterior thorax for lifts, heaves, or thrusts; check for the apical impulse; palpate over the anterior thorax.

Inspection provides information about respiratory effort; palpation helps detect musculoskeletal inflammation.

43. Assess respiratory excursion and tactile fremitus (as the patient repeats the word "ninety-nine").

Respiratory excursion indicates lung expansion; assessing tactile fremitus provides information about content of lungs (vibrations increase over consolidated or fluid-filled areas).

44. Percuss over the anterior thorax.

Percussion over the lung fields helps identify the density and location of the lungs, diaphragm, and other anatomic structures.

45. **Auscultate the lungs through the anterior thorax as the patient breathes slowly and deeply through the mouth.**

Lung auscultation helps to detect abnormal fluid or mucus accumulation as well as obstructed passageways.

46. Inspect the breasts and axillae with the patient's hands resting on both sides of the body, placed on the hips, and then raised above the head.

This technique evaluates the general condition of the breasts and helps to identify any abnormalities.

continues

Performing a Head-to-Toe Physical Assessment (continued)

ACTION   **RATIONALE**

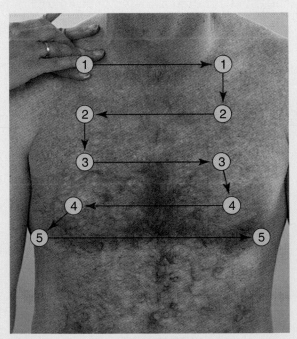

Action 40: Sequence for auscultating posterior thorax.

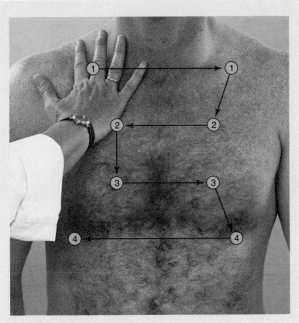

Action 42: Sequence for palpating anterior thorax.

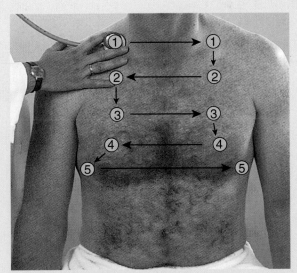

Action 44: Sequence for percussing anterior thorax.

Action 45: Sequence for auscultating anterior thorax.

47. Palpate the axillae with the patient's arms resting against the side of the body; palpate the breasts and nipples with the patient lying supine.

Palpating the axillae helps to detect nodular enlargement and other abnormalities; palpating the breasts evaluates the consistency and elasticity of breast tissue and nipples.

continues

ACTION

RATIONALE

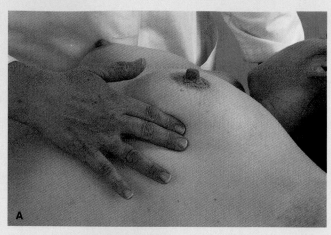

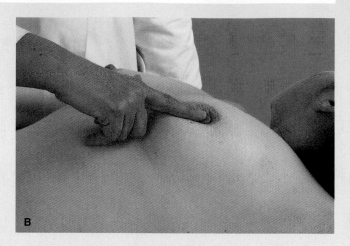

Action 47: Palpating the breasts (**A**) and nipples (**B**).   (Photos by B. Proud.)

48. **Inspect the neck for jugular vein distention with patient lying supine with the head of the bed raised to a 45-degree angle.**

This technique helps to detect right-sided heart pressure.

49. **Palpate the precordium for the apical impulse; auscultate the aortic, pulmonic, tricuspid, and mitral areas and Erb's point for heart sounds.**

Precordium palpation helps evaluate the size and location of the left ventricle; auscultation evaluates heart rate and rhythm and helps detect abnormal heart sounds.

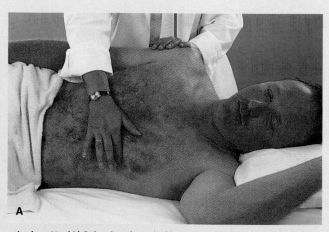

Aortic area

Pulmonic area

Erb's point

Tricuspid area

Mitral (apical) area

Midsternum

Midclavicular line

Action 49: (**A**) Palpating the apical impulse with the fingerpad. (**B**) Traditional areas of auscultation.
(Photos © B. Proud.)

continues

Performing a Head-to-Toe Physical Assessment (continued)

ACTION	RATIONALE
50. Assess the abdomen by observing contour, inspecting for skin characteristics, symmetry, contour, peristalsis, and pulsations.	Observation determines the shape of the abdomen; inspection helps detect an incisional or umbilical hernia or abnormality due to bowel obstruction.
51. **Visualize the four quadrants. Auscultate all four quadrants before percussing or palpating.**	Auscultation detects the presence of bowel sounds indicating peristalsis. Performing auscultation first prevents percussion and palpation from interfering with findings.
52. Percuss from below the right breast to the inguinal area down the right midclavicular line; percuss in a similar fashion on the left; percuss the area over the symphysis pubis.	Percussion on the right side helps evaluate the size of the liver; on the left side, it helps to evaluate the spleen; percussion over the symphysis pubis helps to evaluate the bladder for fullness.

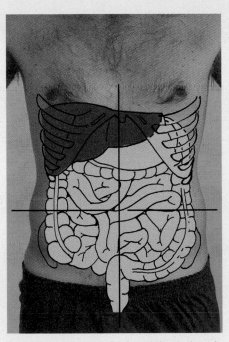

Action 50: Visualizing the four abdominal quadrants. (Photo by B. Proud.)

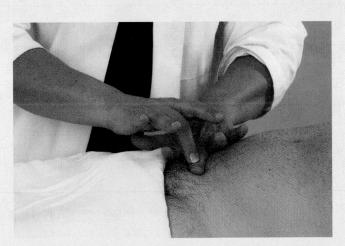

Action 52: Percussing the area over the symphysis pubis. (Photo by B. Proud.)

53. Palpate all four abdominal quadrants.	Palpation provides information about the location, size, and condition of the underlying structures.
54. Palpate for the kidneys on each side of the abdomen. Palpate the liver at the right costal border. Palpate for the spleen at the left costal border. **If the patient reports abdominal pain, assess for rebound tenderness last by palpating deeply in the area of the pain and then releasing suddenly. If rebound tenderness is present, avoid continued palpation of the abdomen.**	Palpation provides information about the overall condition of these organs. Rebound tenderness indicates peritoneal irritation such as from appendicitis. This assessment is performed last because it can cause pain and muscle spasm that could interfere with the rest of the examination. Continued palpation with rebound tenderness could lead to rupture of the appendix.

continues

ACTION   **RATIONALE**

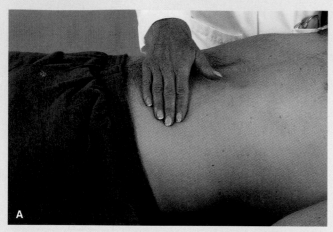

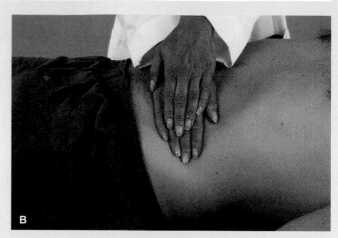

Action 53: Palpating the abdomen: **(A)** Light palpation; **(B)** Deep palpation.   (Photo by B. Proud.)

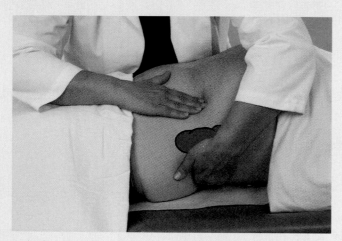

Action 54: Palpating the kidney.   (Photo by B. Proud.)

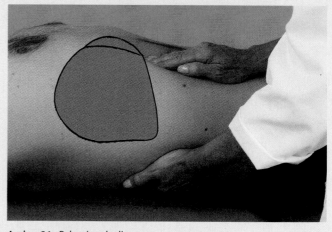

Action 54: Palpating the liver.   (Photo by B. Proud.)

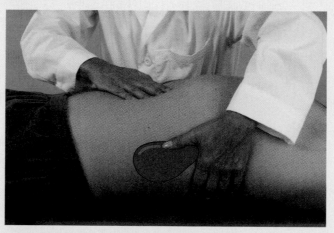

Action 54: Palpating the spleen.   (Photo by B. Proud.)

continues

ACTION   **RATIONALE**

55. **Palpate and auscultate the femoral pulses in the groin.**   This technique assesses vascular patency.

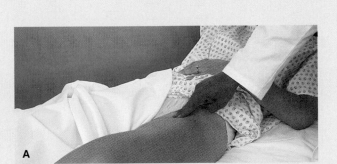
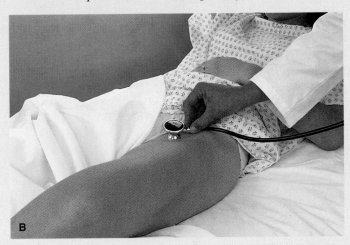

Action 55: Palpating (**A**) and auscultating (**B**) the femoral pulses.   (Photos © B. Proud.)

56. Inspect the external genitalia and rectal area. Have client hold his penis during inspection.   This technique evaluates the general condition of the genitalia and rectal area and helps to identify any abnormalities.

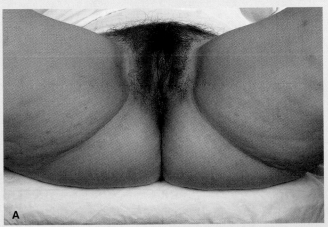
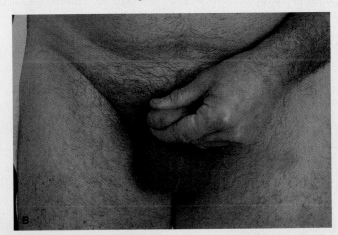
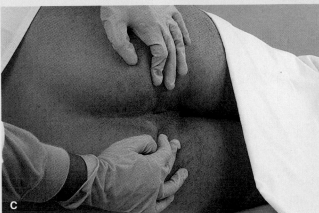

Action 56: Inspecting the female external genitalia (**A**), the male external genitalia (**B**), and the rectal area (**C**).
(Photos A and B by B. Proud.)

continues

Performing a Head-to-Toe Physical Assessment (continued)

ACTION	RATIONALE
57. Examine the arms. Observe the skin and muscle mass.	Observation of the skin provides information about hydration and circulation; observation of muscle mass provides information about injuries and neuromuscular function.
58. Ask patient to extend arms forward and then rapidly turn palms up and down.	This maneuver tests proprioception and cerebellar function.
59. Place your hands on the patient's upturned forearms while the patient pushes up against resistance. Then place your hands under the forearms while the patient pushes down.	This technique checks the muscle strength of the extremities.
60. Inspect and palpate the fingers, wrists, and elbow joints; palpate the hands. Check skin turgor.	Inspection and palpation provide information about deformities, tenderness, or pain; palpating the hands provides information about circulation. Checking skin turgor provides information about hydration status.

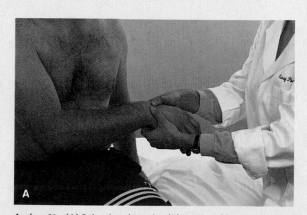
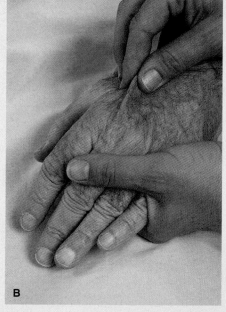

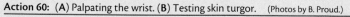
Action 60: (A) Palpating the wrist. (B) Testing skin turgor.   (Photos by B. Proud.)

ACTION	RATIONALE
61. Palpate the radial and brachial pulses.	Pulse palpation helps to evaluate peripheral vascular status.
62. **Inspect the color, shape, and condition of the nails; check for capillary refill.**	These techniques provide data about the integumentary, cardiovascular, and respiratory systems.
63. Have the patient squeeze two of your fingers placed in the palm of the hand.	This maneuver tests the muscle strength of the hands.
64. Examine the legs. Inspect the legs and feet for color, lesions, varicosities, hair growth, nail growth, edema, and muscle mass.	Inspection provides information about peripheral vascular function.
65. Test for pitting edema in the pretibial area.	This technique reveals information about excess interstitial fluid.

continues

Performing a Head-to-Toe Physical Assessment (continued)

ACTION	RATIONALE

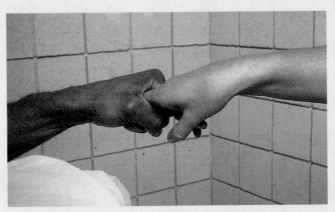

Action 63: Testing grip. Patient squeezes nurse's index and middle fingers.

66. Palpate for pulses and skin temperature at the posterior tibial, dorsalis pedis, and popliteal areas.	Pulses and skin temperature provide information about the patient's peripheral vascular status.
67. Have the patient perform the straight leg test with one leg at a time.	This test checks for vertebral disk problems.
68. Palpate for crepitus as the patient abducts and adducts the hip; repeat on the other side.	This maneuver assesses range of motion and provides information about joint problems.
69. Ask the patient to raise the thigh against the resistance of your hand; next have the patient push outward against the resistance of your hand; then have the patient pull backward against the resistance of your hand. Repeat on the opposite side.	These measures help test the motor strength of the upper and lower legs.

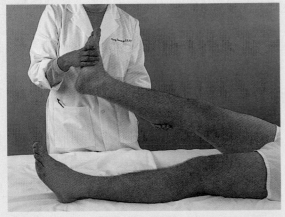

Action 67: Performing straight leg test.   (Photo © B. Proud.)

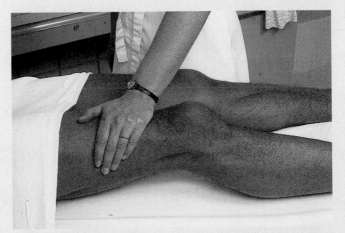

Action 69: Testing motor strength of upper leg. Patient attempts to raise thigh against nurse's resistance.

continues

ACTION

RATIONALE

70. Assess the patient's deep tendon reflexes (DTRs).

   These tests evaluate the brachioradialis, biceps, triceps, patellar, and Achilles DTRs, respectively.

   a. Place your fingers above the patient's wrist and tap them with a reflex hammer; repeat on the other arm.
   b. Place your fingers over the antecubital area and tap with a reflex hammer; repeat on the other side.
   c. Place your fingers over the triceps tendon area and tap with a reflex hammer; repeat on the other side.
   d. Tap just below the patella with a reflex hammer; repeat on the other side.
   e. Tap over the Achilles tendon area with reflex hammer; repeat on the other side.

71. Stroke the sole of the patient's foot with the end of a reflex hammer handle or other hard object such as a key; repeat on the other side.

   This test elicits the Babinski reflex with plantarflexion of all toes.

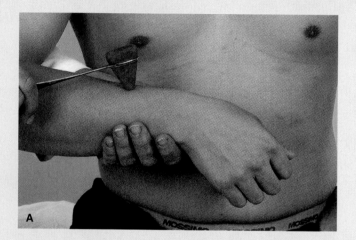
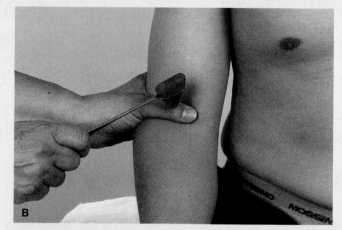
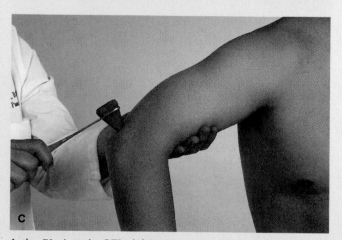
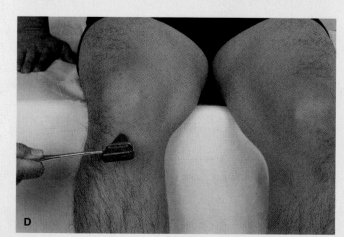

Action 70: Assessing DTRs: (**A**) Brachioradialis. (**B**) Biceps. (**C**) Triceps. (**D**) Patellar.

Performing a Head-to-Toe Physical Assessment (continued)

ACTION	RATIONALE

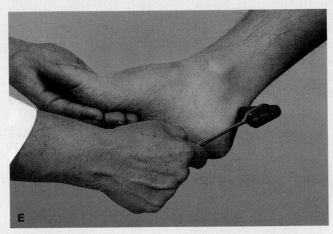

Action 70: *(Continued)* **(E)** Achilles'.   (Photos by B. Proud.)

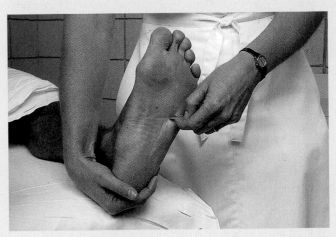

Action 71: Testing Babinski reflex.

72. Ask patient to dorsiflex and then plantarflex both feet against resistance.

These measures test foot strength and range of motion.

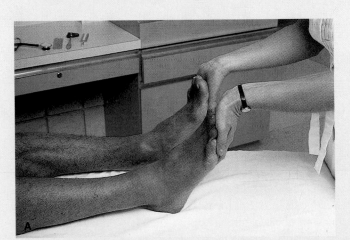 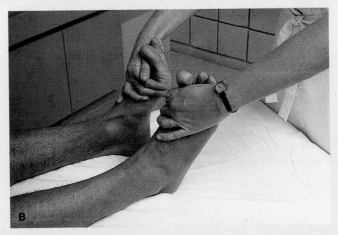

Action 72: Testing ankle flexion and dorsiflexion. The patient first pushes the balls of the feet against resistance of the nurse's hands (**A**), then attempts to pull against nurse's resistance (**B**).

73. Using your finger or applicator, trace a one-digit number on the patient's palm and ask him or her to identify the number. Place a familiar object such as a key in the patient's hand and ask him or her to identify the object.

These tests evaluate tactile discrimination.

74. Observe the patient as he or she walks with a regular gait, on the toes, on the heels, and then heel to toe.

This procedure evaluates cerebellar and motor function.

75. Perform the Romberg's test; ask the patient to stand straight with both eyes closed and both arms extended with palms up.

This test checks cerebellar functioning and evaluates balance and coordination.

76. Document significant normal and abnormal findings in an organized manner according to the related body systems.

Documentation provides for communication and continuity of care.

continues

Performing a Head-to-Toe Physical Assessment (continued)

ACTION	RATIONALE

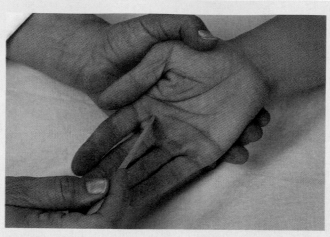

Action 73: Testing tactile discrimination. (Photo by B. Proud.)

EVALUATION

The expected outcome is met when the patient participates in the physical assessment and demonstrates decreased anxiety.

Unexpected Situations and Associated Interventions

- *While you are testing a patient's visual acuity, the patient tells you he can't see anything without his glasses:* Stop the test, instruct the patient to put on his glasses, and then resume testing.
- *When assessing a patient's lungs, you hear short, high-pitched popping sounds on inspiration:* Ask the patient to cough and auscultate again. If the sounds remain, suspect fine crackles, which may indicate restrictive disease such as pneumonia or heart failure. Notify the physician.

Special Considerations

- Always warm equipment such as a stethoscope before using it to prevent chilling the patient.
- If appropriate, complete assessment of upper extremities after examining the thorax.
- Ensure that a patient wears corrective lenses (if needed) when testing visual acuity.
- In a dark-skinned person, cerumen may be dark orange or brown; a fair-skinned person usually has yellow cerumen.
- In a pregnant woman, expect to see enlarged breasts with darkened nipples and areolae and purplish linear streaks. A pregnant patient also may discharge colostrum from the nipple.
- Avoid percussing or palpating the spleen of a patient if there is suspicion of splenic engorgement or injury.

Infant and Child Considerations

- When examining the head of an infant, inspect and gently palpate the fontanels and sutures.
- Lymph nodes may be palpable in children under age 12.
- Use a flashlight to inspect an infant's or toddler's nostrils; a nasal speculum is too sharp.
- An infant's nose is usually slightly flattened.
- For a child under age 8, do not assess the frontal sinuses; they are usually too small to assess.
- When performing an otoscopic exam on a young child, pull the pinna down and back.

continues

Performing a Head-to-Toe Physical Assessment (continued)

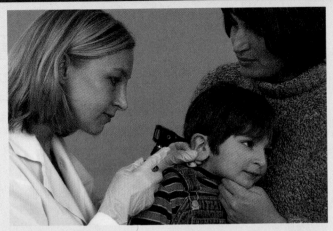

Performing an otoscopic examination on a young child. The pinna is pulled down and back.   (Photo by B. Proud.)

- Note the number of teeth in a child; a child may have up to 20 temporary teeth.
- Measure an infant's chest circumference at the nipple line.
- Auscultate a child's lungs before performing other assessment techniques that may cause crying.
- Expect to hear breath sounds that are harsher or more bronchial than those of an adult.
- Avoid anterior thorax chest percussion in an infant because it is often unreliable due to the infant's small chest size.
- Be alert for functional heart murmurs in children.
- Avoid percussion or palpation of the spleen in a child.
- Use Ortolani's maneuver to assess hip abduction and adduction in an infant.
- Expect to elicit Babinski's sign in children age 2 and younger.

Older Adult Considerations

- Look for a thin, grayish ring in the cornea (arcus senilis). This is normal in an older adult.
- When percussing the thorax, note any hyperresonance; this may be normal due to age-related hyperinflation of the lung tissue.

Collecting a Venous Blood Sample by Venipuncture

A venipuncture is used to obtain a venous blood sample. A venipuncture involves piercing a vein with a needle and collecting blood in a syringe or evacuated tube. Typically, venipuncture is performed using the antecubital fossa, but if necessary it can be performed on a vein in the dorsal forearm, the dorsum of the hand, or another accessible location. Do not use the inner wrist because of the high risk for damage to underlying structures. Although laboratory personnel usually perform this procedure in the hospital setting, nurses may need to perform this skill occasionally.

Equipment

- Tourniquet
- Gloves
- Syringe or evacuated tubes and needle holder
- Antimicrobial swab such as alcohol or povidone–iodine pads
- 20G or 21G needle for the forearm or 25G needle for the wrist, hand, and ankle, and for children
- Color-coded collection tubes containing appropriate additives
- Labels
- Laboratory request form and laboratory biohazard transportation bag
- Gauze pads (2×2)
- Adhesive bandage

ASSESSMENT

Review the patient's medical record and physician order for the blood specimens to be obtained. Ensure that the necessary laboratory request form has been completed. Assess the patient for any allergies (e.g., iodine). Ask the patient about any previous laboratory testing that he or she may have had, including any problems, such as difficulty with venipuncture, fainting, or complaints of dizziness, lightheadedness, or nausea. Assess the patient's anxiety level and understanding about the reasons for the blood test.

NURSING DIAGNOSIS

Determine the related factors for the nursing diagnoses based on the patient's current status. An appropriate nursing diagnosis is Anxiety. Other appropriate nursing diagnoses may include:

- Deficient Knowledge
- Fear
- Risk for Injury
- Risk for Infection

Many other nursing diagnoses also may require the use of this skill.

OUTCOME IDENTIFICATION AND PLANNING

The expected outcome to achieve when collecting a venous blood specimen is that the specimen will be obtained without the patient experiencing undue anxiety and injury. Other outcomes may be appropriate depending on the patient's nursing diagnosis.

IMPLEMENTATION

ACTION	RATIONALE
1. Gather the necessary supplies. If you are using evacuated tubes (Vacutainer), open the needle packet, attach the needle to its holder, and select the appropriate tubes. If you are using a syringe, attach the appropriate needle to it. Choose a syringe large enough to hold all the blood required for the test. Label all collection tubes clearly with the patient's name and room number, the physician's name, the date and time of collection, and your initials (since you will be the person performing the venipuncture).	Organization facilitates efficient performance of the procedure. Proper labeling reduces the risk for error.

continues

Collecting a Venous Blood Sample by Venipuncture (continued)

ACTION

RATIONALE

2. Perform hand hygiene and put on gloves.

Hand hygiene and gloves reduce the risk of microorganism transmission.

3. Confirm the patient's identity. Tell the patient you are about to collect a blood sample and explain the procedure. Ask the patient if he or she has ever felt faint, sweaty, or nauseated when having blood drawn.

Patient identification validates the accuracy of the procedure. Explaining the procedure helps reduce anxiety. Determining previous experiences aids in identifying potential problems.

4. If the patient is on bed rest, ask him or her to lie in a supine position, with the head slightly elevated and arms at the sides. Ask an ambulatory patient to sit in a chair and support the arm securely on an armrest or table.

Proper positioning provides the patient with support and stabilizes the extremity, thereby facilitating the venipuncture.

5. Assess the veins to determine the best puncture site. Observe the skin for the vein's blue color, or palpate the vein for a firm rebound sensation.

Using the best site reduces the risk of injury to the patient.

6. **Tie a tourniquet 5 cm proximal to the area chosen by pulling the ends tightly in the opposite directions.** Tuck one end beneath the other.

By impeding venous return to the heart while still allowing arterial flow, a tourniquet produces venous dilation. If arterial perfusion remains adequate, you will be able to feel the radial pulse. Tucking one end beneath the other allows for quick and easy removal of the tourniquet by pulling on one of the free ends.

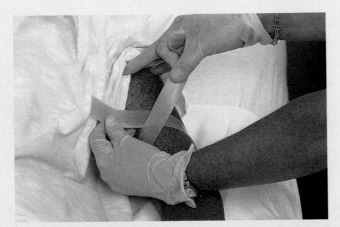

Action 6: Tying the tourniquet.

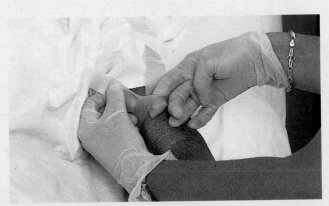

Action 6: Tucking one end under the other.

7. If the tourniquet fails to dilate the vein, have the patient open and close the fist a few times. Then ask the patient to close the fist as you insert the needle and to open it again when the needle is in place.

Opening and closing the fist aids in venous distention.

8. Clean the venipuncture site with the antimicrobial swab per agency policy, wiping in a circular motion spiraling outward. If using alcohol, apply it with friction for 30 seconds or until the final pad comes away clean. Allow the skin to dry before performing the venipuncture.

Using a circular motion ensures that cleaning occurs from the least to most contaminated area and avoids introducing potentially infectious skin flora into the vessel during the procedure. Previously cleaned area is not contaminated again. Allowing the skin to dry maximizes antimicrobial action and prevents contact of the substance with the needle on insertion, thereby reducing the sting associated with insertion.

continues

ACTION

RATIONALE

9. Press just below the venipuncture site with your thumb, drawing the skin taut.

Applying pressure helps immobilize the vein.

10. **Position the needle holder or syringe with the needle bevel up and the shaft parallel to the path of the vein and at a 30-degree angle to the arm.** Insert the needle into the vein.

Positioning the needle at the proper angle reduces the risk of puncturing through the vein.

   a. If using a syringe, look for venous blood to appear in the hub; withdraw the blood slowly, pulling the plunger of the syringe gently to create steady suction until you obtain the required sample.

   a. Pulling the plunger too forcibly may collapse the vein.

   b. If using a needle holder and an evacuated tube, grasp the holder securely to stabilize it in the vein, and push down on the collection tube until the needle punctures the rubber stopper. Blood will flow into the tube automatically.

   b. A vacuum is created with the collection tube, allowing blood to flow into the tube.

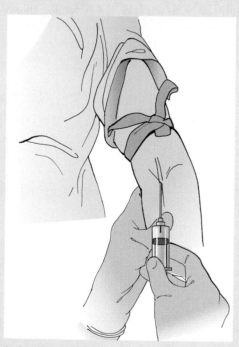

Action 10: Performing the venipuncture.

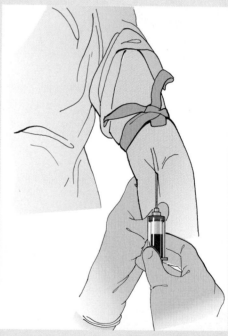

Action 10: Observing blood flowing into the collection tube.

11. **Remove the tourniquet as soon as blood flows adequately.**

Tourniquet removal helps to prevent stasis and hemoconcentration, which can impair test results.

12. Continue to fill the required tubes, removing one and inserting another. Gently rotate each tube as you remove it.

Filling the required tubes ensures that the sample is accurate. Gentle rotation helps to mix the additive with the sample.

continues

Collecting a Venous Blood Sample by Venipuncture (continued)

ACTION	RATIONALE
13. After you have drawn the sample, place a gauze pad over the puncture site and slowly and gently remove the needle from the vein. **When using an evacuated tube, remove the specimen tube from the needle holder to release the vacuum before withdrawing the needle from the vein.**	Slow, gentle needle removal prevents injury to the vein.
14. Apply gentle pressure to the puncture site for 2 to 3 minutes or until bleeding stops.	This prevents bleeding and extravasation into the surrounding tissue, which can cause a hematoma.
15. After bleeding stops, apply an adhesive bandage.	The bandage protects the site and aids in applying pressure.
16. If you have used a syringe, transfer the sample to a collection tube.	For accurate results, the specimen must be placed into the proper collection tubes.
17. Place the specimen tubes inside the biohazard transport bag and handle carefully. Avoid foaming.	Use of a biohazard bag reduces the risk of microorganism exposure and transmission; foaming can cause hemolysis and skew the results.
18. Check the venipuncture site to see if a hematoma has developed.	Development of a hematoma requires further intervention.
19. Discard syringes, needles, and used gloves in the appropriate containers. Perform hand hygiene.	Proper disposal and hand hygiene reduce the risk of microorganism exposure and transmission.
20. Record the date, time, and site of the venipuncture; the name of the test; the time the sample was sent to the laboratory; the amount of blood collected; the patient's temperature; and any adverse reactions to the procedure.	Documentation provides communication and promotes continuity of care.

6/10/06   0945   Blood specimen for CBC with differential obtained from right antecubital space. Approximately 8 cc of blood collected and sent to laboratory.—C. Lewis, RN

Action 20: Documentation.

EVALUATION

The expected outcome is achieved when the blood specimen is obtained and the patient reports a decrease in anxiety. Other outcomes may include: patient states reason for blood test; patient verbalizes minor if any complaint of pain at venipuncture site; and patient exhibits no signs and symptoms of injury at venipuncture site.

Unexpected Situations and Associated Interventions

- *After applying the tourniquet, you have trouble finding a distended vein:* Have the patient make a fist and pump it intermittently, or try tapping the skin over the vein several times. If unsuccessful, remove the tourniquet and try lowering the patient's arm to allow blood to pool in the veins. If necessary, apply warm compresses for about 10 minutes before reapplying the tourniquet.
- *The patient has large, distended, highly visible veins:* Perform venipuncture without a tourniquet to minimize the risk for hematoma.
- *Patient has a clotting disorder or is receiving anticoagulant therapy:* Maintain firm pressure on the venipuncture site for at least 5 minutes after withdrawing the needle to prevent hematoma formation.

continues

Collecting a Venous Blood Sample by Venipuncture (continued)

- *A hematoma develops at the venipuncture site:* Apply pressure until you are sure bleeding has stopped (about 5 minutes). Then obtain an order for warm soaks to promote absorption of the hematoma and provide comfort. Document size and appearance of hematoma and effectiveness of pressure application and warm soaks.
- *Patient reports feeling lightheaded and says she is going to faint:* Stop the venipuncture. If the patient is in bed, have the patient lie flat and elevate the feet. If the patient is in a chair, have the patient put her head between her knees. Encourage the patient to take slow, deep breaths. Call for assistance and stay with the patient. Obtain vital signs if possible.

Special Considerations

- If using povidone–iodine to prepare the venipuncture site, do not wipe off the povidone–iodine with alcohol; alcohol cancels the effect of povidone–iodine.
- If the flow of blood into the collection tube or syringe is sluggish, leave the tourniquet in place longer, but always remove it before withdrawing the needle. Don't leave the tourniquet on for more than 3 minutes.
- Use safety-engineered blood collection sets to prevent needlesticks.
- Never collect a venous sample from an arm that is being used for intravenous therapy or blood administration because this may affect test results. Do not collect a venous sample from an infection site because this may introduce pathogens into the vascular system. Avoid collecting blood from edematous areas, arteriovenous shunts, an upper extremity on the same side as a previous lymph node dissection, and sites of previous hematomas or vascular injury.
- Avoid using leg veins for venipuncture, if possible, because this increases the risk of thrombophlebitis. Some facilities require a physician's order to collect blood from a leg or foot vein. Check your facility's policies.

Infant and Child Considerations

- The veins of infants and children are smaller and more fragile, necessitating the use of smaller-gauge needles.
- Scalp vein (or "butterfly") needles maybe appropriate for obtaining blood in infants and small children.
- Alternative sites for venipuncture in infants and small children include the scalp, hand, and foot.

Older Adult Considerations

- The veins of an older adult are fragile and may collapse easily. In addition, the skin is less elastic and may be more difficult to pull taut.

Obtaining a Blood Specimen for Culture and Sensitivity

Normally bacteria-free, blood is susceptible to infection through infusion lines as well as from thrombophlebitis, infected shunts, and bacterial endocarditis due to prosthetic heart valve replacements. Bacteria may also invade the vascular system from local tissue infections through the lymphatic system and the thoracic duct.

Blood cultures are performed to detect bacterial invasion (bacteremia) and the systemic spread of such an infection (septicemia) through the bloodstream. In this procedure, a laboratory technician, physician, or nurse collects a venous blood sample by venipuncture at the patient's bedside and then transfers it into two bottles, one containing an anaerobic medium and the other an aerobic medium. The bottles are incubated, encouraging any organisms that are present in the sample to grow in the media. Blood cultures allow identification of about 67% of pathogens within 24 hours and up to 90% within 72 hours.

Although some authorities consider the timing of culture collections debatable and possibly irrelevant, others advocate drawing three blood samples at least 1 hour apart. The first of these should be collected at the earliest sign of suspected bacteremia or septicemia. To check for suspected bacterial endocarditis, three or four samples may be collected at 5- to 30-minute intervals before starting antibiotic therapy.

Equipment

- Tourniquet
- Gloves
- Alcohol or povidone–iodine pads
- 10-mL syringe for an adult
- Three or four 20G 1″ needles
- Two or three blood culture bottles (50-mL bottles for adults), with sodium polyethanol sulfonate added (one aerobic bottle containing a suitable medium, such as Trypticase soy broth with 10% carbon dioxide atmosphere; one anaerobic bottle with prereduced medium; and possibly one hyperosmotic bottle with 10% sucrose medium)
- Laboratory request form
- Laboratory biohazard transport bags
- 2×2 gauze pads
- Small adhesive bandages
- Labels

ASSESSMENT

Review the patient's medical record and the physician's order for the number and type of blood cultures to be obtained. Ensure that the necessary laboratory request form has been completed. Assess the patient for signs and symptoms of infection, including vital signs, and note any antibiotic therapy being administered. Inspect any insertion sites for invasive monitoring or incisions for indications of infection. Question the patient about any allergies (e.g., iodine). Ask the patient about any previous blood culture testing that he or she may have had, including any problems (e.g., difficulty with venipuncture, fainting, complaints of dizziness, lightheadedness, or nausea). Assess the patient's anxiety level and understanding about the reasons for the blood culture.

NURSING DIAGNOSIS

Determine the related factors for the nursing diagnoses based on the patient's current status. An appropriate nursing diagnosis is Anxiety. Other appropriate nursing diagnoses may include:

- Hyperthermia
- Deficient Knowledge
- Fear
- Risk for Injury
- Risk for Infection

Many other nursing diagnoses also may require the use of this skill.

continues

OUTCOME IDENTIFICATION AND PLANNING

The expected outcome to achieve when obtaining a blood culture is that the specimen will be obtained without the patient experiencing undue anxiety and injury. Other outcomes may be appropriate depending on the patient's nursing diagnosis.

IMPLEMENTATION

ACTION	RATIONALE
1. Tell the patient you need to collect a series of blood samples to check for infection. Explain the procedure, including that the procedure usually requires three blood samples collected at different times.	Explanation helps ease anxiety and promote cooperation.
2. Perform hand hygiene and put on gloves.	Hand hygiene and gloving reduce the risk of infection transmission.
3. Tie a tourniquet 5 cm proximal to the area chosen, clean the site with an alcohol or a povidone–iodine pad, and perform the venipuncture (see Skill 2-2).	Venipuncture at a properly prepared site is necessary to obtain the blood sample.
4. Withdraw approximately 10 mL of blood from an adult and complete the venipuncture.	An adequate amount of blood is necessary to provide a viable specimen.
5. Wipe the diaphragm tops of the culture bottles with a povidone–iodine pad and allow to dry.	Wiping the tops of the culture bottles prevents contamination of the specimen.
6. Change the needle on the syringe used to draw the blood. Inject 5 mL of blood into each bottle.	Changing the needle maintains sterility and reduces the risk of contamination of the sterile culture bottles.
7. Label the culture bottles with the patient's name and room number, physician's name, and date and time of collection. Indicate the suspected diagnosis and the patient's temperature, and note on the laboratory request form any recent antibiotic therapy.	Proper labeling and identification ensure accurate reporting of results.
8. Place the samples in the laboratory biohazard transport bag and send the samples to the laboratory immediately.	Use of a biohazard bag reduces the risk of microorganism exposure and transmission.
9. Discard syringes, needles, and gloves in appropriate containers. Perform hand hygiene and record the date and time of blood sample collection, name of the test, amount of blood collected, number of bottles used, patient's temperature, and adverse reactions to the procedure.	Proper disposal of equipment and supplies and hand hygiene reduces the risk of microorganism transmission. Documentation promotes communication and continuity of care.

6/6/06   1710   Patient's temperature increased to 104.2°F. Patient very lethargic, pale, diaphoretic, with cool clammy skin. Bradycardic with pulse rate of 56 beats per minute and hypotensive with blood pressure of 90/50 mm Hg. Physician notified. Blood cultures × 3 ordered and obtained.—B. Pearson, RN

Action 9: Documentation.

EVALUATION

The expected outcome is achieved when the patient demonstrates decreased anxiety with the collection of the blood cultures. Other outcomes may include: patient states reason for blood cultures; patient's vital signs are within acceptable parameters; patient demonstrates a reduction in the temperature and other signs of infection; and patient exhibits no signs and symptoms of injury at the venipuncture site.

continues

SKILL 2-3   Obtaining a Blood Specimen for Culture and Sensitivity (continued)

Unexpected Situations and Associated Interventions	• *Your patient has had one set of blood cultures obtained but now requires another set. You expect to obtain the blood cultures from the patient's right antecubital site. When you are applying the tourniquet, the patient tells you, "That's where they got blood the last time":* Clarify if the patient is referring to the last set of blood cultures or other blood specimens. If the site was used for the previous blood cultures, use another site. If the site was used for routine blood specimens, ask the patient if the site is causing discomfort; if it is, choose another site for the venipuncture. If not, prepare the site for venipuncture.
Special Considerations	• The size of the culture bottles may vary according to facility policy, but the sample dilution should always be 1:10. • Avoid using existing blood lines for cultures unless the sample is drawn when the line is inserted or catheter sepsis is suspected. • If anaerobic and aerobic blood cultures are ordered, obtain the anaerobic cultures first.
Infant and Child Considerations	• Use a 6-mL syringe for a child and 20-mL culture bottles for infants and children. • Draw only 2 to 6 mL of blood from a child for each culture, and put 2 mL into each 20-mL pediatric culture bottle.

■ Developing Critical Thinking Skills

1. When obtaining the history from Mr. Lincoln, he reports having a stuffed-up nose, postnasal drip, and a cough that sometimes produces mucus. He has smoked about one and a half packs of cigarettes a day for the past 20 years. Which areas of his physical examination would be most important?
2. The physician orders routine blood work for Lois Felker. She tells you that the last time she had blood drawn, a lump formed at the spot where the needle was inserted. What should you do?
3. Bobby Williams is suspected of having appendicitis. Which aspects of the physical examination would the nurse use to help confirm this diagnosis?

Bibliography

Andresen, G. (1998). Assessing the older patient. *RN, 61*(3), 46–56.

Bickley, L. (2002). *Bates guide to physical examination and history taking* (8th ed.). Philadelphia: Lippincott Williams & Wilkins.

Calfee, D. P., & Farr, B. M. (2002). Comparison of four antiseptic preparations for skin in the prevention of contamination of percutaneously drawn blood cultures: A randomized trial. *Journal of Clinical Microbiology, 40*(5):1660–1665.

Darovic, G. (1997). Assessing pupillary responses. *Nursing, 27*(2), 49.

Faria, S. (1999). Assessment of peripheral arterial pulses. *Home Care Provider, 4*(4), 140–141.

Heath, H., & White, I. (2001). Sexuality and older people: An introduction to nursing assessment. *Nursing Older People, 13*(4), 29–31.

Incredibly easy! Interpreting abnormal abdominal sounds. (2000). *Nursing, 30*(6), 28.

Jackson, R., Alghareeb, M., Alaradi, I., & Tomi, Z. (1999). The diagnosis of skin disease. *Dermatology Nursing, 11*(4), 275, 278–283.

Lyneham, J. (2001). Physical examination (abdomen, thorax and lungs): A review. *Australian Journal of Advanced Nursing, 18*(3), 31.

Nursing procedures (4th ed). (2004). Philadelphia: Lippincott Williams & Wilkins.

Watson, R. (2001). Assessing the musculoskeletal system in older people. *Nursing Older People, 13*(5), 29–30.

Weber, K., & Kelley, J. (2003). *Health assessment in nursing* (2nd ed.). Philadelphia: Lippincott Williams & Wilkins.

Safety

This chapter will help you develop some of the skills related to safety issues for monitoring and intervention necessary to care for the following patients:

Megan Lewis, an 18-month-old who has an IV access in her left forearm

Kevin Mallory, a 35-year-old professional body builder admitted with a severe closed head injury. He is intubated and is constantly reaching for his endotracheal tube.

John Frawley, a 72-year-old diagnosed with Alzheimer's disease who continues to try to get out of bed after falling and breaking a hip

Learning Outcomes

After studying this chapter the reader should be able to:

1. Apply cloth wrist restraints correctly and safely.
2. Apply a vest restraint correctly and safely.
3. Apply elbow restraints correctly and safely.
4. Use leather restraints correctly and safely.

Key Terms

incident report: documentation that describes any injury or potential for injury sustained by a patient in a healthcare agency

restraints: device used to limit movement or immobilize a patient

Safety and security

Safety and security are basic human needs. Safety is a paramount concern that underlies all nursing care, and patient safety is a responsibility of all healthcare providers. Safety is a focus in all healthcare facilities as well as the home, workplace, and community. Many safety concerns are universal for all age groups, but there are unique safety considerations for each developmental stage. Nursing strategies that identify potential hazards and promote wellness evolve from an awareness of factors that affect safety in the environment.

This chapter will cover the skills to assist the nurse in monitoring and intervening for patients with issues involving safety. Please look over the summary boxes and Figure 3-1 to assist you in understanding the skills related to safety.

BOX 3-1 Nursing Interventions to Prevent Falls in a Healthcare Facility

- Complete a risk assessment.
- Indicate risk for falling on patient's door and chart.
- Keep bed in low position.
- Keep wheels on bed and wheelchair locked.
- Leave call bell within patient's reach.
- Instruct patient regarding use of call bell.
- Answer call bells promptly.
- Leave a night light on.
- Eliminate all physical hazards in the room (clutter, wet areas on the floor).
- Provide nonskid footwear.
- Leave water, tissues, bedpan/urinal within patient's reach.
- Document and report any changes in patient's cognitive status to the physician and other nurses at the change of shift.
- Use alternative strategies when necessary instead of restraints.
- As a last resort, use the least restrictive restraint according to agency policy.
- If restraint is applied, assess patient at the required intervals.

BOX 3-2 Choosing Alternatives to Restraints

- Determine whether behavior pattern exists.
- Provide pain relief.
- Involve family in patient's care.
- Reduce noise.
- Check environment for hazards.
- Use night light.
- Identify door of room (eg, use balloon, sign, patient's picture, ribbon).
- Use an alarm system (eg, bed or position-sensitive alarms).
- Allow restless patient to walk after ensuring that environment is safe.
- Use a large plant or piece of furniture as a barrier to limit wandering from designated area.
- Use low-height beds.
- Place floormats on each side of bed.
- Use therapeutic touch.
- Play music or video selections of patient's choice.
- Use pillows wedged against the side of the chair to keep patient positioned safely.
- Use full-length body pillows.
- Assist with toileting at frequent intervals.
- Arrange for a bedside commode.
- Make the environment as homelike as possible.
- Provide a warm beverage.
- Provide comfortable rocking chairs.
- Allow patient to assist staff with simple tasks.
- Encourage daily exercise.
- Investigate possibility of discontinuing bothersome treatment devices (eg, intravenous line, catheter, feeding tube).

BOX 3-3 R-E-S-T-R-A-I-N-T Acronym

The following R-E-S-T-R-A-I-N-T protocol is an effective device when dealing with confused patients in an acute care setting:

- **R**espond to the present, not the past. The patient's current condition, not his or her past history, must determine the need for restraints. This includes assessment of physical condition and mental and behavior status.
- **E**valuate the potential for injury. Determine whether the patient is at increased risk for harming self or others.
- **S**peak with family members or caregivers. Ask them for insights into the patient's behavior, and enlist their help in making a decision.
- **T**ry alternative measures first. Also, investigate the patient's medication regimen and attempt to discuss options with the patient.
- **R**eassess the patient to determine whether alternatives are successful. Agency policy dictates the frequency of assessments and documentation.
- **A**lert the physician and the patient's family if restraints are indicated. Agency policy, JCAHO, and state and federal guidelines require an order from a physician or other healthcare professional licensed to prescribe in the state. The order should include the type of restraint, justification, criteria for removal, and intended duration of use.
- **I**ndividualize restraint use. Choose the least restrictive device.
- **N**ote important information on the chart. Document the date and time the restraint is applied, the type of restraint, alternatives that were attempted and their results, and notification of the patient's family and physician. Include frequency of assessment, your findings, regular intervals when the restraint is removed, and nursing interventions.
- **T**ime-limit the use of restraints. Release the patient from the restraint as soon as he or she is no longer a risk to self or others. Restraints should be used no longer than 24 hours on nonpsychiatric patients. After 24 hours, a new order is required (DiBartolo, 1998).

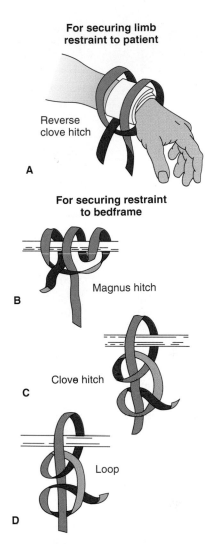

FIGURE 3-1 Appropriate quick-release ties. *For securing limb restraint to patient:* (**A**) Reverse clove hitch. *For securing restraint to bed frame:* (**B**) Magnus hitch. (**C**) Clove hitch. (**D**) Loop.

SKILL 3-1

Applying Cloth Restraint to an Extremity

Cloth restraints are used to prevent a patient from removing lines, dressings, or any other therapeutic treatments or to prevent patients from getting out of bed or chairs. Cloth restraints can be applied to the hands, wrists, waist, torso, or ankles. Restraints should be used only after less restrictive methods have failed. The vest restraint is discussed in Skill 3-2.

Equipment

- Restraint
- Padding, if necessary, for bony prominences

continues

Applying Cloth Restraint to an Extremity (continued)

ASSESSMENT

Assess the patient's physical condition and for the potential for injury to self or others. If the patient is confused and might remove lines or devices needed to sustain life, this would be considered a potential for injury to self. If the patient has had a stroke and cannot move the left arm, a restraint may be needed only on the right arm. Inspect the skin on the extremity where the restraint will be applied. If the skin is injured or an intravenous (IV) line is inserted in the area, extra padding such as rolled gauze may need to be applied to prevent further injury from the restraint. Consider using another form of restraint if the restraint may cause further injury. Assess capillary refill in the digits of the extremities to which the restraint is to be applied. This helps to determine the circulation in the extremity before applying the restraint.

**NURSING
DIAGNOSIS**

Determine the related factors for nursing diagnoses based on the patient's current status. An appropriate nursing diagnosis is Risk for Injury. Other appropriate nursing diagnoses may include:

- Risk for Impaired Skin Integrity
- Risk for Aspiration
- Wandering

**OUTCOME
IDENTIFICATION
AND PLANNING**

The expected outcome to achieve when applying cloth restraints to the extremities is that the patient is contained by the cloth restraint, remains free of injury, and does not interfere with any lines, dressings, or other therapeutic equipment. Other outcomes that may be appropriate include the following: the skin is not injured where the restraint is applied; the patient does not injure himself or herself due to the restraints; and the patient's family will demonstrate an understanding about the need for restraints and what they can do to help.

IMPLEMENTATION

ACTION	RATIONALE
1. Determine need for restraints. Assess patient's physical condition, behavior, and mental status.	Restraints should be used only as a last resort when alternative measures have failed and the patient is at increased risk for harming himself or others.
2. Confirm agency policy for application of restraints. **Secure a physician's order, and ensure that the order has been obtained within the past 24 hours.**	Policy protects the patient and the nurse and specifies guidelines for application as well as type of restraint and duration. **Joint Commission on Accreditation of Healthcare Organizations (JCAHO) standards require that a new order for restraints must be written every 24 hours.**
3. Explain reason for use to patient and family. Clarify how care will be given and needs will be met. Explain that restraint is a temporary measure.	Explanation to patient and family may lessen confusion and anger and provide reassurance. A clearly stated agency policy on application of restraints should be available for patient and family to read. In a long-term care facility, the family must give consent before a restraint is applied.
4. Perform hand hygiene.	Hand hygiene deters the spread of microorganisms.
5. Apply restraints according to manufacturer's directions: a. Choose the least restrictive type of device that allows the greatest possible degree of mobility. b. Pad bony prominences. c. **For a restraint applied to an extremity, ensure that two fingers can be inserted between the restraint and patient's wrist or ankle. If the restraint is applied around the torso or abdomen a hand or fist should fit under the restraint.** Maintain restrained extremity in normal anatomic position.	Proper application prevents injury. a. Proper application ensures that there is no interference with patient's respiration and circulation. b. This provides minimal restriction. c. Padding prevents skin breakdown.

continues

Applying Cloth Restraint to an Extremity (continued)

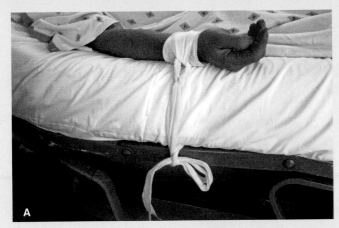

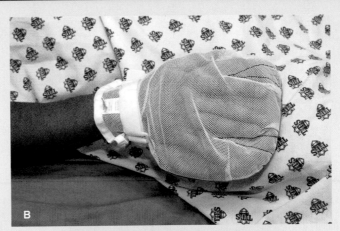

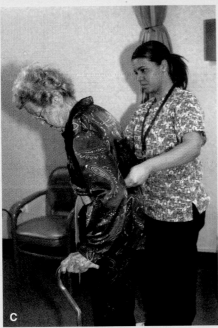

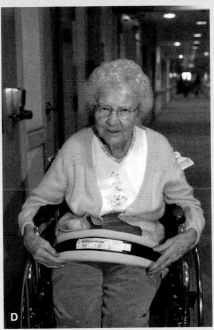

Action 5: (**A**) Cloth wrist restraint. (**B**) Netted hand mitt. (**C**) Roll belt. (**D**) Lap belt.

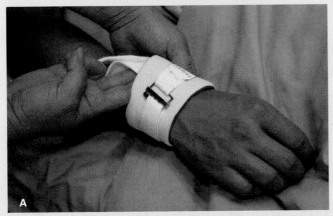

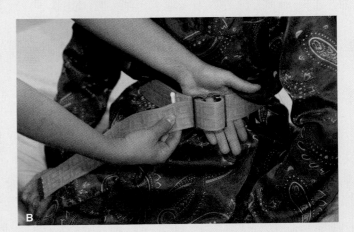

Action 5c: Inserting two fingers under (**A**) wrist restraint and (**B**) roll belt.

continues

ACTION

RATIONALE

d. **Use appropriate tie for all restraints.**

d. This lessens possibility of contracture or musculo-skeletal injury.

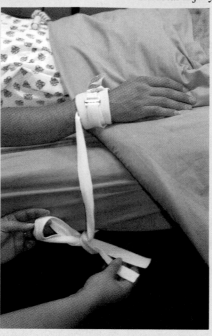

Action 5e: Tying restraint to bed frame.

e. **Fasten restraint to bed frame and not side rail. Site should not be readily accessible to patient.**

e. A quick-release knot ensures that restraint will not tighten when pulled and can be removed quickly in an emergency. Securing the restraint to a side rail may injure the patient when the side rail is lowered. Tying restraint out of patient's reach promotes security.

6. **Remove restraint at least every 2 hours, or according to agency policy and patient need.**
   a. Check for signs of decreased circulation or impaired skin integrity.

Removal allows nurse to assess patient and reevaluate need for restraint.

   a. Improperly applied restraints may cause skin tears, abrasions, or bruises. Decreased circulation may result in paleness, coolness, decreased sensation, tingling, numbness, or pain in extremity.

   b. Perform range-of-motion exercises before reapply-ing restraint.

   b. Exercise increases circulation in restrained extremity.

7. Reassure patient at regular intervals. **Keep call bell within easy reach.**

Reassurance demonstrates caring and provides opportunity for sensory situation as well as ongoing assessment and evaluation. Patient can use call bell to summon assistance quickly.

8. Assess for signs of sensory deprivation, such as in-creased sleeping, daydreaming, anxiety, panic, and hallucinations.

Use of restraints may decrease environmental stimulation and result in sensory deprivation.

9. Perform hand hygiene.

Hand hygiene deters the spread of microorganisms.

continues

Applying Cloth Restraint to an Extremity (continued)

ACTION

10. Document reason for restraining patient, alternative measures attempted before applying restraint, date and time of application, type of restraint, times when removed, and result and frequency of nursing assessment. Obtain a new order after 24 hours if restraints are still necessary.

RATIONALE

Careful documentation supports use of restraints, alternative measures to ensure safety, and assessment data. JCAHO recommends a 24-hour restraint limit for all nonpsychiatric patients.

> 7/10/06   0830   Patient disoriented and combative. Attempting to remove tracheostomy and indwelling urinary catheter. Sitting at bedside, patient continued to tug at catheter and pull on tracheostomy. Family unwilling to sit with patient. Wrist restraints applied bilaterally as ordered.—K. Urhahn, RN
>
> 7/10/06   1030   Patient continues to be disoriented and combative. Wrist restraints removed for 30 minutes during patient's bath; skin intact, passive and active range of motion completed. Wrist restraints reapplied.—K. Urhahn, RN

Action 10: Documentation.

EVALUATION

The expected outcomes are met when the patient remains free of injury to self or others; circulation to extremity remains adequate, skin integrity is not impaired under the restraint; and family is aware of rationale for restraints.

Unexpected Situations and Associated Interventions

- *Patient has an IV catheter in the right wrist and is trying to remove drain from wound:* The left wrist may have a cloth restraint applied. Due to the IV in the right wrist, alternative forms of restraints should be tried, such as a cloth mitt or an elbow restraint.
- *Patient cannot move left arm:* Do not apply restraint to an extremity that is immobile. If patient cannot move the extremity, there is no need to apply a restraint. Restraint may be applied to right arm after obtaining a physician's order.

Special Considerations

- Do not position patient flat in a supine position with wrist restraints. If patient vomits, aspiration may occur.
- Cloth extremity restraints, commonly called wrist restraints (although they may be applied to the ankle), come in different sizes. Check restraint for correct size before applying. If restraint is too large, patient may free the extremity. If restraint is too small, circulation may be affected.
- Consider keeping a pair of scissors with emergency supplies in case the restraints cannot be untied quickly.

SKILL 3-2   Applying a Vest Restraint

Vest restraints are a form of cloth restraint that go around the patient's torso. With vest restraints, patients can move their extremities but cannot get out of the chair or bed.

Equipment
- Vest restraint
- Additional padding

ASSESSMENT

Assess patient's behavior and need for vest restraint. Inspect patient's torso for any wounds or therapeutic devices that may be affected by the vest. Wounds or therapeutic devices may need to be padded before applying the vest. Also assess the patient's respiratory effort. If applied incorrectly, the vest can restrict the patient's ability to breathe.

NURSING DIAGNOSIS

Determine the related factors for nursing diagnoses based on the patient's current status. An appropriate nursing diagnosis is Risk for Injury. Other appropriate nursing diagnoses may include:

- Risk for Impaired Skin Integrity
- Wandering

OUTCOME IDENTIFICATION AND PLANNING

The expected outcome to achieve when applying a vest restraint is that the patient is contained by the vest restraint and does not fall. Other outcomes that may be appropriate include the following: the skin is not injured where the restraint is applied; the patient does not injure himself or herself due to the restraints; and the patient's family understands the need for restraints and what they can do to help.

IMPLEMENTATION

ACTION	RATIONALE
1. Determine the need for restraints. Assess patient's physical condition, behavior, and mental status.	Restraints should be used only as a last resort when alternative measures have failed, and the patient is at increased risk for harming himself or herself or others.
2. Confirm agency policy for application of restraints. **Secure a physician's order. Ensure that the order has been obtained within the past 24 hours.**	Policy protects the patient and the nurse and specifies guidelines for application as well as type of restraint and duration. **JCAHO standards require that a new order for restraints must be written every 24 hours.**
3. Explain reason for restraint use to patient and family. Clarify how care will be given and needs will be met. Explain that restraint is a temporary measure.	Explanation to patient and family may lessen confusion and anger and provide reassurance. A clearly stated agency policy on application of restraints should be available for patient and family to read. In a long-term care facility, the family must give consent before a restraint is applied.
4. Perform hand hygiene.	Hand hygiene deters the spread of microorganisms.
5. Apply restraints according to manufacturer's directions:	Proper application ensures that there is no interference with patient's respiration. The U.S. Food and Drug Administration advises manufacturers to place "front" and "back" labels on vest restraints and that correct size be used.
a. Choose the correct size of the least restrictive type of device that allows the greatest possible degree of mobility.	a. This provides minimal restriction.
b. Pad bony prominences or therapeutic devices that may be affected by the vest.	b. Padding prevents skin breakdown and damage to therapeutic devices.
c. Assist patient to a sitting position, if not contraindicated.	c. This will assist the nurse in helping the patient into the vest.

continues

Applying a Vest Restraint (continued)

ACTION   **RATIONALE**

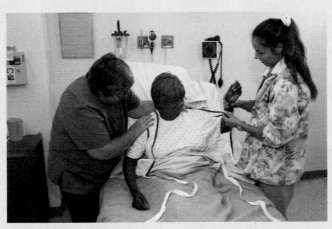

Action 5d: Applying vest restraint with V opening in front.

d. **Place vest on patient over gown, with flaps crisscrossing over the abdomen if appropriate. The V opening should be on the patient's front.**

e. Pull the tabs secure. **Ensure that there are no wrinkles in the vest behind the patient.**

d. Placing the V in the back may cause the patient to choke.

e. Wrinkles in the vest behind the patient may lead to skin impairment.

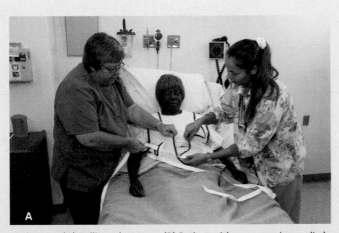
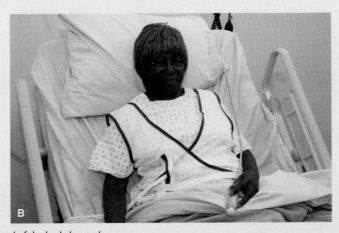

Action 5e: (A) Pulling tabs secure. (B) Patient with vest restraint applied and head of the bed elevated.

f. **Insert fist between restraint and patient to ensure that breathing is not constricted. Assess respirations after restraint is applied.**

g. **Use appropriate tie for all restraints.**

f. This prevents impaired respirations.

g. A quick-release knot ensures that the restraint will not tighten when pulled and can be removed quickly in an emergency.

continues

SKILL 3-2   Applying a Vest Restraint (continued)

ACTION	RATIONALE
h. **Fasten restraint to bed frame, not side rail. Place bed height in low position.** If patient is in a wheelchair, lock the wheels and place the restraints under the arm rests and tie behind the chair. Site should not be readily accessible to the patient.	h. Securing restraint to a side rail may cause patient injury when the side rail is lowered. If patient were to get out of restraint, a low bed height may prevent patient injury. Tying restraint out of patient's reach promotes security.

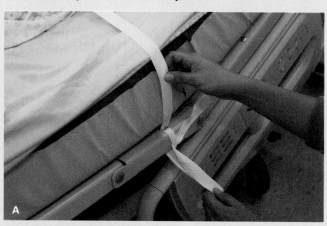
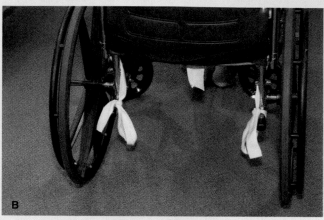

Action 5h: (A) Fastening restraint to bed frame. **(B)** Vest restraint tied to back of wheelchair.

6. **Remove restraint at least every 2 hours, or according to agency policy and patient need. Check for any signs of respiratory difficulties.**	Removal allows nurse to assess patient and reevaluate need for restraint.
7. Reassure patient at regular intervals. **Keep call bell within easy reach for patient.**	Reassurance demonstrates caring and provides opportunity for sensory stimulation as well as ongoing assessment and evaluation. Patient can use call bell to summon assistance quickly.
8. Assess for signs of sensory deprivation, such as increased sleeping, daydreaming, anxiety, panic, and hallucinations.	Use of restraints may decrease environmental stimulation and result in sensory deprivation.
9. Perform hand hygiene.	Hand hygiene deters the spread of microorganisms.
10. Document reason for restraining patient, alternative measures attempted before applying restraint, date and time of application, type of restraint, times when removed, and result and frequency of nursing assessment. Obtain a new order after 24 hours if restraints are still necessary.	Careful documentation supports use of restraints, alternative measures to ensure safety, and assessment data. JCAHO recommends a 24-hour time limit for use of restraints in nonpsychiatric patients.

9/30/06   2130   Patient continues to attempt to get out of bed without assistance. Vest restraint applied at night as ordered when family leaves. Bed height low; side rails up × 2.—K. Urhahn, RN

9/30/06   2300   Vest removed; skin intact; patient ambulated to restroom with assistance. Patient requested to ambulate to kitchen for snack; patient assisted to kitchen; graham crackers and milk obtained. Patient returned to bed and vest reapplied after snack. —K. Urhahn, RN

Action 10: Documentation.

continues

SKILL
3-2 **Applying a Vest Restraint** (continued)

EVALUATION	The expected outcomes are met when the patient remains free of injury; the restraints prevent injury to the patient or others; respirations are easy and effortless; skin integrity is maintained under the restraint; and the family demonstrates understanding of the rationale for using the restraints.

Unexpected Situations and Associated Interventions	• *Patient slides down and neck is caught in restraint:* Immediately release restraint. Determine alternate methods for restraining. • *Patient slides down and out of restraint:* Apply smaller vest restraint. Vest restraints come in various sizes, and the patient should not be able to slide out of vest. • *Patient is exhibiting signs of respiratory distress:* Release vest. Vest may be applied too tightly and cause difficulty with chest expansion.
Special Considerations	• Consider keeping a pair of scissors with emergency supplies in case the restraints cannot be untied quickly.

SKILL
3-3 **Applying an Elbow Restraint**

Elbow restraints are generally used on infants and children. They prevent the child from bending the elbows and reaching incisions or therapeutic devices. The child can move all joints and extremities except the elbow.

Equipment	• Elbow restraint • Padding as necessary
ASSESSMENT	Assess patient's behavior and need for restraint. Check circulation in the hands and fingers. The restraint should not decrease circulation. Measure the distance from the patient's shoulder to wrist to determine which size of elbow restraint to apply.
NURSING DIAGNOSIS	Determine the related factors for nursing diagnoses based on the patient's current status. Appropriate nursing diagnoses may be Risk for Injury or Risk for Impaired Skin Integrity.
OUTCOME IDENTIFICATION AND PLANNING	The expected outcome to achieve when applying an elbow restraint is that the patient cannot reach and interfere with dressings, incisions, or therapeutic devices. Other outcomes that may be appropriate include the following: the skin remains intact where the restraint is applied; the patient does not injure himself or herself due to the restraints; and the patient's family demonstrates understanding of the need for restraints and what they can do to help.

IMPLEMENTATION

ACTION	RATIONALE
1. Determine the need for restraints. Assess patient's physical condition, behavior, and mental status.	Restraints should be used only as a last resort when alternative measures have failed, and the patient is at increased risk for harming himself or herself or others.
2. Confirm agency policy for application of restraints. Secure a physician's order. **Ensure that the physician's order has been obtained within the past 24 hours.**	Policy protects the patient and the nurse and specifies guidelines for application as well as type of restraint and duration. **JCAHO standards require that a new order for restraints must be written every 24 hours.**

continues

SKILL 3-3 Applying an Elbow Restraint (continued)

ACTION	RATIONALE
3. Explain reason for use of restraint to patient and family. Clarify how care will be given and needs will be met. Explain that restraint is a temporary measure.	Explanation to patient and family may lessen confusion and anger and provide reassurance. A clearly stated agency policy on application of restraints should be available for patient and family to read. In a long-term care facility, the family must give consent before a restraint is applied.
4. Perform hand hygiene.	Hand hygiene deters the spread of microorganisms.
5. Apply restraints according to manufacturer's directions:	Proper application ensures that there is no interference with patient's circulation.
a. Choose the least restrictive type of device that allows the greatest possible degree of mobility.	a. This provides minimal restriction.
b. Pad bony prominences. If patient has an infusion or dressing on arm, extra padding may be applied.	b. Padding prevents skin breakdown and may protect IV infusion or dressing.
c. Spread elbow restraint out flat. Place middle of elbow restraint behind patient's elbow. **The restraint should not extend below the wrist or place pressure on the axilla.**	c. Elbow restraint should be placed in middle of arm to ensure that child cannot bend the elbow. Child should be able to move wrist. Pressure on the axilla may lead to skin impairment.
d. **Wrap restraint snugly around patient's arm, but make sure that two fingers can easily fit under restraint.**	d. Wrapping snugly ensures that child will not be able to remove the device. Being able to insert two fingers helps to prevent impaired circulation from restraint.

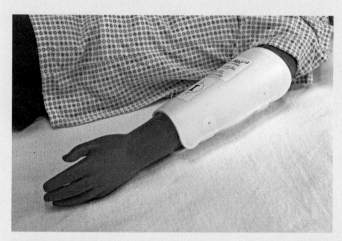

Action 5: Child with elbow restraint in place.

e. Wrap Velcro straps around restraint.	e. Velcro straps will prevent child from removing restraint.
f. Apply restraint to opposite arm if patient can move arm.	f. Bilateral elbow restraints are needed if patient can move both arms.
g. Thread Velcro strap from one elbow restraint across the back and into the loop on the opposite elbow restraint.	g. Strap across the back prevents child from wiggling out of elbow restraints.
h. **Assess circulation to fingers and hand.**	h. Circulation should not be impaired from elbow restraint.

continues

Applying an Elbow Restraint (continued)

ACTION	RATIONALE
6. **Remove restraint at least every 2 hours, or according to agency policy and patient need.**	Removal allows nurse to assess patient and reevaluate need for restraint.
a. Check for signs of decreased circulation or impaired skin integrity.	a. Improperly applied restraints may cause skin tears, abrasions, or bruises. Decreased circulation may result in paleness, coolness, decreased sensation, tingling, numbness, or pain in extremity.
b. Perform range-of-motion exercises before reapplying.	b. Exercise increases circulation in the restrained extremity and will prevent the elbow from becoming stiff.
7. Reassure patient at regular intervals. **Keep call bell within easy reach of patient.**	Reassurance demonstrates caring and provides opportunity for sensory stimulation as well as ongoing assessment and evaluation. Children old enough to use call bell can use it to summon assistance quickly.
8. Assess for signs of sensory deprivation, such as increased sleeping, daydreaming, anxiety, inconsolable crying, and panic.	Use of restraints may decrease environmental stimulation and result in sensory deprivation.
9. Perform hand hygiene.	Hand hygiene deters the spread of microorganisms.
10. Document reason for restraining patient, alternative measures attempted before applying the restraint, date and time of application, type of restraint, times when removed, and result and frequency of nursing assessment. Obtain a new order after 24 hours if restraints are still necessary.	Careful documentation supports use of restraints, alternative measures to ensure safety, and assessment data.

9/1/06   0800   Elbow restraints removed while a.m. care performed (45 minutes). Patient moving arms appropriately. Continues to pick at colostomy bag. Distraction techniques used to no avail. Child removes abdominal binder when applied.—K. Urhahn, RN

9/1/06   0855   Skin intact and warm. Elbow restraints reapplied. Will remove when family arrives at bedside or every 2 hours as per policy.—K. Urhahn, RN

Action 10: Documentation.

EVALUATION

The expected outcome is met when the restraint prevents injury to self or others. In addition, the child cannot bend the elbow; skin integrity is maintained under the restraint; and the family demonstrates an understanding of the rationale for the elbow restraint.

Unexpected Outcomes and Associated Interventions

- *Skin breakdown is noted on elbows:* Ensure that restraints are being removed routinely for at least 30 minutes and a skin inspection is done. If restraints are still needed, a padded dressing may be applied under the elbow restraint.
- *Patient cries when elbow is moved:* Restraints need to be removed more frequently, with active and/or passive range of motion. If elbow is not moved, it will become stiff and painful.

SKILL 3-4 Applying Leather Restraints

Leather restraints are used whenever cloth restraints are not strong enough to restrain the patient. Leather restraints come in a locking and a nonlocking type. If using the locking type, ensure that the key is available at all times. In an emergency situation, leather locking restraints cannot be cut easily.

Equipment
- Restraint
- Padding, if necessary, for bony prominences

ASSESSMENT

Assess the patient's physical condition and potential for injury to self or others. If the patient has had a stroke and cannot move one arm, a restraint may be needed only on the other arm. If the patient is confused and might remove lines or devices needed to sustain life, this would be considered a potential for injury to self. Inspect the skin on the extremity where the restraint will be applied. If the skin is injured or an IV is inserted in the area, extra padding, such as roller gauze, may be needed to prevent injury from the restraint. Assess capillary refill in the digits of the extremities to which the restraint is to be applied. This helps to determine the circulation in the extremity before applying the restraint.

NURSING DIAGNOSIS

Determine the related factors for nursing diagnoses based on the patient's current status. An appropriate nursing diagnosis is Risk for Injury. Other appropriate nursing diagnoses may include:

- Risk for Impaired Skin Integrity
- Risk for Aspiration

OUTCOME IDENTIFICATION AND PLANNING

The expected outcome to achieve when applying leather restraints is that the patient is contained by the leather restraint and does not cause harm to self or others. Other outcomes that may be appropriate include the following: the patient does not interfere with any lines, dressings, or other therapeutic equipment; the skin is not injured where the restraint is applied; and the patient's family will demonstrate an understanding about the need for restraints and what they can do to help.

IMPLEMENTATION

ACTION	RATIONALE
1. Determine the need for restraints. Assess patient's physical condition, behavior, and mental status.	Restraints should be used only as a last resort when alternative measures have failed, and the patient is at increased risk for harming himself or herself or others.
2. Confirm agency policy for application of restraints. Secure a physician's order. **Ensure that the physician's order has been obtained within the past 24 hours.**	Policy protects the patient and the nurse and specifies guidelines for application as well as type of restraint and duration. **JCAHO standards require that a new order for restraints must be written every 24 hours.**
3. Explain reason for restraint use to patient and family. Clarify how care will be given and needs will be met. Explains that restraint is a temporary measure.	Explanation to patient and family may lessen confusion and anger and provide reassurance. A clearly stated agency policy on application of restraints should be available for patient and family to read. In a long-term care facility, the family must give consent before a restraint is applied.
4. Perform hand hygiene.	Hand hygiene deters the spread of microorganisms.
5. Apply restraints according to manufacturer's directions:	Proper application ensures that there is no interference with patient's circulation.
a. Pad bony prominences.	a. This protects the skin and prevents breakdown.
b. **For restraint applied to extremity, ensure that two fingers can be inserted between restraint and patient's wrist or ankle.**	b. This prevents impaired circulation to extremity.

continues

Applying Leather Restraints (continued)

ACTION	RATIONALE
c. Maintain restrained extremity in normal anatomic position.	c. This lessens possibility of contracture or musculoskeletal injury.
d. **If using locking leather restraints, ensure that key is available at all times.**	d. Leather restraints cannot be cut easily in an emergency situation. Key must be available to release patient quickly if needed.
e. **Fasten restraint to bed frame, not side rail.** Leather restraints have leather straps with buckles to secure to the bed frame. Site should not be readily accessible to the patient.	e. Securing restraint to a side rail may cause injury to patient if side rail is lowered. Securing restraint out of patient's reach promotes security.

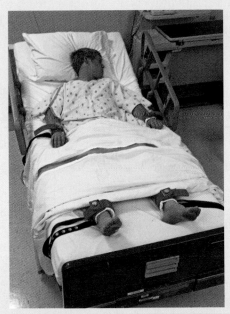

Action 5: Patient secured in leather restraints on all four extremities.

6. **Remove restraint at least every 2 hours, or according to agency policy and patient need. Take care when releasing patient from restraint that neither patient nor nurse is harmed. Consider releasing one extremity at a time.**	Removal allows nurse to assess patient and reevaluate need for restraint. Removing one restraint at a time may be safer for nurse.
a. **Check for signs of decreased circulation or impaired skin integrity.**	a. Improperly applied restraints may cause skin tears, abrasions, or bruises. Decreased circulation may result in paleness, coolness, decreased sensation, tingling, numbness, or pain in extremity.
b. **Perform range-of-motion exercises before reapplying.**	b. Exercise increases circulation in the restrained extremity.
7. Reassure patient at regular intervals. **Keep call bell within easy reach.**	Reassurance demonstrates caring and provides opportunity for sensory situation as well as ongoing assessment and evaluation. Patient can use call bell to summon assistance quickly.
8. Assess for signs of sensory deprivation, such as increased sleeping, daydreaming, anxiety, panic, and hallucinations.	Use of restraints may decrease environmental stimulation and result in sensory deprivation.

continues

SKILL 3-4   Applying Leather Restraints (continued)

ACTION	**RATIONALE**
9. Perform hand hygiene.	Hand hygiene deters the spread of microorganisms.
10. Document reason for restraining patient, alternative measures attempted before applying restraint, date and time of application, type of restraint, times when removed, and result and frequency of nursing assessment. Obtain a new order after 24 hours if restraints are still necessary.	Careful documentation supports use of restraints, alternative measures to ensure safety, and assessment data. JCAHO recommends a 24-hour time limit for restraint use in nonpsychiatric patients.

9/13/06   0100   Patient threatening to injure self and others. De-escalating attempts to no effect; security called; patient subdued and placed in four-point leather restraints as ordered. Key kept in room at all times; patient placed on right side.—K. Urhahn, RN

9/13/06   0200   With security at bedside, extremities released one at time and range of motion performed; skin intact and warm; patient continuing to threaten harm to others.
—K. Urhahn, RN

Action 10: Documentation.

EVALUATION

The expected outcome is met when the patient remains free of injury due to the application of restraints. In addition, injury to others is prevented; circulation to extremity remains adequate; skin integrity remains intact under the restraint; and the family verbalizes an awareness of the rationale for restraint use.

Unexpected Outcomes and Associated Interventions

- *Patient is continually pulling on leather restraints and causing injury to extremities:* Notify physician. Patient may need sedation. Talk with patient to see if there is anything that can be done to help him or her relax.
- *Nurse is afraid for own safety when releasing restraints for inspection and range of motion:* Call for assistance. For their own safety, nurses should have assistance when releasing a combative or agitated patient from leather restraints.

Special Considerations

- Do not position patient flat in a supine position with wrist restraints. If patient vomits, aspiration may occur.
- Have the key for locking leather restraints readily available at all times.

■ Developing Critical Thinking Skills

1. Megan Lewis, an 18-month-old with an IV access in her left forearm, is continually picking at the IV and dressing. What restraints would be appropriate for Megan?
2. Kevin Mallory, a 35-year-old body builder with a closed head injury, is extremely strong. The nurse is afraid that he will rip the cloth restraints and extubate himself. What other type of restraints could the nurse try?
3. John Frawley, a 72-year-old patient with Alzheimer's disease, continually tries to get out of bed without assistance. He has an unsteady gait and has broken one hip due to a fall. What is the least restrictive restraint for John?

Bibliography

Alexander, N., & Edelberg, H. (2002). Assessing mobility and preventing falls in older patients. *Patient Care, 36*(2), 19–29.

Bernardo, L. (2002). Emergency nurses' role in injury prevention. *Emergency Nursing, 37*(1), 135–142.

Brenner, Z., & Duffy-Durnin, K. (1998). Toward restraint-free care. *American Journal of Nursing, 98*(12), 16F–16I.

Carlson, D. (1998). Uncovering the clues of child abuse. *Nursing, 28*(11), 32hn10–11.

Carroll, M., Morin, K., Hayes, E., & Carter, S. (1999). Assessing students' perceived threats to safety in the community. *Nurse Educator, 24*(1), 31–35.

Centers for Disease Control and Prevention (2001). *Injury fact book: 2001–2002,* Atlanta: Author.

Centers for Disease Control and Prevention (2003). *Injury mortality reports, 1999–2000.* Available on-line: *http://webapp.cdc.gov/sasweb/ncipc/mortrate10.html.*

Covinsky, K. E., Kahana, E., Kahana, B., et al. (April 1, 2001). History and mobility exam index to identify community-dwelling elderly persons at risk of falling. *Journal of Gerontology, 56*(4):253M–259.

Crawley-Coha, T. (2002). Childhood injury: a status report, part 2. *Journal of Pediatric Nursing, 17*(2), 133–136.

DiBartolo, V. (1998). 9 steps to effective restraint use. *RN, 61*(12), 23–24.

Dunn, K. (2001). The effect of physical restraints on fall rates in older adults who are institutionalized. *Journal of Gerontological Nursing, 27*(10), 40–48.

Eliopoulos, C. (2003). *Gerontological nursing* (5th ed.). Philadelphia: Lippincott Williams & Wilkins.

Gentleman, B., & Malozemoff, W. (2001). Falls and feelings: Description of a psychosocial group nursing intervention. *Journal of Gerontological Nursing, 27*(10), 35–39.

Gerard, M. (2000). Domestic violence: How to screen & intervene. *RN, 63*(12), 52–56.

Grenier-Sennlier, C., Lombard, Jeny-Loper, Maillet-Gouret, et al. (2002). Designing adverse event prevention programs using quality management methods: The case of falls in hospitals. *International Journal of Quality Health Care, 14*(5), 419–426.

Hayes, L. (2000). Poison emergency? *Nursing, 30*(9), 34–39.

Joint Commission on Accreditation of Healthcare Organizations. (1998). *1998 hospital accreditation standards.* Oakbrook Terrace, IL: Author.

Kimbell, S. (2001). Before the fall. *Nursing, 31*(8), 44–45.

London, M., Ladewig, P., Ball, J., et al. (2003). *Maternal-newborn & child nursing.* Upper Saddle River, NJ: Prentice Hall.

Mace, S., Gerardi, M., Dietrick, A., et al. (2001). Injury prevention and control in children. *Annals of Emergency Medicine, 38*(4), 405–413.

Melillo, K., & Futrell, M. (1998). Wandering and technology devices. *Journal of Gerontological Nursing, 24*(8), 32–38.

Mulryan, K., Cathers, P., & Fagin, A. (2000). Protecting the child. *Nursing, 30*(7), 39–45.

Napierkowski, D. (2002). Using restraints with restraint. *Nursing, 32*(11), 58–62.

North American Nursing Diagnosis Association. (2003). *NANDA nursing diagnoses: Definitions & classifications 2003–2004.* Philadelphia: Author.

Partridge, R., Virk, A. & Antosia, R. (1998) Causes and patterns of injury from ladder falls. *Academic Emergency Medicine, 5*(1), 31–34.

Rawsky, E. (1998). Review of literature on falls among the elderly. *Image—The Journal of Nursing Scholarship, 30*(1), 47–52.

Sullivan, G. (1999). Minimizing your risk in patient falls. *RN, 62*(4), 69–72.

Taft, C., Michalide, A., & Taft, A. *Child passengers at risk in America: A national study of car seat misuse.* Washington, DC: National SAFE KIDS Campaign, February 1999.

Talerico, K., & Capezuti, E. (2001). Myths and facts about side rails. *American Journal of Nursing, 101*(7), 43–48.

Teret, S., et al. (1998). Making guns safer. *Issues in Science and Technology, 14*(4), 37–40.

Todd, J. (2002). When bed isn't a safe haven. *Nursing, 32*(12), 82.

U.S. Census Bureau (2002). *Statistical Abstract of the United States, 2002* (122nd ed.). Washington, DC: Author.

Asepsis and Infection Control

Focusing on Patient Care

This chapter will help you develop some of the skills related to asepsis and infection control necessary to care for the following patients:

Joe Wilson is scheduled to undergo a cardiac catheterization later this morning.

Sheri Lawrence has been ordered to have an indwelling urinary catheter inserted and is at risk for a nosocomial infection.

Edgar Barowski is suspected of having tuberculosis and requires infection control precautions.

Learning Outcomes

After studying this chapter, the reader should be able to:

1. Perform hand hygiene.
2. Prepare a sterile field.
3. Don and remove sterile gloves.
4. Use personal protective equipment, including surgical mask, particulate respirator, protective goggles, and protective gown.

Key Terms

medical asepsis: clean technique; involves procedures and practices that reduce the number and transfers of pathogens

nosocomial infection: hospital-acquired infection

standard precautions: precautions used in the care of all hospitalized individuals regardless of their diagnosis or possible infection status; these precautions apply to blood, all body fluids, secretions and excretions (except sweat), nonintact skin, and mucous membranes

surgical asepsis: sterile technique; involves practices used to render and keep objects and areas free from microorganisms

transmission-based precautions: precautions used in addition to Standard Precautions for patients in hospitals who are suspected of being infected with pathogens that can be transmitted by airborne, droplet, or contact routes; these precautions encompass all the diseases or conditions previously listed in the disease-specific or category-specific classifications

A major concern for all health practitioners is the danger of spreading microorganisms from person to person and from place to place. Microorganisms are naturally present in almost all environments. Some are beneficial, but some are not. Some are considered harmless, while others are not. Moreover, in certain situations, normally harmless microorganisms can be detrimental.

Groups working toward a microorganism-safe environment include government agencies at the international, national, state, and local levels; health personnel; and individuals. Such efforts include mass immunization programs, laws concerning safe sewage disposal, regulations for the control of communicable diseases, and hospital infection surveillance programs. In addition, medical science continues to grapple with problems related to organisms that have become increasingly virulent and drug resistant and with problems related to patients who are immunologically compromised. Prevention of infection is a major focus for nurses. As primary caregivers, nurses are involved in identifying, preventing, controlling, and teaching the patient about infection. Use of the nursing process can prove critical in breaking the cycle of infection.

This chapter will cover skills to assist the nurse in preventing the spread of infection. Please look over the summary boxes at the beginning of this chapter for a quick review of critical knowledge to assist you in understanding the skills related to asepsis and infection control measures.

BOX 4-1 Basic Principles of Medical Asepsis in Patient Care

- Practice good hand hygiene techniques (see Box 4-3).
- Carry soiled items, including linens, equipment, and other used articles, away from the body to prevent them from touching the clothing.
- Do not place soiled bed linen or any other items on the floor, which is grossly contaminated. It increases contamination of both surfaces.
- Avoid having patients cough, sneeze, or breathe directly on others. Provide patients with disposable tissues, and instruct them, as indicated, to cover their mouth and nose to prevent spread by airborne droplets.
- Move equipment away from you when brushing, dusting, or scrubbing articles. This helps prevent contaminated particles from settling on your hair, face, and uniform.
- Avoid raising dust. Use a specially treated or a dampened cloth. Do not shake linens. Dust and lint particles constitute a vehicle by which organisms may be transported from one area to another.
- Clean the least soiled areas first and then move to the more soiled ones. This helps prevent having the cleaner areas soiled by the dirtier areas.
- Dispose of soiled or used items directly into appropriate containers. Wrap items that are moist from body discharge or drainage in waterproof containers, such as plastic bags, before discarding into the refuse holder so that handlers will not come in contact with them.
- Pour liquids that are to be discarded, such as bath water, mouth rinse, and the like, directly into the drain to avoid splattering in the sink and onto you.
- Sterilize items that are suspected of containing pathogens. After sterilization, they can be managed as clean items if appropriate.
- Use personal grooming habits that help prevent spreading microorganisms. Shampoo your hair regularly; keep your fingernails short and free of broken cuticles and ragged edges; do not wear false nails; and do not wear rings with grooves and stones that may harbor microorganisms.
- Follow guidelines conscientiously for infection control or barrier techniques as prescribed by the agency.

BOX 4-2 Basic Principles of Surgical Asepsis

- Only a sterile object can touch another sterile object. Unsterile touching sterile means contamination has occurred.
- Open sterile packages so that the first edge of the wrapper is directed away from the worker to avoid the possibility of a sterile surface touching unsterile clothing. The outside of the sterile package is considered contaminated. Opening a sterile package is shown and described in Skill 4-2.
- Avoid spilling any solution on a cloth or paper used as a field for a sterile setup. The moisture penetrates the sterile cloth or paper and carries organisms by capillary action to contaminate the field. A wet field is considered contaminated if the surface immediately below it is not sterile.
- Hold sterile objects above waist level. This will ensure keeping the object within sight and preventing accidental contamination.
- Avoid talking, coughing, sneezing, or reaching over a sterile field or object. This helps to prevent contamination by droplets from the nose and the mouth or by particles dropping from the worker's arm.
- Never walk away from or turn your back on a sterile field. This prevents possible contamination while the field is out of the worker's view.
- All items brought into contact with broken skin, used to penetrate the skin to inject substances into the body, or used to enter normally sterile body cavities should be sterile. These items include dressings used to cover wounds and incisions, needles for injection, and tubes (catheters) used to drain urine from the bladder.
- Use dry, sterile forceps when necessary. Forceps soaked in disinfectant are not considered sterile.
- Consider the outer 1" edge of a sterile field to be contaminated.
- Consider an object contaminated if you have any doubt as to its sterility.

BOX 4-3 Hand Hygiene (Handwashing or Use of Alcohol-Based Hand Rubs)

- Hand hygiene refers to the washing of the hands with soap and water *or* the use of an alcohol-based hand rub.
- When hands are visibly soiled, before eating, and after using a restroom, wash hands with soap and water.
- If hands are not visibly soiled, an alcohol-based hand rub may used.
- The use of gloves does not eliminate the need for hand hygiene; the use of hand hygiene does not eliminate the need for gloves.
- Hand hygiene should be done:
  - Before and after contact with each patient
  - Before donning sterile gloves
  - Before performing any invasive procedure, such as placement of a peripheral vascular catheter
  - After accidental contact with body fluids or excretions, mucous membranes, nonintact skin, and wound dressings, even if hands are not visibly soiled
  - When moving from a contaminated body site to a clean body site during patient care
  - After contact with inanimate objects near the patient
  - After removal of gloves.

BOX 4-4 Hand Hygiene Using an Alcohol-Based Handrub

- Apply product to the palm of one hand, using the amount of product recommended on the package. (It will vary according to the manufacturer.)
- Rub hands together, making sure to cover all surfaces of the hands and fingers, including in between the fingers.
- Continue rubbing until the hands are dry.

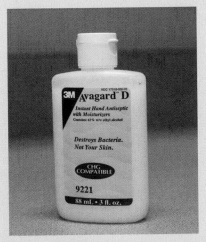

Alcohol-based hand rub

SKILL 4-1   Hand Hygiene

Nurses and other healthcare workers have a key role in reducing the spread of disease, minimizing complications, and reducing adverse outcomes for their patients. Limiting the spread of microorganisms is accomplished by breaking the chain of infection. The most important tool you have against the spread of disease is performing proper hand hygiene. The term "hand hygiene" is now preferred and applies to handwashing with plain soap and water; use of antiseptic hand rubs, including alcohol-based products; or surgical hand antisepsis (Centers for Disease Control and Prevention [CDC], 2002). The CDC has reinforced the previous guideline that hand washing is the most effective way to help prevent the spread of organisms. However, it has looked at the use of other agents, and the guidelines now include the routine use of alcohol-based hand rubs when the nurse's hands are not visibly soiled.

Equipment

- Non-antimicrobial or antimicrobial soap (if in bar form, soap must be placed on a soap rock)
- Paper towels
- Oil-free lotion (optional)

ASSESSMENT

Assess hands for any visible soiling. If hands are visibly soiled, proceed with washing the hands with soap and water. If hands are not visibly soiled, the caregiver has the option of washing hands with soap and water or using an alcohol-based hand rub.

NURSING DIAGNOSIS

Determine the related factors for the nursing diagnoses based on the patient's current status. An appropriate nursing diagnosis is Risk for Infection. Many other nursing diagnoses also may require the use of this skill.

OUTCOME IDENTIFICATION AND PLANNING

The expected outcome to achieve when performing hand washing is that the hands will be free of visible soiling. Other outcomes may be appropriate depending on the specific nursing diagnosis identified for the patient.

IMPLEMENTATION

ACTION	RATIONALE
1. Gather the necessary supplies. Stand in front of the sink. Do not allow your clothing to touch the sink during the washing procedure.	The sink is considered contaminated. Clothing may carry organisms from place to place.
2. Remove jewelry, if possible, and secure in a safe place. A plain wedding band may remain in place.	Removal of jewelry facilitates proper cleansing. Microorganisms may accumulate in settings of jewelry. If jewelry was worn during care, it should be left on during handwashing.

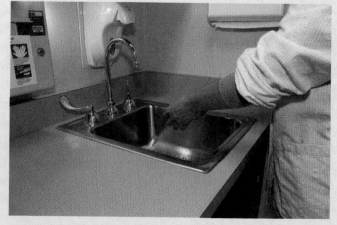

Action 1: Standing in front of sink.

continues

ACTION	RATIONALE
3. Turn on water and adjust force. Regulate the temperature until the water is warm.	Water splashed from the contaminated sink will contaminate clothing. Warm water is more comfortable and is less likely to open pores and remove oils from the skin. Organisms can lodge in roughened and broken areas of chapped skin.
4. Wet the hands and wrist area. Keep hands lower than elbows to allow water to flow toward fingertips.	Water should flow from the cleaner area toward the more contaminated area. Hands are more contaminated than forearms.

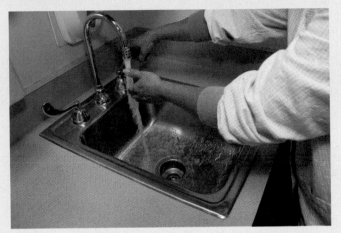

Action 3: Turning on the water at the sink.

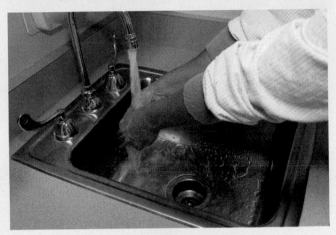

Action 4: Wetting hands to the wrist.

5. Use about 1 teaspoon liquid soap from dispenser or rinse bar of soap and lather thoroughly. Cover all areas of hands with the soap product. Rinse soap bar again and return to soap dish.	Rinsing the soap before and after use removes the lather, which may contain microorganisms.

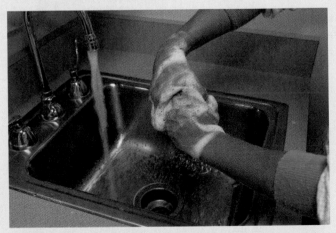

Action 5: Lathering hands with soap and rubbing with firm circular motion.

6. With firm rubbing and circular motions, wash the palms and backs of the hands, each finger, the areas between the fingers, the knuckles, wrists, and forearms. **Wash at least 1" above area of contamination.** If hands are not visibly soiled, wash to 1" above the wrists.	Friction caused by firm rubbing and circular motions helps to loosen dirt and organisms that can lodge between the fingers, in skin crevices of knuckles, on the palms and backs of the hands, and on the wrists and forearms. Cleaning less contaminated areas (forearms and wrists) after hands are clean prevents spreading microorganisms from the hands to the forearms and wrists. *continues*

ACTION

RATIONALE

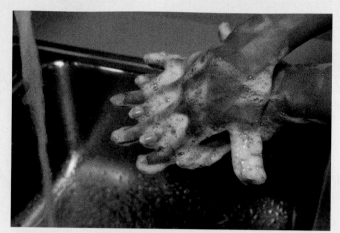

Action 6: Washing areas between fingers.

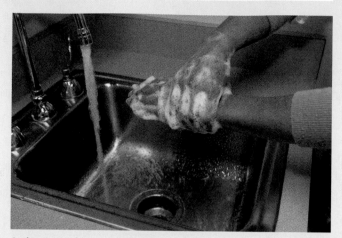

Action 6: Washing to 1 inch above the wrist.

7. Continue this friction motion for at least 15 seconds.

8. Use fingernails of the opposite hand or a clean orange-wood stick to clean under fingernails.

9. Rinse thoroughly with water flowing toward fingertips.

Length of hand washing is determined by degree of contamination.

Area under nails has a high microorganism count, and organisms may remain under the nails, where they can grow and be spread to others.

Running water rinses microorganisms and dirt into the sink.

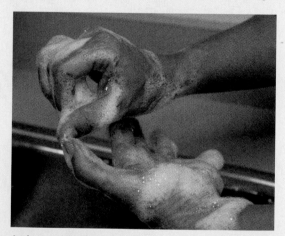

Action 8: Using fingernails to clean under nails of opposite hand.

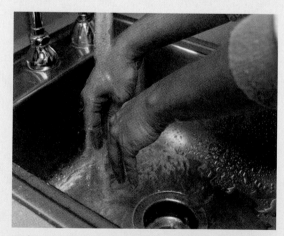

Action 9: Rinsing hands under running water with water flowing toward fingertips.

10. Pat hands dry, beginning with the fingers and moving upward toward forearms, with a paper towel and discard it immediately. Use another clean towel to turn off the faucet. Discard towel immediately without touching other clean hand.

11. Use oil-free lotion on hands if desired.

Patting the skin dry prevents chapping. Dry hands first because they are considered the cleanest and least contaminated area. Turning the faucet off with a clean paper towel protects the clean hands from contact with a soiled surface.

Oil-free lotion helps to keep the skin soft and prevents chapping. It is best applied after patient care is complete and from small, personal containers. Oil-based lotions should be avoided because they can cause deterioration of gloves.

continues

SKILL 4-1   Hand Hygiene (continued)

EVALUATION

The expected outcome is met when the hands are free of visible soiling. Inspect hands; if there is no visible soiling of hands, proceed to next task because the outcome has been achieved. However, if visible soiling is left on hands, repeat handwashing steps.

Special Considerations

- An antimicrobial soap product is recommended for use with hand washing before participating with an invasive procedure and after exposure to blood or body fluids. The length of the scrub will vary based on need.
- Liquid or bar soap, granules, or leaflets are all acceptable forms of non-antimicrobial soap.

SKILL 4-2   Preparing a Sterile Field

A sterile field is created to provide a surgically aseptic workspace. It should be considered a restricted area. A sterile drape may be used to establish a sterile field or to extend the sterile working area. The sterile drape should be waterproof on one side, with that side placed down on the work surface. After establishing the sterile field, other sterile items needed, including solutions, are added. Sterile items and sterile gloved hands are the only objects allowed in the sterile field. If the area is breached, the entire sterile field is considered contaminated.

Equipment

- Sterile wrapped drape or commercially prepared sterile package
- Package of sterile gloves if needed (consider obtaining two packages in case contamination occurs)
- Additional sterile supplies, such as dressings, containers, or solution as needed

ASSESSMENT

Assess the situation to determine the necessity for creating a sterile field. Then assess the area in which the sterile field is to be prepared. Move any unnecessary equipment out of the immediate vicinity.

NURSING DIAGNOSIS

Determine the related factors for the nursing diagnoses based on the patient's current status. Appropriate nursing diagnoses may include:

- Risk for Infection
- Ineffective Protection
- Anxiety

In addition, other nursing diagnoses also may require the use of this skill.

OUTCOME IDENTIFICATION AND PLANNING

The expected outcome to achieve when preparing a sterile field is that the sterile field is created without evidence of contamination and the patient remains free of exposure to potential infection-causing microorganisms.

IMPLEMENTATION

ACTION	RATIONALE
1. Explain the procedure to the patient and perform hand hygiene.	An explanation encourages patient cooperation and reduces apprehension. Hand hygiene deters the spread of microorganisms
2. Check that sterile wrapped drape or package is dry and unopened. Also note expiration date, making sure that the date is still valid.	Moisture contaminates a sterile package. Expiration date indicates period that package remains sterile.

continues

SKILL 4-2   Preparing a Sterile Field (continued)

ACTION	RATIONALE

3. Select a work area that is waist level or higher.

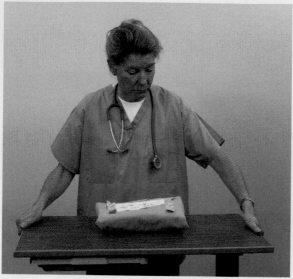

Action 3: Positioning bedside table at waist level, with sterile package on table.

4. a. If appropriate or necessary, open sterile wrapped drape, agency-wrapped sterile package, or commercially prepared sterile package. For sterile wrapped drape, open outer covering. Remove sterile drape, lifting it carefully by its corners. Gently shake open, hold away from your body, and lay drape on selected work area.

   b. Place agency-wrapped or commercially prepared package in center of work area. **Touching outer surface only, carefully reach around item and fold topmost flap of wrapper away from you.** Open right and left flap before grasping the nearest flap and opening toward you.

Work area is within sight. Bacteria tend to settle, so there is less contamination above the waist.

a. Outer 1″ (2.5 cm) of drape is considered contaminated. Any item touching this area is also considered contaminated.

b. Proper placement prevents contamination by reaching across sterile field. Touching outer side of wrapper maintains sterile field.

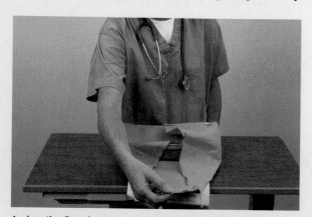

Action 4b: Opening top most flap of sterile package.

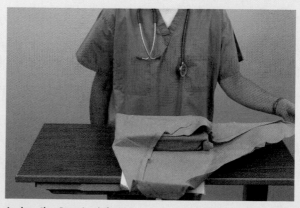

Action 4b: Opening left side.

continues

Preparing a Sterile Field (continued)

ACTION

RATIONALE

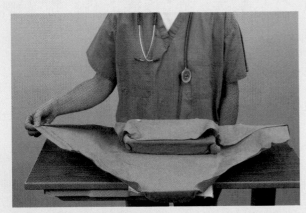

Action 4b: Opening right side.

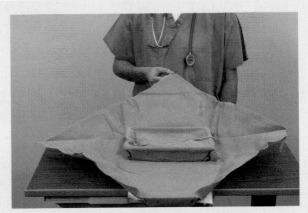

Action 4b: Opening bottom corner toward the body.

5. Place additional sterile items on field as needed.

When Adding a Sterile Item to a Sterile Field

6. a. Hold agency-wrapped item in one hand with top flap opening away from you. With other hand unfold top flap and both sides. Keeping a secure hold on item, **grasp the corners of the wrapper and pull back toward wrist, covering hand and wrist.**

b. If commercially packaged item has an unsealed corner, hold package in one hand and pull back on top cover with other hand. If edge is partially sealed, use both hands to carefully peel apart.

7. Drop sterile item onto sterile field from a 6″ (15 cm) height or add item to field from the side. Be careful to avoid dropping onto the 1″ border.

8. Discard wrapper.

Sterile field is maintained.

a. Only sterile surface and item are exposed before dropping onto sterile field.

b. Contents remain uncontaminated by hands.

Wrapper does not contaminate sterile field. Any items landing on 1″ border are considered contaminated.

A neat work area promotes proper technique.

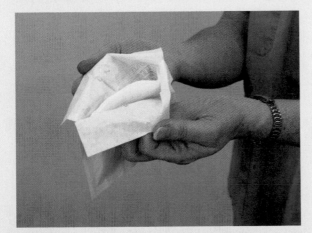

Action 6b: Using both hands and gently pulling apart.

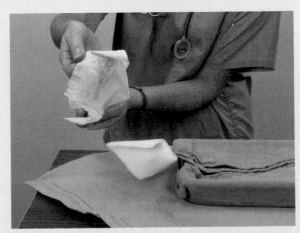

Action 7: Dropping sterile item onto sterile field.

continues

SKILL 4-2

Preparing a Sterile Field (continued)

ACTION	RATIONALE

When Pouring a Sterile Solution

9. Obtain appropriate solution and check expiration date.

10. Open solution container according to directions and **place cap on table with edges up.**

11. If bottle has previously been opened, "lip" it by pouring a small amount of solution into waste container.

Once opened, a bottle should be labeled with date and time. Solution remains sterile for 24 hours once opened.

Sterility of inside cap is maintained.

This cleanses the lip of the bottle.

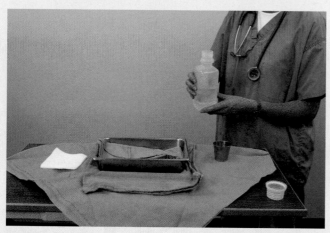

Action 10: Opening bottle of sterile solution without contaminating the cap.

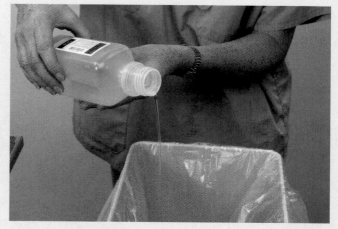

Action 11: Pouring off a small amount of solution into a trash receptacle.

12. Hold bottle outside the edge of the sterile field with the label side facing the palm of your hand and prepare to pour from a height of 4″ to 6″ (10 to 15 cm). The tip of the bottle should never touch a sterile container or dressing.

Label remains dry, and solution may be poured without reaching across sterile field. Minimal splashing occurs from that height. Accidentally touching the tip of the bottle to a container or dressing contaminates them both.

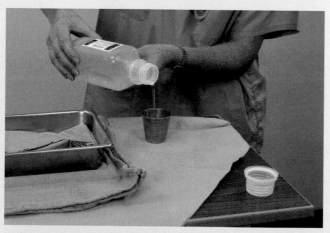

Action 12: Pouring solution into sterile container.

13. Pour required amount of solution steadily into sterile container positioned at side of sterile field. **Avoid splashing any liquid.**

14. Touch only the outside of the lid when recapping.

Moisture contaminates sterile field.

Solution remains uncontaminated.

continues

Preparing a Sterile Field (continued)

EVALUATION   The expected outcome is met when the sterile field is prepared without contamination and the patient has remained free of exposure to potentially infectious microorganisms.

Unexpected Situations and Associated Interventions

- *A part of the sterile field becomes contaminated:* When any portion of the sterile field becomes contaminated, discard all portions of the sterile field and start over.
- *You realize you are missing a supply:* Call for help. Do not leave the sterile field unattended. If you are not able to visualize the sterile field at all times, it is considered contaminated.
- *The patient touches your hands or the sterile field:* If the patient touches your hands and nothing else, you may remove your contaminated gloves and don new, sterile gloves. It is always a good idea to bring two pairs of sterile gloves into the room. If the patient touches the sterile field, discard the supplies and prepare a new sterile field. If the patient is confused, it is a good idea to have someone assist you by holding the patient's hands or reinforcing what is happening.

Donning and Removing Sterile Gloves

While working within a sterile field, sterile gloves must be used. Donning, using, and disposing of sterile gloves requires a specific skill. When applying and wearing sterile gloves, keep your hands above waist level and away from nonsterile surfaces. Any item or hand that goes below your waist is considered contaminated. If this happens, replace your gloves or the item immediately. Also be prepared to replace your gloves if they develop an opening or tear, the integrity of the material becomes compromised, or the gloves come in contact with any unsterile surface or unsterile item. It is a good idea to bring an extra pair of gloves when you gather your supplies. That way, if the first pair is contaminated in some way and needs to be replaced, you won't have to leave the procedure to get a new pair.

Equipment
- Sterile gloves of the appropriate size

ASSESSMENT   Assess the situation to determine the necessity for sterile gloves. In addition, check the patient's chart for information about a possible latex allergy. Also, question the patient about any history of allergy, including latex allergy or sensitivity and signs and symptoms that have occurred. If the patient has a latex allergy, anticipate the need for latex-free gloves.

NURSING DIAGNOSIS   Determine the related factors for the nursing diagnoses based on the patient's current status. An appropriate nursing diagnosis is Risk for Infection. Other nursing diagnoses that may be appropriate include:

- Ineffective Protection
- Risk for Latex Allergy Response

Many other nursing diagnoses also may require the use of this skill.

OUTCOME IDENTIFICATION AND PLANNING   The expected outcome to achieve when donning and removing sterile gloves is that the gloves are applied and removed without contamination. Other outcomes that may be appropriate include the following: the patient remains free of exposure to infectious microorganisms; the patient does not exhibit signs and symptoms of a latex allergy response.

continues

SKILL 4-3   Donning and Removing Sterile Gloves (continued)

IMPLEMENTATION

ACTION	RATIONALE
1. Perform hand hygiene.	Hand hygiene deters the spread of microorganisms. Gloves are easier to don when hands are dry.
2. Place sterile glove package on clean, dry surface at or above your waist.	Moisture could contaminate the sterile gloves. Any sterile object held below the waist is considered contaminated.
3. Open the outside wrapper by carefully peeling the top layer back. Remove inner package, handling only the outside of it.	This maintains sterility of gloves in inner packet.
4. Carefully open the inner package using the flaps and expose the sterile gloves with the cuff end closest to you.	The inner surface of the package is considered sterile. The outer 1″ border of the inner package is considered contaminated.

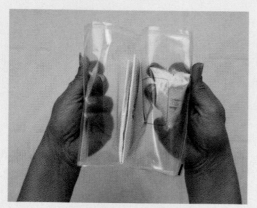

Action 3: Pulling top layer of outside wrapper back.

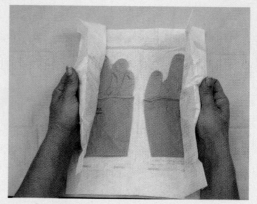

Action 4: Using flaps on the inner package.

5. With the thumb and forefinger of nondominant hand, grasp the folded cuff of the sterile glove for dominant hand.	Unsterile hand touches only inside of glove. Outside remains sterile.
6. Lift and hold glove up and off the inner package with fingers down. **Be careful it does not touch any unsterile object.**	Glove is contaminated if it touches unsterile object.

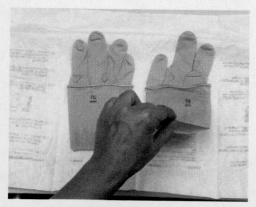

Action 5: Grasping cuff of glove for dominant hand.

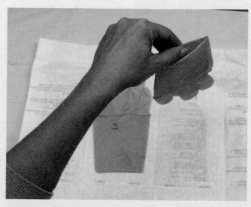

Action 6: Lifting glove from package.

continues

Donning and Removing Sterile Gloves (continued)

ACTION

RATIONALE

7. Carefully insert dominant hand palm up into glove and pull glove on.

8. Holding thumb outward, slide fingers of gloved hand under cuff of remaining glove and lift glove upward.

Attempting to turn upward with unsterile hand may result in contamination of sterile glove.

Thumb is less likely to become contaminated if held outward.

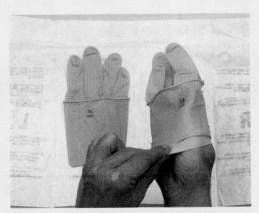

Action 7: Inserting dominant hand into glove.

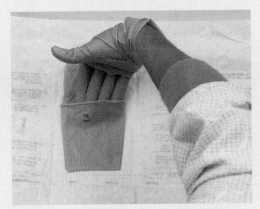

Action 8: Sliding fingers under cuff of glove for non-dominant hand.

9. Carefully insert nondominant hand into glove. **Adjust gloves on both hands, touching only sterile areas with other sterile areas.**

Sterile surface touching sterile surface prevents contamination.

To Remove Gloves

10. Using dominant hand, grasp other glove near cuff end and remove by inverting it, keeping the contaminated area on the inside. Continue to hold onto glove.

Contaminated area does not come in contact with hands or wrists.

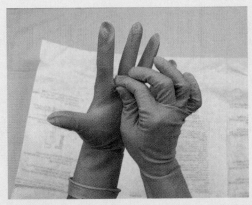

Action 9: Inserting nondominant hand into glove and adjusting gloves.

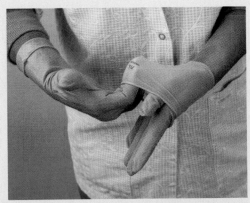

Action 10: Grasping glove near cuff end with other hand and pulling it off.

continues

SKILL 4-3   Donning and Removing Sterile Gloves (continued)

ACTION	RATIONALE
11. Slide fingers of ungloved hand inside the remaining glove. Grasp glove on inside and remove by turning inside-out over hand and other glove.	Contaminated area does not come in contact with hands or wrists.
12. Discard gloves in appropriate container and perform hand hygiene.	Hand hygiene reduces the spread of microorganisms.

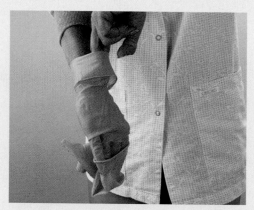

Action 11: Sliding ungloved fingers under glove on opposite hand and pulling glove off.

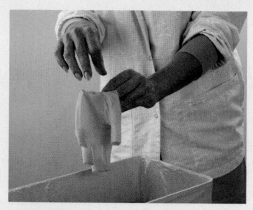

Action 12: Discarding gloves into appropriate receptacle.

EVALUATION

The expected outcome is met when gloves are donned without any contamination. Other expected outcomes are met when the patient remains free of exposure to potential infection-causing microorganisms and does not exhibit any signs and symptoms of a latex allergy response.

Unexpected Situations and Associated Interventions

- *Contamination occurs during donning of the sterile gloves:* Discard gloves and open new package of sterile gloves.
- *A hole or tear is noticed in one of the gloves:* Discard gloves and open new package of sterile gloves.
- *A hole or tear is noticed in one of the gloves during the procedure:* Stop procedure. Remove damaged gloves. Wash hands or perform hand hygiene (depending on whether soiled or not) and don new sterile gloves.
- *Patient has a latex allergy:* Obtain latex-free sterile gloves.

Using Personal Protective Equipment

Personal protective equipment (PPE) refers to any equipment and supplies furnished for the purpose of protecting patients and healthcare workers. This equipment includes clean (unsterile) and sterile gloves, impervious gowns, surgical and high-efficiency particulate air (HEPA) masks, N95 disposable masks, face shields, protective eyewear, surgical caps, shoe covers, and splashguards.

Understanding the potential contamination hazards related to the patient's diagnosis and condition and the institutional policies governing PPE is very important. It is always your responsibility to enforce the proper wearing of PPE during patient care for members of the healthcare team.

Equipment

- Gloves
- Mask (surgical or particulate respirator)
- Gown
- Protective eyewear (does not include eyeglasses)

Depending on the institution's policy, equipment for PPE may vary.

ASSESSMENT

Assess the situation to determine the necessity for PPE. In addition, check the patient's chart for information about a diagnosed infection or communicable disease. Determine the possibility of exposure to blood and body fluids and identify the necessary equipment to prevent exposure. Refer to the infection control manual provided by your facility.

NURSING DIAGNOSIS

Determine the related factors for the nursing diagnoses based on the patient's current status. An appropriate nursing diagnosis is Risk for Infection. Many other nursing diagnoses also may require the use of this skill, including the following:

- Ineffective Protection
- Deficient Knowledge
- Bowel Incontinence
- Diarrhea
- Total Urinary Incontinence
- Impaired Skin Integrity

OUTCOME IDENTIFICATION AND PLANNING

The expected outcome to achieve when using PPE is that the transmission of microorganisms is contained. Other outcomes that may be appropriate include the following: patient remains free of exposure to potentially infectious microorganisms; patient verbalizes information about the rationale for use of PPE; episodes of bowel or urinary incontinence or diarrhea are controlled; and drainage from skin breakdown is contained.

IMPLEMENTATION

ACTION	RATIONALE
1. Check physician's order for type of precautions and review precautions in infection control manual.	Mode of transmission or organism determines type of precautions required.
2. Plan nursing activities before entering patient's room.	Organization facilitates performance of task and adherence to precautions.
3. Provide instruction about precautions to patient, family members, and visitors.	Explanation encourages cooperation of patient and family and reduces apprehension about precaution procedures.
4. Perform hand hygiene.	Hand hygiene deters the spread of microorganisms.

5. Put on gown, gloves, mask, and protective eyewear, if recommended as precaution.
  a. Tie gown securely at neck and waist. Obtain waterproof gown if soiling is likely.
  b. Use clean disposable gloves. If worn with gown, draw glove cuffs over gown sleeves.
	Use of PPE interrupts chain of infection and protects patient and nurse. Gown should protect entire uniform. Gloves protect hands and wrists from microorganisms. Masks protect nurse or patient from droplet nuclei and large-particle aerosols. Eyewear protects mucous membranes in the eye from splashes. *continues*

Using Personal Protective Equipment (continued)

ACTION   **RATIONALE**

c. Place mask strap around head or tie mask securely, fitting it to the face.

d. Use eyewear with protection on side of face or face shields.

e. Alternatively, a combination of a mask and eye barrier device may be used.

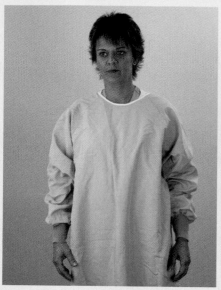

Action 5a: Gown tied at waist and neck.

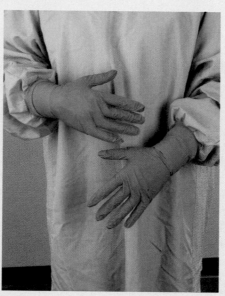

Action 5b: Cuffs of gloves placed over gown sleeves.

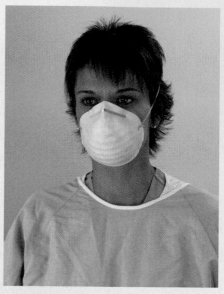

Action 5c: Mask placed on after gown and gloves.

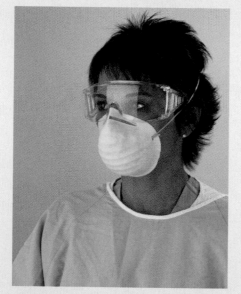

Action 5d: Eyewear placed on after gown, gloves, and mask.

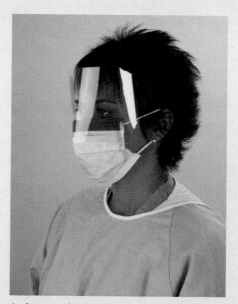

Action 5e: Alternative mask and eye barrier combination.

continues

SKILL 4-4

Using Personal Protective Equipment (continued)

ACTION

6. When patient care is completed, **untie waist strings of gown, then remove gloves as follows:**
   a. **Grasp outside of one glove and turn inside out to remove.** Keep removed glove in the palm of gloved hand.
   b. Insert fingers of ungloved hand inside cuff of remaining glove.
   c. Grasp glove, pulling it off the hand and over the other glove. Drop in appropriate container.

RATIONALE

Waist strings of gown are considered contaminated. Gloves have been involved in patient care and are most soiled. Ungloved hand is clean and should not touch contaminated areas.

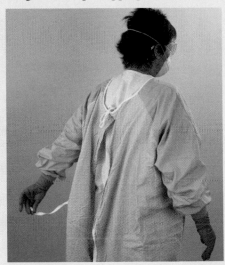

Action 6a: Untying gown at waist.

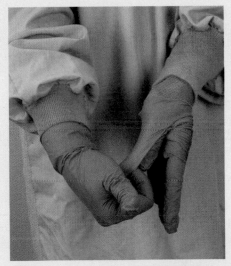

Action 6a: Pulling outside of glove on one hand, turning it inside out.

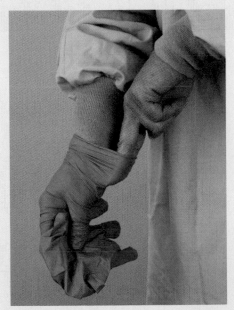

Action 6b: Inserting fingers of ungloved hand inside cuff of other glove.

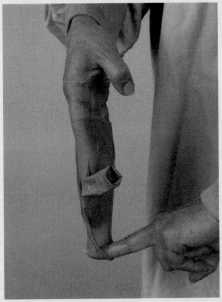

Action 6c: Pulling glove off the hand and over the other glove.

continues

ACTION

RATIONALE

7. After gloves are removed, remove mask:
    a. For a surgical mask: untie mask and drop by strings into waste container. For a mask with an elastic strap: lift strap from behind head and drop by strap into waste container.
    b. For a particulate respirator: use hand to hold respirator in place. Pull bottom strap up and over head. Pull top strap over head. Remove respirator from face and save for future use (HEPA mask) or discard according to manufacturer's directions (disposable mask).

This method prevents mask or respirator from falling off face onto floor.

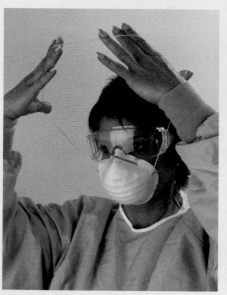

Action 7a: Lifting elastic strap of mask from behind head.

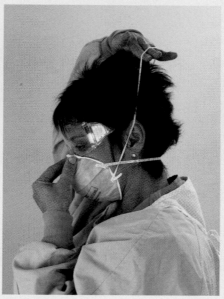

Action 7b: Grabbing bottom of respirator strap and pulling over head.

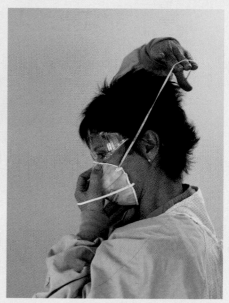

Action 7b: Pulling top strap of respirator mask over head.

8. Remove gown.
    a. Untie neck strings of gown. **Remove gown without touching outside of gown by keeping one hand up and under the gown cuff and using this protected hand to pull the opposite sleeve down and off.**
    b. Use ungowned arm and hand to grasp gown from inside and remove from remaining arm. Remove gown and turn inside out and drop in appropriate container.

Neck strings are considered clean. Outside of gown is contaminated.

continues

Using Personal Protective Equipment (continued)

ACTION   RATIONALE

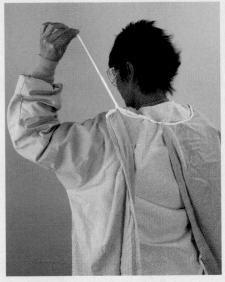

Action 8a: Untying neck strings.

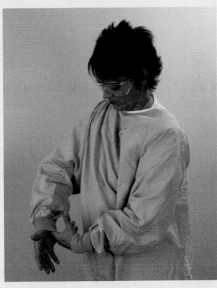

Action 8a: With one had protected inside gown, pulling opposite sleeve down and off.

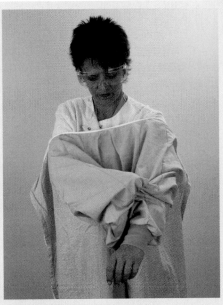

Action 8b: Grasping inside of gown to remove from remaining arm.

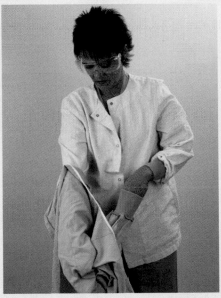

Action 8b: Removing gown by turning inside out.

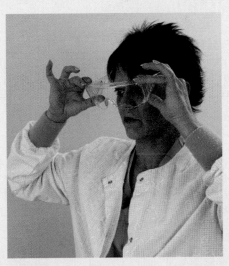

Action 9: Removing eyewear.

9. Remove eyewear last and clean according to agency policy.

10. Perform hand hygiene.

Eyewear is reusable.

Hand hygiene prevents spread of microorganisms.

continues

EVALUATION

The expected outcome is met when the transmission of microorganisms is contained, protecting the patient and nurse from the spread of microorganisms. Other expected outcomes are met when patient is not exposed to potentially infectious microorganisms; patient verbalizes information about the rationale for use of PPE; episodes of bowel or urinary incontinence or diarrhea are controlled; and drainage from skin breakdown is contained.

Unexpected Situations and Associated Interventions

- *You did not realize the need for protective equipment at beginning of task:* Stop task and obtain appropriate protective wear.
- *You are accidentally exposed to blood and body fluids:* Stop task and immediately follow agency protocol for exposure, including reporting the exposure.

■ Developing Critical Thinking Skills

1. While preparing the sterile table in the cardiac catheterization lab for Joe Wilson, you realize that you did not obtain a sterile bowl. How can you obtain a sterile bowl?
2. While you are donning sterile gloves in preparation for an indwelling urinary catheter insertion, your patient, Sheri Lawrence, moves her leg. You do not *think* that Sheri's leg touched the glove, but you are not positive. What should you do?
3. Edgar Barowski's son is visiting and asks you why the masks that are outside Edgar's room are different from the ones that people wear in the operating room. What should you tell Edgar's son?

Bibliography

Centers for Disease Control and Prevention (2000). Monitoring hospital-acquired infections to promote patient safety—US, 1990–1999. *Morbidity and Mortality Weekly Report, 49*(08), 149–153.

Centers for Disease Control and Prevention (2002). Guidelines for hand hygiene in health-care settings. *Morbidity and Mortality Weekly Report, 51*(RR16), 1–45.

Duffy, J. (2002). Nosocomial infections: Important acute care nursing-sensitive outcomes indicators. *AACN Clinical Issues, 13*(3), 358–366.

Girard, N. (2003). OR masks: safe practice or habit? *AORN Journal, 77*(1), 12–15.

Graves, P., & Twomey, C. (2002). The changing face of hand protection. *AORN Journal, 76*(2), 248–264.

Saiman, L., Lerner, A., Saal, L., et al. (2002). Banning artificial nails from health care settings. *American Journal of Infection Control, 30*(4), 252–254.

Winslow, E., & Jacobson, A. (2000). Can a fashion statement harm the patient? *American Journal of Infection Control, 100*(9), 63, 65.

Worthington, K. (2002). Are your medical gloves really protecting you? Take an active role in purchasing the right glove for the job. *American Journal of Infection Control, 102*(10), 108.

Medications

This chapter will help you develop some of the skills needed to safely administer medications to the following patients:

Cooper Jackson, age 2, does not want to take his ordered oral antibiotic.

Erika Jenkins, age 20, is extremely afraid of needles and is at the clinic for her birth control injection.

Jonah Dinerman, age 63, was recently diagnosed with diabetes and needs to be taught how to give himself insulin injections.

Learning Outcomes

After studying this chapter, the reader should be able to:

1. Safely administer medications through various routes
2. Prepare medications for administration in a safe manner
3. Locate different sites for a subcutaneous injection
4. Locate different sites for an intramuscular injection
5. Determine size of needle and syringe needed for intradermal, subcutaneous, or intramuscular injection

Key Terms

ampule: a glass flask that contains a single dose of medication for parenteral administration

inhalation: route to administer medications directly into the lungs or airway passages

intradermal injection: injection placed just below the epidermis; sites commonly used are the inner surface of the forearm, the dorsal aspect of the upper arm, and the upper back

intramuscular injection: injection placed into muscular tissue; sites commonly used are the ventrogluteal, vastus lateralis, deltoid, and dorsogluteal muscles

intravenous route: route to administer medications directly into the vein or venous system; the most dangerous route of medication administration

subcutaneous injection: injection placed between the epidermis and muscle, into the subcutaneous tissue; sites commonly used are the outer aspect of the upper arm, the abdomen, the anterior aspects of the thigh, the upper back, and the upper ventral or dorsogluteal area

sublingually: under the tongue

vial: a glass bottle with a self-sealing stopper through which medication is removed

Medication administration is a basic nursing function that involves skillful technique and consideration of the patient's development and safety. The nurse administering medications needs a knowledge base about drugs, including drug names, preparations, classifications, adverse effects, and physiologic factors that affect drug action.

The nursing process can be applied to the fundamental nursing skill of medication administration. Assessment includes a comprehensive medication history as well as ongoing assessments of the patient's response during and after drug therapy. Nursing diagnoses are developed from the assessment data. Patient-centered outcomes are evaluated after implementation of the plan of care, tailored to the patient's needs.

This chapter will cover skills that the nurse needs to safely administer medications via several routes. Please look over the summary boxes in the beginning of this chapter for a quick review of critical knowledge to assist you in understanding the skills related to medication administration.

BOX 5-1 Five Rights of Administration

To prevent medication errors, always check the Five Rights of Medication Administration:

1. Right patient
2. Right medication
3. Right dosage
4. Right route
5. Right time

BOX 5-2 Clarifying Orders

Another way to prevent medication errors is always to clarify a medication order that is:

- Illegible
- Incomplete
- Incorrect route or dosage
- Not expected for patient's current diagnosis

BOX 5-3 Know Your Medications

Before administering any unfamiliar medications, know the following:

- Mode of action and purpose of medication (making sure that this medication is appropriate for the patient's diagnosis)
- Side effects of and contraindications for medication
- Antagonist of medication
- Safe dosage range for medication
- Interactions with other medications
- Precautions to take prior to administration
- Proper administration technique

BOX 5-4 Needle/Syringe Selection Technique

- When looking at a needle package, the first number is the gauge or diameter of the needle (eg, 18, 20) and the second number is the length in inches (eg 1, 1½).
- As the gauge number becomes larger, the size of the needle becomes smaller: for instance, a 24-gauge needle is smaller than an 18-gauge needle.
- When giving an injection, the viscosity of the medication directs the choice of gauge (diameter). A thicker medication such as a hormone is given through a bigger needle, such as a 20 gauge. A thinner-consistency medication, such as morphine, is given through a smaller needle, such as a 24 gauge.
- The length of the needle is directed by the size of the patient, the selected insertion site, and the tissue you are trying to reach. An intramuscular injection in an emaciated person would require a shorter needle than the same injection in an obese patient.
- Generally, a 1½" needle is sufficient for an intramuscular injection in an adult and a 1" needle is sufficient for a

child. A ⁵/₁₆" to 1" needle is generally used for subcutaneous injections.
- The size of the syringe is directed by the amount of medication to be given. If the amount is less than 1 mL, use a 1-mL syringe to administer the medication. In a 1-mL syringe, the amount of medication may be rounded to the 100th decimal place. In syringes larger than 1 mL, the amount is rounded to the 10th decimal place. If the amount of medication to be administered is less than 3 mL, use a 3-mL syringe. If the amount of medication is equal to the size of the syringe (eg, 1 mL and using a 1-mL syringe), you may go up to the next size syringe to prevent awkward movements when deploying the plunger.
- When administering insulin, the size of syringe and strength of insulin should coincide. U50 insulin should be administered with a syringe calibrated for U50 insulin to prevent medication errors.

continues

BOX 5-4 **Needle/Syringe Selection Technique** *(continued)*

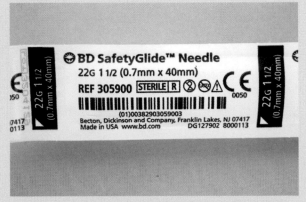

Needle package showing first number (gauge or diameter of needle) and second number (length of the needle in inches).

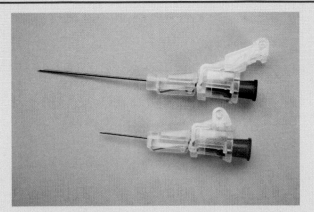

Different needle sizes: a 24-gauge needle and an 18-gauge needle.

BOX 5-5 **Subcutaneous Injections**

- Subcutaneous injections should contain no more than 1 mL of fluid in one insertion site.
- The normal angle for insertion for a subcutaneous injection is 45 to 90 degrees. This angle depends on the length of the needle and the amount of adipose tissue the patient has. An emaciated patient would probably require a 45-degree angle of insertion, while an obese patient may require a 90-degree angle.
- Subcutaneous injection sites include:
  - Outer aspect of upper arm
  - Abdomen
  - Anterior aspects of thigh
  - Upper back
  - Upper ventral or dorsogluteal area
- Insertion site selection depends on patient's preference, nurse's preference, and type of medication to be administered.

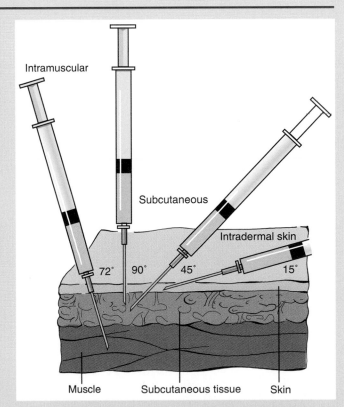

Comparison of the angles of insertion for intramuscular, subcutaneous, and intradermal injections.

continues

BOX 5-5 **Subcutaneous Injections** *(continued)*

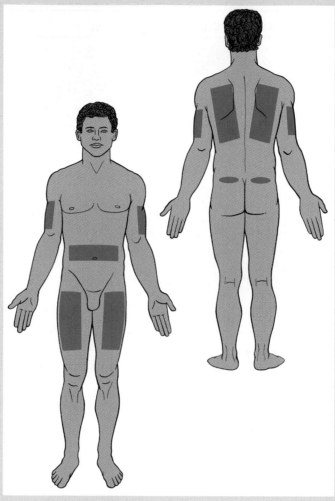

Subcutaneous injection sites.

BOX 5-6 Intramuscular Site Selection

- Intramuscular injections should contain no more than 3 to 5 mL. The smaller the muscle being injected, the smaller the amount should be.
- The normal angle of insertion for an intramuscular injection is 72 to 90 degrees. This angle depends on the length of the needle and the amount of adipose tissue the patient has (see Box 5-3).
- Intramuscular injection sites include:
  - Vastus lateralis
  - Ventrogluteal
  - Deltoid
  - Dorsogluteal

- Insertion site selection depends on:
  - Amount of medication
  - Viscosity of medication
  - Age of patient/development of muscle tissue
  - Preference of patient and nurse
  - Ability of patient to assume position needed for injection
- The ventrogluteal site is the most frequently recommended IM injection site for patients over 7 months old because the muscle is well developed and the site is free of nerves and blood vessels and easily identifiable by bony landmarks.

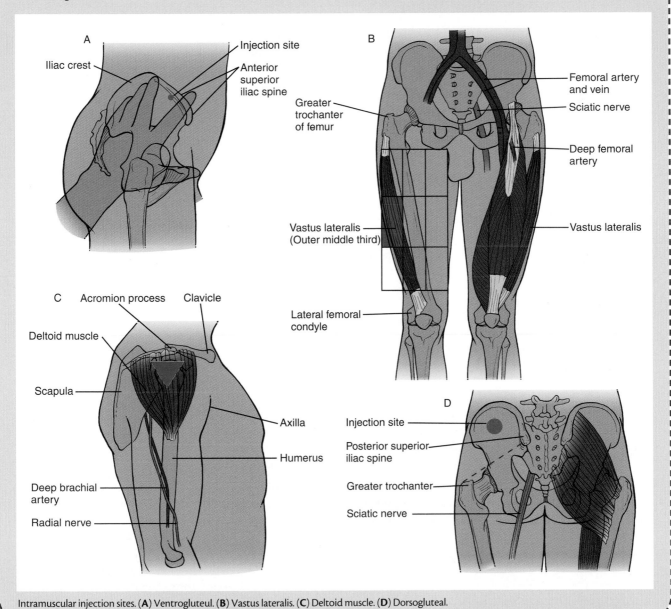

Intramuscular injection sites. (**A**) Ventrogluteul. (**B**) Vastus lateralis. (**C**) Deltoid muscle. (**D**) Dorsogluteal.

SKILL 5-1 Administering Oral Medications

The oral route is the most commonly used route. Drugs given orally are intended for absorption in the stomach and small intestine.

Equipment
- Medication in disposable cup or oral syringe
- Liquid with straw if not contraindicated
- Medication cart or tray
- Medication Kardex or computer-generated MAR

ASSESSMENT

Assess the patient's ability to swallow medications. If the patient cannot swallow, is NPO, or is experiencing nausea or vomiting, the medication should be withheld, the physician notified, and proper documentation completed. Assess the patient's knowledge of the medication. If the patient has a knowledge deficit about the medication, this may be the appropriate time to begin education about the medication. If the medication may affect the patient's vital signs, assess them before administration. If the medication is for pain relief, assess the patient's pain level before and after administration.

NURSING DIAGNOSIS

Determine related factors for the nursing diagnoses based on the patient's current status. Appropriate nursing diagnoses may include:
- Impaired Swallowing
- Risk for Aspiration
- Anxiety
- Deficient Knowledge
- Noncompliance

OUTCOME IDENTIFICATION AND PLANNING

The expected outcome to achieve when administering an oral medication is that the patient will swallow the medication. Other outcomes that may be appropriate include the following: the patient will not aspirate; the patient has decreased anxiety; and the patient understands and complies with the medication regimen.

IMPLEMENTATION

ACTION	RATIONALE
1. Gather equipment. Check each medication order against the original physician's order according to agency policy. Clarify any inconsistencies. Check the patient's chart for allergies.	This comparison helps to identify errors that may have occurred when orders were transcribed. The physician's order is the legal record of medication orders for each agency.
2. Know the actions, special nursing considerations, safe dose ranges, purpose of administration, and adverse effects of the medications to be administered.	This knowledge aids the nurse in evaluating the therapeutic effect of the medication in relation to the patient's disorder and can also be used to educate the patient about the medication.
3. Perform hand hygiene.	Hand hygiene prevents the spread of microorganisms.
4. Move the medication cart to the outside of the patient's room or prepare for administration in the medication area.	Organization facilitates error-free administration and saves time.
5. Unlock the medication cart or drawer.	Locking of the cart or drawer safeguards each patient's medication supply. Hospital accrediting organizations require medication carts to be locked when not in use.
6. **Prepare medications for one patient at a time.**	This prevents errors in medication administration.
7. Select the proper medication from the drawer or stock and compare with the Kardex or order. Check expiration dates and perform calculations if necessary.	Comparison of medication to physician's order reduces errors in medication administration. This is the first safety check. Verify calculations with another nurse if necessary.

continues

SKILL 5-1   Administering Oral Medications (continued)

ACTION

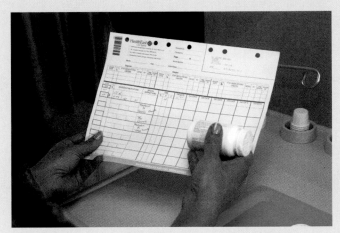

Action 7: Comparing medication with Kardex or order.

a. Place unit dose-packaged medications in a dispos-able cup. **Do not open wrapper until at the bedside.** Keep narcotics and medications that require special nursing assessments in a separate container.
b. When removing tablets or capsules from a bottle, pour the necessary number into the bottle cap and then place the tablets in a medication cup. Break only scored tablets, if necessary, to obtain the proper dosage. Do not touch tablets with hands.
c. Hold liquid medication bottles with the label against the palm. Use the appropriate measuring device when pouring liquids, and read the amount of med-ication at the bottom of the meniscus at eye level. Wipe the lip of the bottle with a paper towel.

8. **Recheck each medication package or preparation with the order as it is poured.**

9. **When all medications for one patient have been pre-pared, recheck once again with the medication order before taking them to the patient.**

10. Transport medications to the patient's bedside care-fully, and keep the medications in sight at all times.

11. **See that the patient receives the medications at the cor-rect time.**

12. **Identify the patient carefully.** There are three correct ways to do this:
    a. Check the name on the patient's identification band.

    b. Ask the patient to state his or her name.

RATIONALE

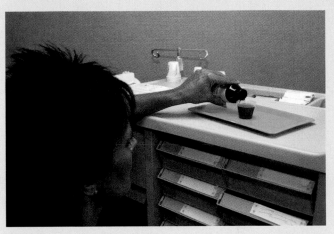

Action 7c: Measuring at eye level.

a. The label is needed for an additional safety check. Pre-requisites to giving certain medications may include as-sessing vital signs and checking laboratory test results.

b. Pouring medication into the cap allows for easy return of excess medication to bottle. Pouring tablets or capsules into the nurse's hand is unsanitary.

c. Liquid that may drip onto the label makes the label diffi-cult to read. Accuracy is possible when the appropriate measuring device is used and then read accurately.

This is a *second* check to guard against a medication error.

This is a *third* check to ensure accuracy and to prevent errors.

Careful handling and close observation prevent accidental or deliberate disarrangement of medications.

Check agency policy, which may allow for administration within a period of 30 minutes before or 30 minutes after designated time.

Identifying the patient is the nurse's responsibility to guard against error.

a. This is the most reliable method. Replace the identifica-tion band if it is missing or inaccurate in any way.

b. This requires a response from the patient, but illness and strange surroundings often cause patients to be confused.

continues

Administering Oral Medications (continued)

ACTION

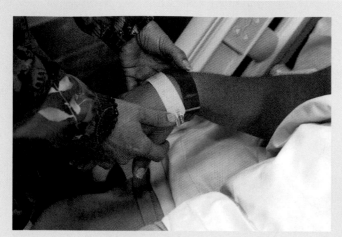

Action 12a: Checking patient identity.

RATIONALE

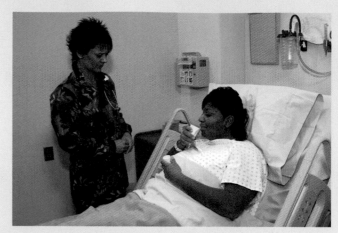

Action 16: Observing patient swallowing medication.

ACTION	RATIONALE

    c. Verify the patient's identification with a staff member who knows the patient.

    c. This is another way to double-check identity. Do not use the name on the door or over the bed, because these may be inaccurate.

13. **Complete necessary assessments before administering medications. Check allergy bracelet or ask patient about allergies. Explain the purpose and action of each medication to the patient.**

Assessment is a prerequisite to administration of medications.

14. Assist the patient to an upright or lateral position.

15. Administer medications:

Swallowing is facilitated by proper positioning. An upright or side-lying position protects the patient from aspiration.

    a. Offer water or other permitted fluids with pills, capsules, tablets, and some liquid medications.

    a. Liquids facilitate swallowing of solid drugs. Some liquid drugs are intended to adhere to the pharyngeal area, in which case liquid is not offered with the medication.

    b. Ask whether the patient prefers to take the medications by hand or in a cup and one at a time or all at once.

    b. This encourages the patient's participation in taking the medications.

    c. If the capsule or tablet falls to the floor, it must be discarded and a new one administered.

    c. This prevents contamination.

    d. Record any fluid intake if intake and output measurement is ordered.

    d. This provides for accurate documentation.

16. **Remain with the patient until each medication is swallowed. Never leave medication at the patient's bedside.**

Unless the nurse has seen the patient swallow the drug, the drug cannot be recorded as administered. The patient's chart is a legal record. Only with a physician's order can medications be left at the bedside.

17. Perform hand hygiene.

Hand hygiene prevents the spread of microorganisms.

18. Record each medication given on the medication chart or record using the required format.

Prompt recording avoids the possibility of accidentally repeating the administration of the drug.

    a. If the drug was refused or omitted, record this in the appropriate area on the medication record and notify the physician.

    a. This verifies the reason medication was omitted and ensures that the physician is aware of the patient's condition.

    b. Recording of administration of a narcotic may require additional documentation on a narcotic record, stating drug count and other specific information.

    b. Controlled substance laws necessitate careful recording of narcotic use. If a computerized medication station is being used, the machine may document needed information upon withdrawal of the medication.

continues

Administering Oral Medications (continued)

ACTION	RATIONALE

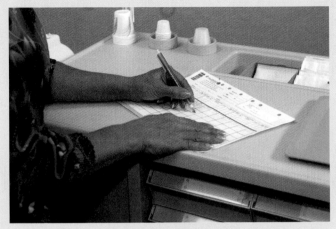

Action 18: Documenting medication administration on CMAR.

> 8/6/06   0835   Mr. Jones complaining of leg pains. Rates pain as an 8/10. 2 Percocet administered.—K. Sanders, RN
>
> 8/6/06   0905   Mr. Jones resting comfortably. Rates leg pain as a 1/10.—K. Sanders, RN
>
> 8/6/06   1300   Mr. Jones refusing to take pain medication. States, "It made me feel woozy last time". Feelings discussed with patient. Patient agrees to take 1 Percocet at this time.—K. Sanders, RN
>
> 8/6/06   1320   Percocet, 1 tablet given P.O. —K. Sanders, RN

Action 19: Documentation.

19. Check on the patient within 30 minutes to verify response to medication.

This provides the opportunity for further documentation and additional assessment of effectiveness of pain relief and adverse effects of medications.

EVALUATION

The expected outcomes are met when the patient swallowed the medication, did not aspirate, has decreased anxiety, and understood and complied with the medication administration.

Unexpected Situations and Associated Interventions

- *Patient feels that medication is lodged in throat:* Offer patient more fluids to drink. If allowed, offer the patient bread or crackers to help move the medication to stomach.
- *It is unclear whether patient swallowed medication:* Check in the patient's mouth, under tongue, and between cheek and gum. Patients may "cheek" medications to avoid taking the medication or to save it for later use. This has been established with many medications, especially antidepressants and pain medication. Patients requiring suicide precautions should be watched closely to ensure that they are not "cheeking" the medication or hiding it in the mouth; they may be trying to accumulate a large amount of medication to take all at once in a suicide attempt. Substance abusers may cheek medication in order to accumulate a large amount to take all at once so that they may feel a high from medication.
- *Patient vomits immediately or shortly after receiving oral medication:* Assess vomit, looking for pills or fragments. Do not readminister medication without notifying physician. If a whole pill is seen and can be identified, physician may ask that medication be administered again. If a pill is not seen or medications cannot be identified, medication should not be readministered so that patient does not receive too large of a dose.
- *Child refuses to take oral medications:* Some medications may be hidden in a small amount of food, such as pudding or ice cream. Do not add to liquid, because medication may alter the taste of liquids; if child then refuses to drink the rest of the liquid, you will not know how much of the medication was ingested. Creativity may be needed when devising ways to administer medications to a child. See below for suggestions.

continues

Administering Oral Medications (continued)

Infant and Child Considerations

- Special devices, such as oral syringes and calibrated nipples, are available in a pharmacy to ensure accurate dose calculations for young children and infants.
- Some creative ways to administer medications to children include: have a "tea party" with medicine cups; place syringe (without needle) or dropper in the space between the cheek and gum and slowly administer the medication; save a special treat for after the medication administration (eg, movie, playroom time, or a special food if allowed).
- The FDA has received reports of infants choking on the plastic caps that fit on the end of syringes when used to administer oral medications. They recommend the following: remove and dispose of caps before giving syringes to patients or families, caution family caregivers to dispose of caps on syringes they buy over the counter, and report any problems with syringe caps to the FDA. Companies have begun to manufacture syringes labeled "oral use" without the caps on them.

Older Adult Considerations

- Elderly patients with arthritis may have difficulty opening childproof caps. On request, the pharmacist can substitute a cap that is easier to open. A rubber band twisted around the cap may provide a more secure grip for older patients.

Home Care Considerations

- Encourage the patient to discard outdated prescription medications.
- Discuss safe storage of medications when there are children and pets in the environment.
- Discuss with parents the difference in over-the-counter medications made for infants and medications made for children. Many times parents do not realize that there are different strengths to the actual medications, leading to under- or over-dosing.
- Encourage patients to carry a card listing all medications, dosage, and frequency in case of an emergency.

Special Considerations

- If the patient questions a medication order or states the medication is different from the usual dose, always recheck and clarify with the original order or physician before giving medication.
- If the patient's level of consciousness is altered or his or her swallowing is impaired, check with the physician to clarify the route of administration or alternative forms of medication. This may also be a solution for a pediatric or a confused patient who is refusing to take a medication.
- Patients with poor vision can request large-type labels on medication containers. A magnifying lens also may be helpful.

SKILL 5-2 Removing Medication From an Ampule

An ampule is a glass flask that contains a single dose of medication for parenteral administration. Because there is no way to prevent airborne contamination of any unused portion of medication after the ampule is opened, if not all the medication is used, the remainder must be discarded. Medication is removed from an ampule after its thin neck is broken.

Equipment
- Sterile syringe and filter needle
- Ampule of medication
- Needle (optional; for medications that are to be given IM, size depends on medication being administered and patient)
- Antimicrobial swab or gauze pad
- Medication Kardex or computer-generated MAR

ASSESSMENT

Assess the medication in the ampule for any particles or discoloration. Assess the ampule for any cracks or chips. Check expiration date before administering the medication.

NURSING DIAGNOSIS

Determine related factors for the nursing diagnoses based on the patient's current status. Appropriate nursing diagnoses may include:
- Risk for Infection
- Risk for Injury

OUTCOME IDENTIFICATION AND PLANNING

The expected outcome to achieve when removing medication from an ampule is that the medication will be removed in a sterile manner and free from glass shards.

IMPLEMENTATION

ACTION	RATIONALE
1. Gather equipment. Check the medication order against the original physician's order according to agency policy.	This comparison helps to identify errors that may have occurred when orders were transcribed.
2. Perform hand hygiene.	Hand hygiene deters the spread of microorganisms.
3. Tap the stem of the ampule or twist your wrist quickly while holding the ampule vertically.	This facilitates movement of medication in the stem to the body of the ampule.
4. **Wrap a small gauze pad or dry antimicrobial swab around the neck of the ampule.**	This protects the nurse's fingers from the glass as the ampule is broken.
5. Use a snapping motion to break off the top of the ampule along the scored line at its neck. Always break away from your body.	This protects the nurse's face and fingers from any shattered glass fragments.
6. **Remove the cap from the filter needle by pulling it straight off. Insert the filter needle into the ampule, being careful not to touch the rim.**	The rim of the ampule is considered contaminated. Use of a filter needle prevents the accidental withdrawing of small glass particles with the medication.
7. Withdraw medication in the amount ordered plus a small amount more (approximately 30%). **Do not inject air into solutions.** Use either of the following methods:	By withdrawing a small amount more of medication, any air bubbles in the syringe can be displaced once the syringe is removed and there will still be ample medication in the syringe.
a. Insert the tip of the needle into the ampule, which is upright on a flat surface, and withdraw fluid into the syringe. **Touch plunger at knob only.**	a. The contents of the ampule are not under pressure; therefore, air is unnecessary and will cause the contents to overflow. Handling plunger at knob only will keep shaft of plunger sterile.

continues

Removing Medication From an Ampule (continued)

ACTION

RATIONALE

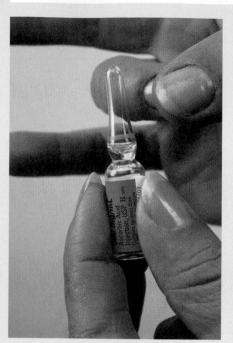

Action 3: Tapping stem of ampule.

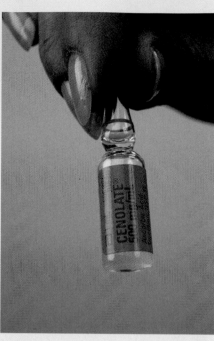

Action 3: Twisting motion of wrist while holding ampule.

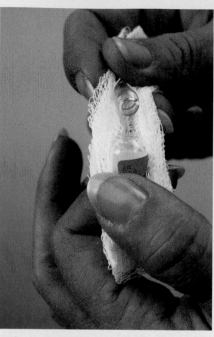

Action 4: Snapping off top of ampule.

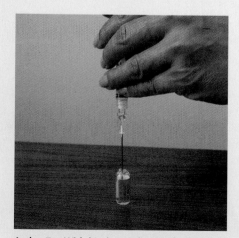

Action 7a: Withdrawing medication from upright ampule.

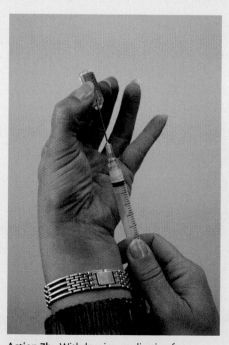

Action 7b: Withdrawing medication from inverted ampule.

continues

Removing Medication From an Ampule (continued)

ACTION	RATIONALE
b. Insert the tip of the needle into the ampule and invert the ampule. Keep the needle centered and not touching the sides of the ampule. Withdraw fluid into syringe. **Touch plunger at knob only.**	b. Surface tension holds the fluids in the ampule when inverted. If the needle touches the sides or is removed and then reinserted into the ampule, surface tension is broken, and fluid runs out. Handling plunger at knob only will keep shaft of plunger sterile.
8. **Wait until the needle has been withdrawn to tap the syringe and expel the air carefully. Do not expel any air bubbles that may form in the solution. Check the amount of medication in the syringe and discard any surplus.**	Ejecting air into the solution increases pressure in the ampule and can force the medication to spill out over the ampule. Ampules may have overfill. Careful measurement ensures that correct dose is withdrawn.
9. Discard the ampule in a suitable container after comparing with the medication Kardex.	Any medication that has not been removed from the ampule must be discarded because there is no way to maintain sterility of contents in an unopened ampule.
10. **Discard the filter needle in a suitable container. If medication is to be given IM or if agency requires the use of a needle to administer medication, attach selected needle to syringe.**	Filter needle used to draw up medication should not be used to administer the medication, to prevent any glass shards from entering the patient. If agency has a needleless IV system, medication is ready to be given.
11. Perform hand hygiene.	Hand hygiene deters the spread of microorganisms.

EVALUATION   The expected outcome is met when the medication is removed from the ampule in a sterile manner and free from glass shards.

Unexpected Situations and Associated Interventions

- *Nurse cuts self while trying to open ampule:* Discard ampule in case contamination has occurred. Bandage wound and retrieve new ampule. Report according to agency policy.
- *All of medication was not removed from the stem and there is not enough medication left in body of ampule for dose:* Retrieve another ampule for the remainder of the dose. Medication should be considered contaminated once neck of ampule has been placed on a nonsterile surface.
- *Nurse injects air into inverted ampule, spraying medication:* Wash hands to remove any medication. If any medication has gotten into eyes, perform an eye irrigation. Retrieve new ampule for medication dose. Report according to agency policy.
- *Medication is drawn up without using a filter needle:* Replace needle with a filter needle. If medication is to be given IM or agency uses a needleless IV system, medication can be injected into a new syringe and then administered to patient.
- *Plunger becomes contaminated before inserted into ampule:* Discard needle and syringe and start over. If plunger is contaminated after medication is drawn into the syringe, it is not necessary to discard and start over. The contaminated plunger will enter the barrel of the syringe when pushing the medication out and will not contaminate the medication.

SKILL 5-3   Removing Medication From a Vial

A vial is a glass bottle with a self-sealing stopper through which medication is removed. For safety in transporting and storing, the single-dose rubber-capped vial is usually covered with a soft metal cap that can be removed easily. The rubber stopper that is then exposed is the means of entrance into the vial.

Equipment
- Sterile syringe and needle (size depends on medication being administered and patient)
- Vial of medication
- Antimicrobial swab
- Second needle (optional)
- Filter needle (optional)
- Medication Kardex or computer-generated MAR

ASSESSMENT

Assess the medication in vial for any discoloration or particles. Check expiration date before administering medication.

NURSING DIAGNOSIS

Determine related factors for the nursing diagnoses based on the patient's current status. An appropriate nursing diagnosis is Risk for Infection.

OUTCOME IDENTIFICATION AND PLANNING

The expected outcome to achieve when removing medication from a vial is withdrawal of the medication into a syringe in a sterile manner.

IMPLEMENTATION

ACTION	RATIONALE
1. Gather equipment. Check medication order against the original physician's order according to agency policy.	This comparison helps to identify errors that may have occurred when orders were transcribed.
2. Perform hand hygiene.	Hand hygiene deters the spread of microorganisms.
3. Remove the metal or plastic cap on the vial that protects the rubber stopper.	The metal or plastic cap prevents contamination of the rubber top.
4. **Swab the rubber top with the antimicrobial swab.**	Antimicrobial swab removes surface bacteria contamination.
5. Remove the cap from the needle by pulling it straight off. (Some agencies recommend use of a filter needle when withdrawing premixed medication from multi-dose vials.) Draw back an amount of air into the syringe that is equal to the specific dose of medication to be withdrawn.	Before fluid is removed, injection of an equal amount of air is required to prevent the formation of a partial vacuum, because a vial is a sealed container. If not enough air is injected, the negative pressure makes it difficult to withdraw the medication. (Use of a filter needle prevents any solid material from being withdrawn through the needle.)
6. Pierce the rubber stopper in the center with the needle tip and inject the measured air into the space above the solution. (Do not inject air into the solution.) The vial may be positioned upright on a flat surface or inverted.	Air bubbled through the solution could result in withdrawal of an inaccurate amount of medication.
7. **Invert the vial and withdraw the needle tip slightly so that it is below the fluid level.**	This prevents air from being aspirated into the syringe.
8. **Draw up the prescribed amount of medication while holding the syringe at eye level and vertically. Be careful to touch the plunger at knob only.**	Holding the syringe at eye level facilitates accurate reading, and the vertical position makes removal of air bubbles from the syringe easy. Handling plunger at knob only will keep shaft of plunger sterile.

continues

Removing Medication From a Vial (continued)

ACTION   RATIONALE

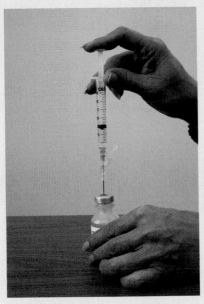

Action 6: Injecting air with vial upright.

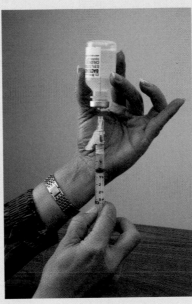

Action 7: Positioning needle tip in solution.

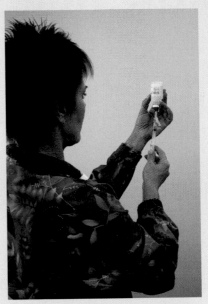

Action 8: Withdrawing medication at eye level.

9. If any air bubbles accumulate in the syringe, tap the barrel of the syringe sharply and move the needle past the fluid into the air space to reinject the air bubble into the vial. Return the needle tip to the solution and continue withdrawal of the medication.

Removal of air bubbles is necessary to ensure accurate dose of medication.

10. After the correct dose is withdrawn, remove the needle from the vial and carefully replace the cap over the needle. If a filter needle has been used to draw up the medication and the medication needs to be administered through a needle, remove the filter needle and replace it with a new needle. (Some agencies recommend changing needles, if needed to administer the medication, before administering the medication.)

This prevents contamination of the needle and protects the nurse against accidental needlesticks. A one-handed recap method may be used as long as care is taken not to contaminate the needle during the process. Filter needle used to draw up medication should not be used to administer the medication to prevent any solid material from entering the patient.

11. **If a multidose vial is being used, label the vial with the date and time opened, and store the vial containing the remaining medication according to agency policy.**

Because the vial is sealed, the medication inside remains sterile and can be used for future injections. Labeling the opened vials with a date and time limits its use after a specific time period.

12. Perform hand hygiene.

Hand hygiene deters the spread of microorganisms.

continues

Removing Medication From a Vial (continued)

ACTION	RATIONALE

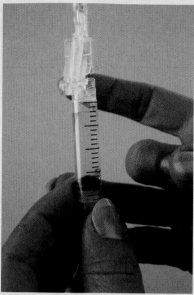

Action 9: Tapping to remove air bubbles.

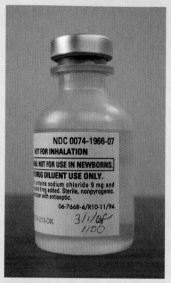

Action 11: Vial with label attached.

EVALUATION

The expected outcome is met when the medication is withdrawn into the syringe in a sterile manner and is ready for administration.

Unexpected Situations and Associated Interventions

- *A piece of rubber stopper is noticed floating in medication in syringe:* Apply a filter needle to the syringe and inject medication into a new syringe. Filter needle should remove any solid material from the medication.
- *As needle attached to syringe filled with air is inserted into vial, the plunger is immediately pulled down:* If possible to withdraw medication, continue steps as explained above. If such a vacuum has formed that this is impossible, remove syringe and inject more air into the vial. This is caused by withdrawal of medication without the addition of air into the vial.
- *Plunger is contaminated before injecting air into vial:* Discard needle and syringe and start over. If plunger is contaminated after medication is drawn into syringe, it is not necessary to discard and start over. The contaminated plunger will enter the barrel of the syringe when pushing the medication out and will not contaminate the medication.

Mixing Insulins in One Syringe

Insulin, a naturally occurring hormone produced by the islets of Langerhans in the pancreas, enables cells to use carbohydrates. Patients with diabetes mellitus type I produce no insulin or produce insulin in insufficient amounts. Several types of insulin are available for use by patients with diabetes mellitus. Insulins vary in their onset and duration of action and are classified as short acting, intermediate acting, and long acting. Many cases of diabetes mellitus are regulated with a combination of two insulins (eg, regular and NPH insulins). Review the duration and peak times of each type of insulin.

Equipment

- Two vials of insulin
- Sterile insulin syringe with 25- to 31-gauge needle
- Antimicrobial swabs
- Medication Kardex or computer-generated MAR

ASSESSMENT

Assess the clarity of each vial of insulin. In the past, clear insulins have been short acting and cloudy insulins have been long acting, but this is no longer the case: there is a new long-acting insulin on the market that is clear. Therefore, it is important to be familiar with each particular insulin's peak and half-life before removing it from the vial.

NURSING DIAGNOSIS

Determine related factors for the nursing diagnoses based on the patient's current status. An appropriate nursing diagnosis is Risk for Infection.

OUTCOME IDENTIFICATION AND PLANNING

The expected outcome to achieve when mixing two different types of insulin in one syringe is that the insulin is appropriately mixed in the syringe in a sterile manner and is ready for administration.

IMPLEMENTATION

ACTION	RATIONALE
1. Gather equipment. Check medication order against the original physician's order according to agency policy.	This comparison helps to identify errors that may have occurred when orders were transcribed.
2. Perform hand hygiene.	Hand hygiene deters the spread of microorganisms.
3. If necessary, remove the cap that protects the rubber stopper on each vial.	The cap protects the rubber top.
4. **If insulin is a suspension (NPH, Lente), roll and agitate the vial to mix it well.**	There is controversy regarding how to mix NPH insulin properly. Some say to roll the vial; others say to shake the vial. Regardless of the method used, it is essential that the suspension be mixed well to avoid administering an inconsistent dose. Regular insulin, which is clear, does not need to be mixed before withdrawal.
5. Cleanse the rubber tops with antimicrobial swabs.	Antimicrobial swab removes surface contamination. It is questionable whether cleaning with alcohol actually disinfects or instead transfers resident bacteria from the hands to another surface. Because it is difficult in a healthcare facility to keep an insulin vial in its original box as recommended, the practice of cleansing with alcohol will most likely continue.
6. Remove cap from needle. Inject air into the modified insulin preparation (eg, NPH insulin). Touch plunger at knob only. Use an amount of air equal to the amount of medication to be withdrawn. **Do not allow needle to touch medication in vial.** Remove needle.	Regular insulin should never be contaminated with NPH or any insulin modified with added protein. Placing air in the NPH insulin first without allowing the needle to contact the insulin ensures that regular insulin is not contaminated with the additional protein in the NPH. Handling plunger by knob only ensures sterility of shaft of plunger.

continues

ACTION   **RATIONALE**

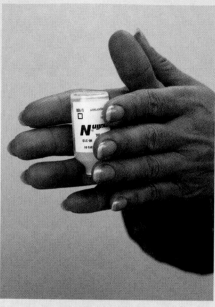

Action 4: Mixing NPH insulin.

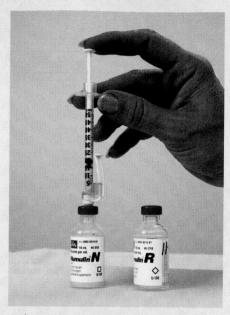

Action 6: Injecting air into modified insulin preparation.

7. Inject air into the regular insulin without additional protein. Use an amount of air equal to the amount of medication to be withdrawn.

An equal amount of air must be injected into the vacuum to allow easy withdrawal of medication.

8. Invert vial of regular insulin and aspirate amount prescribed. Invert and then remove needle from vial.

Regular insulin that contains no additional protein is not contaminated by insulin that contains globulin or protamine.

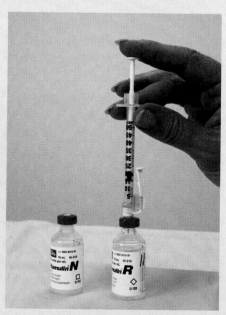

Action 7: Injecting air into regular insulin.

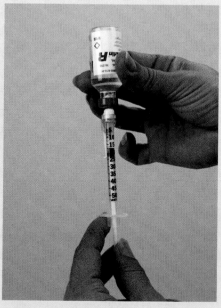

Action 8: Withdrawing regular insulin.

continues

Mixing Insulins in One Syringe (continued)

ACTION	RATIONALE
9. Cleanse the rubber top of the modified insulin vial. Insert the needle into this vial, invert it, and withdraw the medication. Carefully replace the cap over the needle.	Previous addition of air eliminates need to create positive pressure. Capping the needle prevents contamination and protects the nurse against accidental needlesticks. A one-handed recap method may be used as long as care is taken to ensure that the needle remains sterile.
10. Store the vials according to agency recommendations.	Insulin need not be refrigerated but must be protected from temperature extremes.
11. Perform hand hygiene.	Hand hygiene deters the spread of microorganisms.

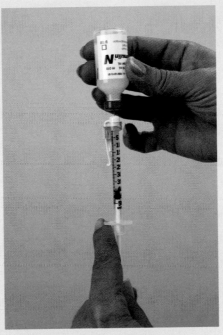

Action 9: Withdrawing modified insulin.

EVALUATION

The expected outcome is met when the insulin is mixed appropriately (in a sterile manner) in the syringe following the steps above and is ready for administration.

Unexpected Situations and Associated Interventions

- *Nurse contaminates plunger before injecting air into insulin vial:* Discard needle and syringe and start over. If plunger is contaminated after medication is drawn into the syringe, it is not necessary to discard and start over. The contaminated plunger will enter the barrel of the syringe when pushing the medication out and will not contaminate the medication.
- *Nurse allows NPH insulin to come in contact with syringe before entering the regular insulin vial:* Discard needle and syringe and start over.
- *Nurse notices that the combined amount is not the ordered amount (eg, nurse has less or more units in combined syringe than ordered):* Discard syringe and start over. There is no way to know for sure which dosage is wrong.
- *Nurse injects regular insulin into NPH vial:* Discard vial and syringe and start over.

continues

Mixing Insulins in One Syringe (continued)

Special Considerations

- An insulin-cartridge pen (the Novolin Pen) is available that allows the patient to dial the correct dose of insulin and press a button to release the dose quickly through a short, fine, 27-gauge needle.
- A type 1 diabetic patient who is visually impaired may find it helpful to use a magnifying apparatus that fits around the syringe.
- Before attempting to explain or demonstrate devices that help low-vision diabetic patients to prepare their medication, attempt to use the device yourself under similar circumstances. To detect any difficulties the patient may experience, practice using the aid with your eyes closed or in a poorly lit room.

Administering an Intradermal Injection

The intradermal route has the longest absorption time of all parenteral routes. For this reason, intradermal injections are used for diagnostic purposes, such as the tuberculin test and tests to determine sensitivity to various substances. The advantage of the intradermal route for these tests is that the body's reaction to substances is easily visible, and degrees of reaction are discernible by comparative study. Intradermal injections are placed just below the epidermis.

Equipment

- Medication
- Sterile syringe and needle (25 to 27 gauge, $\frac{1}{4}''$ to $\frac{5}{8}''$ long)
- Antimicrobial swab
- Disposable gloves
- Acetone and 2×2 sterile gauze square (optional)
- Medication Kardex or computer-generated MAR

ASSESSMENT

Assess the patient for any allergies. Assess the site on the patient where the injection is to be given; it should not be given in broken or open skin. Avoid areas that are highly pigmented and hairy. Assess the patient's knowledge of reason for injection. This may provide an opportune time for patient education.

NURSING DIAGNOSIS

Determine related factors for the nursing diagnoses based on the patient's current status. Appropriate nursing diagnoses may include:

- Deficient Knowledge
- Risk for Allergy Response
- Anxiety

OUTCOME IDENTIFICATION AND PLANNING

The expected outcome to achieve when administering an intradermal injection is appearance of a wheal or blister at the site of injection. Other outcomes that may be appropriate include the following: the patient understands the rationale for the injection; the patient experiences no allergy response; the patient refrains from rubbing the site; and the patient's anxiety is decreased.

IMPLEMENTATION

ACTION	RATIONALE
1. Assemble equipment and check the physician's order.	This ensures that the patient receives the right medication at the right time by the proper route. Many intradermal drugs are potent allergens and may cause a significant reaction if given in an incorrect dose.

continues

SKILL
5-5
Administering an Intradermal Injection (continued)

ACTION	RATIONALE
2. Explain the procedure to the patient.	Explanation encourages cooperation and reduces apprehension.
3. Perform hand hygiene. Don disposable gloves.	Hand hygiene deters the spread of microorganisms. Gloves act as a barrier and protect the nurse's hands from accidental exposure to blood during the injection procedure.
4. If necessary, withdraw medication from an ampule or vial as described in Skills 5-2 and 5-3.	
5. Select an area on the inner aspect of the forearm that is not heavily pigmented or covered with hair. The upper chest and upper back beneath the scapulae also are sites for intradermal injections.	The forearm is a convenient and easy location for introducing an agent intradermally. Hair or lesions at the injection site may interfere with assessments of skin changes at the site.
6. Cleanse the area with an antimicrobial swab while wiping with a firm, circular motion and moving outward from the injection site. Allow the skin to dry. If the skin is oily, clean the area with a pledget moistened with acetone.	Pathogens on the skin can be forced into the tissues by the needle. Introducing alcohol into tissues irritates the tissues and is uncomfortable for the patient. Acetone is effective for removing oily substances from the skin.
7. Remove the needle cap with the nondominant hand by pulling it straight off.	Taut skin provides an easy entrance into intradermal tissue.
8. Use the nondominant hand to spread the skin taut over the injection site.	The cap protects the needle from contact with microorganisms. This technique lessens the risk of an accidental needlestick.
9. **Place the needle almost flat against the patient's skin, bevel side up, and insert the needle into the skin so that the point of the needle can be seen through the skin. Insert the needle only about ⅛″ with entire bevel under the skin.**	Intradermal tissue is entered when the needle is held as nearly parallel to the skin as possible and is inserted about ⅛″.
10. Slowly inject the agent while watching for a small wheal or blister to appear. If none appears, withdraw the needle to ensure bevel is in interdermal tissue.	If a small wheal or blister appears, the agent is in the intradermal tissue.
11. Once the agent has been injected, withdraw the needle quickly at the same angle that it was inserted.	Withdrawing the needle quickly and at the angle at which it entered the skin minimizes tissue damage and discomfort for the patient.

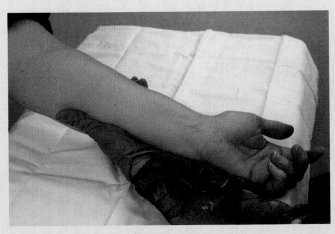

Action 8: Holding forearm skin taut.

continues

SKILL 5-5   Administering an Intradermal Injection (continued)

ACTION

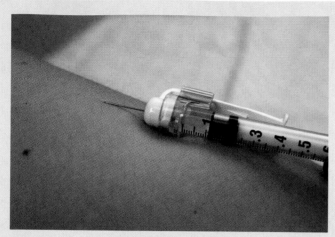

Action 9: Inserting the needle almost level with the skin.

12. **Do not massage area after removing needle. Tell patient not to rub or scratch site.**

13. Do not recap the used needle. Discard the needle and syringe in the appropriate receptacle.

14. Assist the patient to a position of comfort.

15. Remove gloves and dispose of them properly. Perform hand hygiene.

16. Chart the administration of the medication as well as the site of administration. Some agencies recommend circling the injection site with ink. Charting may be documented on CMAR, including location.

17. Observe the area for signs of a reaction at ordered intervals, usually at 24 to 72 hours. Inform the patient of this inspection.

RATIONALE

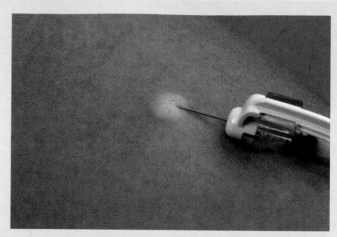

Action 10: Observing for wheal while injecting medication.

Massaging the area where an intradermal injection is given may interfere with test results by spreading medication to underlying subcutaneous tissue.

Proper disposal of the needle protects the nurse from accidental injection. Most accidental puncture wounds occur when recapping needles.

This provides for the well-being of the patient.

Hand hygiene deters the spread of microorganisms.

Accurate documentation is necessary to prevent medication error. Circling the injection site easily identifies the site of the intradermal injection and allows for careful observation of the exact area.

With many intradermal injections, the nurse will need to look for a localized reaction in the area of the injection.

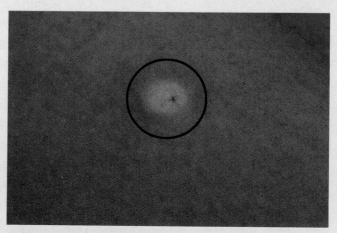

Action 16: Marking injection site.

continues

SKILL 5-5 Administering an Intradermal Injection (continued)

EVALUATION

The expected outcomes are met when the nurse notes a wheal or blister at site of injection; patient understood the rationale for the injection; the patient experienced no allergy response; the patient does not rub or scratch the site; and the patient's anxiety is decreased.

Unexpected Situations and Associated Interventions

- *Nurse does not note wheal or blister at site of injection:* Medication has been injected subcutaneously. Nurse may need to obtain order to repeat procedure.
- *Medication leaks out of injection site before needle is withdrawn:* Needle was inserted less than ⅛". Nurse may need to obtain order to repeat procedure.
- *Nurse sticks self with needle before injection:* Discard needle and syringe appropriately. Follow agency policy regarding needlestick injury. Prepare new syringe with medication and administer to patient. Complete appropriate paperwork and follow agency's policy regarding needlesticks.
- *Nurse sticks self with needle after injection:* Follow agency's policy regarding needlestick injuries. Discard needle and syringe appropriately. Complete the appropriate paperwork. Do not document needlestick in patient's notes.
- *After or during injection, the patient pulls away from the needle before medication is delivered fully:* Remove and appropriately discard needle. Attach a new needle to the syringe and administer the remaining medication.

Special Considerations

- Since the needle is entering only the dermal portion of tissue, where there are no large blood vessels, aspiration (pulling back on the plunger) is not recommended for an intradermal injection.
- Some agencies recommend administering intradermal injections with the bevel down instead of the bevel up.

SKILL 5-6 Administering a Subcutaneous Injection

Subcutaneous tissue lies between the epidermis and the muscle. Because there is subcutaneous tissue all over the body, various sites are used for subcutaneous injections. These sites are the outer aspect of the upper arm, the abdomen (from below the costal margin to the iliac crests), the anterior aspects of the thigh, the upper back, and the upper ventral or dorsogluteal area (see Box 5-5). This route is used to administer insulin, heparin, and certain immunizations. If needed, review the specifics of the particular medication before administrating.

Equipment

- Medication
- Sterile syringe and needle (size depends on medication being administered and patient)
- Antimicrobial swabs
- Disposable gloves
- Medication Kardex or computer-generated MAR
- Cotton balls or dry sponge (optional)

ASSESSMENT

Assess the patient for any allergies. Assess the patient's knowledge of the medication. If the patient has a knowledge deficit about the medication, this may be an appropriate time to begin education about the medication. Assess the area where injection is to be given. Subcutaneous injections should not be given into areas of skin that are broken or open.

NURSING DIAGNOSIS

Determine related factors for the nursing diagnoses based on the patient's current status. Appropriate nursing diagnoses may include:

- Deficient Knowledge
- Acute Pain
- Anxiety
- Risk for Allergy Response

continues

Administering a Subcutaneous Injection (continued)

OUTCOME IDENTIFICATION AND PLANNING

The expected outcome to achieve when administering a subcutaneous injection is that the patient receives medication via the subcutaneous route. Other outcomes that may be appropriate include the following: the patient understands the reason for the procedure and has minimal pain, decreased anxiety, and no allergic response.

IMPLEMENTATION

ACTION	RATIONALE
1. Assemble equipment and check the physician's order.	This ensures that the patient receives the right medication at the right time by the proper route.
2. Explain the procedure to the patient.	Explanation encourages patient cooperation and reduces apprehension.
3. Perform hand hygiene.	Hand hygiene deters the spread of microorganisms.
4. If necessary, withdraw medication from an ampule or vial as described in Procedures 5-2 and 5-3.	
5. Identify the patient carefully by checking the identification band on the patient's wrist and asking the patient his or her name. Close the curtain to provide privacy. Don disposable gloves.	It is the nurse's responsibility to guard against error. Gloves act as a barrier and protect the nurse's hands from accidental exposure to blood during the injection procedure.
6. Have the patient assume a position appropriate for the most commonly used sites. See Box 5-5. a. Outer aspect of upper arm: the patient's arm should be relaxed and at the side of the body. b. Anterior thighs: the patient may sit or lie with the leg relaxed. c. Abdomen: the patient may lie in a semirecumbent position.	Injection into a tense extremity causes discomfort.
7. Locate the site of choice according to directions given in Box 5-5. Ensure that the area is not tender and is free of lumps or nodules.	Good visualization is necessary to establish the correct location of the site and avoid damage to tissues. Nodules or lumps may indicate a previous injection site where absorption was inadequate.
8. Clean the area around the injection site with an antimicrobial swab. Use a firm, circular motion while moving outward from the injection site. Allow area to dry.	Friction helps to clean the skin. A clean area is contaminated when a soiled object is rubbed over its surface.
9. Remove the needle cap with the nondominant hand, pulling it straight off.	The cap protects the needle from contact with microorganisms. This technique lessens the risk of an accidental needlestick.
10. Grasp and bunch the area surrounding the injection site or spread the skin at the site.	This provides for easy, less painful entry into the subcutaneous tissue. The decision to pinch or spread tissue at the injection site depends on the size of the patient. If the patient is thin, skin needs to be bunched to create a skin fold.

continues

Administering a Subcutaneous Injection (continued)

ACTION

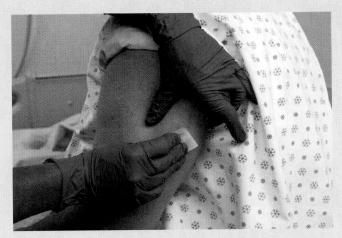

Action 8: Cleaning injection site.

11. **Hold the syringe in the dominant hand between the thumb and forefinger. Inject the needle quickly at an angle at 45 to 90 degrees, depending on the amount and turgor of the tissue and the length of the needle, as shown.**

12. After the needle is in place, release the tissue. If you have a large skin fold pinched up, ensure that the needle stays in place as the skin is released. Immediately move your nondominant hand to steady the lower end of the syringe. Slide your dominant hand to the tip of the barrel.

13. **Aspirate, if recommended, by pulling back gently on the plunger of the syringe to determine whether the needle is in a blood vessel. If blood appears, the needle should be withdrawn, the medication syringe and needle discarded, and a new syringe with new medication prepared. *Do not aspirate when giving insulin or any form of heparin.***

RATIONALE

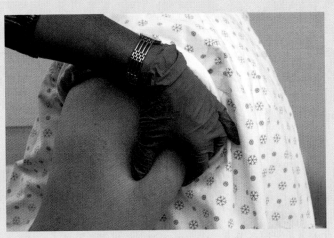

Action 10: Bunching tissue around injection site.

Inserting the needle quickly causes less pain to the patient. Subcutaneous tissue is abundant in well-nourished, well-hydrated people and spare in emaciated, dehydrated, or very thin persons. For a thin person, it is best to insert the needle at a 45-degree angle.

Injecting the solution into compressed tissues results in pressure against nerve fibers and creates discomfort. If there is a large skin fold, the skin may retract away from the needle. The nondominant hand secures the syringe and allows for smooth aspiration.

Discomfort and possibly a serious reaction may occur if a drug intended for subcutaneous use is injected into a vein. Heparin is an anticoagulant and may cause bruising if aspirated. Because the insulin needle is so small, aspiration after insulin has proved unreliable in predicting needle placement.

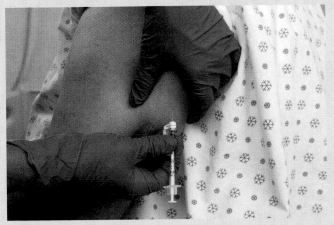

Action 11: Inserting needle.

continues

Administering a Subcutaneous Injection (continued)

ACTION	RATIONALE
14. If no blood appears, inject the solution slowly.	Rapid injection of the solution creates pressure in the tissues, resulting in discomfort.
15. Withdraw the needle quickly at the same angle at which it was inserted.	Slow withdrawal of the needle pulls the tissues and causes discomfort. Applying countertraction around the injection site helps to prevent pulling on the tissue as the needle is withdrawn. Removing the needle at the same angle at which it was inserted minimizes tissue damage and discomfort for the patient.

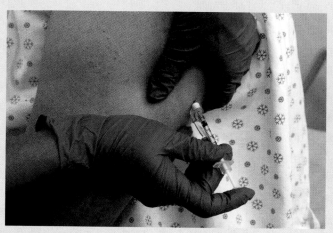

Action 14: Injecting medication.

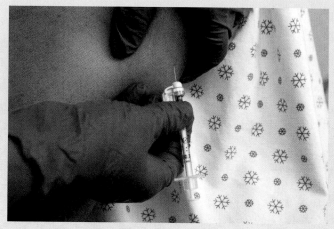

Action 15: Withdrawing needle.

16. Massage the area gently with cotton ball or dry swab. **Do not massage a subcutaneous heparin or insulin injection site.** Apply a small bandage if needed.	Massaging helps to distribute the solution and hastens its absorption. Massaging the site of a heparin injection causes additional bruising. Massaging after an insulin injection may contribute to unpredictable absorption of the medication.

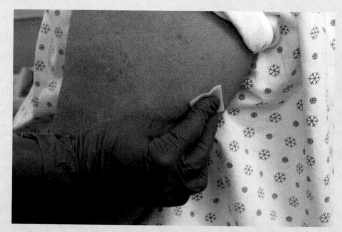

Action 16: Massaging injection site.

continues

Administering a Subcutaneous Injection (continued)

ACTION	RATIONALE
17. Do not recap the used needle. Discard the needle and syringe in the appropriate receptacle.	Proper disposal of the needle protects the nurse from accidental injection. Most accidental puncture wounds occur when recapping needles.
18. Assist the patient to a position of comfort.	This provides for the well-being of the patient.
19. Remove gloves and dispose of them properly. Perform hand hygiene.	Hand hygiene deters the spread of microorganisms.
20. Chart the administration of the medication, including the site of administration. This charting can be done on CMAR.	Accurate documentation is necessary to prevent medication error.
21. Evaluate the response of the patient to the medication within an appropriate time frame.	Reaction to medication given by the parenteral route may occur within 15 to 30 minutes after injection.

EVALUATION   The expected outcomes are met when the patient has received the medication via the subcutaneous route; understands the reason for the procedure; experienced minimal pain; has decreased anxiety; and has had no allergic response.

Unexpected Situations and Associated Interventions

- *When skin fold is released, needle pulls out of skin:* Remove and appropriately discard needle. Attach new needle to syringe and administer injection.
- *Patient refuses to let nurse administer medication in another location:* Explain the rationale behind rotating injection sites. Discuss other available injection sites with patient. If patient will still not allow injection in another area, administer medication to patient, document patient's refusal and discussion, and notify physician.
- *Nurse sticks self with needle before injection:* Discard needle and syringe appropriately. Follow the agency's policy regarding needlesticks. Prepare a new syringe with medication and administer to patient. Complete appropriate paperwork.
- *Nurse sticks self with needle after injection:* Discard needle and syringe appropriately. Follow agency's policy regarding needlesticks. Complete appropriate paperwork. Do not document needlestick in patient's notes.
- *After or during injection, patient pulls away from needle before medication is delivered fully:* Remove and appropriately discard needle. Attach a new needle to syringe and administer remaining medication.

Infant and Child Considerations

- Do not tell a child that an injection will not hurt. Describe the feel of the injection as a pinch or a sting. A child who believes you have been dishonest with him or her is less likely to cooperate with future procedures.

Older Adult Considerations

- Many elderly patients have less adipose tissue. Adjust the angle of the needle accordingly. You do not want to inadvertently give a subcutaneous medication intramuscularly.

Home Care Considerations

- According to the American Diabetes Association, reuse of insulin syringes in the home setting appears safe. Once the needle is dull, it should be discarded (usually after 2 to 10 uses).

SKILL 5-7   Administering an Intramuscular Injection

The intramuscular route is often used for drugs that are irritating because there are few nerve endings in deep muscle tissue. If a sore or inflamed muscle is entered, however, the muscle may act as a trigger area, and severe referred pain often results. It is best to palpate a muscle before injection. Select a site that does not feel tender to the patient and where the tissue does not contract and become firm and tense. Avoid nodules, lumps, and scars.

Absorption occurs as in subcutaneous administration but more rapidly because of the greater vascularity of muscle tissue. The amount of 5 mL is considered the maximum to be given in one site for an adult with well-developed muscles, although the patient's size and the site used (eg, deltoid muscle) may necessitate smaller injection (Nicoll & Hesby, 2002).

An important point in the administration of an intramuscular injection is the selection of a safe site away from large nerves, bones, and blood vessels (see Box 5-6). When care is not taken, common complications include abscesses, necrosis and skin slough, nerve injuries, lingering pain, and periostitis (inflammation of the membrane covering a bone).

The sites for injecting intramuscular medications should be rotated when therapy requires repeated injections. The sites described in this skill may all be used on a rotating basis. Whatever pattern of rotating sites is used, a description of it should appear in the patient's plan of nursing care.

Equipment

- Disposable gloves
- Medication
- Sterile syringe and needle (size depends on medication being administered and patient)
- Antimicrobial swab
- Dry sponge
- Medication Kardex or computer-generated MAR

ASSESSMENT

Assess the patient for any allergies. Assess the patient's knowledge of the medication. If the patient has a knowledge deficit about the medication, this may be an appropriate time to begin education about the medication. Assess the area where the injection is to be given. Intramuscular injections should not be given into areas of skin that are broken or open. If the medication is for pain, assess the patient's level of pain. If the medication may affect the patient's vital signs or laboratory test results, check them before administering the medication.

NURSING DIAGNOSIS

Determine related factors for the nursing diagnoses based on the patient's current status. Appropriate diagnoses may include:

- Deficient Knowledge
- Acute Pain
- Risk for Allergy Response
- Anxiety
- Risk for Injury
- Risk for Impaired Skin Integrity

OUTCOME IDENTIFICATION AND PLANNING

The expected outcome to achieve when administering an intramuscular injection is that the patient receives the medication via the intramuscular route. Other outcomes that may be appropriate include the following: the patient understands the reasons for the injection; has minimal pain; has no allergy response; has decreased anxiety; and experiences no injury; and patient's skin remains intact.

continues

Administering an Intramuscular Injection (continued)

IMPLEMENTATION

ACTION	RATIONALE
1. Assemble equipment and check the physician's order.	This ensures that the patient receives the right medication at the right time by the proper route.
2. Explain procedure to patient.	Explanation encourages cooperation and alleviates apprehension.
3. Perform hand hygiene.	Hand hygiene deters the spread of microorganisms.
4. If necessary, withdraw medication from an ampule or vial as described in Procedures 5-2 and 5-3.	
5. Do not add air to the syringe.	The addition of air to the syringe is potentially dangerous and may result in an overdose of medication.
6. Identify the patient carefully. There are three correct ways to do this: a. Check the name on the patient's identification badge. b. Ask the patient his or her name. c. Verify the patient's identification with a staff member who knows the patient.	Identifying the patient is the nurse's responsibility to guard against error. a. This is the most reliable method. Replace the identification band if it is missing or inaccurate in any way. b. This requires a response from the patient, but illness and strange surroundings often cause patients to be confused. c. This is another way to double-check identity. Do not use the name on the door or over the bed, because these may be inaccurate.
7. Provide for privacy. Have the patient assume a position appropriate for the site selected, and encourage the patient to relax. a. Ventrogluteal: the patient may lie on the back or side with the hip and knee flexed. b. Vastus lateralis: the patient may lie on the back or may assume a sitting position. c. Deltoid: the patient may sit or lie with arm relaxed. d. Dorsogluteal: the patient may lie prone with toes pointing inward or on the side with the upper leg flexed and placed in front of the lower leg.	Injection into a tense muscle causes discomfort.

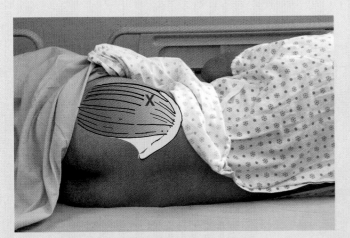

Action 7a: Positioning for ventrogluteal site injection.

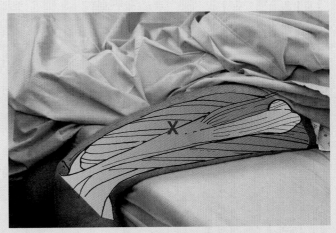

Action 7b: Positioning for vastus lateralis site injection.

SKILL 5-7   Administering an Intramuscular Injection (continued)

ACTION	RATIONALE

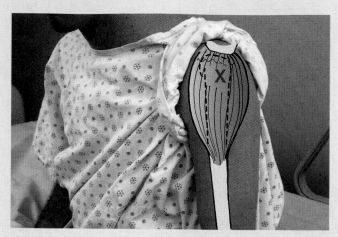

Action 7c: Positioning for deltoid muscle site injection.

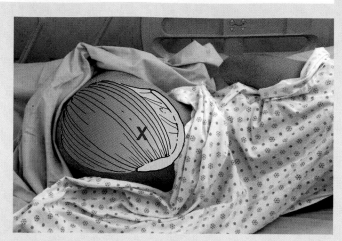

Action 7d: Positioning for dorsogluteal site injection.

8. Locate the site of choice according to directions given in Box 5-6. Ensure that the area is nontender and free of lumps or nodules. Don disposable gloves.

Good visualization is necessary to establish the correct location of the site and avoid damage to tissues. Nodules or lumps may indicate a previous injection site where absorption was inadequate. Gloves act as a barrier and protect the nurse's hands from accidental exposure to blood during the injection procedure.

9. Clean the area thoroughly with an antimicrobial swab, using friction. Allow to dry.

Pathogens present on the skin and antimicrobial agent can be forced into the tissues by the needle.

10. Remove the needle cap by pulling it straight off.

The cap protects the needle from contact with microorganisms. This technique lessens the risk of an accidental needlestick and also prevents inadvertently unscrewing the needle from the barrel of the syringe.

11. Displace the skin in a Z-track manner by pulling to one side or spread the skin at the site using your nondominant hand.

This makes the tissue taut and minimizes discomfort. Using the Z-track method prevents seepage of the medication into the needle track and is less painful.

12. Hold the syringe in your dominant hand between the thumb and forefinger. Quickly dart the needle into the tissue at a 90-degree angle.

A quick injection is less painful. Inserting the needle at a 90-degree angle facilitates entry into muscle tissue.

13. As soon as the needle is in place, use your nondominant hand to hold the lower end of the syringe. Slide your dominant hand to the tip of the barrel.

This acts to steady the syringe and allows for smooth aspiration.

14. **Aspirate by slowly (for at least 5 seconds) pulling back on the plunger to determine whether the needle is in a blood vessel. If blood is aspirated, discard the needle, syringe, and medication, prepare a new sterile setup, and inject another site.**

Discomfort and possibly a serious reaction may occur if a drug intended for intramuscular use is injected into a vein. Allowing slow aspiration facilitates backflow of blood even if needle is in a small, low-flow blood vessel.

continues

Administering an Intramuscular Injection (continued)

ACTION

RATIONALE

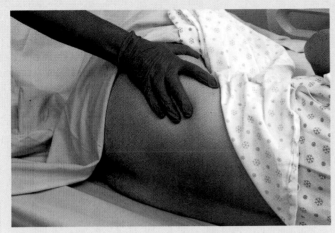

Action 11: Spreading the skin at ventrogluteal site.

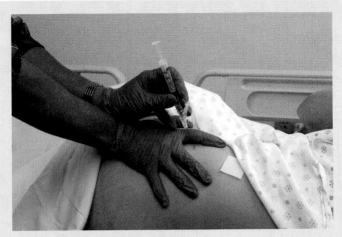

Action 12: Darting needle into the tissue.

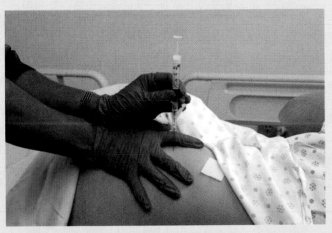

Action 12: Inserting needle in the ventrogluteal site.

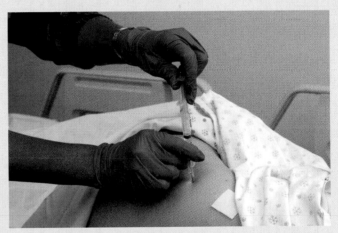

Action 14: Aspirating.

15. If no blood is aspirated, inject the solution slowly (10 seconds per mL of medication).

16. Remove needle slowly and steadily. Release displaced tissue if Z-track technique was used.

17. Apply gentle pressure at the site with a small, dry sponge.

18. Do not recap used needle. Discard needle and syringe in appropriate receptacle.

19. Assist patient to position of comfort. Encourage patient to exercise extremity used for injection if possible.

20. Remove gloves and dispose of them properly. Perform hand hygiene.

Injecting slowly helps to reduce discomfort by allowing time for solution to disperse in the tissues.

Slow withdrawal allows the medication to begin to diffuse through the muscle. Releasing displaced skin seals medication in the tissues.

Light pressure causes less trauma and irritation to the tissues. Massaging can force medication into subcutaneous tissues.

Proper disposal of needle protects nurse from accidental injection. Most accidental puncture wounds occur when recapping needles.

Exercise promotes absorption of medication.

Hand hygiene deters the spread of microorganisms.

continues

SKILL 5-7 Administering an Intramuscular Injection (continued)

ACTION   **RATIONALE**

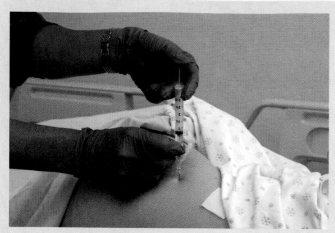

Action 15: Injecting medication.

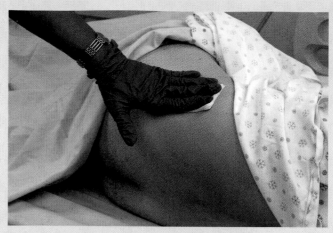

Action 17: Applying pressure at the injection site.

21. Chart the administration of the medication, including the site of administration. This may be documented on the CMAR.

Accurate documentation is necessary to prevent medication error.

22. Evaluate patient's response to medication within an appropriate time frame. Assess site, if possible, within 2 to 4 hours after administration.

Reaction to medication given by the parenteral route is a possibility. Visualization of the site also allows for assessment of any untoward effects.

EVALUATION

The expected outcomes are met when the patient has received the medication via the intramuscular route; understood the reasons for injection; had minimal pain; experienced no allergy response; has decreased anxiety; and experienced no injury; and patient's skin remained intact.

Unexpected Situations and Associated Interventions

- *Nurse sticks self with needle before injection:* Discard needle and syringe appropriately. Follow the agency's policy regarding needlesticks. Prepare a new syringe with medication and administer to the patient. Complete appropriate paperwork.
- *Nurse sticks self with needle after injection:* Discard needle and syringe appropriately. Follow the agency's policy regarding needlesticks. Complete appropriate paperwork. Do not document needlestick in the patient's notes.
- *After or during injection, patient pulls away from needle before medication is delivered fully:* Remove and discard needle appropriately. Attach a new needle to syringe and administer remaining medication in a new site.
- *While injecting needle into patient, nurse hits patient's bone:* Withdraw and discard the needle. Apply new needle to syringe and administer in alternate site. Document incident in patient's notes. Notify physician. May need to complete incident report.

Infant and Child Considerations

- Safe administration of an intramuscular injection into an infant's vastus lateralis muscle may require use of a 1″ needle rather than the commonly used ⅝″ needle. A 1″ needle consistently allows penetration into the muscle and safe administration of the medication.

Adding Medications to an IV Solution Container

Medications may be added to the patient's infusion solution. The recommended procedure is for the pharmacist to add the prescribed drug to a large volume of IV solution, but sometimes the drug is added in the nursing unit, in which case sterile technique must be maintained.

When medication is administered by continuous infusion, the patient receives it slowly and over a long period. Although sometimes this can be an advantage when it is desirable to give the medication slowly, it is a disadvantage when the patient needs to receive the drug more quickly. Also, if for some reason all of the solution cannot be infused, the patient will not receive the prescribed amount of the medication. The patient receiving medication by a continuous IV infusion should be checked for possible adverse effects at least every hour.

Equipment
- Medication prepared in a syringe with a 19- to 21-gauge needle, blunt needle or needleless device (follow agency policy)
- IV fluid container (bag or bottle)
- Antimicrobial swab
- Label to be attached to the IV container
- Medication Kardex or computer-generated MAR

ASSESSMENT

Assess the patient for allergies. Assess the patient's knowledge of the medication. If patient has a knowledge deficit, this may be an appropriate time to begin education about the medication.

NURSING DIAGNOSIS

Determine related factors for the nursing diagnoses based on the patient's current status. Appropriate nursing diagnoses may include:
- Risk for Injury
- Risk for Allergy Response
- Risk for Infection
- Deficient Knowledge
- Anxiety

OUTCOME IDENTIFICATION AND PLANNING

The expected outcome to achieve when adding medications to an IV solution container is that the medication is added to an adequate amount of IV solution and mixed appropriately. Other outcomes that may be appropriate include the following: medication is delivered to the patient in a safe and effective way; patient experiences no allergy response; patient remains infection free; and patient understands and experiences decreased anxiety regarding medication infusion.

IMPLEMENTATION

ACTION	RATIONALE
1. Gather all equipment. Check the medication order with the physician's order and that medication is compatible with IV fluid. Take equipment to patient's bedside.	Checking the order ensures that the patient receives the correct medication at the correct time and in the right manner. Compatibility of medication and solution prevents complications. Having equipment available saves time and facilitates performance of the task.
2. Perform hand hygiene.	Hand hygiene deters the spread of microorganisms.
3. Identify patient by checking identification band on patient's wrist and asking patient his or her name. Check for any allergies patient may have.	This ensures that the medication is given to the right person.
4. Explain procedure to patient.	Explanation allays patient anxiety.

continues

SKILL 5-8   Adding Medications to an IV Solution Container (continued)

ACTION

5. Add the medications to the IV solution that is infusing:
   a. **Check that the volume in the bag or bottle is adequate.**
   b. Close the IV clamp.

   c. Clean the medication port with an antimicrobial swab.
   d. Steady the container and uncap the needle or needleless device and insert it into the port. Inject the medication.
   e. Remove the container from the IV pole and gently rotate the solutions.
   f. Rehang the container, open the clamp, and readjust the flow rate.
   g. **Attach the label to the container so that the dose of medication that has been added is apparent.**

RATIONALE

   a. The volume should be sufficient to dilute the drug
   b. This prevents backflow directly to the patient of improperly diluted medication.
   c. This deters entry of microorganisms when the port is punctured.
   d. This ensures that the needle or needleless device enters the container and medication can be dispersed into the solution.
   e. This mixes the medication with the solution.
   f. This ensures the infusion of the IV with the medication at the prescribed rate.
   g. This confirms that the prescribed dose of medication has been added to the IV solution.

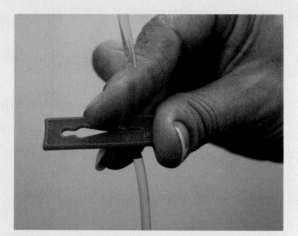

Action 5b: Closing the IV clamp.

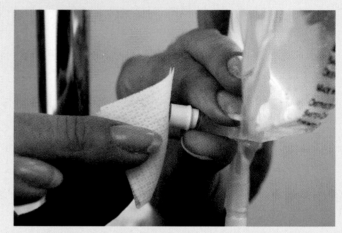

Action 5c: Cleaning the medication port.

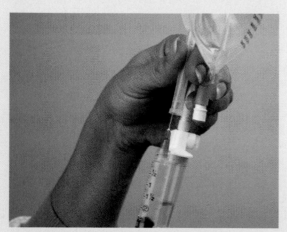

Action 5d: Steadying bag and uncapping needle.

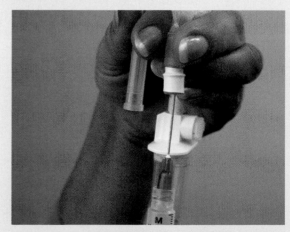

Action 5d: Inserting needle into port.

continues

SKILL 5-8 | Adding Medications to an IV Solution Container (continued)

ACTION	RATIONALE

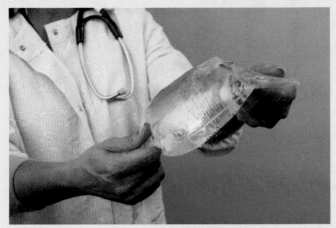

Action 5e: Rotating solution to distribute medication.

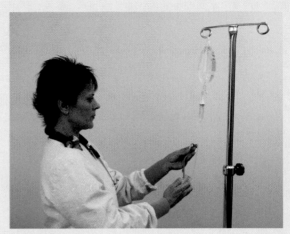

Action 5f: Readjusting flow rate.

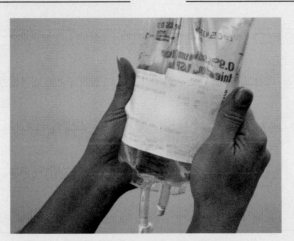

Action 5g: Labeling container to show medication.

ACTION	RATIONALE
6. Add the medication to the IV solution before the infusion:	
a. Carefully remove any protective cover and locate the injection port. Clean with an antimicrobial swab.	a. This deters entry of microorganisms when the needle punctures the port.
b. Uncap the needle or needleless device and insert into the port. Inject the medication.	b. This ensures that the needle enters the container and that medication can be dispersed into the solution.
c. Withdraw and insert the spike into the proper entry site on the bag or bottle.	c. This punctures the seal in the IV bag or bottle.
d. With tubing clamped, gently rotate the IV solution in the bag or bottle. Hang the IV.	d. This mixes the medication with the solution.
e. **Attach the label to the container so that the dose of medication that has been added is apparent.**	e. This confirms that the prescribed dose of medication has been added to the IV solution.
7. Dispose of equipment according to agency policy.	This prevents inadvertent injury from the equipment.
8. Perform hand hygiene.	Hand hygiene deters the spread of microorganisms.
9. Chart the addition of medication to the IV solution. This may be done on the CMAR.	Accurate documentation is necessary to prevent medication errors.
10. Evaluate the patient's response to medication within the appropriate time frame.	Patients require careful observation because medications given by the IV route may have a rapid effect.

continues

SKILL 5-8   Adding Medications to an IV Solution Container (continued)

EVALUATION

The expected outcomes are met when the medication is added to an adequate amount of IV solution and mixed appropriately; patient received the medication in a safe and effective way; patient experienced no allergy response; patient experienced no infection; patient understood reasons for procedure; and patient experienced decreased anxiety regarding medication infusion.

Unexpected Situations and Associated Interventions

- *There is not enough IV solution in container:* Obtain new IV fluid from medication station and add medication. Remove current IV bag and replace with newly admixed IV fluid. (Some institutions would prefer that the pharmacy mix any new bags so that the process may be done in a sterile environment.)
- *Nurse realizes that wrong medication or wrong amount of medication was added to the IV bag:* Immediately stop infusion. Assess patient for any distress and notify physician. Follow agency policy for medication error. Remove bag of IV fluids and replace with IV containing ordered medication.
- *Nurse sticks self with needle while trying to inject medication into port:* Discard syringe and needle. Prepare new syringe with medication.
- *Needle goes through side of medication injection port:* Discard syringe, needle, and current bag of IV solution. Replace with newly admixed IV fluid. (Some institutions would prefer pharmacy mix any new bags so that the process may be done in a sterile environment.)

SKILL 5-9   Adding a Bolus IV Medication to an Existing IV

A medication can be administered as an IV bolus or push. This involves a single injection of a concentrated solution administered directly into an IV line.

Equipment

- Antimicrobial swab
- Watch with second hand, or stopwatch
- Disposable gloves
- Medication prepared in a syringe with needless device or 23- to 25-gauge, 1″ needle (if needleless system in use, needle is not needed).
- Medication Kardex or computer-generated MAR

ASSESSMENT

Assess patient's IV site, noting any swelling, coolness, leakage of fluid from IV site, or pain. If fluids are infusing through the IV, assess fluid's compatibility with medication to be administered and determine rate at which medication is to be given. Assess patient for allergies. Assess patient's knowledge of medication. If patient has a knowledge deficit, this may be an appropriate time to begin education about the medication.

NURSING DIAGNOSIS

Determine related factors for the nursing diagnoses based on the patient's current status. Appropriate nursing diagnoses may include:

- Acute Pain
- Risk for Allergy Response
- Deficient Knowledge
- Risk for Infection
- Anxiety

Adding a Bolus IV Medication to an Existing IV (continued)

OUTCOME IDENTIFICATION AND PLANNING

The expected outcome to achieve when adding a bolus IV medication to an existing IV is that the IV bolus is given safely. Other outcomes that may be appropriate include the following: patient experiences no or minimal discomfort; patient experiences no allergy response; patient is knowledgeable about medication being added by bolus IV; patient remains infection free; and patient has no, or decreased, anxiety.

IMPLEMENTATION

ACTION	RATIONALE
1. Bring equipment to patient's bedside. Check the medication order with the physician's order. Check a drug resource to clarify whether medication needs to be diluted before administration.	Having equipment available saves time and facilitates performance of the task. Checking the order ensures that the patient receives the correct medication at the correct time and in the right manner.
2. Explain procedure to patient.	Explanation allays patient anxiety.
3. Perform hand hygiene. Don clean gloves.	Hand hygiene deters the spread of microorganisms. Gloves protect the nurse from exposure to bloodborne pathogens.
4. Identify patient by checking the identification band on patient's wrist and asking patient his or her name.	This ensures that medication is given to right person.
5. **Assess IV site for presence of inflammation or infiltration.**	IV medication must be given directly into a vein for safe administration.
6. Select injection port on tubing that is closest to venipuncture site. Clean port with antimicrobial swab.	Using port closest to needle insertion site minimizes dilution of medication. Cleaning deters entry of microorganisms when port is punctured.
7. Uncap syringe. Steady port with your nondominant hand while inserting needleless device or needle into center of port.	This supports injection port and lessens risk for accidentally dislodging IV or entering port incorrectly.

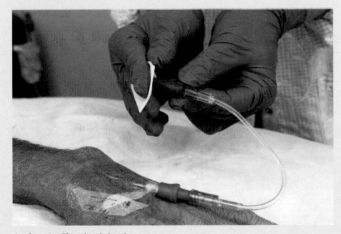

Action 6: Cleaning injection port.

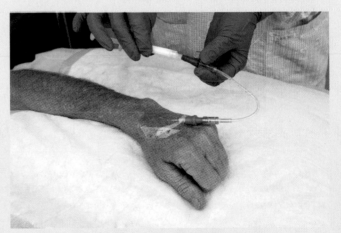

Action 7: Inserting needleless system into port.

8. Move your nondominant hand to section of IV tubing directly behind or just distal to injection port. Fold tubing between your fingers to temporarily stop flow of IV solution.	This minimizes dilution of IV medication with IV solution.
9. Pull back slightly on plunger just until blood appears in tubing. If no blood appears, medication may still be administered while assessing IV insertion site for signs of infiltration.	This ensures injection of medication into a vein.

continues

ACTION	RATIONALE
10. Inject medication at recommended rate (see Special Considerations below).	This delivers correct amount of medication at proper interval according to manufacturer's directions.

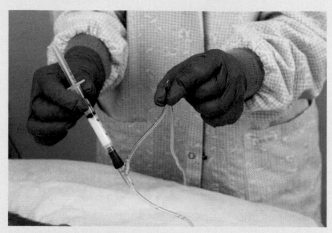

Action 8: Interrupting IV flow.

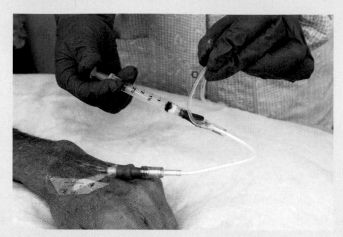

Action 10: Injecting medication while interrupting IV flow.

11. Remove needle. Do not cap it. Release tubing and allow IV to flow at proper rate.	This prevents accidental needlestick.
12. Dispose of syringe in proper receptacle.	Proper disposal prevents accidental injury and spread of microorganisms.
13. Remove gloves and perform hand hygiene.	Hand hygiene deters spread of microorganisms.
14. Chart administration of the medication. This may be done on the CMAR.	Accurate documentation is necessary to prevent medication errors.
15. Evaluate patient's response to medication within appropriate time frame.	Patient requires careful observation because medications given by IV bolus injection may have a rapid effect.

EVALUATION

The expected outcomes are met when the patient receives the medication via an IV bolus; had no, or minimal, discomfort; experienced no allergy response; understood rationale for medication added by bolus IV; experienced no infection; and experienced decreased anxiety.

Unexpected Situations and Associated Interventions

- *Upon assessing patient's IV site before administering medication, nurse notes that IV has infiltrated:* Stop IV fluid and remove IV from extremity. Restart IV in a different location. Continue to monitor new IV site as medication is administered.
- *While administering medication, nurse notes a cloudy, white substance forming in IV tubing:* Stop IV from flowing and stop administering medication. Clamp IV at site nearest to patient. Tubing will need to be flushed thoroughly to get rid of any remaining precipitate. Check literature regarding incompatibilities of medications.
- *While nurse is administering medication, patient begins to complain of pain at IV site:* Stop medication. Assess IV site for any signs of infiltration or phlebitis. You may want to flush the IV with normal saline to check for patency. If the IV site appears within normal limits, resume medication administration at a slower rate.

continues

SKILL 5-9 — Adding a Bolus IV Medication to an Existing IV (continued)

Special Considerations

- Agency policy may recommend the following variations when injecting a bolus IV medication:
  - Release folded tubing after each increment of the drug has been administered at prescribed rate to facilitate delivery of medication.
  - Use a syringe with 1 mL normal saline to flush tubing after an IV bolus is delivered to ensure that residual medication in tubing is not delivered too rapidly.
- Consider how fast IV fluid is flowing to determine whether a flush of normal saline is in order after administering medication. If IV fluid is flowing less than 50 mL per hour, it may take medication up to 30 minutes to reach patient. This depends on what type of tubing is being used in the agency.
- If the IV is a small gauge (22 to 24 gauge) placed in a small vein, a blood return may not occur even if IV is intact. Also, patient may complain of stinging and pain at site while medication is being administered due to irritation of vein. Placing a warm pack over vein or slowing the rate may relieve discomfort.

SKILL 5-10 — Administering IV Medications by Piggyback, Mini-infusion Pump, or Volume-Control Administration Set

Medications can be administered by intermittent IV infusion. The drug is mixed with a small amount of the IV solution (50 to 100 mL) and administered over a short period at the prescribed interval (eg, every 4 hours). Needleless devices (recommended by the Centers for Disease Control and Prevention and the Occupational Safety and Health Administration) prevent needlesticks and provide access to the primary venous line. Either blunt-ended cannulas or recessed connection ports may be used.

A patient with an IV line in place can receive the solution containing the medication by way of a piggyback setup, a mini-infusion pump, or a volume-control administration set (eg, Pediatrol or Volutrol). The IV piggyback delivery system requires the intermittent or additive solution to be placed higher than the primary solution container. An extension hook provided by the manufacturer provides for easy lowering of the main IV container. The port on the primary IV line has a back-check valve that automatically stops the flow of the primary solution, allowing the secondary or piggyback solution to flow when connected. Because manufacturers' designs vary, check the directions carefully for the systems used in your agency. The nurse is responsible for calculating and manually adjusting the flow rate of the IV intermittent infusion or regulating the infusion with an infusion pump or controller.

The mini-syringe pump for intermittent infusion is battery operated and allows medication mixed in a syringe to be connected to the primary line and delivered by mechanical pressure applied to the syringe plunger.

Medications can also be placed in a controlled-volume administration set for intermittent IV infusion. The medication is diluted with a small amount of solution and administered through the patient's IV line. This type of equipment is also used for infusing solutions into children and older patients when the volume of fluid infused must be monitored carefully.

continues

Administering IV Medications by Piggyback, Mini-infusion Pump, or Volume-Control Administration Set (continued)

Equipment

- Medication Kardex or computer-generated MAR

For Piggyback or Mini-infusion Pump:

- Gloves (optional)
- Medication prepared in labeled piggyback set or syringe (5 to 100 mL)
- Secondary infusion tubing (microdrip or macrodrip)
- Needleless device, stopcock, or sterile needle (21- to 23-gauge)
- Antimicrobial swab
- Tape
- Metal or plastic hook
- Mini-infusion pump
- Date label for tubing

For Volume-Control Set:

- Gloves (optional)
- Volume-control set (eg, Volutrol, Buretrol, Burette)
- Medication (in vial or ampule)
- Syringe with needleless device attached or a 20- or 21-gauge needle
- Antimicrobial swab
- Medication label

ASSESSMENT

Assess patient for allergies. Assess patient's knowledge of the medication. If patient has a knowledge deficit, this may be an appropriate time to begin education about the medication. Assess patient's IV site, noting any swelling, coolness, leaking of fluid from IV site, or pain. If fluids are infusing through the IV, assess the fluid's compatibility with the medication to be administered.

NURSING DIAGNOSIS

Determine related factors for the nursing diagnoses based on the patient's current status. Appropriate nursing diagnoses include:

- Acute Pain
- Risk for Allergy Response
- Risk for Infection
- Deficient Knowledge

OUTCOME IDENTIFICATION AND PLANNING

The expected outcome to achieve when administering IV medications by piggyback, volume-control administration set, or mini-infusion pump is that the medication is delivered via the parenteral route. Other outcomes that may be appropriate include the following: patient experiences no or minimal discomfort; patient experiences no allergy response; patient remains infection free; and patient understands the rationale for medication administration.

IMPLEMENTATION

ACTION	RATIONALE
1. Gather equipment and bring to patient's bedside. Check the medication order against the original physician's order according to agency policy.	Having equipment available saves time and facilitates performance of the task. Checking the order ensures that the patient receives the correct medication at the correct time and in the right manner.

continues

SKILL 5-10

Administering IV Medications by Piggyback, Mini-infusion Pump, or Volume-Control Administration Set (continued)

ACTION	RATIONALE
2. Identify patient by checking identification band on patient's wrist and asking patient his or her name.	This ensures that the medication is given to the right person.
3. Explain procedure to patient.	Explanation allays patient anxiety.
4. Perform hand hygiene and don gloves.	Hand hygiene deters the spread of microorganisms. Gloves protect the nurse when connecting setup to an existing IV.
5. **Assess IV site for presence of inflammation or infiltration.**	Medication must be administered directly into a vein that is not inflamed to avoid injuring surrounding tissue.

Using Piggyback Infusion

6. Attach infusion tubing to piggyback set containing diluted medication. Place label on tubing with appropriate date and attach needle or needleless device to end of tubing according to manufacturer's directions. Open clamp and prime tubing. Close clamp.	This removes air from tubing and preserves sterility of setup. Tubing for piggyback setup may be used for 48 to 72 hours, depending on agency policy.
7. **Hang piggyback container on IV pole, positioning it higher than primary IV according to manufacturer's recommendations.** Use metal or plastic hook to lower primary IV.	Position of container influences flow of IV fluid into primary setup.
8. Use antimicrobial swab to clean appropriate port.	This deters entry of microorganisms when piggyback setup is connected to port.
9. Connect piggyback setup to: a. Needleless port b. Stopcock: turn stopcock to "open" position	a&b. Needleless systems and stopcock setup eliminate the need for a needle and are recommended by the Centers for Disease Control and Prevention.
c. Primary IV line: uncap needle and insert into secondary IV port closest to top of primary tubing. Use strip of tape to secure secondary set tubing to primary infusion tubing. Primary line is left unclamped if port has a backflow valve.	c. Tape stabilizes needle in infusion port and prevents it from slipping out. Backflow valve in primary line secondary port stops flow of primary infusion while piggyback solution is infusing. Once completed, backflow valves opens and flow of primary solution resumes.
10. Open clamp on piggyback set and regulate flow at prescribed delivery rate or set for secondary infusion on infusion pump. Monitor medication infusion at periodic intervals.	Delivery over a 30- to 60-minute interval is usually a safe method of administering IV medication. It is important to verify the safe administration rate for each drug to prevent adverse effects.
11. Clamp tubing on piggyback set when solution is infused. Follow agency policy regarding disposal of equipment.	This reduces risk for contaminating primary IV setup.
12. Readjust flow rate of primary IV.	Piggyback medication administration may interrupt normal flow rate of primary IV. Rate readjustment may be necessary.

continues

ACTION

RATIONALE

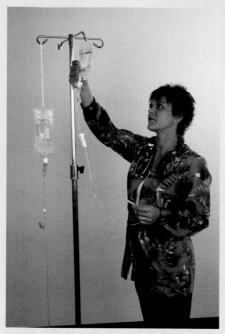

Action 7: Positioning piggyback container on IV pole.

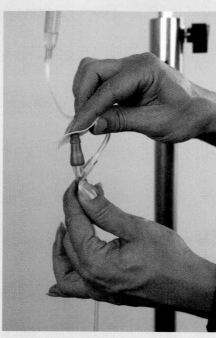

Action 8: Cleaning injection port.

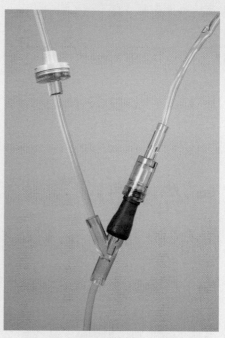

Action 9: Connecting piggyback setup to needleless port.

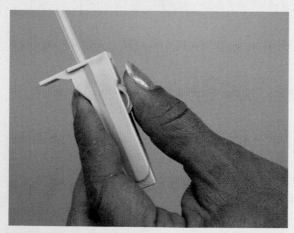

Action 10: Adjusting primary IV fluid to administer piggyback.

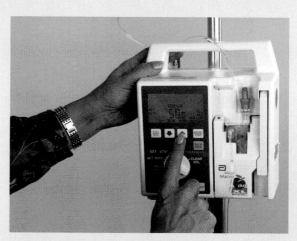

Action 10: Adjusting pump rate.

Using a Mini-infusion Pump

13. Connect prepared syringe to mini-infusion tubing.

Special tubing connects prepared medication to primary IV line.

14. Fill tubing with medication by applying gentle pressure to syringe plunger.

This removes air from tubing.

15. Insert syringe into mini-infusion pump according to manufacturer's directions.

Syringe must fit securely in pump apparatus for proper operation.

continues

SKILL 5-10

Administering IV Medications by Piggyback, Mini-infusion Pump, or Volume-Control Administration Set (continued)

ACTION	RATIONALE
16. Use antimicrobial swab to cleanse appropriate connector. Connect mini-infusion tubing to appropriate connector, as in Action 9.	This deters entry of microorganisms when piggyback setup is connected to port. Proper connection allows IV medication to flow into primary line.
17. Program pump to begin infusion. Set alarm if recommended by manufacturer.	Pump delivers medication at controlled rate. Alarm is recommended for use with IV lock apparatus.
18. Recheck flow rate of primary IV once pump has completed delivery of medication.	Normal flow rate of primary IV may have been altered by mini-infusion pump.

Using a Volume-Control Administration Set

19. Withdraw medication from vial or ampule into prepared syringe. See Skill 5-2 or 5-3.	The correct dose is prepared for dilution in the IV solution.
20. Open clamp between IV solution and volume-control administration set or secondary setup. Follow manufacturer's instructions and fill with desired amount of IV solution. Close clamp.	This dilutes the medication in the minimal amount of solution. Reclamping prevents the continued addition of fluid to the volume to be mixed with medication.

Action 20: Bag with volume control set and tubing.

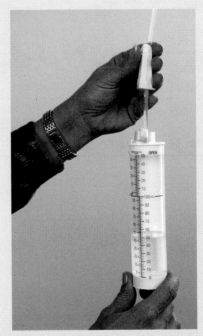

Action 20: Adjusting clamp between bag and volume control set.

21. Use antimicrobial swab to clean injection port on secondary setup.	This deters entry of microorganisms when needle punctures port.
22. Remove clamp and insert needle or blunt needleless device into port while holding syringe steady. Inject medication. Mix gently with IV solution.	This ensures that medication is evenly mixed with solution.

continues

SKILL
5-10 Administering IV Medications by Piggyback, Mini-infusion Pump, or Volume-Control Administration Set (continued)

ACTION	RATIONALE
23. Open clamp below secondary setup and regulate at pre-scribed delivery rate. Monitor medication infusion at periodic intervals.	Delivery over a 30- to 60-minute interval is a safe method of administering IV medication.
24. **Attach the medication label to the volume-control device.**	This prevents medication error.
25. Place syringe with uncapped needle in designated container.	Proper disposal of needle protects the nurse against accidental injection. Most accidental puncture wounds occur when recapping needles.

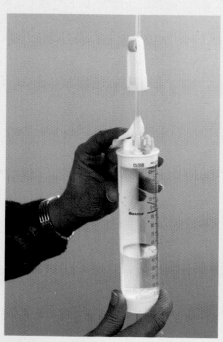

Action 21: Cleaning injection port.

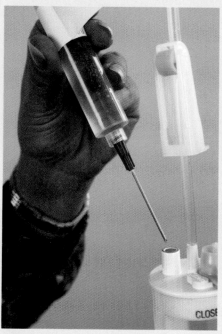

Action 22: Holding syringe steady while inserting blunt needleless device into port and injecting medication.

26. Perform hand hygiene.	Hand hygiene deters the spread of microorganisms.
27. Chart administration of medication after it has been infused. This can be done on the CMAR.	Accurate documentation is necessary to prevent medication errors.
28. Evaluate patient's response to medication within appropriate time frame.	Patient requires careful observation because medications given by the parenteral route may have a rapid effect.

continues

Administering IV Medications by Piggyback, Mini-infusion Pump, or Volume-Control Administration Set (continued)

ACTION   RATIONALE

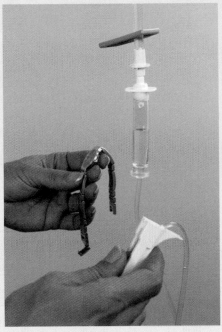

Action 23: Adjusting flow rate of primary fluid.

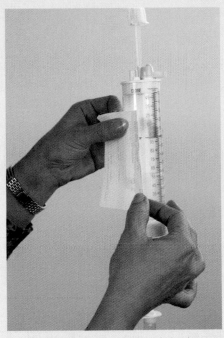

Action 24: Applying medication label to burette.

EVALUATION

The expected outcomes are met when the patient has received the medication via the parenteral route; experienced no, or minimal, discomfort; experienced no allergy response; and experienced no infection; and the patient understood the rationale for medication administration.

Unexpected Situations and Associated Interventions

- *Upon assessing the IV site before administering medication, the nurse notes that the IV has infiltrated:* Stop IV fluid and remove the IV from the extremity. Restart the IV in a different location. Continue to monitor the new IV site as medication is administered.
- *While administering medication, the nurse notes a cloudy, white substance forming in the IV tubing:* Stop the IV from flowing and stop administering the medication to prevent precipitate from entering the patient's circulation. Clamp the IV at the site nearest to the patient. The tubing will need to be flushed thoroughly to rid of any remaining precipitate. Always check the literature regarding incompatibilities of medications before administering.
- *While nurse is administering medication, the patient begins to complain of pain at the IV site:* Stop the medication. Assess the IV site for any signs of infiltration or phlebitis. You may want to flush the IV with normal saline to check for patency. If the IV site appears within normal limits, resume medication administration at a slower rate.

Infant and Child Considerations

- Small infants and children with fluid restrictions may not tolerate the added IV fluid needed for administration with piggyback or volume-control systems. For these children, consider using the mini-infusion pump.

A heparin or saline lock, or intermittent venous access device, is used for patients who require intermittent IV medication but not a continuous IV infusion. This device consists of a needle or catheter connected to a short length of tubing capped with a sealed injection port. After the catheter is in place in the patient's vein, the catheter and tubing are anchored to the patient's arm so that the catheter remains in place until the patient no longer requires the repeated IV medication.

An IV lock allows the patient more freedom than a continuous IV infusion. The patient is connected to the IV line when it is time to receive the medication and disconnected when the medication is completed. A saline flush rather than a heparin flush is used in many agencies to maintain the patency of the lock. Using saline eliminates any possible systemic effects on coagulation, development of a heparin allergy, and drug incompatibility that may occur when a heparin solution is used. The intermittent infusion is not started until the nurse confirms IV placement. The saline lock is flushed after the infusion is completed to clear the vein of any medication. Positive pressure is used when flushing a saline lock to prevent clot formation in the catheter.

Equipment

- Medication
- Saline vial
- Sterile syringe (two) with needleless device or 25-gauge needle
- Antimicrobial swabs
- Watch with second hand or stopwatch feature
- Gloves (optional)
- Medication Kardex or computer-generated MAR

For Bolus Injection:

- Sterile syringe (two) with needleless device

For Intermittent IV Delivery

- Needleless device or 25-gauge needle
- IV setup with needleless device attached to tubing or a 25-gauge needle
- Adhesive tape (optional)

ASSESSMENT

Assess the patient for allergies. Assess the patient's knowledge of the medication. If patient has a knowledge deficit, this may be an appropriate time to begin education about the medication. Assess the patient's IV site, noting any swelling, coolness, leaking of fluid from IV site, or pain.

NURSING DIAGNOSIS

Determine related factors for the nursing diagnoses based on the patient's current status. Appropriate nursing diagnoses may include:

- Acute Pain
- Risk for Allergy Response
- Risk for Infection
- Deficient Knowledge

OUTCOME IDENTIFICATION AND PLANNING

The expected outcome to achieve when introducing drugs through a heparin or IV lock using the saline flush is that the medication is delivered via the parenteral route. Other outcomes that may be appropriate include the following: patient experiences no or minimal discomfort; patient experiences no allergy response; patient experiences no infection; and patient understands the rationale for medication administration.

continues

IMPLEMENTATION

ACTION	RATIONALE
1. Assemble equipment and check physician's order.	This ensures that the patient receives the right medication at the right time by the proper route.
2. Identify patient by checking identification band on patient's wrist and asking patient his or her name. Explain procedure to patient.	This ensures that the right patient is receiving the medication. Explanation alleviates the patient's apprehension about IV drug administration.
3. Perform hand hygiene.	Hand hygiene deters the spread of microorganisms.
4. Withdraw 1 to 2 mL of sterile saline from the vial into the syringe as described in Skill 5-3.	Using saline eliminates concerns about drug incompatibilities and the effect on systemic circulation that exists with heparin.
5. Don clean gloves and prepare to administer medication.	Gloves protect the nurse's hands from contact with the patient's blood.
6. **For Bolus IV Injection:**	
a. **Check drug package for correct injection rate for IV push route.**	a. Using the correct injection rate prevents speed shock from occurring.
b. Clean port of lock with antimicrobial swab.	b. Cleaning removes surface bacteria at the lock entry site.
c. Stabilize port with your nondominant hand and insert needleless device or needle of syringe of normal saline into port.	c. This allows for careful insertion into the center circle of the lock.

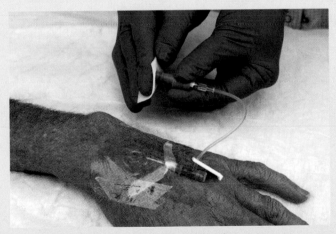

Action 6b: Cleaning port with antimicrobial swab.

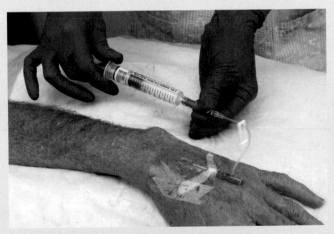

Action 6c: Inserting syringe with blunt needle into port.

d. Aspirate gently and check for blood return (blood return does not always occur even though lock is patent).	d. Blood return usually indicates that the catheter is in the vein.
e. Gently flush with 1 mL of normal saline. Remove syringe.	e. Saline flush ensures that the IV line is patent. A patient's complaint of pain or resistance to the flush detected by the nurse may indicate that the IV line is not patent.
f. Insert needleless device or needle of syringe with medication into port and gently inject medication, using a watch to verify correct injection rate. **Do not force the injection if resistance is felt.** If the lock is clogged, it must be changed. Remove medication syringe and needle when administration is complete.	f. Easy installation of medication usually indicates that the lock is still patent and in the vein. If force is used against resistance, a clot may break away and cause a blockage elsewhere in the body.

continues

SKILL 5-11   Introducing Drugs Through a Heparin or IV Lock Using the Saline Flush (continued)

ACTION

RATIONALE

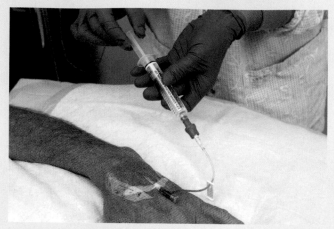

Action 6d: Aspirating for blood return.

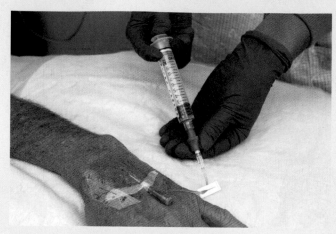

Action 6e: Flushing saline lock.

g. Remove syringe with medication from port. Stabilize port with your nondominant hand and insert needleless device or needle of syringe of normal saline into port. **Slowly flush reservoir with 1 to 2 mL of sterile saline using positive pressure.** To gain positive pressure, you can either clamp the IV tubing as you are still flushing the last of the saline into the IV or remove the syringe as you are still flushing the remainder of the saline into the IV. Remove syringe and discard uncapped needles and syringes in the appropriate receptacle. Remove gloves and discard appropriately.

g. Positive pressure prevents blood from backing into IV catheter and causing the IV to clot off.

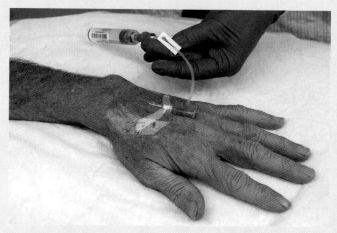

Action 6g: Clamping IV.

7. **For Drug Administration via an Intermittent Delivery System:**

a. Use a drug resource book to check for the correct flow rate of the medication (the usual is 30 to 60 minutes).

b. Connect infusion tubing to medication setup according to manufacturer's directions using sterile technique. Hang IV setup on pole. Open clamp and allow solution to clear IV tubing of air. Reclamp tubing.

c. Attach needleless connector or sterile 25-gauge needle to end of infusion tubing.

d. Clean port of lock with antimicrobial swab.

e. Stabilize port with your nondominant hand and insert needleless device or needle of syringe of normal saline into port.

a. Using the correct injection rate prevents speed shock from occurring.

b. This removes air from the tubing and preserves the sterility of the setup.

c. A small-gauge needle prevents damage to the lock.

d. Cleaning removes surface bacteria at the lock entry site.

e. This allows for careful insertion into the port.

continues

Introducing Drugs Through a Heparin or IV Lock Using the Saline Flush (continued)

ACTION   **RATIONALE**

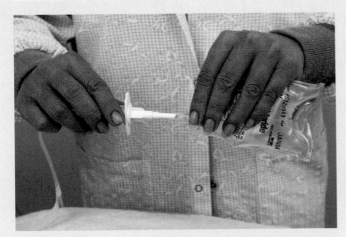

Action 7b: Spiking bag with tubing.

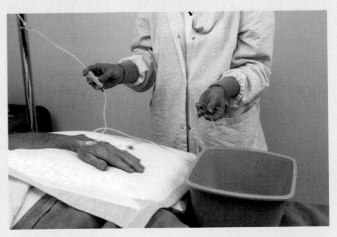

Action 7b: Priming tubing.

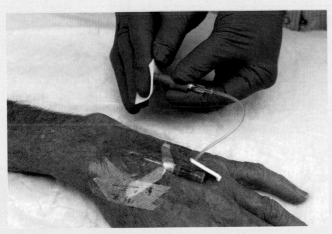

Action 7d: Cleaning port with antimicrobial swab.

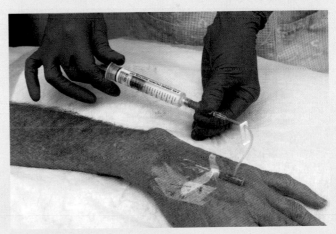

Action 7e: Inserting syringe into port.

f. Aspirate gently and check for blood return (blood return does not always occur even though lock is patent).

g. Gently flush with 1 mL of normal saline. Remove syringe.

h. Insert blunt needleless device or needle attached to tubing into port. If necessary, secure with tape.

i. Open clamp and regulate flow rate or attach to IV pump or controller according to manufacturer's directions. Close clamp when infusion is complete.

j. Remove needleless connector or needle from lock. Carefully replace uncapped, used needle or needleless device with a new sterile one. Allow medication setup to hang on pole for future use according to agency policy. Stabilize port with your nondominant hand and insert needleless device or needle of syringe of normal saline into the port. **Slowly flush the reservoir with 1 to 2 mL of sterile saline using positive pressure.**

f. Blood return usually indicates that the catheter is in the vein.

g. Saline flush ensures that the IV line is patent.

h. Tape secures the needle in the lock port.

i. This ensures that the patient receives the medication at the correct rate.

j. This prevents possible needlestick with contaminated needle. Agency policy specifies length of time for safe use of IV infusion tubing. Saline clears the line of medication with less of the systemic effects of the heparin flush. Positive pressure prevents blood from backing into IV catheter and causing the IV to clot off.

continues

SKILL
5-11

Introducing Drugs Through a Heparin or IV Lock Using the Saline Flush (continued)

ACTION	RATIONALE

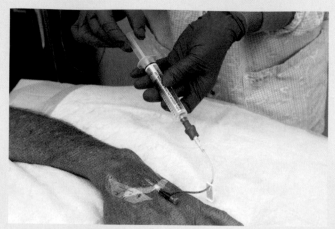

Action 7f: Aspirating for blood return.

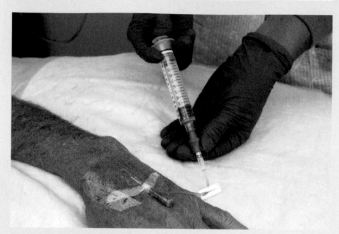

Action 7g: Flushing saline lock.

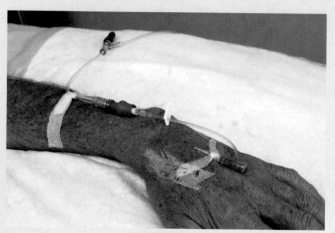

Action 7h: Attaching tubing to saline lock.

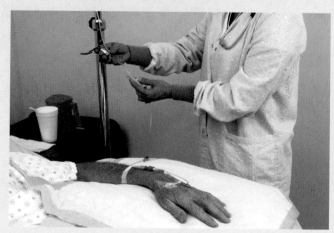

Action 7i: Regulating flow rate manually.

To gain positive pressure, you can either clamp the IV tubing as you are still flushing the last of the saline into the IV or remove the syringe as you are still flushing the remainder of the saline into the IV. Remove syringe and discard uncapped needles and syringes in appropriate receptacle. Remove gloves and discard appropriately.

8. Perform hand hygiene.

9. Check injection site and IV lock at least every 8 hours and administer a small amount of saline (2 to 3 mL) if medication is not given at least every 8 to 12 hours.

10. **Change heparin lock at least every 72 to 96 hours or according to agency policy.** A lock that is not patent should be changed immediately.

11. Chart administration of medication or saline flush.

Hand hygiene deters the spread of microorganisms.

This ensures patency of system for continuing injections.

Changing a heparin lock regularly and having it free of clotted blood reduces dangers of infection and emboli in the circulating blood.

Accurate documentation is necessary to prevent medication error.

continues

SKILL 5-11   Introducing Drugs Through a Heparin or IV Lock Using the Saline Flush (continued)

ACTION	RATIONALE

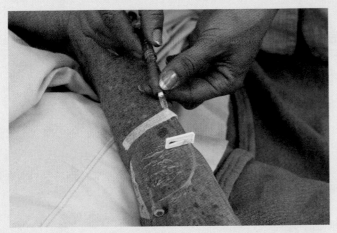

Action 7i: Removing tubing from lock.

EVALUATION

The expected outcomes are met when the patient has received the medication via the parenteral route; experienced no or minimal discomfort; experienced no allergy response; remains infection free; and understood the rationale for medication administration.

Unexpected Situations and Associated Interventions

- *Upon assessing the IV site before administering medication, nurse notes that the IV has infiltrated:* Stop IV fluid and remove IV from extremity. Restart IV in a different location. Continue to monitor new IV site as medication is administered.
- *While nurse is administering medication, patient begins to complain of pain at the IV site:* Stop the medication. Assess the IV site for any signs of infiltration or phlebitis. You may want to flush the IV with normal saline to check for patency. If the IV site appears within normal limits, resume medication administration at a slower rate.
- *Nurse notes white, cloudy particles forming in lock during medication administration:* Stop administering the medication. Remove needle or needleless device from lock. Insert needle or needleless device attached to empty syringe and pull back on plunger, attempting to remove any fluid remaining in lock. If unable to pull back fluid, change lock on IV before resuming medication administration. Entire IV setup and lock may need to be changed.
- *As nurse is attempting to access lock, needle or tip of syringe touches patient's arm:* Discard needle and syringe. Prepare new dose for administration.

Special Considerations

- Some agencies recommend the use of single-dose saline vials without preservative in the solution. Preservatives may be linked to an increased incidence of phlebitis with heparin locks.

Infant and Child Considerations

- If the volume of medication being administered is small (<1.0 mL), always include the amount of flush solution as part of the total amount to be injected and take this into account when determining how fast to push a medication. For example, if the medication is to be injected at a rate of 1.0 mL per minute and the total amount of solution to be injected is 2.25 mL (0.25 mL medication volume plus 2.0 mL saline flush solution volume equals 2.25 ml), then the medication would be injected over a period of 2 minutes 15 seconds.

SKILL 5-12   Applying a Transdermal Patch

The transdermal route is being used more frequently to deliver medication. This involves application to the skin of a disk or patch that contains medication intended for daily use or for longer intervals. Transdermal patches are commonly used to deliver hormones, narcotic analgesics, and nicotine. Medication errors have occurred when patients applied multiple patches at once or failed to remove the overlay on the patch that exposes the skin to the medication. Narcotic analgesic patches are associated with the most adverse drug effects. Clear patches have a cosmetic advantage but can be difficult to find on the patient's skin when they need to be removed or replaced. Despite a slow onset of action, transdermal drug patches maintain consistent serum drug levels.

Equipment
- Medication
- Gloves
- Scissors (optional)
- Washcloth, soap and water
- Medication Kardex or computer-generated MAR

ASSESSMENT

Assess the patient for allergies. Assess the skin at the location where the patch will be applied. Transdermal patches should not be placed on irritated or broken skin. Check the manufacturer's instructions for location of the patch. Assess the patient for any old patches. A new transdermal patch should not be placed until old patches have been removed. Assess the patient's knowledge about the medication. If the patient has a knowledge deficit, now may be an appropriate time for education.

NURSING DIAGNOSIS

Determine related factors for the nursing diagnoses based on the patient's current status. Appropriate nursing diagnoses may include:
- Risk for Allergy Response
- Deficient Knowledge
- Risk for Impaired Skin Integrity

OUTCOME IDENTIFICATION AND PLANNING

The expected outcome to achieve when applying a transdermal patch is that the medication is delivered successfully via the transdermal route. Other outcomes that may be appropriate include the following: patient experiences no allergy response; patient understands the rationale for medication administration; patient's skin remains free from injury.

IMPLEMENTATION

ACTION	RATIONALE
1. Bring equipment to patient's bedside. Check medication order against original physician's order according to agency policy.	Having equipment available saves time and facilitates performance of task. Checking the orders ensures that patient receives the correct medication at the correct time and in the right manner.
2. Identify patient by checking identification band on patient's wrist and asking patient his or her name. Ask patient about any allergies.	This ensures that the medication is given to the right person.
3. Explain procedure to patient.	Explanation allays patient anxiety.
4. Perform hand hygiene and don gloves.	Hand hygiene deters the spread of microorganisms. Gloves protect the nurse when handling the medication on the transdermal patch.

continues

SKILL 5-12   Applying a Transdermal Patch (continued)

ACTION	RATIONALE
5. Assess patient's skin where patch is to be placed, looking for any signs of irritation or breakdown. Find place that does not have a large amount of hair. **If patient has a large amount of hair on chest or back, scissors may be used to trim hair.** Do not shave hair.	Transdermal patches should not be placed on skin that is irritated or broken down. Hair can prevent the patch from sticking to the skin. Shaving has been shown to cause small cuts on the skin's surface that may lead to infection.
6. **Remove any old transdermal patches from the patient's skin.** Gently wash the area where the old patch was with soap and water.	Leaving old patches on patient while applying new ones may lead to delivery of a toxic level of the drug. Washing area with soap and water removes all traces of medication in that area.
7. Remove cover of patch without touching adhesive side. Put patch on patient's skin, pressing firmly with palm of hand for 10 seconds.	Touching the adhesive side may alter the amount of medication left on the patch. Pressing firmly for 10 seconds ensures that the patch stays on the patient's skin.
8. On transdermal patch, write your initials, date, and time.	This prevents medication error by ensuring that old patches are removed.

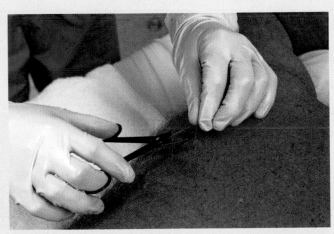

Action 5: Trimming excess hair using scissors.

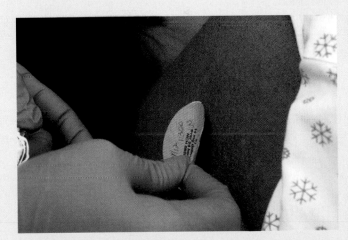

Action 6: Removing old patch.

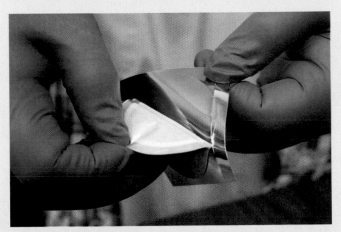

Action 7: Removing backing from patch.

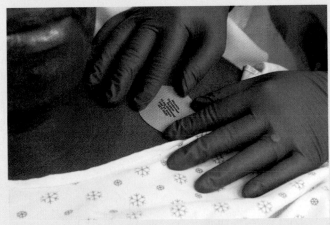

Action 7: Applying pressure to transdermal patch.

continues

ACTION	RATIONALE

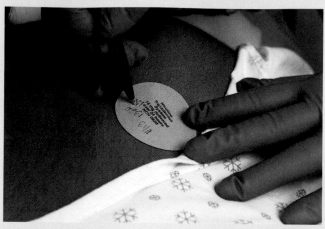

Action 8: Transdermal patch with date and time of application and nurse's initials.

9. Remove gloves and perform hand hygiene.

Hand hygiene deters the spread of microorganisms.

10. Chart site of patch administration. This may be done on the CMAR.

Accurate documentation is necessary to prevent medication errors.

11. Evaluate patient's response to medication within appropriate time frame.

Patient needs to be evaluated to ensure that patch is delivering drug appropriately and that patient is not experiencing any adverse effects.

EVALUATION

The expected outcomes are met when the patient has received the medication via the transdermal patch; experienced no allergic response; and understood rationale for medication administration; and patient's skin has remained intact.

Unexpected Situations and Associated Interventions

- *Nurse did not wear gloves while applying transdermal patch:* Immediately perform good hand hygiene. The nurse may feel the effects of the medication if any came into contact with his or her skin.
- *Nurse finds more than one old transdermal patch while applying new transdermal patch:* Remove all old patches of the same kind; remember that more than one medication may be delivered via transdermal patch. Check physician orders to ensure that patient is still receiving medication. Failure to remove old transdermal patches is considered a medication error in some institutions. Follow agency policy regarding paperwork for medication errors.
- *When removing an old transdermal patch, nurse notes skin underneath is erythematous and swollen:* Wash skin with soap and water and assess patient for any latex or adhesive allergies. Discuss with patient whether patch site has been rotated. Notify physician before applying a new patch.

Instilling Eyedrops

Eyedrops are instilled for their local effects, such as for pupil dilation or constriction when examining the eye, for treating an infection, or to help control intraocular pressure (for patients with glaucoma). The type and amount of solution depend on the purpose of the instillation.

Equipment
- Gloves
- Medication
- Tissue, washcloth
- Medication Kardex or computer-generated MAR

ASSESSMENT

Assess the patient for allergies. Assess the affected eye for any drainage, erythema, or swelling. Assess the patient's knowledge of medication. If patient has a knowledge deficit, this may be an appropriate time to begin education about the medication.

NURSING DIAGNOSIS

Determine related factors for the nursing diagnoses based on the patient's current status. Appropriate nursing diagnoses may include:
- Risk for Allergy Response
- Risk for Injury
- Deficient Knowledge

OUTCOME IDENTIFICATION AND PLANNING

The expected outcome to achieve when administering eyedrops is that the medication is delivered successfully into the eye. Other outcomes that may be appropriate include the following: patient experiences no allergy response; patient's eye remains free from injury; and patient understands the rationale for medication administration.

IMPLEMENTATION

ACTION	RATIONALE
1. Bring equipment to patient's bedside. Check medication order against original physician's order according to agency policy.	Having equipment available saves time and facilitates performance of task. Checking the order ensures that the patient receives the correct medication at the correct time and in the right manner.
2. Identify patient by checking identification band on patient's wrist and asking patient his or her name. Ask patient about any allergies.	This ensures that the medication is given to the right person.
3. Explain procedure to patient.	Explanation allays patient anxiety.
4. Perform hand hygiene and don gloves.	Hand hygiene deters the spread of microorganisms. Gloves protect the nurse when coming in contact with drainage from eyes (solution or tears).
5. Offer tissue to patient.	Solution and tears may spill from the eye during the procedure.
6. **Cleanse the eyelids and eyelashes of any drainage with a washcloth moistened with normal saline solution, proceeding from the inner canthus to the outer canthus. Use each area of the washcloth only once.**	Debris can be carried into the eye when the conjunctival sac is exposed. By using each area of washcloth once and going from the inner canthus to the outer canthus, debris is kept away from the lacrimal duct.
7. Tilt patient's head back slightly. The head may be turned slightly to the affected side.	Tilting patient's head back slightly makes it easier to reach the conjunctival sac. This should be avoided if the patient has a cervical spine injury. Turning the head to the affected side helps to prevent solution or tears from flowing toward the opposite eye.

continues

SKILL 5-13 Instilling Eyedrops (continued)

ACTION	RATIONALE

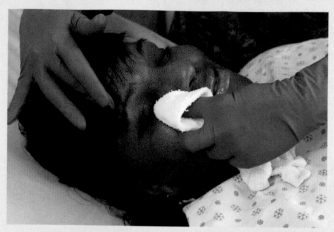

Action 6: Cleaning lids and lashes from inside of eye to outside.

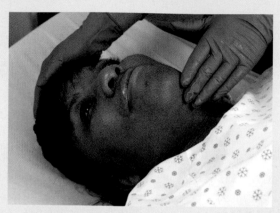

Action 7: Positioning patient for eyedrops.

8. Remove cap from medication bottle, being careful to not touch the inner side of the cap.

Touching the inner side of the cap may contaminate the bottle of medication.

9. Invert the monodrip plastic container that is commonly used to instill eyedrops. Have patient look up and focus on something on the ceiling.

By having the patient look up and focus on something else, the procedure is less traumatic.

10. Place thumb or two fingers near margin of lower eyelid immediately below eyelashes, and exert pressure downward over bony prominence of cheek. Lower conjunctival sac is exposed as lower lid is pulled down.

The eyedrop should be placed in the conjunctival sac, not directly on the eyeball.

11. **Hold dropper close to eye, but avoid touching eyelids or lashes. Squeeze container and allow prescribed number of drops to fall in lower conjunctival sac.**

Touching the eye, eyelids, or lashes can contaminate the medication in the bottle; startle the patient, causing blinking; or injure the eye. Do not allow medication to fall onto cornea. This may injure the cornea or cause the patient to have an unpleasant sensation.

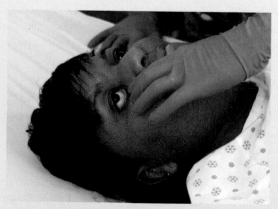

Action 10: Holding eye in position.

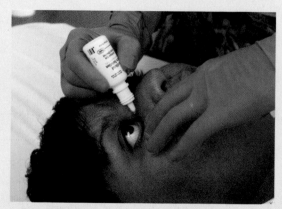

Action 11: Administering eyedrops.

continues

Instilling Eyedrops (continued)

ACTION	RATIONALE
12. Release lower lid after eyedrops are instilled. Ask patient to close eyes gently.	This allows the medication to be distributed over the entire eye.
13. Apply gentle pressure over inner canthus to prevent eyedrops from flowing into tear duct.	This minimizes the risk of systemic effects from the medication.

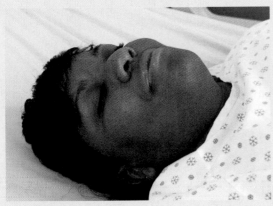

Action 12: Eyes closed.

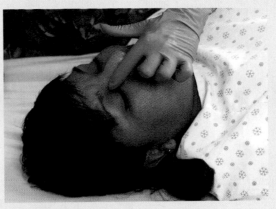

Action 13: Applying pressure.

14. Instruct patient not to rub affected eye.	This prevents injury and irritation to eye.
15. Remove gloves and perform hand hygiene.	Hand hygiene deters the spread of microorganisms.
16. Chart administration of medication. This may be done on the CMAR.	Accurate documentation is necessary to prevent medication errors.
17. Evaluate patient's response to medication within appropriate time frame.	The patient needs to be evaluated for any adverse affects from the medication.

EVALUATION

The expected outcomes are met when the patient has received the eyedrops; experienced no adverse affects, including allergy response or injury; and understood the rationale for the medication administration.

Unexpected Situations and Associated Interventions

- *Drop is placed on eyelid or outer margin of eyelid due to patient blinking or moving:* Do not count this drop in total number of drops administered. Allow the patient to regain composure and proceed with application of medication.
- *Nurse cannot open eyelids due to dried crust and matting of eyelids:* Place a warm wet washcloth over the eye and allow it to remain there for approximately 3 minutes. You may need to repeat this procedure if there is a large amount of matting.
- *Bottle comes in contact with eyeball when applying medication:* Bottle is contaminated; discard appropriately. Notify pharmacy or retrieve new bottle for oncoming shift.

Infant and Child Considerations

- To apply eyedrops in a small child, two or more people may be needed to restrain the child. Make sure the child does not reach up to the eye for fear of jabbing the medication bottle into the eye.

Administering an Eye Irrigation

Eye irrigation is performed to remove secretions or foreign bodies or to cleanse and soothe the eye. Whenever irrigating one eye, care should be taken so that the overflowing irrigation fluid does not contaminate the other eye.

Equipment

- Sterile irrigating solution (warmed to 37°C [98.6°F])
- Sterile irrigation set (sterile container and irrigating or bulb syringe)
- Emesis basin or irrigation basin
- Washcloth
- Waterproof pad
- Towel
- Disposable gloves
- Medication Kardex or computer-generated MAR

ASSESSMENT

Assess the patient's knowledge of the procedure. If patient has a knowledge deficit about the procedure, this may be an appropriate time to begin patient education. Assess the patient's level of consciousness to determine whether the patient will cooperate with the procedure.

NURSING DIAGNOSIS

Determine related factors for the nursing diagnoses based on the patient's current status. Appropriate nursing diagnoses may include:

- Deficient Knowledge
- Noncompliance
- Risk for Injury
- Acute Pain

OUTCOME IDENTIFICATION AND PLANNING

The expected outcome to achieve when administering eye irrigation is that the eye is cleansed successfully. Other outcomes that may be appropriate include the following: patient understands the rationale for the procedure and is able to participate willingly; patient's eye remains free from injury; and patient remains free from pain.

IMPLEMENTATION

ACTION	RATIONALE
1. Explain procedure to patient.	Explanation facilitates cooperation and reassures patient.
2. Assemble equipment at patient's bedside.	This provides for an organized approach to the task.
3. Perform hand hygiene.	Hand hygiene deters the spread of microorganisms.
4. Have patient sit or lie with head tilted toward side of affected eye. Protect patient and bed with a waterproof pad.	Gravity aids flow of solution away from unaffected eye and from inner canthus of affected eye toward outer canthus.
5. Don disposable gloves. Clean lids and lashes with washcloth moistened with normal saline or the solution ordered for the irrigation. Wipe from inner canthus to outer canthus. Use a different corner of washcloth with each wipe.	Materials lodged on lids or in lashes may be washed into eye. This cleaning motion protects nasolacrimal duct and other eye.
6. Place curved basin at cheek on side of affected eye to receive irrigating solution. If patient is sitting up, ask him or her to support the basin.	Gravity aids flow of solution.
7. Expose lower conjunctival sac and hold upper lid open with your nondominant hand.	Solution is directed into lower conjunctival sac because cornea is sensitive and easily injured. This also prevents reflex blinking.

continues

Administering an Eye Irrigation (continued)

ACTION

RATIONALE

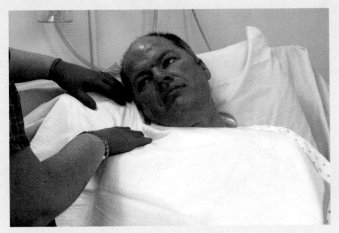

Action 4: Patient positioned for eye irrigation.

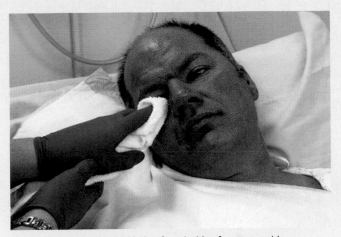

Action 5: Cleaning lids and lashes from inside of eye to outside.

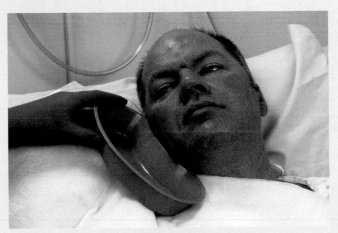

Action 6: Basin in place to catch irrigating fluid.

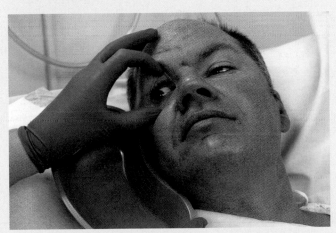

Action 7: Holding eyelid in position.

8. **Hold irrigator about 2.5 cm (1″) from eye. Direct flow of solution from inner to outer canthus along conjunctival sac.**

This minimizes the risk for injury to the cornea. Directing solution toward the outer canthus helps to prevent the spread of contamination from the eye to the lacrimal sac, the lacrimal duct, and the nose.

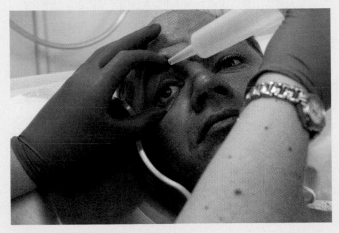

Action 8: Preparing to irrigate eye.

continues

SKILL 5-14   Administering an Eye Irrigation (continued)

ACTION	RATIONALE
9. Irrigate until the solution is clear or all the solution has been used. **Use only enough force to remove secretions gently from the conjunctiva. Avoid touching any part of the eye with the irrigating tip.**	Directing solutions with force may cause injury to the tissues of the eye as well as to the conjunctiva. Touching the eye is uncomfortable for the patient and may cause damage to the cornea.
10. Have patient close eye periodically during procedure.	Movement of the eye when the lids are closed helps to move secretions from the upper to the lower conjunctival sac.
11. Dry area after irrigation with gauze sponge. Offer towel to patient if face and neck are wet.	Leaving the skin moist after irrigation is uncomfortable for the patient.
12. Remove gloves and perform hand hygiene.	Hand hygiene deters the spread of microorganisms.
13. Chart the irrigation, appearance of eye, drainage, and patient's response.	This provides accurate documentation.

7/25/03   2210   Irrigation of left eye performed using 1000 mL of sterile water. The sclera of the eye remains reddened. Periorbital area remains slightly edematous. Prior to irrigation thick, yellow liquid was draining from eye. After irrigation no drainage is present. Patient tolerated procedure with little discomfort. Is refusing pain medication at this time. Rates pain as a 1/10.—K. Sanders, RN

Action 13: Documentation.

EVALUATION

The expected outcomes are met when the eye has been irrigated successfully; the patient understood the rationale for the procedure and complied with the procedure; the eye was not damaged; and the patient experienced minimal discomfort.

Unexpected Situations and Associated Interventions

- *Patient complains of a large amount of pain during procedure:* Stop the procedure and notify the physician. Physician may need to check for any foreign objects such as glass before proceeding with irrigation.
- *Patient cannot keep the eye open during the procedure:* Nurse may need assistance to help patient keep the eye open.

Instilling Eardrops

Drugs are instilled into the auditory canal for their local effect. They are used to soften wax, relieve pain, apply local anesthesia, destroy organisms, or destroy an insect lodged in the canal, which can cause almost intolerable discomfort. If the ear canal has swollen to the point that medication cannot pass, a long piece of cotton material called a wick is inserted so that one end is near the middle ear and the other end is external. This cotton acts as a wick to help medication get to the inner ear.

The tympanic membrane separates the external ear from the middle ear. Normally, it is intact and closes the entrance to the middle ear completely. If it is ruptured or has been opened by surgical intervention, the middle ear and the inner ear have a direct passage to the external ear. When this occurs, instillations should be performed with the greatest of care to prevent forcing materials from the outer ear into the middle ear and the inner ear. Sterile technique is used to prevent infection.

Equipment

- Medication (warmed to 37°C [98.6°F])
- Tissue
- Cotton ball (optional)
- Gloves (optional)
- Washcloth (optional)
- Medication Kardex or computer-generated MAR

ASSESSMENT

Assess the affected ear for any drainage or tenderness. Assess the patient for allergies. Assess the patient's knowledge of medication. If the patient has a knowledge deficit about the medication, this may be an appropriate time to begin education.

NURSING DIAGNOSIS

Determine related factors for the nursing diagnoses based on the patient's current status. Appropriate nursing diagnoses may include:

- Deficient Knowledge
- Anxiety
- Acute Pain
- Risk for Allergy Response

OUTCOME IDENTIFICATION AND PLANNING

The expected outcome to achieve when administering eardrops is that drops are administered successfully. Other outcomes that may be appropriate include the following: patient understands the rationale for the ear drop instillation and has decreased anxiety; patient remains free from pain; and patient experiences no allergy response.

IMPLEMENTATION

ACTION	RATIONALE
1. Bring equipment to patient's bedside. Check physician's order.	Having equipment available saves time and facilitates performance of task. Checking the order ensures that the patient receives the correct medication at the correct time and in the right manner.
2. Identify patient by checking identification band on patient's wrist and asking patient his or her name. Ask patient regarding any medication allergies.	This ensures that the medication is given to the right person.
3. Explain procedure to patient.	Explanation allays patient anxiety.
4. Perform hand hygiene and don gloves (gloves are to be worn if drainage is present).	Hand hygiene deters the spread of microorganisms. Gloves protect the nurse when coming in contact with drainage from ear.

continues

ACTION	RATIONALE
5. Offer tissue to patient.	Solution may spill from the ear during the procedure and run toward the eye.
6. Cleanse external ear of any drainage with cotton ball or washcloth moistened with normal saline.	Debris and drainage may prevent some of the medication from entering the ear canal.
7. Place patient on unaffected side in bed, or if ambulatory, have patient sit with head well tilted to the side so that affected ear is uppermost.	This positioning prevents the drops from escaping from the ear.
8. Draw up amount of solution needed in dropper. Do not return excess medication to stock bottle. A prepackaged monodrip plastic container may also be used.	Risk for contamination is increased when medication is returned to the stock bottle.
9. **Straighten auditory canal by pulling cartilaginous portion of pinna up and back in an adult and down and back in an infant or a child younger than 3 years.**	Pulling on the pinna as described helps to straighten the canal properly for ear drop instillation.

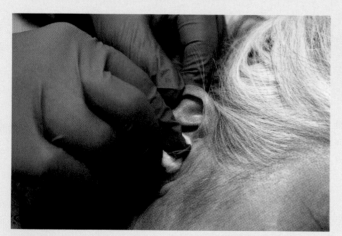

Action 6: Cleaning external ear.

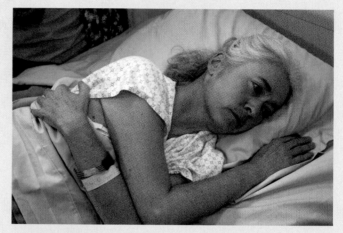

Action 7: Adult positioned for ear drop instillation.

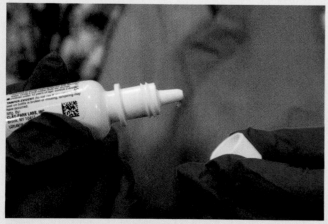

Action 8: Prepackaged ear drop solution.

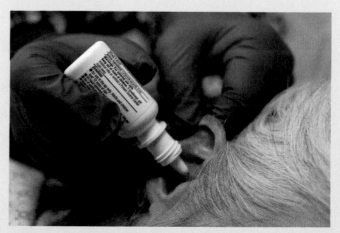

Action 9: Technique for administering ear drops in adult.

continues

SKILL 5-15 Instilling Eardrops (continued)

ACTION	RATIONALE

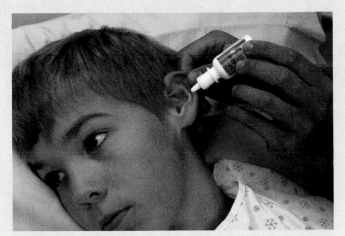

Action 9: Technique for administering ear drops in child over 3 years old.

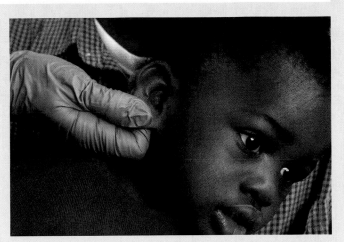

Action 9: Technique for administering eardrops in child under 3 years old.

10. Hold dropper in ear with its tip above auditory canal. For an infant or an irrational or confused patient, protect dropper with a piece of soft tubing to help prevent injury to ear.

By holding the dropper in the ear, the majority of medication will enter the ear canal. The hard tip of the dropper can damage the tympanic membrane if it is jabbed into the ear.

11. **Allow drops to fall on side of canal.**

It is uncomfortable for the patient if drops fall directly onto the tympanic membrane.

12. Release pinna after instilling drops, and have patient maintain the position to prevent escape of medication.

Medication should remain in ear canal for at least 5 minutes.

13. Gently press on tragus a few times.

Pressing on tragus causes medication from canal to move toward tympanic membrane.

14. If ordered, loosely insert a cotton ball into ear canal.

Cotton ball can help prevent medication from leaking out of ear canal.

15. Remove gloves and perform hand hygiene.

Hand hygiene deters the spread of microorganisms.

16. Document medication administration and any drainage from ear noted. Documentation may be done on CMAR.

This provides accurate documentation and helps to prevent medication errors.

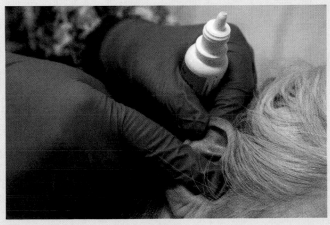

Action 13: Applying pressure to tragus.

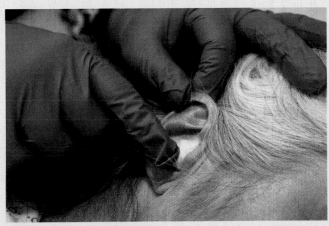

Action 14: Cotton ball inserted in ear.

continues

SKILL 5-15 Instilling Eardrops (continued)

EVALUATION

The expected outcomes are met when the patient has received the eardrops successfully; understood the rationale for ear drop instillation and exhibited no or decreased anxiety; experienced no or minimal pain; and experienced no allergy response.

Unexpected Situations and Associated Interventions

- *Medication runs from ear into eye:* Notify physician and check with the pharmacy. Eye irrigation (Skill 5-14) may need to be performed.
- *Patient complains of extreme pain when nurse presses on tragus:* Allow patient to press on tragus. If pain is too much, this part may be deferred.

Infant and Child Considerations

- Distraction techniques, such as TV or a quiet toy, may be helpful when attempting to keep a child quiet for 5 minutes. Reading to the child may not be appropriate because the child's hearing may be compromised during medication administration.

SKILL 5-16 Administering an Ear Irrigation

Irrigations of the external auditory canal are ordinarily performed for cleaning purposes or for applying heat to the area. Typically, normal saline solution is used, although an antiseptic solution may be indicated for local action. To prevent pain, the irrigation solution should be at least at room temperature. An irrigation syringe is used in most instances. An irrigating container with tubing and an ear tip may also be used, especially if the purpose of the irrigation is to apply heat to the area.

Equipment

- Prescribed irrigating solution (warmed to 37°C [98.6°F])
- Irrigation set (container and irrigating or bulb syringe)
- Waterproof pad
- Emesis basin
- Cotton-tipped applicators
- Disposable gloves (optional)
- Cotton balls
- Medication Kardex or computer-generated MAR

ASSESSMENT

Assess the ear for any drainage or pain. Assess the patient's knowledge of the procedure.

NURSING DIAGNOSIS

Determine related factors for the nursing diagnoses based on the patient's current status. Appropriate nursing diagnoses may include:

- Acute Pain
- Deficient Knowledge

OUTCOME IDENTIFICATION AND PLANNING

The expected outcome to achieve when performing ear irrigation is that the irrigation is administered successfully. Other outcomes that may be appropriate include the following: patient remains free from pain, and patient understands the rationale for the procedure.

continues

SKILL 5-16   Administering an Ear Irrigation (continued)

IMPLEMENTATION

ACTION	RATIONALE
1. Explain procedure to patient.	Explanation facilitates cooperation and provides reassurance for the patient.
2. Bring equipment to patient's bedside. Check physician's order.	This provides for an organized approach to the task.
3. Perform hand hygiene.	Hand hygiene deters the spread of microorganisms.
4. Have patient sit up or lie with head tilted toward side of affected ear. Protect patient and bed with a waterproof pad. Have patient support basin under the ear to receive the irrigating solution.	Gravity causes the irrigating solution to flow from the ear to the basin.
5. Clean pinna and meatus at auditory canal as necessary with moistened cotton-tipped applicators dipped in warm tap water or the irrigating solution.	Materials lodged on the pinna and at the meatus may be washed into the ear.
6. Fill bulb syringe with warm solution. If an irrigating container is used, allow air to escape from tubing.	Air forced into the ear canal is noisy and therefore unpleasant for the patient.

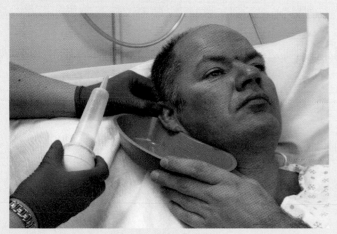

Action 4: Adult positioned for ear irrigation.

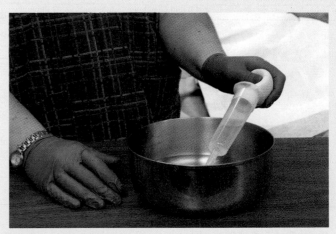

Action 6: Filling a bulb syringe.

7. Straighten auditory canal by pulling pinna down and back for an infant or child up to 3 years of age and up and back for an adult.	Straightening the ear canal allows solution to reach all areas of the canal easily.
8. **Direct a steady, slow stream of solution against the roof of the auditory canal, using only enough force to remove secretions. Do not occlude the auditory canal with the irrigating nozzle. Allow solution to flow out unimpeded.**	Directing the solution at the roof of the canal helps prevent injury to the tympanic membrane. Continuous in-and-out flow of the irrigating solution helps to prevent pressure in the canal.
9. When irrigation is complete, place cotton ball loosely in auditory meatus and have patient lie on side of affected ear on a towel or absorbent pad.	The cotton ball absorbs excess fluid, and gravity allows the remaining solution in the canal to escape from the ear.
10. Perform hand hygiene.	Hand hygiene deters the spread of microorganisms.
11. Chart irrigation, appearance of drainage, and patient's response.	This provides accurate documentation.
12. Return in 10 to 15 minutes and remove cotton ball and assess drainage.	Drainage or pain may indicate injury to the tympanic membrane.

continues

ACTION   **RATIONALE**

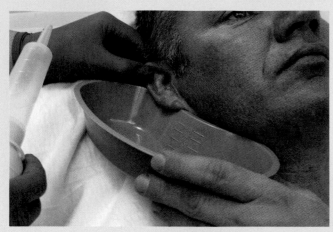

Action 7: Straightening the ear canal for irrigation in adult.

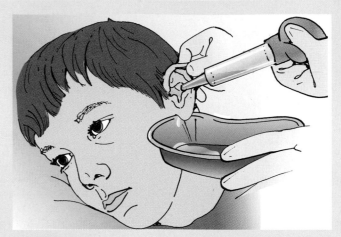

Action 7: Straightening the ear canal for irrigation in child over 3 years old.

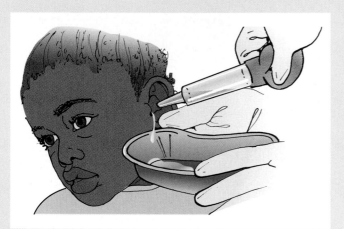

Action 7: Straightening the ear canal for irrigation in child under 3 years old.

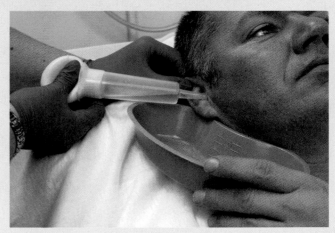

Action 8: Instilling irrigation fluid.

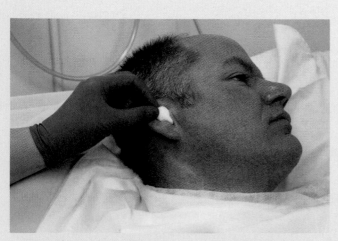

Action 9: Placing cotton ball in ear.

7/25/03   Irrigation of AS done with 100 mL of warmed normal saline. No drainage noted from ear canal. Patient tolerated procedure without discomfort. Rates ear pain as a 0/10.
—K. Sanders, RN

Action 11: Documentation.

continues

Administering an Ear Irrigation (continued)

EVALUATION

The expected outcomes are met when the ear canal has been irrigated successfully; patient experienced no or minimal pain or discomfort; and patient understood the rationale for the ear irrigation procedure.

Unexpected Situations and Associated Interventions

- *Patient complains of a large amount of pain during irrigation:* Stop the irrigation. Check the temperature of the solution. If the solution has cooled, rewarm it and try again. If the patient still complains of pain, stop the irrigation and notify the physician.

Instilling Nose Drops

Nasal instillations are used to treat allergies, sinus infections, and nasal congestion. Medications with a systemic effect, such as vasopressin, may also be prepared as a nasal instillation. The nose is normally not a sterile cavity, but because of its connection with the sinuses, medical asepsis should be observed carefully when using nasal instillations.

Equipment

- Medication
- Gloves
- Tissue
- Medication Kardex or computer-generated MAR

ASSESSMENT

Assess the patient for allergies. Assess the patient's knowledge of medication. If the patient has a knowledge deficit about the medication, this may be an appropriate time to begin education. Assess the nares for any drainage or broken skin.

NURSING DIAGNOSIS

Determine related factors for the nursing diagnoses based on the patient's current status. Appropriate nursing diagnoses may include:

- Deficient Knowledge
- Risk for Allergy Response
- Risk for Impaired Skin
- Acute Pain

OUTCOME IDENTIFICATION AND PLANNING

The expected outcome to achieve when instilling nose drops is that the medication is administered successfully. Other outcomes that may be appropriate include the following. patient understands the rationale for the nose drop instillation; patient experiences no allergy response; patient's skin remains intact; patient experiences no, or minimal, pain.

IMPLEMENTATION

ACTION	RATIONALE
1. Bring equipment to patient's bedside. Check physician's order.	Having equipment available saves time and facilitates performance of task. Checking the order ensures that the patient receives the correct medication at the correct time and in the right manner.
2. Identify patient by checking identification band on patient's wrist and asking patient his or her name. Also ask patient regarding any medication allergies.	This ensures that the medication is given to the right person.
3. Explain procedure to patient.	Explanation allays patient anxiety.

continues

Instilling Nose Drops (continued)

ACTION	RATIONALE
4. Perform hand hygiene and don gloves (gloves are to be worn if drainage is present).	Hand hygiene deters the spread of microorganisms. Gloves protect the nurse when coming in contact with drainage from nose.
5. **Provide patient with paper tissues and ask patient to blow his or her nose.**	Blowing the nose clears the nasal mucosa prior to medication administration.
6. Have patient sit up with head tilted well back. If patient is lying down, tilt head back over a pillow.	These positions allow the solution to flow well back into the nares. Do not tilt head if patient has a cervical spine injury.
7. Draw sufficient solution into dropper for both nares. Do not return excess solution to a stock bottle.	Returning solution to a stock bottle increases the risk for contamination of the stock bottle.

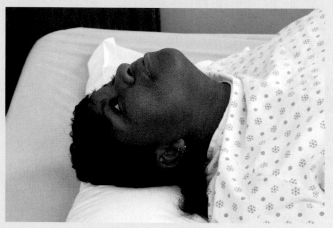

Action 6: Patient positioned for nose drops.

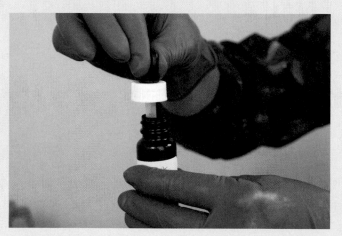

Action 7: Drawing up nose drops.

8. Hold tip of nose up and place dropper just inside naris, about one third of an inch. Instill prescribed number of drops in one naris and then into the other. Protect dropper with a piece of soft tubing if patient is an infant or young child. Avoid touching naris with dropper.	The soft tubing will protect the patient's nares from injury during administration of medication. Touching the naris may cause the patient to sneeze and will contaminate the dropper.

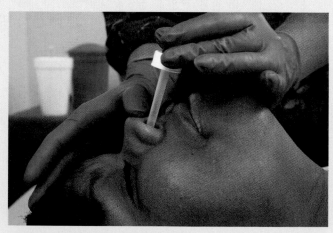

Action 8: Administering nose drops.

continues

SKILL 5-17 Instilling Nose Drops (continued)

9. Have patient remain in position with head tilted back for a few minutes.

Tilting the head back prevents the escape of the medication.

10. Document medication administration and any drainage from nose noted. Documentation may be done on the CMAR.

This provides accurate documentation and helps to prevent medication errors.

EVALUATION

The expected outcomes are met when the patient has received the nose drops successfully; understood the rationale for nose drop instillation; and experienced no allergy response; patient's skin remained intact; and patient experienced no, or minimal, pain or discomfort.

Unexpected Situations and Associated Interventions

- *Patient sneezes immediately after receiving nose drops:* Do not repeat the dosage, because you cannot determine how much medication was actually absorbed.

SKILL 5-18 Inserting a Vaginal Suppository or Cream

Creams, foams, and tablets can be applied intravaginally using a narrow, tubular applicator with an attached plunger. Suppositories that melt when exposed to body heat are also administered by vaginal insertion. Suppositories should be refrigerated for storage.

Ask the patient to void before inserting the medication. Position the patient so that she is lying on her back with the knees flexed. Maintain privacy with draping. Adequate light should be available to visualize the vaginal opening.

Equipment

- Medication
- Washcloth
- Gloves
- Medication Kardex or computer-generated MAR

ASSESSMENT

Assess the patient for allergies. Assess the patient's knowledge of the medication. If patient has a knowledge deficit about the medication, this may be an appropriate time to begin education. Assess the patient's perineal area for any drainage or broken skin.

NURSING DIAGNOSIS

Determine related factors for the nursing diagnoses based on the patient's current status. Appropriate nursing diagnoses may include:

- Deficient Knowledge
- Risk for Allergy Response
- Risk for Impaired Skin Integrity
- Acute Pain
- Anxiety

OUTCOME IDENTIFICATION AND PLANNING

The expected outcome to achieve when inserting a vaginal suppository or cream is that the medication is administered successfully. Other outcomes that may be appropriate include the following: patient understands the rationale for the vaginal instillation; patient experiences no allergy response; patient's skin remains intact; patient experiences no, or minimal, pain; and patient experiences minimal anxiety.

continues

SKILL
5-18   Inserting a Vaginal Suppository or Cream (continued)

IMPLEMENTATION

ACTION	RATIONALE
1. Bring equipment to patient's bedside. Check physician's order.	Having equipment available saves time and facilitates performance of task. Checking the order ensures that the patient receives the correct medication at the correct time and in the right manner.
2. Identify patient by checking identification band on patient's wrist and asking patient his or her name. Ask patient regarding any medication allergies.	This ensures that the medication is given to the right person.
3. Explain procedure to patient. Provide privacy.	Explanation allays patient anxiety.
4. Perform hand hygiene and don gloves.	Hand hygiene deters the spread of microorganisms. Gloves protect the nurse when coming in contact with drainage from vagina.
5. Fill vaginal applicator with prescribed amount of cream, or have suppository ready.	This ensures the correct dosage of medication will be administered.

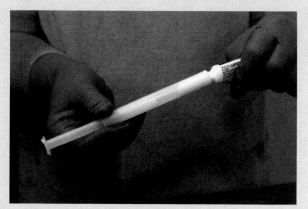

Action 5: Filling vaginal applicator with cream.

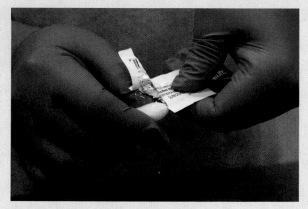

Action 6: Lubricating suppository.

6. Lubricate applicator with water, as necessary. A suppository may be lubricated with a water-soluble gel.

Ordinarily lubrication is unnecessary, but it may be used to reduce friction while inserting the applicator or suppository.

7. **Spread labia well with fingers, and clean area at vaginal orifice with washcloth and warm water, using a different corner of the washcloth with each stroke. Wipe from above orifice downward toward sacrum (front to back).**

These techniques prevent contamination of vaginal orifice with debris surrounding anus.

Administering Vaginal Cream With Applicator

8. Introduce applicator gently in a rolling manner while directing it downward and backward.

This follows the normal contour of the vagina for its full length.

9. After applicator is properly positioned, labia may be allowed to fall in place if necessary to free the hand for manipulating plunger. Push plunger to its full length and then gently remove applicator with plunger depressed.

Pushing the plunger will gently deploy the cream into the vaginal orifice.

continues

SKILL 5-18

Inserting a Vaginal Suppository or Cream (continued)

ACTION

RATIONALE

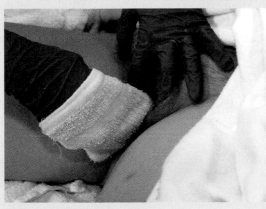

Action 7: Performing perineal care.

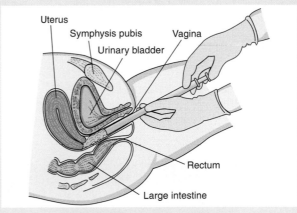

Action 8: Inserting vaginal cream using an applicator.

Inserting a Vaginal Suppository

10. Insert suppository well into vagina.

11. **Ask patient to remain in supine position for 5 to 10 minutes after insertion.**

12. Offer patient a perineal pad to collect drainage.

13. Remove gloves and perform hand hygiene.

14. Document medication administration, any drainage from vagina, and condition of skin in perineal area. Medication documentation may be performed on the CMAR.

If suppository is not adequately inserted into vagina, suppository may become dislodged and lie in perineal area.

This gives the medication time to be absorbed in the vaginal cavity.

As medication heats up, some medication may leak from vaginal orifice.

Hand hygiene deters the spread of microorganisms.

This provides accurate documentation and helps prevent medication errors.

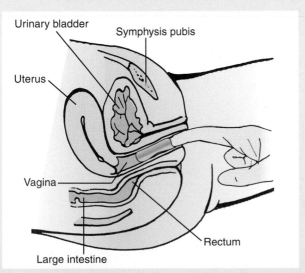

Action 10: Inserting suppository.

7/23/06 2300   Monistat vaginal suppository administered as ordered. Small amount of curdlike, white discharge noted from vagina. Perineal skin remains erythematous. Patient states, "It doesn't itch as much."
—K. Sanders, RN

Action 14: Documentation.

continues

SKILL 5-18 Inserting a Vaginal Suppository or Cream (continued)

EVALUATION

The expected outcomes are met when the patient has received vaginal medication successfully; patient understood the rationale for the medication administration; patient experienced no allergy response; patient's skin remained intact; patient experienced no or minimal discomfort; and patient experienced no or minimal anxiety.

Unexpected Situations and Associated Interventions

- *Upon assessing patient after administering a vaginal suppository, nurse notes the suppository is not in the vagina but instead is between the labia:* Don gloves and reinsert the suppository, ensuring that it is inserted fully.

SKILL 5-19 Applying an Insulin Pump

Some medications may be administered continuously via the subcutaneous route. One example of this is insulin.

Equipment

- Insulin pump
- Pump syringe
- Vial of insulin
- Sterile infusion set
- Insertion (triggering) device
- Needle (24 or 22 gauge, or blunt-ended needle)
- Antimicrobial swab (two)
- Sterile nonocclusive dressing
- Medication Kardex or computer-generated MAR

ASSESSMENT

Assess the patient for allergies. Assess the patient's knowledge of the medication. If the patient has a knowledge deficit, this may be an appropriate time to begin education about the medication. Assess skin in the area where the pump is to be applied. The pump should not be placed on skin that is irritated or broken down. The pump should be moved every 2 to 3 days.

NURSING DIAGNOSIS

Determine related factors for the nursing diagnoses based on the patient's current status. Appropriate nursing diagnoses may include:

- Deficient Knowledge
- Risk for Allergy Response
- Risk for Impaired Skin Integrity
- Acute Pain

OUTCOME IDENTIFICATION AND PLANNING

The expected outcome to achieve when inserting applying an insulin pump is that the device is attached successfully and medication is administered. Other outcomes that may be appropriate include the following: patient understands the rationale for the pump attachment; patient experiences no allergy response; patient's skin remains intact; and patient experiences no or minimal pain.

SKILL 5-19   Applying an Insulin Pump (continued)

IMPLEMENTATION

ACTION	RATIONALE
1. Bring equipment to patient's bedside. Check physician's order.	Having equipment available saves time and facilitates performance of task. Checking the order ensures that the patient receives the correct medication at the correct time and in the right manner.
2. Identify patient by checking identification band on patient's wrist and asking patient his or her name.	This ensures that the medication is given to the right person.
3. Explain procedure to patient. Provide privacy.	Explanation allays patient anxiety.
4. Perform hand hygiene.	Hand hygiene deters the spread of microorganisms.
5. Attach blunt-ended needle or small-gauge needle to syringe. Follow Skill 5-3 to remove insulin from vial. Remove enough insulin to last patient 2 to 3 days, plus 30 units for priming tubing.	Patient will wear pump for up to 3 days without changing syringe or tubing.
6. Attach sterile tubing to syringe. Push plunger of syringe until insulin is coming from introducer needle. **Check for any bubbles in tubing.**	Removing all air from tubing ensures that patient receives the correct dose of insulin.

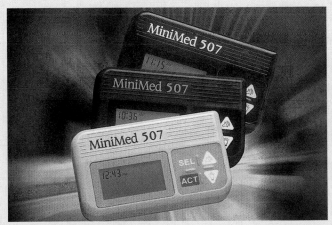

Action 1: MiniMed insulin pump.

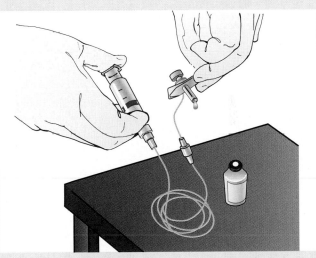

Action 6: Priming insulin pump tubing.

7. Program pump according to manufacturer's recommendations following physician's orders. Open pump and place syringe in compartment according to manufacturer's directions. Close pump.	Syringe must be placed in pump correctly for delivery of insulin.
8. Activate insertion device. Place needle between prongs of insertion device with sharp edge facing out. Push insertion set down until click is heard.	To ensure correct placement of insulin pump needle, insertion device must be used.
9. Put on gloves. Clean area around injection site with antimicrobial swab. Use a firm, circular motion while moving outward from insertion site. Allow antiseptic to dry.	Friction helps to clean the skin.

continues

ACTION	RATIONALE

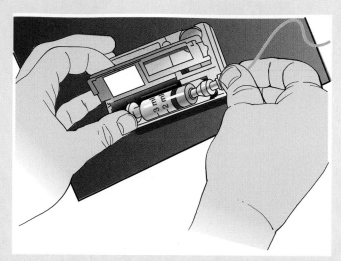

Action 7: Placing syringe in compartment according to manufacturer's directions.

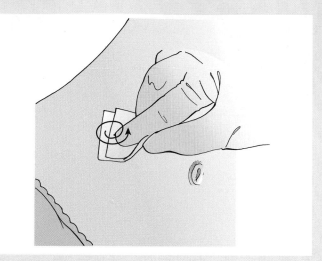

Action 9: Cleaning area before insertion.

10. Remove paper from adhesive backing. Remove needle guard. Pinch skin at insertion site, press insertion device on site, and press release buttons to insert needle. Remove triggering device.

11. **While holding needle hub, turn it a quarter-turn and remove needle. Discard appropriately.**

To ensure delivery of insulin into subcutaneous tissue, a skin fold is made with a pinch *before* insertion of the medication.

The actual metal needle is removed and a plastic stylet is left in place to deliver the medication. If needle hub is not rotated, the stylet may be removed as well.

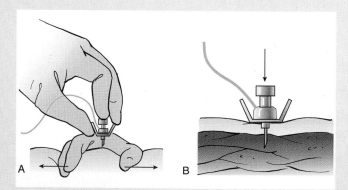

Action 10: Inserting needle into abdomen.

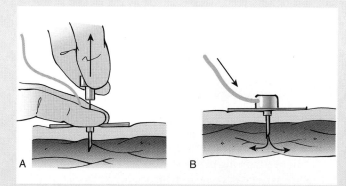

Action 11: Removing needle from insulin pump.

12. Apply sterile occlusive dressing over insertion site. Attach the pump to patient's clothing.

13. Remove gloves. Perform hand hygiene.

14. Document type of insulin, pump settings, insertion site, and any teaching done with patient.

Pump can be dislodged easily if not attached securely to patient.

Hand hygiene deters the spread of microorganisms.

This provides accurate documentation and helps to prevent medication errors.

continues

SKILL 5-19 Applying an Insulin Pump (continued)

ACTION	RATIONALE
15. Evaluate patient's response to medication within appropriate time frame.	Patient needs to be evaluated to ensure that pump is delivering drug appropriately and that patient is not suffering any adverse affects caused by the medication.

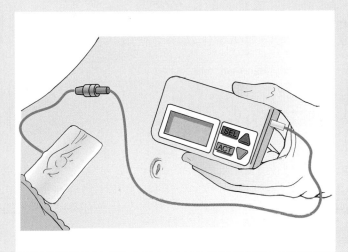

Action 12: MiniMed insulin pump attached.

7/22/05   Insulin pump inserted by patient on LVQ of abdomen with minimal assistance. Pump filled with 300 units (3 mL) of lispro insulin. Pump settings at 1 unit per hour. Patient would like to insert pump next time without assistance.—K. Sanders, RN

Action 14: Documentation.

EVALUATION

The expected outcomes are met when the patient has received insulin from the attached pump successfully without hypo- or hyperglycemic effects noted; patient understood the rationale for the pump attachment; patient experienced no allergy response; patient's skin remained intact; and patient experienced no or minimal pain.

Unexpected Situations and Associated Interventions

- *After pump is attached to patient, a large amount of air is noted in tubing:* Remove pump from patient. Obtain new sterile tubing with insertion needle. Prime tubing and reinsert.
- *Patient must rotate site more frequently than every 2 to 3 days due to insulin usage:* Check manufacturer's recommendations. Most pumps are initially set in a smaller mode but can be changed for a large amount of insulin delivery.
- *Patient is refusing to rotate site at least every 3 days:* Inform patient that absorption of medication decreases after 3 days, which may increase his or her need for insulin. Rotating sites prevents this decrease in absorption from developing.
- *Nurse notes that insertion site is now erythematous:* Remove the stylet, obtain a new pump setup, and insert in another site at least 1″ from old site.
- *Occlusive dressing will not stick due to perspiration:* Apply deodorant around insertion site but not over insertion site.

■ Developing Critical Thinking Skills

1. When entering Cooper Jackson's room with the antibiotic, the nurse asks Cooper's mother about any medication allergies that Cooper may have. The mother says, "The only medication that Cooper is allergic to is penicillin. It made it hard for him to breathe the last time he received it." The nurse notes that the ordered medication is a cephalosporin. Should the nurse administer the medication? What is the best technique to administer liquid medication to an uncooperative 20-month-old? Thirty minutes after receiving an oral medication, Cooper vomits. Should the nurse readminister the medication?

2. What are some ways that the nurse can make Erika Jenkins feel more relaxed about receiving her injection? What should the nurse do if Erika moves and dislodges the needle during the injection or if Erika tenses her muscles so tightly that the needle does not penetrate the skin?

3. What are some priority points that the nurse needs to discuss with Jonah Dinerman, who has type I diabetes, if the education needs to be completed in a short time?

Bibliography

Abrams, A. (2001). *Clinical drug therapy* (6th ed.). Philadelphia: Lippincott Williams & Wilkins.

Ahmed, D., & Fecik, S. (2000). MAOIs: Still here, still dangerous. *American Journal of Nursing, 100*(2), 29–30.

Carroll, P. (2003). Medication errors: The bigger picture. *RN, 66*(1), 52–58.

Eisenhauer, L., Nichols, L., Spencer, R., & Bergan, F. (1998). *Clinical pharmacology and nursing management* (5th ed.). Philadelphia: Lippincott Williams & Wilkins.

Fain, J. (2002). Delivering insulin round the clock. *Nursing, 32*(8), 54–56.

Fleming, D. (1999). Challenging traditional insulin injection practices. *American Journal of Nursing, 99*(2), 72–74.

Haddad, A. (2001). Ethics in action. *RN, 64*(9), 25–28.

Jech, A. (2001). The next step in preventing med errors. *RN, 64*(4), 46–49.

Johanson, L. (2001). Complacency can kill. *RN, 64*(8), 49–50.

Karch, A., & Karch, F. (2001). Let the user beware. *American Journal of Nursing, 101*(2), 25.

Karch, A., & Karch, F. (2001). Take part in the solution: How to report medication errors. *American Journal of Nursing, 101*(10), 25.

Katsma, D., & Katsma, R. (2000). The myth of the 90°-angle intramuscular injection. *Nurse Educator, 25*(1), 34–37.

Koschel, M. (2001). Question of practice: Filter needles. *American Journal of Nursing, 101*(1), 75.

Kuhn, M. (1998). *Pharmacotherapeutics: a nursing process approach* (4th ed.). Philadelphia: F. A. Davis.

McConnell, E. (2001). Clinical do's & don'ts: Instilling eyedrops. *Nursing, 31*(9), 17.

McKenry, L., & Salerno, E. (2002). *Pharmacology in nursing* (21st ed.). St. Louis: C. V. Mosby.

Morris, M. (2002). When a phone order differs from the written one. *RN, 65*(1), 71.

Nicoll, L., & Hesby, A. (2002). Intramuscular injection: An integrative research review and guideline for evidence-based practice. *Applied Nursing Research, 16*(2), 149–162.

North American Nursing Diagnosis Association. (2002). *Nursing diagnoses: definitions and classification 2002–2003*. Philadelphia: Author.

Pope, B. (2002). How to administer subcutaneous and intramuscular. *Nursing, 32*(1), 50–51.

Trooskin, S. (2002). Low-technology, cost-efficient strategies for reducing medication errors. *American Journal of Infection Control, 30*(6), 351–354.

Wentz, J., Karch, A., & Karch, F. (2000). You've caught the error, now how do you fix it? *American Journal of Nursing, 100*(9), 24.

Winland-Brown, J., & Valiante, J. (2000). Effectiveness of different medication management approaches on elders' medication adherence. *Outcomes Management for Nursing Practice, 4*(4), 172–176.

Wolf, Z., Serembus, J., & Beitz, J. (2001). Clinical inference of nursing students concerning harmful outcomes after medication errors. *Nurse Educator, 26*(6), 268–270.

Perioperative Nursing

This chapter will help you develop the skills related to safe perioperative nursing care for the following patients:

Josie McKeown, a 2-day-old girl who needs surgery to correct a heart defect

Tatum Kelly, a 28-year-old woman having outpatient surgery for breast reduction

Dorothy Gibbs, an 81-year-old woman having surgery to remove a bowel obstruction

Learning Outcomes

After studying this chapter the reader should be able to:

1. Provide safe care for the preoperative patient.
2. Provide safe care for the postoperative patient.
3. Apply a forced air warming device.

Key Terms

anesthetic: medication that produces such states as narcosis (loss of consciousness), analgesia, relaxation, and loss of reflexes

atelectasis: incomplete expansion or collapse of a part of the lungs

conscious sedation/analgesia: type of anesthesia used for short procedures; the intravenous administration of sedatives and analgesics raises the pain threshold and produces an altered mood and some degree of amnesia, but the patient maintains cardiorespiratory function and can respond to verbal commands

elective surgery: surgery that is recommended but can be omitted or delayed without catastrophe

embolus: foreign body or air in the circulatory system

emergency surgery: surgery that must be performed immediately to save the person's life or a body organ

hemorrhage: excessive blood loss due to the escape of blood from blood vessels

hypovolemic shock: shock due to a decrease in blood volume

perioperative nursing: wide variety of nursing activities carried out before, during, and after surgery

perioperative period: time frame consisting of the preoperative phase (starts with decision that surgery is necessary and lasting until the patient is transferred to the operating room), the intraoperative phase (starts from the arrival in the operating room until transfer to the recovery room) and the postoperative phase (begins with transfer to recovery room and lasts until complete recovery from surgery)

pneumonia: inflammation or infection of the lungs

thrombophlebitis: inflammation in a vein associated with thrombus formation

A wide range of illnesses and injuries may require treatment that includes some type of surgical intervention. Surgery may be planned or unplanned, major or minor, invasive or noninvasive and may involve any body part or system. A surgical procedure of any extent is a stressor that requires physical and psychosocial adaptations for both the patient and the family. The patient's recovery from a surgical procedure requires skillful and knowledgeable nursing care whether the surgery is done on an outpatient basis or in the hospital.

Nursing care provided for the patient before, during, and after surgery is called perioperative nursing. All phases of the nursing process are used to make assessments and provide interventions to promote the recovery of health, prevent further injury or illness, and facilitate coping with alterations in physical structure and function. This chapter will cover the skills to assist the nurse in providing safe perioperative nursing care to the patient. Please look over the summary tables and boxes at the beginning of this chapter for a quick review of critical knowledge to assist you in understanding the skills related to perioperative nursing care.

TABLE 6-1 **Classification of Surgical Procedures**

Classification	Purpose	Examples
Based on Urgency		
Elective: Delay of surgery has no ill effects; can be scheduled in advance based on patient's choice	• To remove or repair a body part • To restore function • To improve health • To improve self-concept	Tonsillectomy, hernia repair, cataract extraction and lens implantation, hemorrhoidectomy, hip prosthesis, scar revision, facelift, mammoplasty
Urgent: Usually done within 24–48 hours	• To remove or repair a body part • To preserve or restore health • To restore function • To prevent further tissue damage	Removal of gallbladder, coronary artery bypass, surgical removal of a malignant tumor, colon resection, amputation
Emergency: Done immediately	• To preserve life (plus purposes listed above)	Control of hemorrhage; repair of trauma, perforated ulcer, intestinal obstruction; tracheostomy
Based on Degree of Risk		
Major: may be elective, urgent, or emergency	• To preserve life • To remove or repair a body part • To restore function • To improve or maintain health	Carotid endarterectomy, cholecystectomy, nephrectomy, colostomy, hysterectomy, radical mastectomy, amputation, trauma repair
Minor: Primarily elective	• To restore function • To remove skin lesions • To correct deformities	Teeth extraction, removal of warts, skin biopsy, dilation and curettage, laparoscopy, cataract extraction, arthroscopy
Based on Purpose		
Diagnostic	• To make or confirm a diagnosis	Breast biopsy, laparoscopy, bronchoscopy, exploratory laparotomy
Ablative	• To remove a diseased body part	Appendectomy, subtotal thyroidectomy, partial gastrectomy, colon resection, amputation
Palliative	• To relieve or reduce intensity of an illness; is not curative	Colostomy, nerve root resection, débridement of necrotic tissue, balloon angioplasties, arthroscopy
Reconstructive	• To restore function to traumatized or malfunctioning tissue • To improve self-concept	Scar revision, plastic surgery, skin graft, internal fixation of a fracture, breast reconstruction
Transplantation	• To replace organs or structures that are diseased or malfunctioning	Kidney, liver, cornea, heart, joints
Constructive	• To restore function in congenital anomalies	Cleft palate repair, closure of atrial–septal defect

TABLE 6-2 Postoperative Assessments and Interventions on Return to the Unit

Factors to Assess	Assessments and Interventions
Vital signs	• Temperature, blood pressure, pulse and respiratory rates • Note, report, and document deviations from preoperative and PACU data as well as symptoms of complications
Color and temperature of skin	• Skin color (pallor, cyanosis), skin temperature, diaphoresis
Level of consciousness	• Orientation to time, place, person • Reaction to stimuli and ability to move extremities
Intravenous fluids	• Type and amount of solution, flow rate, security and patency of tubing • Infusion site
Surgical site	• Dressing and dependent areas for drainage (color, amount, consistency) • Drains and tubes; be sure they are intact, patent, and properly connected to drainage systems.
Other tubes	• Indwelling urinary catheter, gastrointestinal suction, and others for drainage, patency, amount of output • Be sure dependent drainage bags are hanging properly and suction drainage is attached and functioning. • If oxygen is ordered, ensure placement of ordered application and flow rate.
Comfort	• Pain (location, duration, intensity), and determine whether analgesics were given in the PACU. • Nausea and vomiting • Cover patient with blanket. • Reorient to room as necessary. • Allow family members to remain with patient after initial assessment is completed.
Position and safety	• Place patient in an ordered position, or • If patient is not fully conscious, place in side-lying position. • Elevate side rails and place bed in low position.

BOX 6-1 Sample Preoperative Teaching: Activities and Events for In-Hospital Surgery

Preoperative Phase
- [ ] Exercises and physical activities
    - [ ] Deep-breathing exercises
    - [ ] Coughing
    - [ ] Incentive spirometry
    - [ ] Turning
    - [ ] Leg exercises
- [ ] Pain management
    - [ ] Meaning of PRN orders for medications
    - [ ] Timing for best effect of medications
    - [ ] Splinting incision
    - [ ] Nonpharmacologic pain management options
- [ ] Visit by anesthesiologist
- [ ] Physical preparation
    - [ ] NPO
    - [ ] Sleeping medication the night before
    - [ ] Preoperative checklist (review items)
- [ ] Visitors and waiting room
- [ ] Transported to operating room by stretcher

Intraoperative Phase
- [ ] Holding area
    - [ ] Skin preparation
    - [ ] Intravenous lines and fluids
    - [ ] Medications
- [ ] Operating room
    - [ ] Operating room bed
    - [ ] Lights and common equipment (eg, cardiac monitor, pulse oximeter, warming device, etc.).
    - [ ] Safety belt
    - [ ] Sensations
    - [ ] Staff

Postoperative Phase
- [ ] Postanesthesia care unit
    - [ ] Frequent vital signs, assessments (eg, orientation, movement or extremities, strength of grasp)
    - [ ] Dressings/drains/tubes/catheters
    - [ ] Intravenous lines
    - [ ] Pain medications/comfort measures
    - [ ] Family notification
    - [ ] Sensations
    - [ ] Airway/oxygen therapy/pulse oximetry
    - [ ] Staff
- [ ] Transfer to unit (on stretcher)
    - [ ] Frequent vital signs
    - [ ] Sensations
    - [ ] Pain medications/nonpharmacologic strategies
    - [ ] NPO, diet progression
    - [ ] Exercises
    - [ ] Early ambulation
    - [ ] Family visits

SKILL 6-1   Preoperative Patient Care: Hospitalized Patient

The preoperative phase consists of the time from when it is decided that surgery is needed until the patient arrives in the operating room. This is a time of assessment and education.

Equipment

- No special equipment needed

ASSESSMENT

Assess patient's medication list, noting when the last dose was taken. Assess patient's intake for the past 24 hours, including when the last meal and beverages were ingested. Remove any jewelry, hairpieces or barrettes, nail polish, retainers, or dentures. Assess for any loose teeth. Review the nursing database, history, and physical examination. Check that the baseline data are recorded.

NURSING DIAGNOSIS

Determine related factors for the nursing diagnosis based on the patient's current status. Appropriate nursing diagnoses may include:

- Anxiety
- Fear
- Deficient Knowledge

OUTCOME IDENTIFICATION AND PLANNING

The expected outcome to achieve when providing preoperative patient care for the hospitalized patient is that the patient will proceed to surgery. Other outcomes that may be appropriate include the following: the patient will be free from anxiety; the patient will be free from fear; and the patient will demonstrate an understanding of the need for surgery and the measures to minimize the postoperative risks associated with surgery.

IMPLEMENTATION

ACTION	RATIONALE
1. **Identify patients for whom surgery is a greater risk, including the following:** a. Very young and elderly patients b. Obese or malnourished patients c. Patients with fluid and electrolyte imbalances d. Patients in poor general health from chronic disease and infectious processes e. Patients taking certain medications (ie, anticoagulants, antibiotics, diuretics, depressants, steroids) f. Patients who are extremely anxious	Identification of high risk status allows for recognition of patients who may be prone to complications after surgery.
2. Review the nursing database, history, and physical examination. Check that the baseline data are recorded; report those that are abnormal.	Review identifies patients who are surgical risks.
3. **Check that diagnostic testing has been completed and results are available; identify and report abnormal results.**	This check may influence the type of surgery performed and anesthetic used, as well as the timing of surgery or the need for additional consultation.
4. Promote optimal nutrition and hydration status as ordered.	This promotes wound healing.

continues

Preoperative Patient Care: Hospitalized Patient (continued)

ACTION	RATIONALE

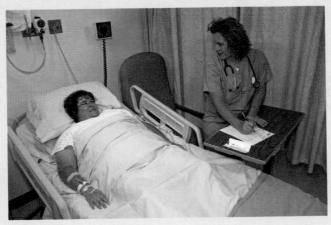

Action 2: Reviewing baseline data and checking forms.

5. **Identify learning needs of patient and family.**

   This enhances surgical recovery and allays anxiety by preparing patients for postoperative convalescence, discharge plans, and self-care.

6. Conduct preoperative teaching regarding coughing and deep-breathing exercises with splinting if necessary.

   Deep-breathing exercises improve lung expansion and volume, help expel anesthetic gases and mucus from the airway, and facilitate the oxygenation of body tissues. Coughing helps remove retained mucus from the respiratory tract. Splinting minimizes pain while coughing or moving.

7. Conduct preoperative teaching regarding respiratory therapy regimens such as incentive spirometry.

   Incentive spirometry improves lung expansion, helps expel anesthetic gases and mucus from the airway, and facilitates oxygenation of body tissues.

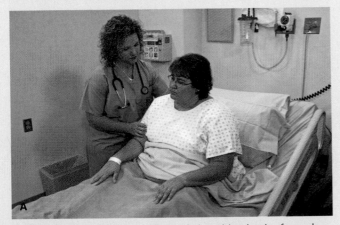

Action 6: Assisting patient to semi-Fowler's position, leaning forward.

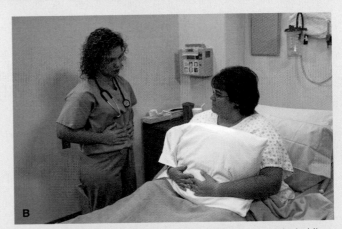

Action 6: Having patient splint a chest or abdominal incision by holding a folded bath blanket or pillow against the incision.

continues

SKILL 6-1   Preoperative Patient Care: Hospitalized Patient (continued)

ACTION   **RATIONALE**

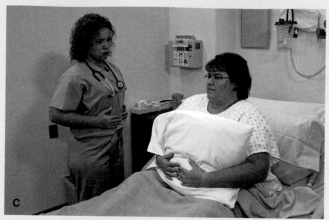

Action 6: Telling patient to take a deep breath and hold it for 3 seconds.

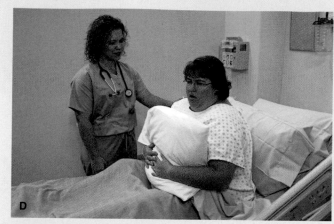

Action 6: Encouraging patient to "hack" out three short coughs after holding breath.

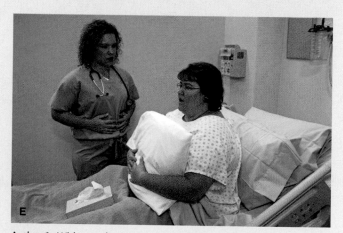

Action 6: With mouth open, patient should take a quick breath.

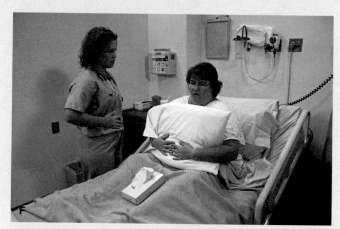

Action 6: Encouraging patient to cough deeply once or twice and then take another deep breath.

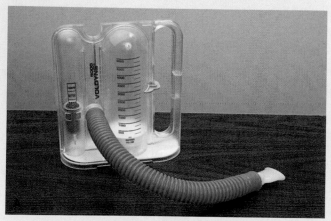

Action 7: An incentive spirometer helps increase lung volume and promotes inflation of the alveoli.

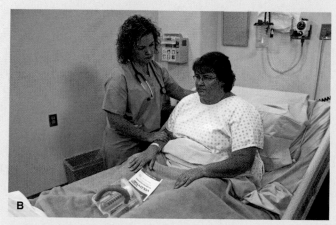

Action 7: Assisting patient to semi-Fowler's position.

continues

ACTION

RATIONALE

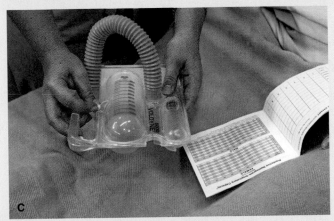

Action 7: Setting the volume goal indicator on the spirometer.

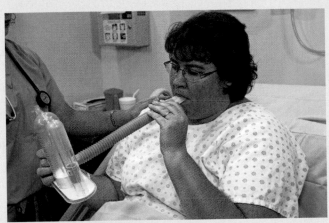

Action 7: Patient holding the device and placing lips around the mouthpiece to create a seal, then taking a deep breath in.

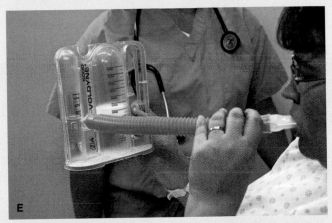

Action 7: The patient can observe progress toward the goal by watching the balls or diaphragm of spirometer elevate or lights go on (depending on equipment used). Have patient repeat exercise 5 to 10 times every 1 to 2 hours while awake.

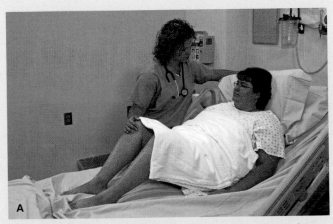

Action 9: Assisting patient to a semi-Fowler's position with knees bent.

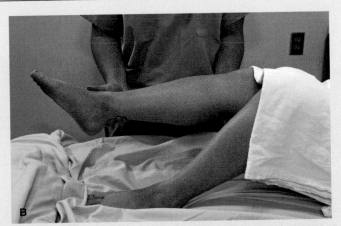

Action 9: Raising patient's right foot and keeping it elevated for a few seconds.

8. Conduct preoperative teaching regarding management of pain after surgery.

9. Conduct preoperative teaching regarding leg exercises.

Using ordered analgesics to minimize pain helps prevent postoperative complications.

Leg exercises promote venous return and decrease complications related to venous stasis.

continues

ACTION   RATIONALE

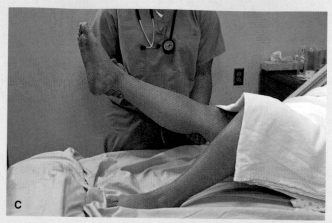

Action 9: Extending the lower portion of the leg.

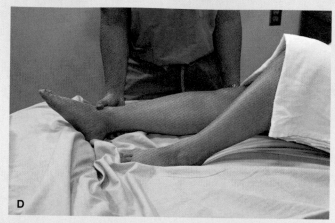

Action 9: Lowering the entire leg to the bed. This exercise is repeated five times with each leg.

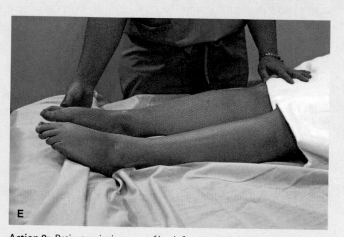

Action 9: Patient pointing toes of both feet toward the foot of the bed, with both legs extended.

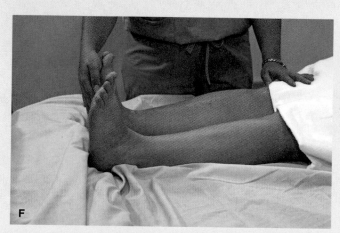

Action 9: Patient pulling toes toward chin, as if a string were attached to them.

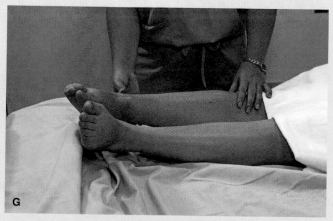

Action 9: Having patient make circles with both ankles, first one way and then the other.

continues

Preoperative Patient Care: Hospitalized Patient (continued)

ACTION	RATIONALE

10. Provide preoperative teaching regarding early ambulation and turning in bed.

11. Provide preoperative teaching regarding postoperative equipment and monitoring devices.

12. Provide preoperative teaching regarding home care requirements.

13. Document findings and instruction given.

Turning and moving in bed helps to minimize pain and prevent postoperative complications.

Documentation ensures communication and continuity of care.

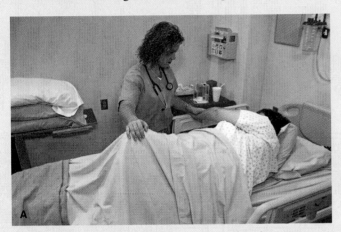

Action 10: Instructing patient to raise one knee and reach across to grasp the side rail on the side of the bed toward which he or she will be turning.

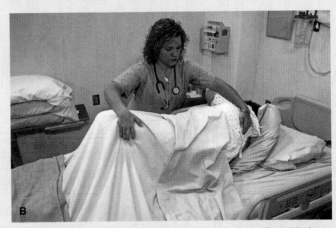

Action 10: Helping patient to roll over while he or she pushes with the bent leg and pulls on the side rail.

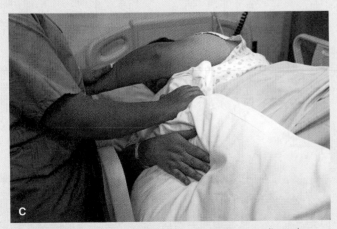

Action 10: Showing patient how to use a small pillow to splint a chest or abdominal incision while turning.

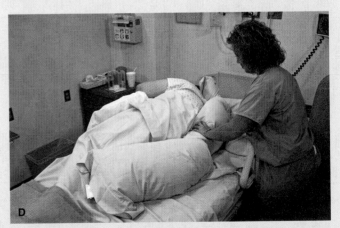

Action 10: After patient is turned, providing support with pillows behind the patient's back.

4/2/06 1030   Patient in for preoperative clinic visit. Patient taught to do incentive spirometry, deep breathing, splinting while coughing, and leg exercises. Patient demonstrated each item and verbalized understanding. Questions answered.—J. Grabbs, RN

Action 13: Documentation.

continues

Preoperative Patient Care: Hospitalized Patient (continued)

ACTION	RATIONALE
Day Before Surgery	
14. Provide emotional support. Answer questions realistically. Provide spiritual assistance if requested. Include family when possible.	This allays family and patient misconceptions and fears.
15. **Follow preoperative fluid and food restrictions.**	This reduces risk for vomiting and aspiration during surgery. Anesthetic agents temporarily depress gastrointestinal function and processes.
16. Prepare for elimination needs during and after surgery.	Anesthetic agents and abdominal surgery interfere with normal elimination function. A urinary catheter inserted preoperatively minimizes risk for inadvertent trauma to bladder during surgery.
17. Attend to patient's special hygiene needs (ie, use of antiseptic cleaning agents to prepare surgical site).	This decreases risk for infection.
18. Provide for adequate rest.	Rest minimizes stress before surgery.
Day of Surgery	
19. **Check that proper identification band is on patient.**	Double-checking ensures identity of patient.
20. Check that preoperative consent forms are signed, witnessed, and correct, that advance directives are in the medical record (as applicable), and that the medical record is in order.	This fulfills legal requirement related to informed consent and educates patient regarding advance directives.
21. **Check vital signs.** Notify physician of any pertinent changes (ie, rise or drop in blood pressure, elevated temperature, cough, symptoms of infection).	This provides baseline data for comparison.
22. Provide hygiene and oral care. **Remind patient of food and fluid restrictions before surgery.**	This promotes comfort and prevents intraoperative complications during anesthesia induction.
23. Continue nutritional and hydration preparation.	This prepares patient for operative procedure.
24. Remove cosmetics, jewelry, nail polish, and prostheses (eg, contact lenses, false eyelashes, dentures, and so forth). Some facilities allow a wedding band to be left in place depending on the type of surgery, provided it is secured to the finger with tape. Reassess for loose teeth.	These interfere with assessment during surgery.

Action 21: Obtaining preoperative vital signs.

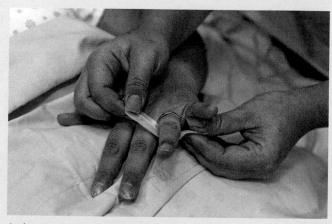

Action 24: Taping wedding band in place.

continues

Preoperative Patient Care: Hospitalized Patient (continued)

ACTION	RATIONALE
17. Place valuables in appropriate area. The hospital safe is most appropriate place for valuables. They should not be placed in narcotics drawer.	This ensures safety of valuables and personal possessions.
18. **Have patient empty bladder and bowel before surgery.**	An empty bladder and bowel minimize risk for injury or complications during and after surgery.
19. Attend to any special preoperative orders.	This prepares patient for operative procedure.
20. Complete preoperative checklist and record of patient's preoperative preparation.	This ensures accurate documentation and communication with perioperative nurse caring for patient.
21. **Administer preoperative medication as prescribed by physician/anesthesia provider.**	Medication reduces anxiety, provides sedation, and diminishes salivary and bronchial secretions.
22. Raise side rails of bed; place bed in lowest position. Instruct patient to remain in bed or on stretcher. If necessary, a safety restraint may be used.	These actions ensure the patient's safety once the preoperative medication has been given.
23. Help move the patient from the bed to the transport stretcher if necessary. Reconfirm patient identification and ensure that all preoperative events and measures are documented.	Helping the patient move prevents injury. Reconfirming patient identity helps to ensure that the correct patient is being transported to surgery.

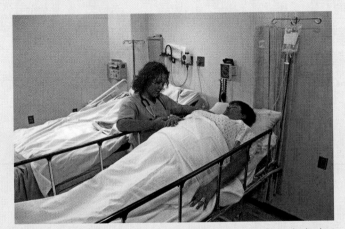

Action 23: Confirming identification after patient moves from the bed to the stretcher.

24. After the patient leaves for the operating room, prepare the room and bed for postoperative care. Anticipate any necessary equipment based on the type of surgery and the patient's history.	Preparing for the patient's return helps to promote efficient care in the postoperative period.

EVALUATION

The expected outcome is met when the patient proceeds to surgery; is prepared for surgery so that he or she is free from anxiety and fear; and demonstrates understanding of the importance of pre- and postoperative instructions.

continues

SKILL 6-1   Preoperative Patient Care: Hospitalized Patient (continued)

Unexpected Situations and Associated Interventions

- *A patient's laboratory results are noted to be abnormal:* Notify physician. Some abnormalities, such as an elevated INR, may postpone the surgery.
- *A patient says to you, "I'm not sure I really want this surgery":* Discuss with the patient why he or she feels this way. Notify physician. Patients should not undergo surgery until they are sure that surgery is what they want.
- *A patient admits he ate "just a little bit" before arriving for his outpatient surgery:* Notify the physician. The patient's surgery may have to be postponed for a few hours to prevent aspiration during surgery.
- *Identification band is not in place:* Ensure identity of patient and obtain new identification band. Patient cannot proceed to surgery without identification band.
- *Consent form is not signed:* Notify physician. It is the physician's responsibility to obtain consent for surgery and anesthesia. The patient should not proceed to surgery without a signed consent form (unless it is an emergency).
- *Patient does not want to remove dentures before surgery, saying, "I never take my dentures out":* Discuss with surgeon or anesthesia provider. Patient may be allowed to go to the preoperative area with dentures and remove the dentures before entering the operating room.
- *Patient refuses to take preoperative medication:* Notify physician before patient goes to operating room. Many medications are necessary to protect the patient pre- or postoperatively.

Infant and Child Considerations

- In many institutions, the parents are allowed to enter the preoperative area with the child. This has been shown to decrease the child's and the parents' anxiety.
- The breastfed infant may be allowed to nurse closer to the time of surgery than a bottle-fed infant would be allowed to have a bottle of formula. Breast milk is easier for the stomach to digest, so the clearance time is shorter than for formula.

SKILL 6-2   Postoperative Care When Patient Returns to Room

Postoperative care facilitates recovery from surgery and supports the patient in coping with physical changes or alterations. Nursing interventions promote physical and psychological health, prevent complications, and teach self-care skills for the patient to use after the hospital stay. After surgery, patients spend time on the postanesthesia care unit (PACU). From the PACU, they are transferred back to their rooms. At this time, nursing interventions focus on actual problems and anticipated problems the patient is at risk for developing.

Equipment

- None needed

ASSESSMENT

A wide variety of factors increase the risk for postoperative complications. Ongoing postoperative assessments and teaching are used to decrease the risk for postoperative complications.

NURSING DIAGNOSIS

Determine the related factors for the nursing diagnosis based on the patient's current status. Appropriate nursing diagnoses may include the following:

- Anxiety
- Risk for Aspiration
- Disturbed Body Image
- Risk for Imbalanced Body Temperature

continues

Postoperative Care When Patient Returns to Room (continued)

- Hypothermia
- Risk for Infection
- Impaired Skin Integrity
- Risk for Perioperative Positioning Injury
- Impaired Physical Mobility
- Acute Pain

Depending on the type and extent of surgery, other nursing diagnoses may apply, such as Ineffective Airway Clearance, Impaired Gas Exchange, Impaired Urinary Elimination, or Deficient Fluid Volume.

**OUTCOME
IDENTIFICATION
AND PLANNING**

The expected outcome to achieve when providing postoperative care to a patient is that the patient will recover from the surgery. Other outcomes that may be appropriate include the following: patient is free from anxiety; patient is comfortable with body image; patient's temperature remains between 36.5° and 37.5°C (97.7° to 99.5°F); patient will remain free from infection; patient will not experience any skin breakdown; patient will regain mobility; and patient will have pain managed appropriately.

IMPLEMENTATION

ACTION	RATIONALE
1. When patient returns from the PACU, obtain a report from the PACU nurse and review the operating room and PACU data. Check the patient's identification. Perform hand hygiene. **Place patient in safe position (semi- or high Fowler's or side-lying). Note level of consciousness.**	Obtaining report ensures accurate communication and promotes continuity of care. A sitting position facilitates deep breathing; the side-lying position with neck slightly extended prevents aspiration and airway obstruction.
2. **Monitor and record vital signs frequently.** Assessment order may vary, but usual frequency includes taking vital signs every 15 minutes the first hour, every 30 minutes the next 2 hours, every hour for 4 hours, and finally every 4 hours.	Comparison with baseline preoperative vital signs may indicate impending shock or hemorrhage.

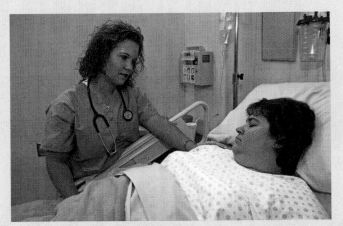

Action 1: Placing the patient in a safe position (high Fowler's or side-lying).

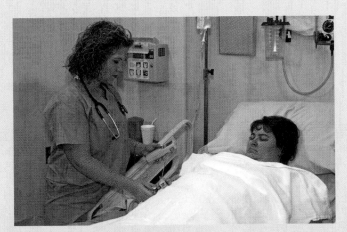

Action 2: Obtaining postoperative vital signs.

Postoperative Care When Patient Returns to Room (continued)

ACTION	RATIONALE
3. Provide for warmth, using blankets as necessary. Assess skin color and condition.	Hypothermia is uncomfortable and may lead to cardiac arrhythmias and impaired would healing.
4. **Check dressings for color, odor, and amount of drainage, and feel under the patient for bleeding.**	Hemorrhage and shock are life-threatening complications of surgery.

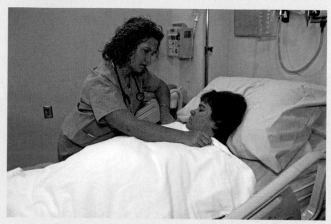

Action 3: Providing comfort and warmth to the patient.

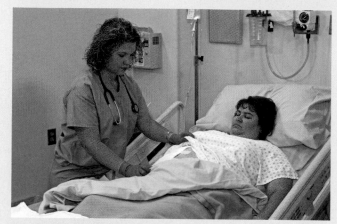

Action 4: Checking the dressings for color, odor, and amount of drainage.

5. **Verify that all tubes and drains are patent and equipment is operative; note amount of drainage in collection device.**	This ensures maintenance of vital functions.
6. Maintain IV infusion at correct rate.	This prevents dehydration and electrolyte imbalances.

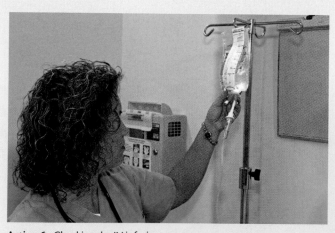

Action 6: Checking the IV infusion.

7. Provide for a safe environment. Keep bed in low position with side rails up. Have call bell within patient's reach.	This prevents accidental injury.
8. Relieve pain by administering medications ordered by physician. Check record to verify if analgesic medication was administered in the PACU.	Analgesics are used for relief of postoperative pain.
9. Record assessments and interventions on chart.	This provides for accurate documentation.

continues

Postoperative Care When Patient Returns to Room (continued)

ACTION	RATIONALE

Ongoing Care

10. Promote optimal respiratory function:

   a. Coughing and deep-breathing
   b. Incentive spirometry
   c. Early ambulation
   d. Frequent position change
   e. Administration of oxygen as ordered

Anesthetic agents may depress respiratory function: patients who have existing respiratory or cardiovascular disease or abdominal or chest incisions or who are obese or elderly or in a poor state of nutrition are at greater risk for respiratory complications.

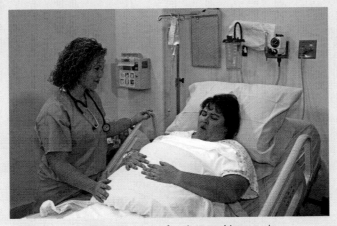

Action 10a: Assisting patient in performing coughing exercises.

11. Maintain adequate circulation, including:

   a. Frequent position changes
   b. Early ambulation
   c. Application of antiembolism stockings or pneumatic compression devices, if ordered by physician
   d. Leg and range-of-motion exercises if not contra-indicated

Preventive measures can improve venous return and circulatory status.

12. **Assess urinary elimination status:**

   a. Promote voiding by offering bedpan at regular intervals.
   b. Monitor catheter drainage if present.
   c. Measure intake and output.

Anesthetic agents and surgical manipulation in the area may temporarily depress bladder tone and response.

13. Promote optimal nutrition status and return of gastro-intestinal function:

   a. Assess for return of peristalsis.
   b. Assist with diet progression.
   c. Encourage fluid intake.
   d. Monitor intake.
   e. Medicate for nausea and vomiting as ordered by physician.

Anesthetic agents and narcotics depress peristalsis and normal functioning of gastrointestinal tract.

14. Promote wound healing by using surgical asepsis; assess condition of wound and any drainage.

Alterations in nutritional, circulatory, and metabolic status may predispose patient to infection and delayed healing.

continues

ACTION	RATIONALE
15. Provide for rest and comfort.	This shortens recovery period and facilitates return to normal function.
16. Provide emotional and spiritual support.	This facilitates individualized care and patient's return to normal health.
17. Document findings and interventions used.	Documentation provides a means of communication and facilitates continuity of care.

4/10/06   1330   Patient's temperature 38.1°C. Incentive spirometry completed × 10 cycles, 750 mL each. Patient deep breathing and coughing without production and turned to right side with HOB elevated.—J. Grabbs, RN

Action 17: Documentation.

EVALUATION

The expected outcome is met when the patient recovers from surgery; is free from anxiety; is comfortable with self-image; has a temperature of 36.5° to 37.5°C (97.7° to 99.5°F); remains free from infection; develops no pressure ulcers or areas of skin breakdown; has a dressing that is clean, dry and intact; can ambulate (if able before surgery); and achieves adequate pain control.

Unexpected Situations and Associated Interventions

- *Vital signs are progressively increasing or decreasing from baseline:* Notify physician. A continued decrease in blood pressure or an increase in heart rate could indicate internal bleeding.
- *Dressing was clean before but now has large amount of fresh blood:* Do not remove dressing. Reinforce dressing with more bandages. Removing the bandage could dislodge any clot that is forming and lead to further blood loss. Notify physician.
- *Patient reports pain that is not relieved by ordered medication:* After fully assessing pain (location, description, alleviating factors, causal factors), notify physician. Pain can be a clue to other problems, such as hemorrhage.
- *Patient is febrile within 12 hours of surgery:* Assist patient with coughing and deep-breathing. If ordered, begin incentive spirometry. A temperature this early after surgery is usually not indicative of infection but rather of atelectasis.
- *Adult patient has a urine output of less than 30 mL per hour:* Unless this is expected, notify physician. Urine output is a good indicator of tissue perfusion. Patient may need more fluid or may need medication to increase blood pressure if it is low.
- *Family members are anxious and want to be with patient:* Allow family members to visit patient briefly. Stress the need for the patient's continued rest.

Special Considerations

- For patients undergoing throat surgery, such as a tonsillectomy, evaluate swallowing pattern. A patient who has had throat surgery and swallows frequently may be bleeding from the incision site.

Applying a Forced-Air Warming Device

Often patients returning from surgery are hypothermic. A more effective way of warming the patient than using warm blankets is application of a forced-air warming device, which circulates warm air around the patient.

Equipment

- Forced-air warming device unit
- Forced-air blanket
- Thermometer

ASSESSMENT

Assess patient's temperature and skin color and perfusion. Patients who are hypothermic are generally pale to dusky and cool to the touch and have decreased peripheral perfusion.

NURSING DIAGNOSIS

Determine the related factors for the nursing diagnosis based on the patient's current status. Appropriate nursing diagnoses may include the following:

- Risk for Imbalanced Body Temperature
- Hypothermia

OUTCOME IDENTIFICATION AND PLANNING

The expected outcome to achieve when applying a forced-air warming device is that the patient will return to and maintain a temperature of 36.5° to 37.5°C (97.7° to 99.5°F). Other outcomes that may be appropriate include the following: skin will become pink and warm, capillary refill will be less than 2 seconds, and patient will not experience shivering.

IMPLEMENTATION

ACTION	RATIONALE
1. Gather equipment. Check physician's order and explain procedure to patient.	Organization facilitates performance of task. Explanation encourages patient cooperation.
2. Perform hand hygiene.	Hand hygiene deters the spread of microorganisms.
3. **Assess patient's temperature, and document.**	Baseline temperature should be documented before the warming device is used.
4. Plug forced-air warming device into electrical outlet. Place blanket over patient, with plastic side up. Keep air hose inlet at foot of bed.	Blanket should always be used with device. Do not place air hose under cotton blankets with airflow blanket. "Hosing" is dangerous and can cause burns to the patient.
5. Securely insert air hose into inlet. Place a lightweight fabric blanket over forced-air blanket. Turn machine on and adjust temperature of air to desired effect.	Air hose must be properly inserted to ensure that it will not fall out. Blanket will help keep warmed air near patient. Adjust air temperature depending on desired patient temperature. If blanket is being used to maintain an already stable temperature, it may be turned down lower than if needed to raise patient's temperature.
6. **Monitor patient's temperature at least every 30 minutes while using the forced-air device. If rewarming a patient with hypothermia, do not raise temperature more than 1°C per hour to prevent a rapid vasodilation effect.**	Monitoring the patient's temperature ensures that the patient does not experience too rapid a rise in body temperature, resulting in vasodilation.
7. Discontinue use of forced-air device once patient's temperature is adequate and patient can maintain the temperature without assistance.	Forced-air device is not needed once patient is warm and stable enough to maintain temperature.

continues

ACTION	RATIONALE
8. Remove device and clean according to agency policy and manufacturer's instructions. Document patient status.	Proper care of equipment helps to maintain function of the device. Documentation provides communication, indicating the effectiveness of the treatment, and promotes continuity of care.

4/23/06   1440   Patient's temperature 35.9°C tympanically. Forced-air warming device applied to patient due to decreased temperature. Device temperature set on medium. Patient's temperature after first 30 minutes 36.0°C tympanically.—J. Grabbs, RN

Action 8: Documentation.

EVALUATION

The expected outcome is met when the patient's temperature returns to the normal range of 36.5° to 37.5°C (97.7° to 99.5°F) and the patient can maintain this temperature; skin is pink and warm; and patient is free from shivering.

Unexpected Situations and Associated Interventions

- *Patient's temperature is increasing more than 1°C per hour:* Decrease temperature of air. If air is down to lowest setting, turn device off. If patient's temperature increases too rapidly, it can lead to a vasodilation effect that will cause the patient to become hypotensive.

■ Developing Critical Thinking Skills

1. Josie has a prophylactic antibiotic ordered to be given "on call to the OR." This means when the preoperative nurses are ready for Josie, they will call and have Josie sent down to this area. When this phone call is received, the nurse is to administer the prescribed medication. However, the phone call comes during a busy period, and the nurse realizes that Josie has been transported down to the preoperative holding area without receiving her dose of prophylactic antibiotics. What should the nurse do?

2. After her surgery, Tatum rates her pain as 8 out of 10. The nurse administers the ordered pain medication. Fifteen minutes later, Tatum is now rating her pain as 9 out of 10 and is beginning to writhe with pain. Tatum has no more ordered pain medications for another hour. What should the nurse do?

3. Dorothy Gibbs returns from surgery with a core temperature of 35.2°C (95.4°F), blood pressure of 128/72 mm Hg, and pulse of 60 beats per minute. Her skin is pale and cool to the touch. A forced-air warming device is placed on Dorothy and the nurse turns the warmer to the highest heat setting. An hour later, the nurse takes Dorothy's vital signs. Her tympanic temperature is 37.8°C (100.0°F), her blood pressure is 82/48 mm Hg, and her pulse is 100 beats per minute. What should the nurse do?

Bibliography

Adams, A. (2001). Preventing surgical site infection: Guidelines at a glance. *Nursing Management, 32*(8) OR Edition, 46.

Agency for Health Care Policy and Research. (1992) *Acute pain management: Operative or medical procedures and trauma. Clinical practice guidelines.* DHHS Pub. No. (AHCPR) 920032. Silver Spring, MD: Author.

Allen, G. (2002). Malnutrition and its effect on wound healing. *AORN Journal, 76*(5), 893.

American Association of Nurse Anesthetists. (2003). CRNA. Available at *www.aana.com/crna.careerqna.asp.*

American Society of PeriAnesthesia Nurses. (1998). *Standards of perianesthesia nursing practice.* Thorofare, NJ: Author.

Arnstein, P. (2002). Optimizing perioperative pain management. *AORN Journal, 76*(5), 812–818.

Association of Operating Room Nurses. (1997). *AORN's Age-Specific Competency Series.* Denver, CO: Author.

Association of Operating Room Nurses. (2002). *AORN standards, recommended practices and guidelines.* Denver, CO: Author.

Borchardt, M. (1999). Review of the clinical pharmacology and use of the benzodiazepines. *Journal of Perianesthesia Nursing, 14*(2), 65–72.

Christie, F. (1998). Pulmonary embolism. *American Journal of Nursing, 98*(11), 36–37.

Collins, N. (2003). Obesity and wound healing. *Advances in Skin & Wound Care: The Journal for Prevention and Healing, 16*(1), 45–47.

Crenshaw, J., & Winslow, E. (2002). Original research: Preoperative fasting: Old habits die hard. *American Journal of Nursing, 102*(5), 36–45.

Goodwin, S. A. (1999). Notes from the American Society of Anesthesiologists meeting. *Journal of Perianesthesia Nursing, 14*(2), 102–105.

Kost, M. (1999). Conscious sedation: Guarding your patient against complications. *Nursing, 29*(4), 34–39.

Noble, K. (1999). PACU: Ensuring a safe experience. *Advance for Nurses, 1*(5), 11–13.

Patton, C. M. (1999). Preoperative nursing assessment of the adult patient. *Seminars in Perioperative Nursing, 8*(1), 42–47.

Pessagno, J. J. (1999). Ambulatory care: Adjusting to the evolution of a changing health care system. *Advances for Nurses, 1*(8), 20–21.

Pessagno, J. J. (2002). Recommended practices for managing the patient receiving local anesthesia. *AORN Journal, 75*(4), 849–852.

Porth, C. M. (2002). *Pathophysiology: Concepts of altered health states* (5th ed.). Philadelphia: Lippincott.

Rothrock, J., Smith, D., & McEwen, D. (Eds.). (2003). *Alexander's care of the patient in surgery* (12th ed.). St. Louis: Mosby.

Promoting Healthy Physiologic Responses

Hygiene

This chapter will help you develop some of the skills related to hygiene necessary to care for the following patients:

Denasia Kerr, a 6-year-old who is on bedrest after surgery and needs her hair washed

Cindy Vortex, age 34, who is in a coma after a car accident and needs her contact lenses removed

Carl Sheen, age 76, who needs help cleaning his dentures

Learning Outcomes

After studying this chapter the reader should be able to:

1. Give a bed bath
2. Apply antiembolism stockings
3. Make an unoccupied bed
4. Make an occupied bed
5. Assist with oral care
6. Provide oral care for a dependent patient
7. Give a bed shampoo
8. Remove and clean contact lenses
9. Assist with a sitz bath
10. Assist a patient with shaving

Key Terms

alopecia: baldness

caries: cavities of the teeth

cerumen: ear wax; consists of a heavy oil and brown pigmentation

dermis: underlying portion of the skin

epidermis: superficial portion of the skin

gingivitis: inflammation of the gingivae (gums)

halitosis: offensive breath

integument: skin

necrosis: death of cells

pediculosis: infestation with lice

plaque: transparent, adhesive coating on teeth consisting of mucin, carbohydrate, and bacteria

podiatrist: one who treats foot disorders; synonym for chiropodist

pyorrhea: extensive inflammation of the gums and alveolar tissues; synonym for periodontitis

sebaceous gland: gland found in the skin that secretes an oily substance called sebum

tartar: hard deposit on the teeth near the gum line formed by plaque buildup and dead bacteria

Measures for personal cleanliness and grooming that promote physical and psychological well-being are called personal hygiene. Personal hygiene practices vary widely among people. The time of day one bathes and how often a person shampoos his or her hair or changes the bed linens and sleeping garments are relatively unimportant. What is important is that personal care be carried out conveniently and frequently enough to promote personal hygiene.

People who are well ordinarily are responsible for their own hygiene. In some cases, the nurse may assist a well person through teaching to develop personal hygiene habits the person may lack. Illness, hospitalization, and institutionalization generally require modifications in hygiene practices. In these situations, the nurse helps the patient to continue sound hygiene practices and can teach the patient and family members, when necessary, regarding hygiene. Nurses assisting patients with basic hygiene should respect individual patient preferences and give only the care that patients cannot or should not provide for themselves.

This chapter will cover the skills to assist the nurse in promoting hygiene. Please look over the summary figure at the beginning of this chapter for a quick review of critical knowledge related to one aspect of hygiene, perineal care.

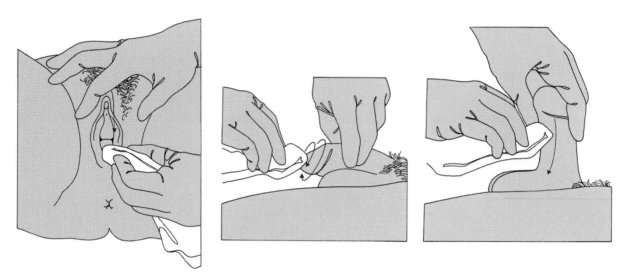

FIGURE 7-1 Performing normal perineal care.

SKILL 7-1   Giving a Bed Bath

A bed bath may be termed a partial bed bath (if the patient is well enough to perform most of the bath and the nurse needs to assist with washing areas that the patient cannot reach easily) or a complete bed bath (if the patient is physically unable to carry out parts of the bath without assistance).

Equipment

- Washbasin
- Bed linen
- Personal hygiene supplies (deodorant, lotion, and others)
- Soap and dish
- Towels (two)
- Washcloths
- Bath blanket

continues

Giving a Bed Bath (continued)

- Gown or pajamas
- Bedpan or urinal
- Laundry bag or cart
- Disposable gloves for anal and perineal care (optional for remainder of bath)

ASSESSMENT

Assess the patient's ability to bathe himself or herself. Allow the patient to do any part of the bath that he or she can do (eg, washing the face) while the nurse does the rest. Assess the patient's skin for dryness, redness, or areas of breakdown, and gather any other appropriate supplies that may be needed as a result.

NURSING DIAGNOSIS

Determine the related factors for the nursing diagnosis based on the patient's current status. Appropriate nursing diagnoses may include:

- Bathing/Hygiene Self-Care Deficit
- Acute Pain
- Ineffective Coping
- Deficient Knowledge
- Risk for Infection
- Disturbed Body Image
- Impaired Skin Integrity
- Risk for Impaired Skin Integrity
- Impaired Social Interaction

OUTCOME IDENTIFICATION AND PLANNING

The expected outcome to achieve when giving a bed bath is that the patient will be clean and fresh. Other outcomes that may be appropriate include the following: patient regains feelings of control by assisting with the bath; patient verbalizes positive body image; and patient demonstrates understanding about the need for cleanliness.

IMPLEMENTATION

ACTION	RATIONALE
1. Discuss procedure with patient and assess patient's ability to assist in the bathing process, as well as personal hygiene preferences. Review chart for any limitations in physical activity.	This discussion promotes reassurance and provides knowledge about the procedure. Dialogue encourages patient participation and allows for individualized nursing care.
2. Bring necessary equipment to the bedside stand or overbed table. Remove sequential compression devices and antiembolism stockings from lower extremities according to agency protocol.	Bringing everything to the bedside conserves time and energy. Arranging items nearby is convenient, saves time, and avoids unnecessary stretching and twisting of muscles on the part of the nurse. Most manufacturers and agencies recommend removal of these devices before the bath to allow for assessment.
3. Close curtains around bed and close door to room if possible.	This ensures the patient's privacy and lessens the risk for loss of body heat during the bath.
4. Offer patient bedpan or urinal.	Voiding or defecating before the bath lessens the likelihood that the bath will be interrupted, because warm bath water may stimulate the urge to void.
5. Perform hand hygiene.	Hand hygiene deters the spread of microorganisms.
6. Raise bed to high position.	Having the bed in a high position prevents strain on the nurse's back.
7. Lower side rail nearer to you and assist patient to side of bed where you will work. Have patient lie on his or her back.	Having the patient positioned near the nurse and lowering the side rail avoid unnecessary stretching and twisting of muscles on the part of the nurse. *continues*

ACTION

RATIONALE

8. Loosen top covers and remove all except the top sheet. Place bath blanket over patient and then remove top sheet while patient holds bath blanket in place. If linen is to be reused, fold it over a chair. Place soiled linen in laundry bag.

The patient is not exposed unnecessarily, and warmth is maintained. If a bath blanket is unavailable, the top sheet may be used in place of the bath blanket.

9. Assist patient with oral hygiene, as necessary. See Skill 7-5.

This helps maintain teeth and gums in good condition, alleviates unpleasant odor and taste, and may improve appetite. Some patients may prefer oral care after the bath.

10. Remove patient's gown and keep bath blanket in place. If patient has an IV line and is not wearing a gown with snap sleeves, remove gown from other arm first. **Lower the IV container and pass gown over the tubing and the container. Rehang the container and check the drip rate.**

This provides uncluttered access during the bath and maintains warmth of the patient. IV fluids must be maintained at the prescribed rate.

11. **Raise side rail.** Fill basin with a sufficient amount of comfortably warm water (43° to 46°C [110° to 115°F]). Change as necessary throughout the bath. Lower side rail closer to you when you return to the bedside to begin the bath.

Side rails maintain patient safety. Warm water is comfortable and relaxing for the patient. It also stimulates circulation and provides for more effective cleansing.

12. Fold the washcloth like a mitt on your hand so that there are no loose ends.

Having loose ends of cloth drag across the patient's skin is uncomfortable. Loose ends cool quickly and feel cold to the patient.

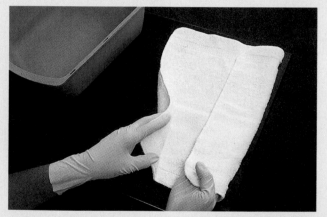

Action 12: Folding washcloth in thirds around hand to make a bath mitt.

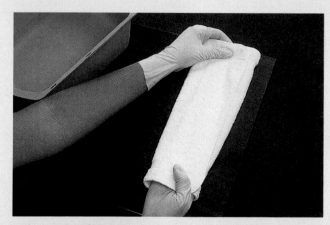

Action 12: Straightening washcloth before folding into mitt.

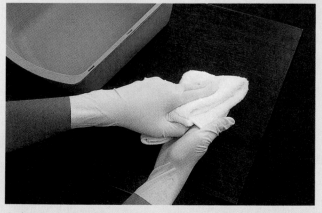

Action 12: Folding ends over and tucking ends under folded washcloth over palm.

continues

ACTION	RATIONALE
13. Lay a towel across patient's chest and on top of bath blanket.	This prevents chilling and keeps bath blanket dry.
14. **With no soap on the washcloth, wipe one eye from the inner part of the eye, near the nose, to the outer part. Rinse or turn the cloth before washing the other eye.**	Soap is irritating to the eyes. Moving from the inner to the outer aspect of the eye prevents carrying debris toward the nasolacrimal duct. Rinsing or turning the washcloth prevents spreading organisms from one eye to the other.
15. Bathe patient's face, neck, and ears, avoiding soap on the face if the patient prefers.	Soap can be drying and may be avoided as a matter of personal preference.
16. Expose patient's far arm and place towel lengthwise under it. Using firm strokes, wash arm and axilla, rinse, and dry.	The towel helps to keep the bed dry. Washing the far side first eliminates contaminating a clean area once it is washed. Gentle friction stimulates circulation and muscles and helps remove dirt, oil, and organisms. Long, firm strokes are relaxing and more comfortable than short, uneven strokes.

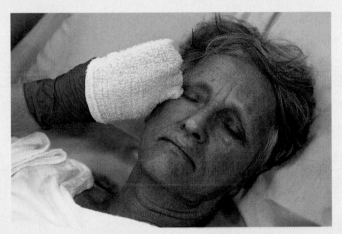

Action 14: Washing from the inner corner of the eye outward.

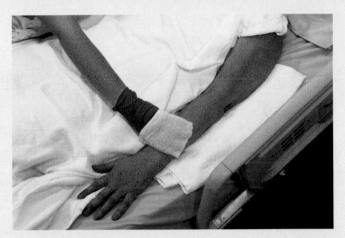

Action 16: Exposing the far arm and washing it.

17. Place a folded towel on the bed next to patient's hand and put basin on it. Soak patient's hand in basin. Wash, rinse, and dry hand.	Placing the hand in the basin of water is an additional comfort measure for the patient. It facilitates thorough washing of the hands and between the fingers and aids removing debris from under the nails.

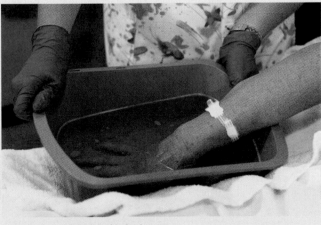

Action 17: Soaking hand in basin.

continues

SKILL 7-1 Giving a Bed Bath (continued)

ACTION	RATIONALE

18. Repeat Actions 16 and 17 for the arm nearer you. (An option for the shorter nurse or one prone to back strain might be to bathe one side of the patient and move to the other side of the bed to complete the bath.)

19. Spread a towel across patient's chest. Lower bath blanket to patient's umbilical area. Wash, rinse, and dry chest. Keep chest covered with towel between the wash and rinse. Pay special attention to skin folds under the breasts.

Exposing, washing, rinsing, and drying one part of the body at a time avoids unnecessary exposure and chilling. Skin-fold areas may be sources of odor and skin breakdown if not cleansed and dried properly.

20. Lower bath blanket to perineal area. Place a towel over patient's chest.

Keeping the bath blanket and towel in place avoids exposure and chilling.

21. Wash, rinse, and dry abdomen. Carefully inspect and cleanse umbilical area and any abdominal folds or creases.

Skin-fold areas may be sources of odor and skin breakdown if not cleansed and dried properly.

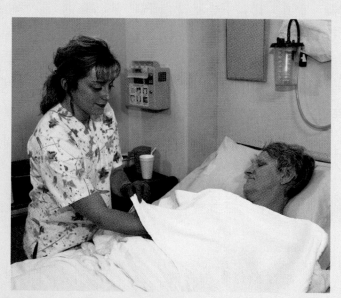

Action 19: Washing the chest area, including the axilla.

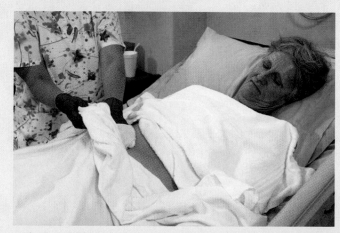

Action 21: Washing the abdomen, with perineal and chest areas covered.

22. Return bath blanket to original position and expose far leg. Place towel under far leg. Using firm strokes, wash, rinse, and dry leg from ankle to knee and knee to groin.

The towel protects linens and prevents the patient from feeling uncomfortable from a damp or wet bed. Washing from ankle to groin with firm strokes promotes venous return.

23. Fold a towel near patient's foot area and place basin on it. Place foot in basin while supporting the ankle and heel in your hand and the leg on your arm. Wash, rinse, and dry, paying particular attention to area between toes.

Supporting the patient's foot and leg helps reduce strain and discomfort for the patient. Placing the foot in a basin of water is comfortable and relaxing and allows for thorough cleaning of the feet and the areas between the toes and under the nails.

continues

Giving a Bed Bath (continued)

ACTION

RATIONALE

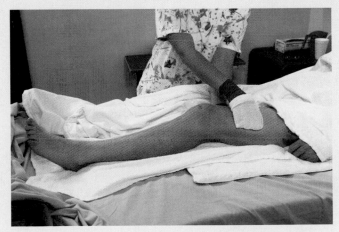

Action 22: Washing and drying far leg, keeping the other leg covered.

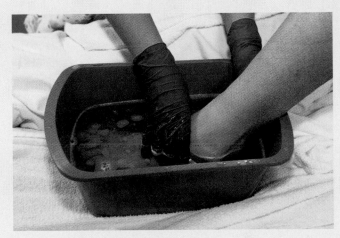

Action 23: Soaking the foot in basin.

24. Repeat Actions 22 and 23 for the other leg and foot.

25. Make sure patient is covered with bath blanket. Change water and washcloth at this point or earlier if necessary. Assist patient onto his or her side.

The bath blanket maintains warmth and privacy. Clean, warm water prevents chilling and maintains patient comfort.

26. Assist patient to prone or side-lying position. Position bath blanket and towel to expose only the back and buttocks.

Positioning the towel and bath blanket protects the patient's privacy and provides warmth.

27. Wash, rinse, and dry back and buttocks area. **Pay particular attention to cleansing between gluteal folds, and observe for any redness or skin breakdown in the sacral area.**

Fecal material near the anus may be a source of microorganisms. Prolonged pressure on the sacral area or other bony prominences may compromise circulation and lead to development of decubitus ulcer.

28. If not contraindicated, give patient a backrub, as described in Chapter 10. Back massage may be given also after perineal care.

A backrub improves circulation to the tissues and is an aid to relaxation. A backrub may be contraindicated in patients with cardiovascular disease or musculoskeletal injuries.

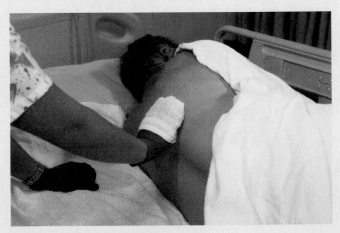

Action 27: Washing the upper back.

continues

ACTION	RATIONALE
29. Refill basin with clean water. Discard washcloth and towel.	The washcloth, towel, and water are contaminated after washing the patient's gluteal area. Changing to clean supplies decreases the spread of organisms from the anal area to the genitals.
30. Clean perineal area or set up patient so that he or she can complete perineal self-care.	Providing perineal self-care may decrease embarrassment for the patient. Effective perineal care reduces odor and decreases the risk for infection through contamination.
31. Help patient put on a clean gown and attend to personal hygiene needs.	This provides for the patient's warmth and comfort.
32. Protect pillow with towel and groom patient's hair.	
33. Change bed linens, as described in Skills 7-3 and 7-4. Remove gloves and perform hand hygiene. Dispose of soiled linens according to agency policy.	These actions deter the spread of microorganisms.
34. Record any significant observations and communication on chart.	A careful record is important for planning and individualizing the patient's care.

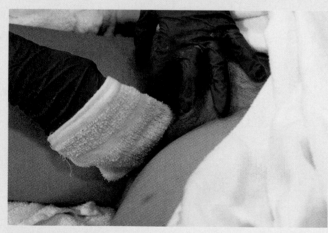

Action 30: Cleansing the perineal area.

7/14/04   Bath done with complete assistance;
reddened area noted on patient's sacral area;
skin care team consultation made.
—C. Stone, RN

Action 34: Documentation.

EVALUATION

The expected outcomes are met when the patient is clean, demonstrates some feeling of control in his or her care; verbalizes an improved body image; and states the importance of cleanliness.

Unexpected Situations and Associated Interventions

- *Patient becomes chilled during bath:* If the room temperature is adjustable, increase it. Another bath blanket may be needed.
- *The patient becomes unstable during the bath:* Critically ill patients often need to be bathed in stages. For instance, the right arm is bathed, and then the patient is allowed to rest for a short period before the left arm is bathed. The amount of rest time needed depends on how unstable the patient is and which parameter is being monitored. If the blood pressure drops when the patient is stimulated, the nurse may watch the blood pressure while bathing the patient and stop when it begins to decrease. Once the blood pressure returns to the previous level, the nurse can begin to bathe the patient again.

continues

Giving a Bed Bath (continued)

Special Considerations

- To remove the gown from a patient with an IV line, take the gown off the uninvolved arm first and then thread the IV tubing and bottle or bag through the arm of the gown. To replace the gown, place the clean gown on the unaffected arm first and thread the IV tubing and bottle or bag from inside the arm of the gown on the involved side. Never disconnect IV tubing to change a gown, because this causes a break in a sterile system and could introduce infection.
- Lying flat in bed during the bed bath may be contraindicated for certain patients. The position may have to be modified to accommodate their needs.

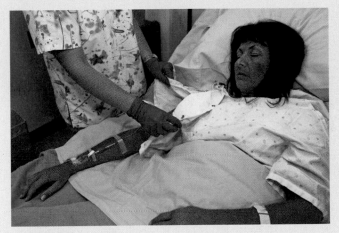

Assisting patient with an IV to put on a new gown.

Infant and Child Considerations

- When bathing an infant or young child, have supplies within easy reach and support or hold the child securely at all times to ensure safety.
- Never leave the child alone.

Older Adult Considerations

- Check the temperature of the water carefully before bathing an older patient, because sensitivity to temperature may be impaired in older persons.
- An older, continent patient may not require a full bed bath with soap and water every day. If dry skin is a problem, water and skin lotion or bath oil may be used on alternate days. If applying lotion, place the lotion dispenser in warm bath water while bathing the patient. This will warm the lotion before it is applied to the patient.

Home Care Considerations

- Evaluate the safety of the bathing area in the home. Tub mats, adhesive strips, grab bars, and shower stools can help prevent falls.

SKILL 7-2

Applying and Removing Antiembolism Stockings

Antiembolism stockings are often used for patients with limited activity to help prevent phlebitis and thrombi formation. Antiembolism stockings help force blood in the superficial veins of the legs to deeper veins, prevent stagnation of blood in the leg veins, and promote venous return to the heart. A physician's order is required for their use.

Equipment

- Elastic stockings (in correct size). *For knee-high stockings:* Measure from heel to popliteal space. Measure circumference of calf at widest point. *For thigh-high stockings:* Measure from heel to gluteal fold. Measure circumference of calf and thigh at widest point.
- Measuring tape
- Talcum powder (optional)

ASSESSMENT

Assess patient's legs for any redness, swelling, warmth, or tenderness that may indicate a deep vein thrombosis. If any of these symptoms is noted, notify physician before applying stockings. Obtain the appropriate measurements for the type of stocking ordered.

NURSING DIAGNOSIS

Determine related factors for the nursing diagnosis based on the patient's current status. Appropriate nursing diagnoses may include:

- Ineffective Peripheral Tissue Perfusion
- Risk for Impaired Skin Integrity
- Excess Fluid Volume
- Risk for Injury

OUTCOME IDENTIFICATION AND PLANNING

The expected outcome to achieve when applying and removing antiembolism stockings is that the stockings will be applied with minimal discomfort to patient. Other outcomes that may be appropriate include the following: edema will decrease in the lower extremities; patient will understand the rationale for stocking application; and patient will remain free of deep vein thrombosis.

IMPLEMENTATION

ACTION	RATIONALE
1. Explain to patient rationale for use of elastic stockings.	Explanation encourages patient cooperation.
2. Perform hand hygiene.	Hand hygiene deters the spread of microorganisms.
3. Assist patient to supine position. If patient has been sitting or walking, have him or her lie down with legs and feet well elevated for at least 15 minutes before applying stockings.	Dependent position of legs encourages blood to pool in the veins.
4. Provide privacy. Expose legs one at a time, and powder lightly unless patient has dry skin. If the skin is dry, a lotion may be used. Powders and lotions are not recommended by some manufacturers.	Powder and lotion reduce friction and make application of stockings easier.
5. Place hand inside stocking and grasp heel area securely. Turn stocking inside-out to the heel area.	Inside-out technique provides for easier application; bunched elastic material can compromise extremity circulation.
6. Ease foot of stocking over foot and heel. Check that patient's heel is centered in heel pocket of stocking.	Wrinkles and improper fit interfere with circulation.

continues

Applying and Removing Antiembolism Stockings (continued)

ACTION   **RATIONALE**

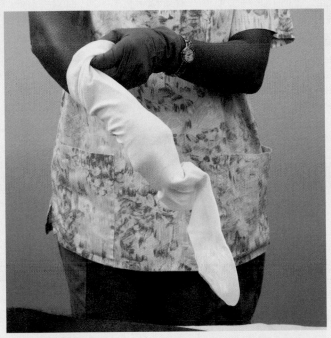

Action 5: Sliding hand into antiembolism stockings.

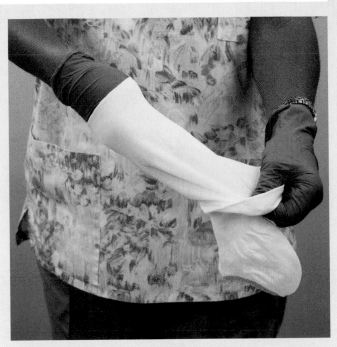

Action 5: Pulling antiembolism stockings inside out.

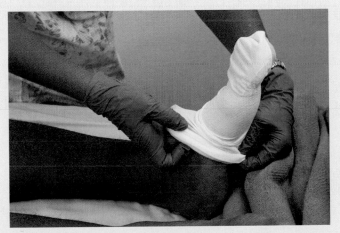

Action 6: Putting foot of stocking on patient.

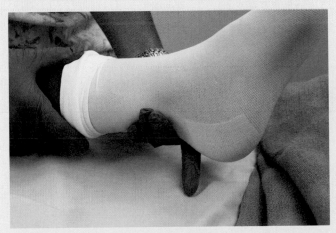

Action 6: Ensuring heel is centered after stocking is on.

7. Using your fingers and thumbs, carefully grasp edge of stocking and pull it up smoothly over ankle and calf until entire stocking is turned right side out. Pull forward slightly on toe section. Repeat for other leg. **Caution patient not to roll stockings partially down.**

8. Perform hand hygiene.

Removing Stockings

9. To remove stocking, grasp top of stocking with your thumb and fingers and smoothly pull stocking off inside-out to heel. Support foot and ease stocking over it.

Easing the stocking carefully into position ensures proper fit of the stocking to the contour of the leg. Rolling stockings may have a constricting effect on veins. Loosening the toe section provides for comfort in that area.

Hand hygiene deters the spread of microorganisms.

This preserves the elasticity and contour of the stocking.

continues

Applying and Removing Antiembolism Stockings (continued)

ACTION	RATIONALE

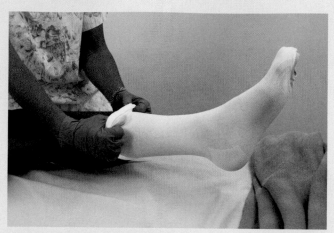

Action 7: Pulling the sock up the leg.

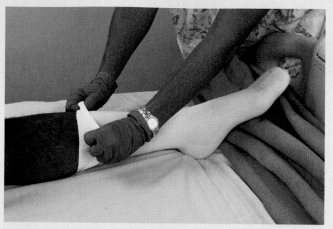

Action 9: Grasping the top of stocking to remove it.

10. **Remove stockings once every shift for 20 to 30 minutes.** Wash and air-dry as necessary (according to manufacturer's directions).

This allows assessment of circulatory status and condition of skin on lower extremity.

11. Record application of elastic stockings as well as assessment of circulatory status and skin condition.

This provides accurate documentation of the procedure.

> 7/22/04   0945   Knee-high antiembolism stockings applied bilaterally. Post tibial and dorsalis pedal pulses +2 bilaterally; capillary refill <2 seconds and skin on toes is pink and warm. Skin on lower extremities is intact bilaterally. —C. Stone, RN

Action 11: Documentation.

EVALUATION

The expected outcome is met when the stockings are applied and removed as indicated. Other outcomes are met when the patient exhibits a decrease in peripheral edema, and the patient can state the reason for using the stockings.

Unexpected Situations and Associated Interventions

- *Patient has large amount of pain with application of stockings:* If pain is expected (eg, if the patient has a leg incision), the patient may be premedicated and the stockings applied once the medication has had time to take effect. If the pain is unexpected, a physician may need to be notified because the patient may be developing a deep vein thrombosis.
- *Patient has an incision on the leg:* When applying and removing stockings, be careful not to hit the incision. If the incision is draining, apply a small bandage to the incision so that it does not drain onto the stockings. If the stockings become soiled by drainage, wash and dry according to instructions.
- *Patient is to ambulate with stockings:* Place skid-resistant socks or slippers on before patient attempts to ambulate.

Special Considerations

- Despite the use of elastic stockings, a patient may develop thrombophlebitis. A unilateral swelling, redness, tenderness, and warmth are possible indicators of thrombophlebitis. A patient may also have a positive Homans' sign (pain on dorsiflexion) with thrombophlebitis.

continues

SKILL 7-2 — Applying and Removing Antiembolism Stockings (continued)

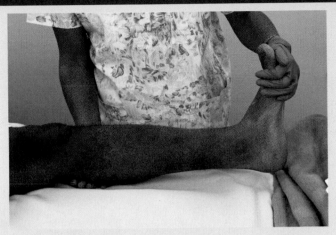

Assessing Homans' sign.

Home Care Considerations

- Make sure that the patient has an extra pair of stockings ordered during hospitalization before discharge (for payment and convenience purposes).
- Stockings may be laundered with other "white" clothing. Avoid excessive bleach. Remove from dryer as soon as "low heat" cycle is complete to avoid shrinkage. Stockings may also be air-dried.

SKILL 7-3 — Making an Unoccupied Bed

If the patient can get out of bed, the bed should be made while it is unoccupied to decrease stress on the patient and the nurse.

Equipment

- Two large sheets (or one large sheet and one fitted sheet)
- Drawsheet (optional)
- Blankets
- Bedspread
- Pillowcases
- Linen hamper or bag
- Bedside chair
- Waterproof protective pad (optional)
- Disposable gloves (for use if linens are soiled)

ASSESSMENT

Before beginning to change linens, inspect the bed for evidence of any body secretions or fluids on the linens. If present, don disposable gloves before changing linens. Also check for any patient belongings that may have accidentally been placed in bed, such as eyeglasses or prayer cloths.

NURSING DIAGNOSIS

Determine the related factors for the nursing diagnosis based on the patient's current status. Many nursing diagnoses may require the use of this skill. Possible nursing diagnoses may include:

- Risk for Impaired Skin Integrity
- Risk for Activity Intolerance
- Impaired Physical Mobility

continues

**OUTCOME
IDENTIFICATION
AND PLANNING**

The expected outcome to achieve when making an unoccupied bed is that the bed linens will be changed without injury to the nurse or patient.

IMPLEMENTATION

ACTION	RATIONALE
1. Perform hand hygiene.	Hand hygiene deters the spread of microorganisms.
2. Assemble equipment and arrange on a bedside chair in the order in which items will be used.	Organization facilitates performance of task.
3. Adjust bed to high position and drop side rails.	Having the bed in the high position and the side rails down reduces strain on the nurse while working.
4. Disconnect call bell or any tubes from bed linens.	Disconnecting devices prevents damage to the devices.
5. Loosen all linen as you move around the bed, from the head of the bed on the far side to the head of the bed on the near side.	Loosening the linen helps prevent tugging and tearing on linen. Loosening the linen and moving around the bed systematically reduce strain caused by reaching across the bed.
6. Fold reusable linens, such as sheets, blankets, or spread, in place on the bed in fourths and hang them over a clean chair.	Folding saves time and energy when reusable linen is replaced on the bed. Folding linens while they are on the bed reduces strain on the nurse's arms. Some agencies change linens only when soiled.
7. **Snugly roll all the soiled linen inside the bottom sheet and place directly into the laundry hamper. Do not place on floor or furniture. Do not hold soiled linens against your uniform.**	Rolling soiled linens snugly and placing them directly into the hamper helps prevent the spread of microorganisms. The floor is heavily contaminated; soiled linen will further contaminate furniture. Soiled linen contaminates the nurse's uniform, and this may spread organisms to another patient.
8. If possible, shift mattress up to head of bed.	This allows more foot room for the patient.
9. Place the bottom sheet with its center fold in the center of the bed and high enough to have a sufficient amount of the sheet to tuck under the head of the mattress.	Opening linens on the bed reduces strain on the nurse's arms and diminishes the spread of microorganisms.

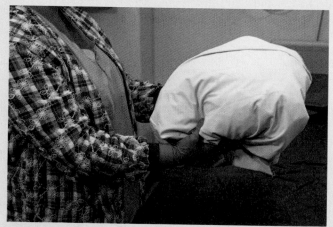

Action 7: Bundling soiled linens in bottom sheet and holding them away from body.

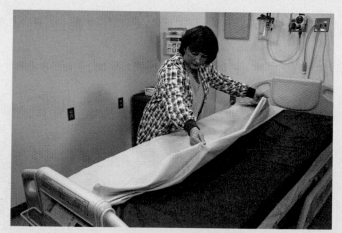

Action 9: Placing clean linens to begin bed making.

10. Place the drawsheet with its center fold in the center of the bed and positioned so it will be located under the patient's midsection. If a protective pad is used, place it over the drawsheet in the proper area. Not all agencies use drawsheets routinely. The nurse may decide to use one.	If the patient soils the bed, drawsheets can be changed without the bottom and top linens on the bed. Having all bottom linens in place before tucking them under the mattress avoids unnecessary moving about the bed. A drawsheet is also an aid when moving the patient in bed.

continues

ACTION   **RATIONALE**

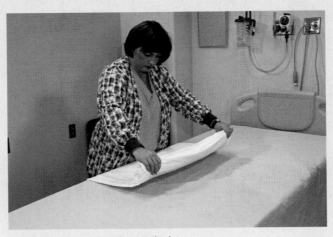

Action 10: Placing drawsheet on bed.

11. Tuck the bottom sheet securely under the head of the mattress on one side of the bed, making a corner according to agency policy. A mitered corner is shown. Using a fitted bottom sheet eliminates the need to miter corners. Tuck the remaining bottom sheet and drawsheet securely under the mattress. (At this point, before moving to the other side of the bed, top linens may be placed on the bed, unfolded, and secured, allowing the entire side of the bed to be completed at one time, as shown in the illustrations.)

Making the bed on one side and then completing the bed on the other side saves time. Having bottom linens free of wrinkles reduces patient discomfort.

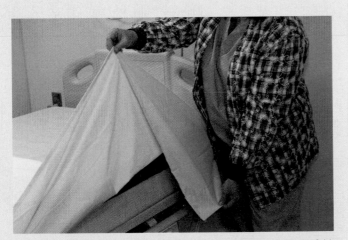

Action 11: Beginning to make mitered corner by creating a triangular fold.

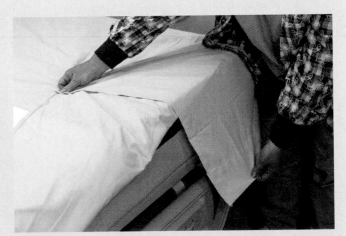

Action 11: Laying triangular fold on top of bed.

continues

ACTION

RATIONALE

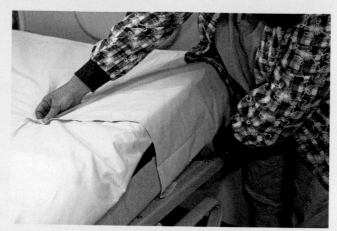

Action 11: Tucking end of sheet under mattress.

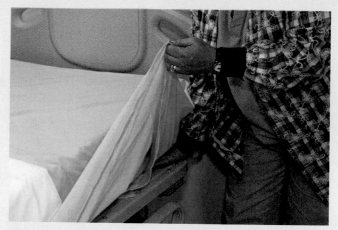

Action 11: Folding triangular linen fold down over side of mattress.

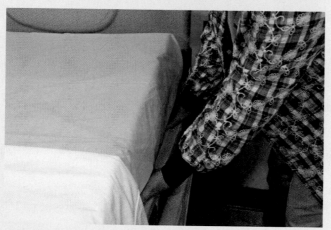

Action 11: Tucking end of triangular linen fold under mattress to complete mitered corner.

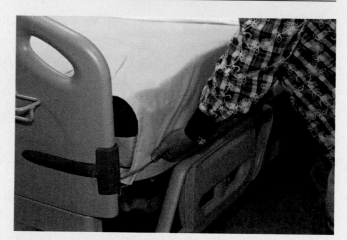

Action 11: Tucking sheet snugly under foot of mattress.

12. Move to the other side of the bed to secure bottom linens. Secure bottom sheet under the head of the mattress and miter the corner. **Pull remainder of sheet tightly and tuck under mattress.** Do the same for drawsheet.

This rids bottom linens of wrinkles, which can cause patient discomfort and promote skin breakdown.

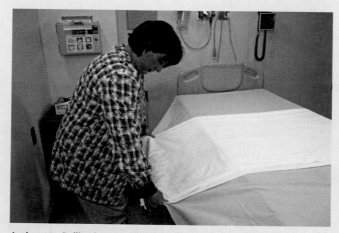

Action 12: Pulling bottom sheet tightly on opposite side of bed.

continues

ACTION

RATIONALE

13. Place the top sheet on the bed with its center fold in the center of the bed and with the top of the sheet placed so that the hem is even with the head of the mattress. Unfold the top sheet in place. Follow same procedure with top blanket or spread, placing the upper edge about 6″ below the top of the sheet.

14. Tuck the top sheet and blanket under the foot of the bed on the near side. Miter the corners.

15. Fold the upper 6″ of the top sheet down over the spread and make a cuff.

Opening linens by shaking them spreads organisms into the air. Holding linens overhead to open them causes strain on the nurse's arms.

This saves time and energy and keeps the top linen in place.

This makes it easier for the patient to get into bed and pull the covers up.

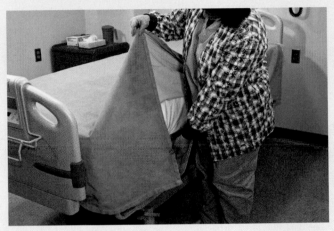

Action 14: Mitering corner of top sheet and spread.

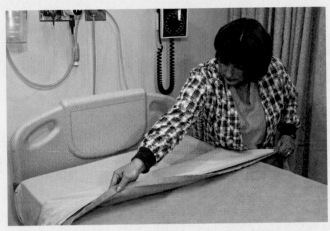

Action 15: Cuffing top linens.

16. Move to the other side of the bed and follow the same procedure for securing top sheets under the foot of the bed and making a cuff.

17. Place the pillows on the bed. Open each pillowcase in the same manner as you opened other linens. Gather the pillowcase over one hand toward the closed end. Grasp the pillow with the hand inside the pillowcase. Keeping a firm hold on the top of the pillow, pull the cover onto the pillow.

18. Place the pillow at the head of the bed with the open end facing toward the window.

Working on one side of the bed at a time saves energy and is more efficient.

Opening linens by shaking them causes organisms to be carried on air currents. Covering the pillow while it rests on the bed reduces strain on the nurse's arms and back.

This provides for a neater appearance.

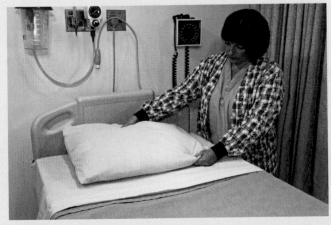

Action 18: Placing pillow on bed.

continues

ACTION	RATIONALE
19. Fan-fold or pie-fold the top linens.	Having linens opened makes it more convenient for the patient to get into bed.
20. **Secure the signal device on the bed according to agency policy.**	The patient will be able to call for assistance as necessary.

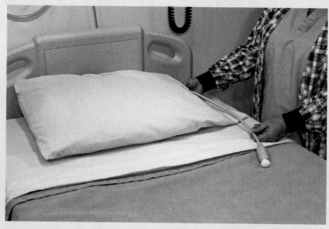

Action 20: Securing signal device to bed.

21. **Adjust bed to low position.**	Having the bed in the low position makes it easier and safer for the patient to get into bed.
22. Dispose of soiled linen according to agency policy. Perform hand hygiene.	This deters the spread of microorganisms.

EVALUATION

The expected outcome is met when the bed linens are changed without any injury to the patient or nurse.

Unexpected Situations and Associated Interventions

- *Drawsheet is not available:* A flat sheet can be folded in half to substitute for a drawsheet, but extra care must be taken to avoid wrinkles in the bed.
- *Patient is frequently incontinent of stool or urine:* More than one protective pad can be placed under the patient to protect the bed, but care must be taken to ensure that the patient is not lying on wrinkles from linens.

Making an Occupied Bed

If the patient cannot get out of bed, the linens may need to be changed with the patient still in the bed. This is termed an "occupied" bed.

Equipment
- Two large sheets (or one large sheet and one fitted sheet)
- Drawsheet (optional)
- Blankets
- Bedspread
- Pillowcases
- Linen hamper or bag
- Bedside chair
- Protective pad (optional)
- Disposable gloves (if linens are soiled)

ASSESSMENT

Before beginning to change linens, check for evidence of any body secretions or fluids on the linens. If present, don disposable gloves before changing linens. Check the bed for any patient belongings that may have accidentally been placed or fallen there, such as eyeglasses or prayer cloths.

NURSING DIAGNOSIS

Determine the related factors for the nursing diagnosis based on the patient's current status. Many nursing diagnoses may require the use of this skill. Possible nursing diagnoses may include:
- Risk for Impaired Skin Integrity
- Risk for Activity Intolerance
- Impaired Physical Mobility
- Impaired Bed Mobility
- Impaired Transfer Ability

Many other nursing diagnoses may require the use of this skill.

OUTCOME IDENTIFICATION AND PLANNING

The expected outcome to achieve when making an occupied bed is that the bed linens are applied without injury to the patient or nurse. Other possible outcomes may include: patient participates in moving from side to side, and patient verbalizes feelings of increased comfort.

IMPLEMENTATION

ACTION	RATIONALE
1. Explain procedure to patient. Check chart for limitations on patient's physical activity.	This facilitates patient cooperation and determines level of activity.
2. Perform hand hygiene.	Hand hygiene deters the spread of microorganisms.
3. Assemble equipment and arrange on bedside chair in the order the items will be used.	Organization facilitates performance of task.
4. Close door or curtain.	This provides for privacy.
5. Adjust bed to high position. Lower side rail nearest you, leaving the opposite side rail up. Place bed in flat position unless contraindicated.	Having the bed in the high position reduces strain on the nurse while working. Having the mattress flat makes it easier to prepare a wrinkle-free bed.
6. Check bed linens for patient's personal items. **Disconnect the call bell or any tubes from bed linens.**	It is costly and inconvenient when personal items are lost. Disconnecting tubes from linens prevents discomfort and accidental dislodging of the tubes.

continues

ACTION	RATIONALE
7. Place bath blanket, if available, over patient. Have patient hold onto bath blanket while you reach under it and remove top linens. Leave top sheet in place if a bath blanket is not used. Fold linen that is to be reused over the back of a chair. Discard soiled linen in laundry bag or hamper.	This provides warmth and privacy.
8. If possible and another person is available to assist, grasp mattress securely and shift it up to head of bed.	This allows more foot room for the patient.
9. Assist patient to turn toward opposite side of the bed, and reposition pillow under patient's head.	This allows the bed to be made on the vacant side.
10. Loosen all bottom linens from head and sides of bed.	This facilitates removal of linens.
11. Fan-fold soiled linens as close to patient as possible.	This makes it easier to remove linens when the patient turns to the other side.

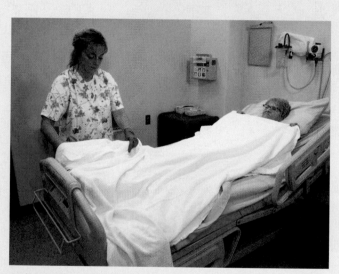

Action 7: Removing top linens from under bath blanket.

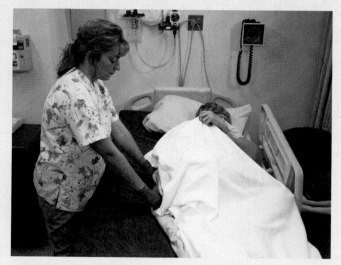

Action 11: Moving soiled linen as close to patient as possible.

12. Use clean linen and make near side of bed following Actions 9, 10, and 11 of Skill 7-3. Fan-fold the clean linen as close to patient as possible.	This positions clean linen to make the side of the bed.
13. Raise side rail. Assist patient to roll over the folded linen in the middle of the bed toward you. Reposition pillow and bath blanket or top sheet. Move to other side of the bed and lower side rail.	This ensures patient safety. The movement allows the bed to be made on the other side. The bath blanket provides warmth and privacy.
14. Loosen and remove all bottom linen. Place in linen bag or hamper. Hold soiled linen away from your uniform.	Proper disposal of soiled linen prevents spread of microorganisms.
15. Ease clean linen from under patient. Pull taut and secure bottom sheet under head of mattress. Miter corners (see Skill 7-3). Pull the side of the sheet taut and tuck under side of mattress. Repeat with drawsheet.	This removes wrinkles and creases in the linens, which are uncomfortable to lie on.
16. Assist patient to return to center of bed. Remove pillow and change pillowcase (see Skill 7-3, Action 17) before replacing, with open end facing toward the window.	This provides for a neater appearance.

continues

ACTION

RATIONALE

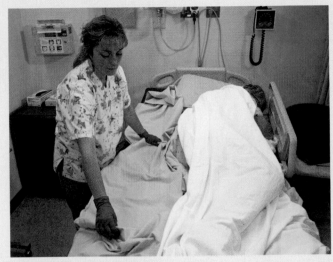

Action 12: Opening and folding clean linens.

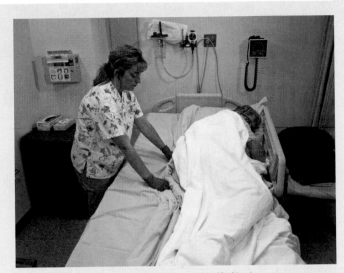

Action 12: Aligning clean bottom sheet on half of bed.

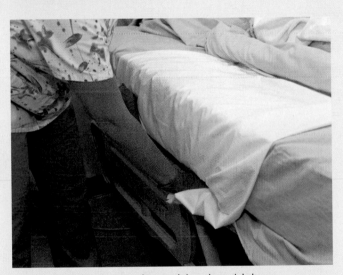

Action 12: Tucking bottom sheet and drawsheet tightly.

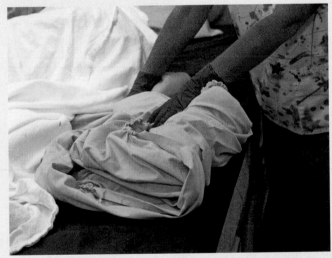

Action 14: Removing soiled bottom linens from other side of bed.

17. Apply top linen so that it is centered and top hems are even with the head of the mattress. Have patient hold onto top linen so bath blanket can be removed.

This allows bottom hems to be tucked securely under the mattress and provides for privacy.

18. Secure top linens under foot of mattress and miter corners. Loosen top linens over patient's feet by grasping them in the area of the feet and pulling gently toward foot of bed.

This provides for a neat appearance. Loosening linens over the patient's feet gives more room for movement.

19. **Raise side rail. Lower bed height and adjust head of bed to a comfortable position. Reattach call bell and drainage tubes.**

This provides for the patient's safety.

20. Dispose of soiled linens according to agency policy. Perform hand hygiene.

This prevents the spread of microorganisms.

continues

ACTION   **RATIONALE**

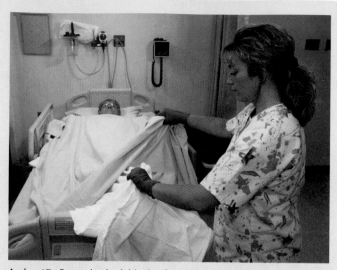

Action 17: Removing bath blanket from under top linens.

EVALUATION

The expected outcome is met when the bed linens are changed and the patient and nurse remain free of injury. In addition, the patient assists in moving from side to side and states feelings of increased comfort after the bed is changed.

Unexpected Situations and Associated Interventions

- *Dirty linens are grossly contaminated with fecal drainage:* Obtain an extra towel or protective pad. Place the pad under and over the soiled linens so that new linens will not be in contact with soiled linens.

Older Adult Considerations

- Using a synthetic sheepskin, a soft bath blanket, or a flannelette blanket as a bottom sheet may solve the problem of "coldness" for elderly patients with vascular problems or arthritis.

Assisting the Patient With Oral Care

Oral care is important not only to prevent dental caries but also to improve the patient's self-image. Oral care should be done at least twice a day for ambulatory patients.

Equipment

- Toothbrush
- Toothpaste
- Emesis basin
- Glass with cool water
- Disposable gloves
- Towel
- Mouthwash (optional)
- Dental floss (optional)
- Denture-cleansing equipment (if necessary)
- Denture cup
- Denture cleaner
- 4 × 4 gauze
- Washcloth or paper towel
- Lip lubricant (optional)

ASSESSMENT

Assess patient's oral cavity and dentition. Look for any caries, sores, or white patches. The white patches may indicate a fungal infection called thrush. Assess patient's ability to perform own care.

NURSING DIAGNOSIS

Determine the related factors for the nursing diagnosis based on the patient's current status. Possible nursing diagnoses may include:

- Ineffective Health Maintenance
- Impaired Oral Mucous Membrane
- Disturbed Body Image
- Deficient Knowledge

OUTCOME IDENTIFICATION AND PLANNING

The expected outcome to achieve when performing oral care is that the patient's mouth and teeth will be clean; the patient will exhibit a positive body image; and the patient will verbalize the importance of oral care.

IMPLEMENTATION

ACTION	RATIONALE
1. Explain procedure to patient.	Explanation facilitates cooperation.
2. Perform hand hygiene. Don disposable gloves if assisting with oral care.	Hand hygiene deters the spread of microorganisms. Gloves protect the nurse from exposure to blood and bloodborne infections.
3. Assemble equipment on overbed table within patient's reach.	Organization facilitates performance of task.
4. Provide privacy for patient.	Patient may be embarrassed if cleansing involves removal of dentures.
5. Lower side rail and assist patient to sitting position if permitted, or turn patient onto side. Place towel across patient's chest. Raise bed to a comfortable working position.	The sitting or side-lying position prevents aspiration of fluids into the lungs. The towel protects the patient from dampness.

continues

ACTION

RATIONALE

6. Encourage patient to brush own teeth, or assist if necessary:

   a. Moisten toothbrush and apply toothpaste to bristles.

   b. Place brush at a 45-degree angle to gum line and brush from gum line to crown of each tooth. Brush outer and inner surfaces. Brush back and forth across biting surface of each tooth.

   c. Brush tongue gently with toothbrush.

   d. Have patient rinse vigorously with water and spit into emesis basin. Repeat until clear. Suction may be used as an alternative for removal of fluid and secretions from mouth.

   a. Water softens the bristles.

   b. This facilitates removal of plaque and tartar. The 45-degree angle of brushing permits cleansing of all surface areas of the tooth.

   c. This removes coating on the tongue. Gentle motion does not stimulate gag reflex.

   d. The vigorous swishing motion helps to remove debris. Suction is appropriate if swallowing reflex is impaired or absent.

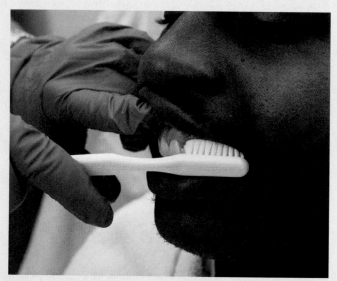

Action 6b: Placing brush at a 45-degree angle to the gum line.

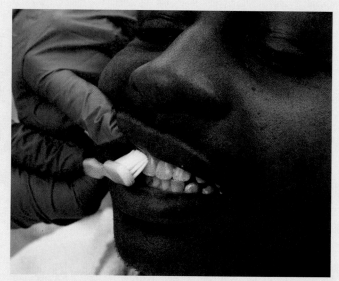

Action 6b: Brushing from the gum line to the crown of each tooth.

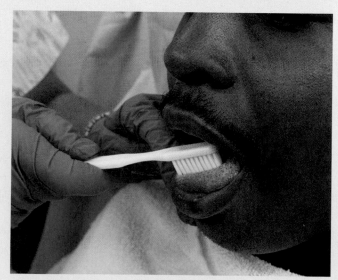

Action 6c: Brushing the tongue.

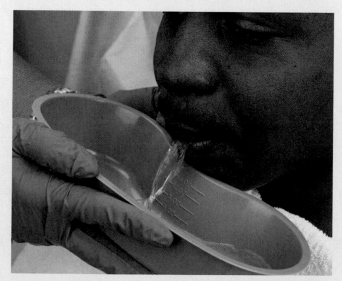

Action 6d: Holding emesis basin for patient to rinse and spit.

continues

Assisting the Patient With Oral Care (continued)

ACTION	RATIONALE
e. Assist patient to floss teeth if necessary.	e. Flossing aids in removal of plaque and promotes healthy gum tissue.
f. Offer mouthwash if patient prefers.	f. Mouthwash leaves a pleasant taste in the mouth.
7. Assist patient with removal and cleansing of dentures if necessary:	
a. Apply gentle pressure with 4 × 4 gauze to grasp upper denture plate and remove. Place it immediately in denture cup. Lift lower dentures using slight rocking motion, remove, and place in denture cup.	a. Rocking motion breaks suction between denture and gum. Using 4 × 4 gauze prevents slippage and discourages spread of microorganisms.

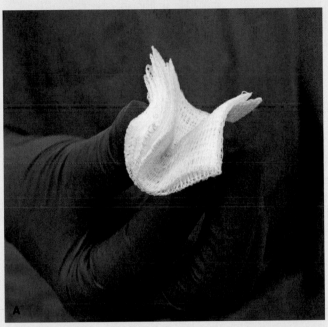

Action 7a: Preparing to remove dentures.

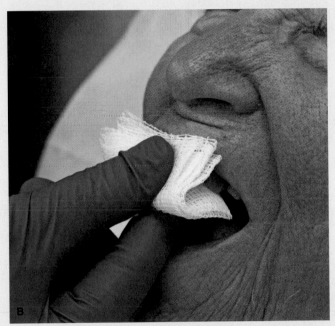

Action 7a: Removing dentures with a gauze sponge.

b. If patient prefers, add denture cleanser to cup with water and follow directions on preparation, or brush all areas thoroughly with toothbrush and paste. **Place paper towels or washcloth in sink while brushing.**	b. Dentures collect food and microorganisms and require daily cleansing. Putting paper towels or a washcloth in the sink protects against breakage.
c. Rinse thoroughly with water and return dentures to patient.	c. Water aids in removal of debris and acts as a cleansing agent.
d. Offer mouthwash so patient can rinse mouth before replacing dentures.	d. Mouthwash leaves a pleasant taste in the mouth and removes food particles, thus permitting proper fit.
e. Apply lubricant to lips if needed.	e. Lubricant prevents cracking and drying of lips.

Flossing Teeth

8. Remove approximately 6″ of dental floss from container or use a plastic floss holder. Wrap the floss around the index fingers, keeping about 1″ to 1.5″ of floss taut between the fingers.	The floss must be held taut to get between the teeth.
9. Insert floss gently between teeth, moving it back and forth downward to the gums.	Trauma to the gums can occur if floss is forced between teeth.

continues

SKILL 7-5   Assisting the Patient With Oral Care (continued)

ACTION

RATIONALE

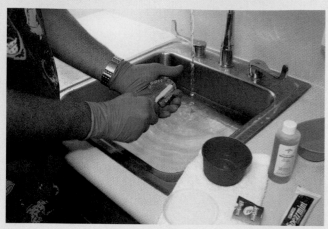

Action 7b: Cleaning dentures at the sink.

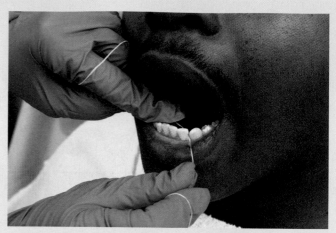

Action 10: Flossing the teeth.

10. Move the floss up and down first on one side of a tooth and then on the side of the other tooth, until the surfaces are clean.

This ensures that the sides of both teeth are cleaned.

11. Repeat Actions 9 and 10 in the spaces between all teeth.

12. Instruct patient to rinse mouth well with water after flossing.

Vigorous rinsing helps to remove food particles and plaque that have been loosened by flossing.

13. Remove equipment and assist patient to a position of comfort. Record any unusual bleeding or inflammation. Raise side rail and lower bed.

This promotes oral hygiene and provides for oral assessment. Elevated side rails and lowered bed position maintain safety for bedridden patients.

14. Remove disposable gloves from inside out and discard appropriately. Perform hand hygiene.

This protects the nurse from contact with any micro-organisms. Hand hygiene deters spread of micro-organisms.

EVALUATION

The expected outcomes are met when the patient receives oral care, experiences little to no discomfort, states mouth feels refreshed, and demonstrates understanding of reasons for proper oral care.

Unexpected Situations and Associated Interventions

- *While cleaning the teeth, you notice a large amount of bleeding from the gum line:* Stop brushing. Allow patient to gently rinse mouth with water and spit into emesis basin. Before brushing again, check most recent platelet level.
- *Patient has braces on teeth:* Brush extra thoroughly. Braces collect food particles.

Infant and Child Considerations

- When assisting small children with oral care, do not use a toothpaste that contains fluoride if the child cannot spit out excess. Excessive amounts of ingested fluoride can lead to a discoloration of the teeth.

SKILL 7-6

Providing Oral Care for the Dependent Patient

Some patients cannot perform their own oral care. When assisting the dependent patient, the nurse may have to protect the patient's airway while performing oral care.

Equipment

- Toothbrush
- Toothpaste
- Emesis basin
- Glass with cool water
- Disposable gloves
- Towel
- Mouthwash (optional)
- Normal saline solution
- Dental floss (optional)
- Denture-cleansing equipment (if necessary)
- Denture cup
- Denture cleaner
- 4 × 4 gauze
- Washcloth or paper towel
- Lip lubricant (optional)
- Sponge toothette or tongue blades padded with 4 × 4 gauze sponges
- Irrigating syringe with rubber tip (optional)
- Suction catheter with suction apparatus (optional)

ASSESSMENT

Assess the patient's level of consciousness and overall ability to assist with oral care and respond to directions. Inspect the patient's oral cavity and teeth. Look for any caries, sores, or white patches. The white patches may indicate a fungal infection called thrush. Assess the patient's ability to perform care.

NURSING DIAGNOSIS

Determine the related factors for the nursing diagnosis based on the patient's current status. Possible nursing diagnoses may include:

- Ineffective Health Maintenance
- Impaired Oral Mucous Membrane
- Disturbed Body Image
- Deficient Knowledge

Other nursing diagnoses also may require the use of this skill.

OUTCOME IDENTIFICATION AND PLANNING

The expected outcome to achieve when performing oral care is that the patient's mouth and teeth will be clean; the patient will participate as much as possible with oral care; the patient will demonstrate improvement in body image; and the patient will verbalize an understanding about the importance of oral care.

IMPLEMENTATION

ACTION	RATIONALE
1. Explain procedure to patient.	Explanation facilitates cooperation.
2. Perform hand hygiene and don disposable gloves.	Hand hygiene and disposable gloves deter the spread of microorganisms.
3. Assemble equipment on overbed table within reach.	Organization facilitates performance of task.
4. Provide privacy for patient. Adjust height of bed to a comfortable position. Lower one side rail and position patient on the side, with head tilted forward. Place towel across patient's chest and emesis basin in position under chin.	The side-lying position with head forward prevents aspiration of fluid into lungs. Towel and emesis basin protects patient from dampness.

continues

ACTION

RATIONALE

5. Open patient's mouth and gently insert a padded tongue blade between back molars if necessary.

A padded tongue blade keeps the mouth open for easier cleaning and prevents the patient from biting the nurse's fingers.

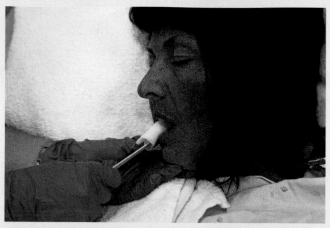

Action 5: Gently inserting padded tongue blade between back molars.

6. If teeth are present, brush carefully with toothbrush and paste. Remove dentures if present and clean before replacing (see Skill 7-5). Use a toothette or gauze-padded tongue blade moistened with normal saline or dilute mouthwash solution to gently cleanse gums, mucous membranes, and tongue.

Toothbrush or padded tongue blade provides friction necessary to clean areas where plaque and tartar accumulate. Hydrogen peroxide is considered an irritant and is not longer recommended. The mechanical action of cleansing is more important than the solution used.

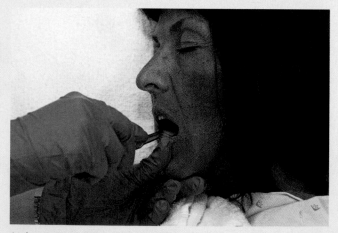

Action 6: Carefully brushing patient's teeth.

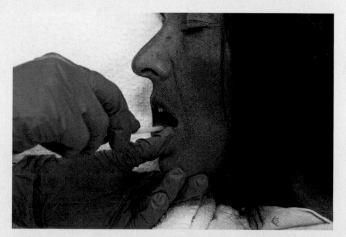

Action 6: Using moistened padded tongue blade to cleanse gums, mucous membranes, and tongue.

7. Use gauze-padded tongue blade dipped in mouthwash solution to rinse the oral cavity. If desired, insert the rubber tip of the irrigating syringe into patient's mouth and rinse gently with a small amount of water. Position patient's head to allow for return of water or use suction apparatus to remove the water from oral cavity.

Rinsing helps cleanse debris from the mouth. Forceful irrigation may cause aspiration.

continues

Providing Oral Care for the Dependent Patient (continued)

ACTION	RATIONALE

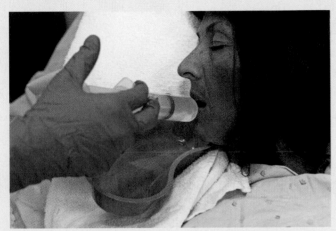

Action 7: Using irrigating syringe and a small amount of water to rinse mouth.

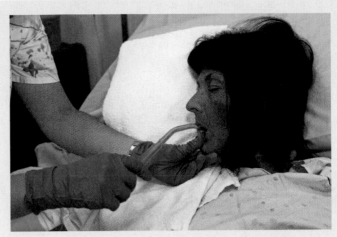

Action 7: Using suction to remove excess fluid.

8. Apply lubricant to patient's lips.

9. Remove equipment and return patient to a position of comfort. Raise side rail and lower bed. **Record any unusual bleeding or inflammation.**

10. Perform hand hygiene.

This prevents drying and cracking of lips.

This promotes oral hygiene and provides for oral assessment. Raised side rail and lowered bed maintain patient safety.

Hand hygiene deters the spread of microorganisms.

> 7/10/04   0945   Oral care done. Small
> amount of bleeding noted from gums after
> using soft-bristled toothbrush. Resolved
> spontaneously when brushing completed.
> —C. Stone, RN

Action 9: Documentation.

EVALUATION

The expected outcomes are met when the patient's oral cavity is clean and patient states or demonstrates improved body image. In addition, the patient verbalizes a basic understanding of the need for oral care if alert and oriented.

Unexpected Situations and Associated Interventions

- *Patient begins to cough and gag during oral care:* Stop performing oral care. Assist patient onto side and remove secretions from mouth with suction.
- *Patient begins to bite on padded tongue blade:* Do not jerk tongue blade out. Wait for patient to relax mouth before removing padded tongue blade.

Special Considerations

- A patient receiving chemotherapy medication may have bleeding gums and extremely sensitive mucous membranes. Use a soft sponge toothette for cleaning, or substitute a salt water rinse (0.5 teaspoon salt in 1 cup of warm water) for brushing of teeth.

SKILL 7-7   Giving a Bed Shampoo

The easiest way to wash a patient's hair is to assist him or her in the shower, but not all patients can take showers. If the patient's hair needs to be washed but the patient is unable or is not allowed to get out of bed, a bed shampoo can be performed.

Equipment

- Pitcher of warm water
- Shampoo
- Conditioner (optional)
- Disposable gloves (optional)
- Protective pad for bed
- Shampoo board
- Bucket
- Towel
- Gown
- Comb or brush
- Blow dryer (optional)

ASSESSMENT

Assess the patient's ability to get out of bed to have his or her hair washed. If the physician's orders allow it and patient is physically able to wash his or her hair in the shower, the patient may prefer to do so. If the patient cannot tolerate being out of bed or is not allowed to do so, perform a bed shampoo. Inspect the patient's scalp for any cuts, lesions, or bumps. Note any flaking, drying, or excessive oiliness.

NURSING DIAGNOSIS

Determine the related factors for the nursing diagnosis based on the patient's current status. An appropriate nursing diagnosis is Bathing/Hygiene Self-Care Deficit. Other nursing diagnosis may include:

- Activity Intolerance
- Impaired Physical Mobility
- Impaired Transfer Ability
- Impaired Social Interaction
- Disturbed Body Image

OUTCOME IDENTIFICATION AND PLANNING

The expected outcome to achieve when giving a bed shampoo is that the patient's hair will be clean. Other outcomes that may be appropriate include the following: the patient will tolerate the shampoo with little to no difficulty; the patient will demonstrate an improved body image, and the patient will state an increase in comfort.

IMPLEMENTATION

ACTION	RATIONALE
1. Gather equipment and place at bedside.	Organization facilitates performance of tasks.
2. Perform hand hygiene. **If you suspect there are any cuts of the scalp or blood in the hair, don disposable gloves.** Lower head of bed.	Hand hygiene deters the spread of microorganisms. Gloves protect the nurse from any pathogens.
3. Remove pillow and place protective pad under patient's head and shoulders.	This protects the sheets from getting wet.
4. **Fill the pitcher with warm water (43° to 46°C [110° to 115°F]).** Place shampoo board underneath patient's head by having patient lift the head.	Warm water is comfortable and relaxing for the patient. It also stimulates circulation and provides for more effective cleansing.

continues

Giving a Bed Shampoo (continued)

ACTION

RATIONALE

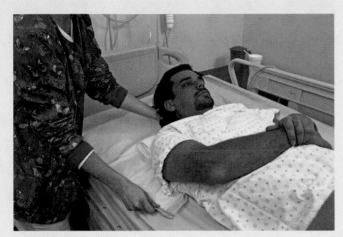

Action 3: Padding head of bed with protective sheets.

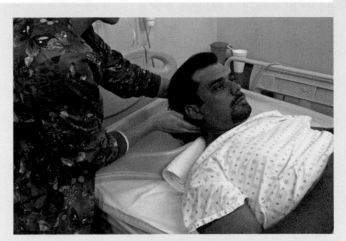

Action 4: Placing patient's head on shampoo board.

5. Place bucket on floor underneath the drain of the shampoo board.

6. Pour pitcher of warm water slowly over patient's head, making sure that all hair is saturated. Refill pitcher if needed.

The bucket will catch the runoff water, preventing a mess on the floor.

By pouring slowly, more hair will become wet, and it is more soothing for the patient.

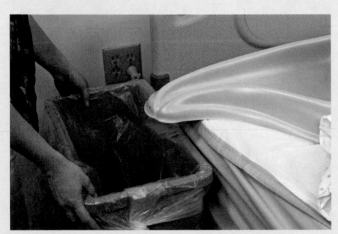

Action 5: Positioning drain container for shampoo board.

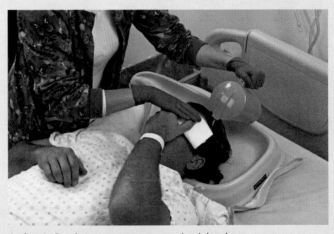

Action 6: Pouring warm water over patient's head.

7. Apply a small amount of shampoo to patient's hair. **Massage deep into the scalp, avoiding any cuts, lesions, or sore spots.**

8. Rinse with warm water (43° to 46°C [110° to 115°F]) until all shampoo is out of hair. Repeat shampoo if necessary.

9. If patient has thick hair or requests, apply a small amount of conditioner to hair and massage throughout. Avoid any cuts, lesions, or sore spots.

10. If bucket is small, empty before rinsing hair. Rinse with warm water (43° to 46°C [110° to 115°F]) until all conditioner is out of hair.

Shampoo will help to remove dirt or oil.

Shampoo left in hair may cause pruritus. If hair is still dirty, another shampoo treatment may be needed.

Conditioner eases tangles and moisturizes hair and scalp.

Bucket may overflow, making mess on floor if not emptied. Conditioner left in hair may cause pruritus.

continues

ACTION

RATIONALE

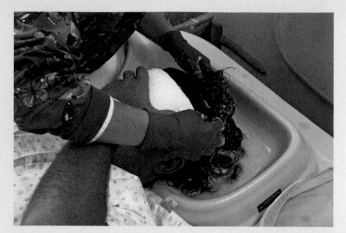

Action 7: Lathering up shampoo.

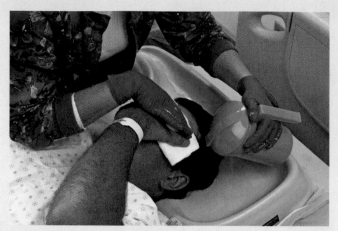

Action 8: Rinsing shampoo from patient's head.

11. Place towel around patient's hair. Remove shampoo board.

12. Pat hair dry, avoiding any cuts, lesions, or sore spots. Remove protective padding but keep one dry protective pad under patient's hair.

This prevents the patient from getting cold.

Patting dry removes any excess water without damaging hair or scalp.

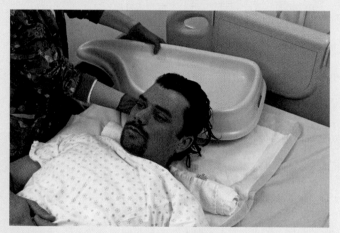

Action 11: Removing shampoo board from bed.

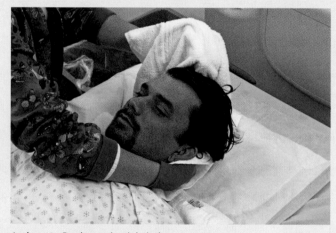

Action 12: Patting patient's hair dry.

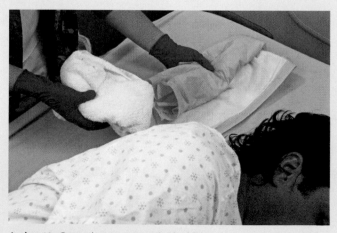

Action 12: Removing wet protective bedding.

continues

Giving a Bed Shampoo (continued)

ACTION	**RATIONALE**
13. Gently brush hair, removing tangles as needed.	Removing tangles helps hair to dry faster. Brushing hair improves patient's self-image.
14. **Blow-dry hair on a cool setting** if allowed and if patient wishes.	Blow-drying hair helps hair to dry faster and prevents patient from becoming chilled.
15. Change patient's gown and remove protective pad.	If patient's gown is damp, patient will become chilled. Protective pad is no longer needed once hair is dry.
16. Remove gloves. Perform hand hygiene.	Hand hygiene deters spread of microorganisms.
17. Document that hair was washed and any cuts or lesions found.	A careful record is important for planning and individualizing the patient's care.

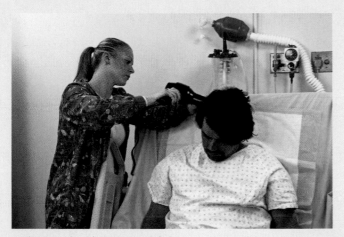

Action 14: Blow-drying patient's hair.

7/4/04   1130   Hair washed. Moderate amount of dried blood in hair noted. 3-cm laceration noted over parietal area. Edges well approximated, sutures intact, and no drainage noted.—C. Stone, RN

Action 15: Documentation.

EVALUATION   The expected outcomes are met when the patient's hair is clean, the patient verbalizes a positive body image, and the patient reports an increase in comfort level.

Unexpected Situations and Associated Interventions
- *Glass is found in hair:* Carefully comb through hair before washing to remove as much glass as possible. Discard glass in appropriate container. When massaging scalp, be alert to signs of pain from the patient; glass could be cutting the patient's head.

Special Considerations
- If the patient has a spinal cord or neck injury, use of the shampoo board may be contraindicated. In this case, a makeshift protection area can be created to wash the patient's hair without using the board. Place a protective pad underneath the patient's head and shoulders. Roll a towel into the bottom of the protective pad and direct the roll into one area so that water will drain into the container.

Removing and Cleaning Contact Lenses

From vision aids to decorative accessories, contact lenses have become very common in young and older people alike. If an unresponsive patient is admitted, a quick check of the eyes can establish if contact lenses are in place. Contact lenses may need to be removed to prevent any complications.

Equipment

- Disposable gloves
- Container for contact lenses (if unavailable, two small sterile containers marked "L" and "R" will suffice)
- Sterile normal saline solution
- Rubber pincer (for removal of soft lenses)
- Suction cup remover (for removal of hard lenses)

ASSESSMENT

Assess both eyes for contact lenses, as some people wear them in only one eye. Assess eyes for any redness or drainage, which may indicate an infection of the eye or an allergic response. Assess for any eye injury. If an injury is present, notify the physician about the presence of the contact lens. Do not try to remove the contact lens in this situation due to the risk for additional eye injury.

NURSING DIAGNOSIS

Determine the related factors for the nursing diagnosis based on the patient's current status. An appropriate nursing diagnosis is Risk for Injury.

OUTCOME IDENTIFICATION AND PLANNING

The expected outcome to achieve when removing contact lenses is that the lenses are removed without trauma to the eye.

IMPLEMENTATION

ACTION	RATIONALE
1. Explain procedure to patient.	Explanation encourages patient cooperation.
2. Perform hand hygiene. Don disposable gloves.	Hand hygiene deters the spread of microorganisms.
3. Assist patient to supine position. Elevate bed. Lower side rail closest to you.	Supine position with the bed raised and the side rail down is the least stressful position for the nurse to remove the contact lens.
4. If containers are not already labeled, do so now. Place 5 mL of normal saline in each container.	Many patients have different prescription strengths for each eye. The saline will prevent the contact from drying out.

Removing Hard Contact Lenses

5. **If the lens is not centered over the cornea, apply gentle pressure on the lower eyelid to center the lens.**	Lens must be over the cornea for easy removal.
6. Gently pull the outer corner of the eye toward the ear.	This breaks the suction between the contact lens and the eye.
7. Position the other hand below the lens and ask patient to blink.	Blinking helps to move the contact out of the eye.

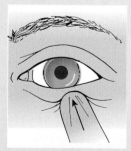

Action 5: Applying gentle pressure to lower eyelid with gloved fingers.

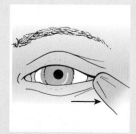

Action 6: Pulling on corner of eye with gloved finger.

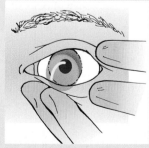

Action 7: Pulling back on eye while other hand is catching the contact lens.

continues

Removing and Cleaning Contact Lenses (continued)

ACTION	RATIONALE

If Patient Cannot Blink

8. Gently spread the eyelids beyond the top and bottom edges of the lens.

   This helps to break the suction between the contact lens and the eye.

9. Gently press the lower eyelid up against the bottom of the lens.

   This helps to begin removal of the contact lens from the eye.

10. After the lens is tipped slightly, move the eyelids toward one another to cause the lens to slide out between the eyelids.

   This helps to remove contact lens from eye.

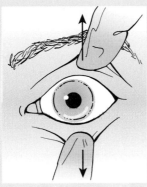 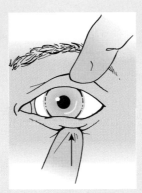 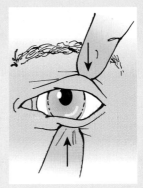

Action 8: Using gloved fingers to spread the eyelids.   Action 9: Applying pressure to lower eyelid.   Action 10: Moving eyelids together.

If a Suction Cup Remover is Available

11. Ensure that contact lens is centered on cornea. Place a drop of sterile saline on the suction cup.

   This ensures that the suction cup is not accidentally placed on the eye. The normal saline helps to form a suction between the device and the lens.

12. Place the suction cup in the center of the contact lens and gently pull the contact lens off the eye.

   The suction cup will adhere to the contact lens to aid in removal from the eye.

13. To remove the suction cup from the lens, slide the lens off sideways.

   This breaks the suction and allows the lens to become free.

For Soft Contact Lenses

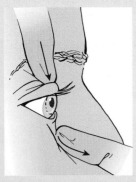

14. Have patient look forward. Retract the lower lid with one hand. Using the pad of the index finger of the other hand, move the lens down to the sclera.

15. Using the pads of the thumb and index finger, grasp the lens with a gentle pinching motion and remove.

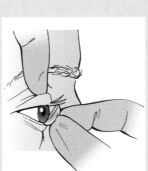

   This helps to break the suction between the contact lens and the eye.

   This removes the lens from the eye.

Action 14: Retracting the lower lid while the other finger moves the lens down.

Action 15: Grasping the lens.

continues

SKILL 7-8   Removing and Cleaning Contact Lenses (continued)

ACTION	RATIONALE

If Rubber Pincer is Available

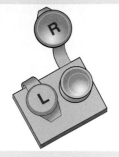

Action 18: Lenses placed in appropriate container.

ACTION	RATIONALE
16. Locate the contact lens and place the rubber pincers in the center of the lens.	This ensures that the pincers are on the lens, not on the eye.
17. Gently squeeze the pincers and remove the lens from the eye.	The pincers should be squeezed gently to prevent injury to the eye or contact lens.
18. Place removed contact lens into the appropriately marked container. Repeat actions to remove other contact lens.	Many patients have different lens prescriptions for both eyes.
19. If patient is awake and has glasses at bedside, offer patient glasses.	Not being able to see clearly creates anxiety.
20. Remove gloves. Perform hand hygiene.	Hand hygiene deters the spread of microorganisms.
21. Document the removal of contact lenses as well as the condition of the eye: drainage, color of sclera, complaints of pain.	A careful record is important for planning and individualizing the patient's care.

> 7/15/04   1045   Contacts removed from eyes without trauma. Sclera white with no drainage from eye. Glasses placed at bedside.—C. Stone, RN

Action 21: Documentation.

EVALUATION

The expected outcome is met when the patient remains free of injury as the contact lenses are removed. Eye exhibits no signs and symptoms of trauma, irritation, or redness.

Unexpected Situations and Associated Interventions

- *The contact lens cannot be removed:* Use tool to remove lens. For hard lenses, the tool has a small suction cup that is placed over the contact lens. For soft lenses, the tool is a small pair of rubber grippers that can be placed over the contact lens to aid in removal.
- *Hard contact is not over cornea:* Place a cotton-tipped applicator over upper eyelid and grasp lid, everting lid over applicator. Examine eye for lens. If lens is not in the upper portion, place finger below eye and gently pull down on lid while having patient look up. When the lens is found, gently slide it over the cornea (Ramponi, 2001). (Soft contacts may be removed from other areas of the eye.)

SKILL
7-9

Assisting with a Sitz Bath

A sitz bath can help relieve pain and discomfort after childbirth or surgery and can increase circulation to the tissues, promoting healing.

Equipment
- Disposable gloves
- Towel
- Disposable sitz bath bowl with water bag

ASSESSMENT

Determine patient's ability to ambulate to the bathroom and maintain sitting position for 15 to 20 minutes. Prior to the sitz bath, inspect perineal/rectal area for swelling, drainage, redness, warmth, and tenderness. Assess bladder fullness and encourage patient to void prior to sitz bath.

NURSING DIAGNOSIS

Determine related factors for the nursing diagnosis based on the patient's current status. Possible nursing diagnoses may include:

- Acute Pain
- Risk for Hypothermia
- Risk for Infection
- Impaired Tissue Integrity

OUTCOME IDENTIFICATION AND PLANNING

The expected outcome to achieve when administering a sitz bath is that the patient will state an increase in comfort. Other outcomes that may be appropriate include the following: the patient will experience a decrease in healing time, maintain normal body temperature, remain free of any signs and symptoms of infection, and exhibit signs and symptoms of healing.

IMPLEMENTATION

ACTION	RATIONALE
1. Explain procedure to patient.	Explanation facilitates cooperation.
2. Perform hand hygiene and don disposable gloves.	Hand hygiene and disposable gloves deter the spread of microorganisms.
3. Assemble equipment in bathroom.	Organization facilitates performance of task.
4. Raise lid of toilet. Place bowl of sitz bath, with drainage ports to rear and infusion port in front, in the toilet. Fill bowl of sitz bath about halfway full with tepid to warm water (37° to 46°C [98° to 115°F]).	Sitz bath will not drain appropriately if placed in toilet backwards. Tepid water can promote relaxation and help with edema; warm water can help with circulation.
5. Clamp tubing on bag. Fill bag with same temperature water as mentioned above. Hang bag above patient's shoulder height on hook or IV pole.	If bag is hung lower, the rate of flow will not be sufficient and water may cool too quickly.
6. Assist patient to sit on toilet. Insert tubing into infusion port of sitz bath. Slowly unclamp tubing and allow sitz bath to fill.	If tubing is placed into sitz bath before patient sits on toilet, patient may trip over tubing. Filling the sitz bath ensures that the tissue is submerged in water.
7. Clamp tubing once sitz bath is full. Instruct patient to open clamp when water in bowl becomes cool. **Ensure that call bell is within reach. Instruct patient to call if she feels light-headed, "spacy," or dizzy or has any problems. Instruct patient not to try standing without assistance.**	Cool water may produce hypothermia. Patient may become light-headed due to vasodilation, so call bell should be within reach.
8. When patient is finished, help patient stand and gently pat bottom dry. Assist patient to bed or chair. Ensure that call bell is within reach.	Patient may be light-headed and dizzy due to vasodilation. Patient should not stand alone, and bending over to dry self may cause patient to fall.

continues

ACTION   **RATIONALE**

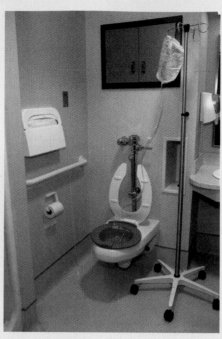

Disposable sitz bath

9. Empty and disinfect sitz bath bowl according to agency policy. Remove gloves and perform hand hygiene.

Proper equipment cleaning and hand hygiene deter the spread of microorganisms.

10. Document the sitz bath, including water temperature, length of bath, and how patient tolerated the bath.

A careful record is important for planning and individualizing the patient's care.

> 7/30/04   1620   Perineum assessed. Epi-
> siotomy mediolateral; edges well approxi-
> mated. Patient assisted to sitz bath. Patient
> took warm water sitz bath (temperature 99°F)
> for 20 minutes. Denies feeling light-headed or
> dizzy. Assisted back to bed after bath. Patient
> states pain level has dropped "from a 5 to a 2."
> —C. Stone, RN

Action 10: Documentation.

EVALUATION   The expected outcomes are met when the patient verbalizes a decrease in pain or discomfort, patient tolerates sitz bath without problems, area remains clean and dry, and patient demonstrates signs of healing.

Unexpected Situations and Associated Interventions

- *Patient complains of feeling light-headed or dizzy during sitz bath:* Stop sitz bath. Do not attempt to ambulate patient by self. Use call light to summon help. Let patient sit on toilet with face up until feeling subsides or help has arrived to assist patient back to bed.
- *Temperature of water is uncomfortable:* The water may be too warm or cold, depending on the patient's preference. If this happens, clamp the tubing, disconnect the water bag, and refill it with water that is comfortable for the patient.

Assisting the Patient to Shave

Shaving for many patients is a daily ritual of hygiene. They may feel disheveled and unclean without shaving. Some patients may need help with shaving.

Equipment
- Shaving cream
- Safety razor
- Towel
- Washcloth
- Bath basin
- Disposable gloves
- Aftershave or lotion (optional)

ASSESSMENT

Assess patient for any bleeding problems. If patient is receiving any anticoagulant such as heparin or warfarin (Coumadin), has received an antithrombolytic agent, or has a low platelet count, consider using an electric razor. Inspect the area to be shaved for any lesions or weeping areas.

NURSING DIAGNOSIS

Determine related factors for the nursing diagnosis based on the patient's current status. Appropriate nursing diagnoses may include:
- Risk for Injury
- Bathing/Hygiene Self-Care Deficit
- Activity Intolerance
- Impaired Physical Mobility

Many other nursing diagnosis may require this skill.

OUTCOME IDENTIFICATION AND PLANNING

The expected outcome to achieve when assisting the patient with shaving is that the patient will be clean, without evidence of hair growth or trauma to the skin. Other outcomes that may be appropriate include the following: the patient tolerates shaving with minimal to no difficulty and the patient verbalizes feelings of improved self-esteem.

IMPLEMENTATION

ACTION	RATIONALE
1. Gather equipment. Explain procedure to patient.	Explanation encourages cooperation. Organization facilitates performance of task.
2. Perform hand hygiene and don disposable gloves.	Hand hygiene deters the spread of microorganisms. Gloves should be worn due to the possibility of contact with blood if the person is cut during shaving.
3. Fill bath basin with warm (43° to 46°C [110° to 115°F]) water. Moisten the area to be shaved with a washcloth.	Warm water is comfortable and relaxing for the patient.
4. Dispense shaving cream into palm of hand. Rub hands together, then apply to area to be shaved in a layer around 0.5″ thick.	Using shaving cream helps to prevent skin irritation and prevents hair from pulling.
5. Using a smooth stroke, begin shaving. Pull the skin taut if necessary. *If shaving the face,* shave with the direction of hair growth in downward, short strokes. *If shaving a leg,* shave against the hair in upward, short strokes.	The skin on the face is more sensitive and needs to be shaved with the direction of hair growth to prevent discomfort.
6. Wash off residual shaving cream.	Shaving cream can lead to irritation if left on the skin.

continues

ACTION	RATIONALE

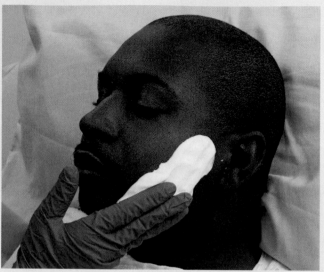

Action 4: Applying shaving cream to face.

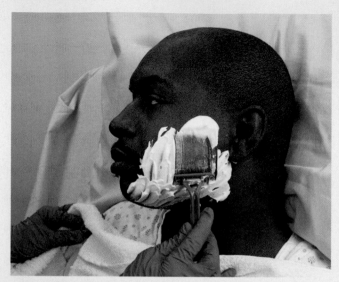

Action 5: Shaving the face.

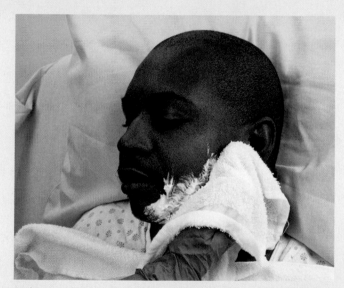

Action 6: Using a wet washcloth to rinse remaining shaving cream off patient.

7. If patient requests, apply aftershave or lotion to area shaved.

Aftershave and lotion can reduce skin irritation.

8. Remove and discard gloves and perform hand hygiene.

Proper glove removal and hand hygiene deter the spread of microorganisms.

continues

<table>
<tr><td>

SKILL 7-10
</td><td>

Assisting the Patient to Shave (continued)
</td></tr>
</table>

EVALUATION The expected outcome is met when the patient exhibits a clean-shaven face without evidence of trauma, irritation, or redness. In addition, the patient verbalizes feeling refreshed and demonstrates improved self-esteem.

Unexpected Situations and Associated Interventions

- *Patient is cut and bleeding during shave:* Apply pressure with gauze or towel to injured area. Do not release pressure for 2 to 3 minutes. After bleeding has stopped, resume shaving. The water basin may need to be rewarmed before washing the shaving cream off.
- *Patient has large amount of hair to be shaved:* If hair is longer, it may need to be trimmed with scissors before shaving to prevent pulling of hair when shaving.

Special Considerations

- *Patient is brought to hospital with full beard:* Do not shave patient's beard without consent unless it is an emergency situation, such as insertion of an endotracheal tube. For this procedure, shave only the area needed and leave the rest of the beard.

■ Developing Critical Thinking Skills

1. Denasia Kerr, the 6-year-old on bedrest, needs her hair shampooed. It is now several days after surgery. How would you accomplish this task?
2. Cindy Vortex is the 34-year-old woman who is now in a coma after a car accident and who is wearing contact lenses. What information would be important to gather before attempting to remove the contact lenses?
3. Carl Sheen, 76 years old, asks you, "How can I clean my dentures with my right hand all tied up with this IV?" How best could you help Mr. Sheen with this hygiene activity while still fostering his independence?

Bibliography

Aiello, A., & Larson, E. (2002). Causal inference: The case of hygiene and health. *American Journal of Infection Control, 30*(8), 503–510.

Cottrell, B. (2003). Vaginal douching. *Journal of Obstetric, Gynecologic, and Neonatal Nursing, 32*(1), 12–18.

Dougherty, J., & Long, C. (2003). Techniques for bathing without a battle. *Home Healthcare Nurse, 21*(1), 38–39.

Dunn, J., Thiru-Chelvam, B., & Beck, C. (2002). Bathing: Pleasure or pain? *Journal of Gerontological Nursing, 28*(11), 6–13.

Fort, C. (2002). Get pumped to prevent DVT. *Nursing, 32*(9), 50–52.

Hayes, J., Lehman, C., & Castonguay, P. (2002). Graduated compression stockings: Updating practice, improving compliance. *MedSurg Nursing, 11*(4), 163–166, 191.

Hess, C. (2003). Managing a diabetic ulcer. *Nursing, 33*(7), 82–83.

Hilgers, J. (2003). Comforting a confused patient. *Nursing, 33*(1), 48–50.

Larson, E. (2002). The 'hygiene hypothesis': How clean should we be? *American Journal of Nursing, 102*(1), 81–89.

Larson, E., Gomez-Duarte, C., Qureshi, K., & Miranda, D. (2001). How clean is the home environment? A tool to assess home hygiene. *Journal of Community Health Nursing, 18*(3), 139–150.

McConnell, E. (2002). Applying antiembolism stockings. *Nursing, 32*(4), 17.

Pauldine, E. (2003). Taking a bite out of Lyme disease. *Nursing, 33*(4), 49–52.

Plummer, S. (2001). Chronic complications. *RN, 64*(5), 34–42.

Ramponi, D. (2001). Eye on contact lens removal. *Nursing, 31*(8), 56–57.

Stewart, K. (2002). Stopping the itch of scabies and lice. *Nursing, 30*(7), 30–31.

Stone, C. (1999). Preventing cerumen impaction in nursing facility residents. *Journal of Gerontological Nursing, 25*(5), 43–45.

Skin Integrity and Wound Care

Focusing on Patient Care

This chapter will help you develop some of the skills related to skin integrity and wound care necessary to care for the following patients:

Lori Downs, a patient with diabetes, is admitted with a chronic ulcer of her left foot.

Tran Nguyen, diagnosed with breast cancer, has had a modified radical mastectomy.

Arthur Lowes has an appointment with his surgeon today for a follow-up examination and removal of surgical staples following a colon resection.

Learning Outcomes

After studying this chapter, the reader should be able to:

1. Remove sutures
2. Remove surgical staples
3. Provide care to a Penrose drain
4. Provide care to a T-tube drain
5. Provide care to a Jackson-Pratt drain
6. Provide care to a Hemovac drain
7. Clean a wound and apply a sterile dressing
8. Collect a wound culture
9. Irrigate a sterile wound
10. Apply a wound vacuum-assisted closure (VAC) system
11. Apply an external heating device
12. Apply a warm sterile compress to an open wound
13. Apply a cooling blanket
14. Apply cold therapy
15. Apply Montgomery straps
16. Apply a saline-moistened dressing
17. Apply a hydrocolloid dressing

Key Terms

approximated wound edges: edges of a wound that are lightly pulled together. Edges appear to be touching; wound appears closed.

dehiscence: accidental separation of wound edges, especially a surgical wound

ecchymosis: discoloration of an area resulting from infiltration of blood into the subcutaneous tissue

edema: accumulation of fluid in the interstitial tissues

epithelialization: stage of wound healing in which epithelial cells move across the surface of a wound; tissue color ranges from the color of "ground glass" to pink

erythema: redness or inflammation of an area as a result of dilation and congestion of capillaries

eschar: a thick, leathery scab or dry crust composed of dead cells and dried plasma

granulation tissue: new tissue that is pink/red and composed of fibroblasts and small blood vessels that fill an open wound when it starts to heal

hypothermia: condition characterized by a body temperature below 96.8°F

ischemia: insufficient blood supply to a body part due to obstruction of circulation

jaundice: condition characterized by yellowness of the skin, whites of eyes, mucous membranes, and body fluids as a result of deposition of bile pigment resulting from excess bilirubin in the blood

maceration: softening of tissue due to excessive moisture

necrosis: localized tissue death

nosocomial infection: infection acquired while receiving healthcare

pathogens: microorganisms that can harm humans

peripheral neuropathy: abnormal condition characterized by inflammation and degeneration of the peripheral nerves. Sensations reported include burning, tingling, numbness, and pins and needles.

pressure ulcer: lesion caused by unrelieved pressure that results in damage to underlying tissue

sinus tract: cavity or channel underneath a wound that has the potential for infection

sterile technique: surgical asepsis; removing all microorganisms to prevent the introduction or spread of pathogens from the environment into a patient

surgical asepsis: removal of all microorganisms to prevent the introduction or spread of pathogens from the environment into a patient

surgical staples: stainless-steel wire used to close a surgical wound

surgical sutures: thread or wire used to stitch parts of the body together

tachycardia: abnormally rapid heart rate, usually above 100 beats per minute in an adult

tunneling: passageway or opening that may be visible at skin level, but with most of the tunnel under the surface of the skin

undermining: areas of tissue destruction underneath intact skin along the margins of a wound

vasoconstriction: narrowing of the lumen of a blood vessel

vasodilation: an increase in the diameter of a blood vessel

The skin is the body's first line of defense. An intact skin surface provides a barrier to harmful microorganisms. A disruption in the normal integrity of the skin is called a wound. This disruption creates a potentially dangerous and possibly life-threatening situation. The patient is at risk for wound complications such as infection, hemorrhage, dehiscence, and evisceration. These complications increase the risk for generalized illness and death, lengthen the time that the patient needs healthcare interventions, and add to healthcare costs.

Caring for wounds is one aspect of nursing care. Nursing responsibilities related to skin integrity included developing an individualized plan of care to assess the patient, to implement and evaluate skills essential to wound care, to identify and prevent complications, and to provide physical and emotional support. These interventions facilitate healing, adaptation, and self-care.

This chapter will cover skills to assist the nurse in providing care related to skin integrity and wounds. Please look over the summary boxes at the beginning of this chapter and those found in Chapter 4 for a quick review of critical knowledge to assist you in understanding the skills related to skin integrity and wound care.

BOX 8-1 **Anatomy and Physiology of Skin and the Integumentary System**

- Skin is the body's largest organ. It provides protective, sensory, and regulatory functions.
- Changes to or disruptions in skin integrity can interfere with the functions of the integumentary system. The body relies heavily on an intact integumentary system for defense against the environment.
- The skin has two major layers, the epidermis and dermis.
- The epidermis depends on the dermis for nutrition. It forms the hair, nails, and glandular structures of the skin.
- The dermis lies under and is thicker than the epidermis. It produces collagen and elastin. It is home for lymphatic vessels and nerve tissues.
- Skin provides protection from injury, infection, and damage from ultraviolet rays. Secretions produced by the skin inhibit the growth of pathogens present on the skin.
- The dilation and constriction of blood vessels in the skin help to regulate body temperature.
- Nerve endings in the skin are sensitive to pain, itch, vibration, heat, and cold.
- The skin makes vitamin D to aid in the absorption of calcium and phosphorus.
- The skin is a large part of a person's body appearance and attractiveness. It contributes to communication through facial expression and appearance.
- Normal skin tones vary among races of people. Skin is normally warm, dry to the touch, and smooth in texture. Normal skin has good elasticity or turgor. As a person ages, turgor normally decreases.

BOX 8-2 **Factors Affecting Integumentary Function**

- Healthy, viable skin requires adequate blood flow. Alterations in circulation can lead to skin that has abnormal color, texture, thickness, moisture, or temperature or skin that becomes ulcerated.
- Healthy skin requires a balanced diet. Deficiencies of protein, calories, or multiple vitamins and minerals result in dull, dry hair and dry, flaky skin. Skin that is not healthy becomes more fragile and susceptible to dysfunction.
- Healthy skin requires personal hygiene practices and the avoidance of certain environmental factors. Lack of cleanliness can hinder skin health because bacteria, sweat, and debris are not removed. Overexposure to ultraviolet radiation can lead to wrinkling, changes in texture and elasticity of the skin, and cancer.
- Lack of moisture can lead to breaks in the integrity of the skin, allowing microorganisms to enter the body.
- Allergic reactions, such as those to foods or poison ivy, and resulting skin inflammation can lead to breaks in the integrity of the skin, allowing microorganisms to enter the body.
- An abnormal growth rate of skin cells, such as psoriasis or melanoma, can disrupt the integrity of the skin.
- Many chronic diseases, such as peripheral vascular disease, can lead to disruption in the integrity of the skin due to diminished delivery of blood and oxygen to the underlying tissues.
- Trauma to the skin, such as from surgical or accidental wounds, can disrupt the integrity of the skin.
- Exposure to excessive heat, electricity, chemicals, and radiation results in injuries that can disrupt the integrity of the skin.

BOX 8-3 **Wound Healing and Complications**

- Wounds heal by primary or secondary intention.
- Wounds healing by primary intention form a clean, straight line with little loss of tissue. The wound edges are well approximated with sutures. These wounds usually heal rapidly with minimal scarring.
- Wounds healing by secondary intention are large wounds with considerable tissue loss. The edges are not approximated. Healing occurs by formation of granulation tissue. These wounds have a longer healing time, a greater chance of infection, and larger scars.
- Wounds healing by primary intention that become infected heal by secondary intention. These wounds generate a greater inflammatory reaction and more granulation tissue. They have large scars and are less likely to shrink to a flat line as they heal.

- Wound complications include infection, hemorrhage, dehiscence, and evisceration. These problems increase the risk for generalized illness, lengthen the time during which the patient needs healthcare interventions, and increase the cost of healthcare, and can result in death.
- Multiple psychological effects can occur as a result of trauma to the integumentary system. Actual and potential emotional stressors are common in patients with wounds. Pain is part of almost every wound. In addition, anxiety and fear play a large role in a patient's recovery from a wound. Many patients must deal with changes in body image, body structure, and function related to a wound.

BOX 8-4 **Wound Assessment**

Wounds are assessed for appearance, size, drainage, pain, presence of sutures, drains, and tubes, and the evidence of complications.

- Assess the wound's appearance by inspecting and palpating. Look for the approximation of the edges and the color of the wound and surrounding area. The edges should be clean and well approximated. Edges may be reddened and slightly swollen for about a week, then closer to normal in appearance. Skin around the wound may be bruised initially. Observe for signs of infection, including increased swelling, redness, and warmth.
- Note the presence of any sutures, drains, and tubes. These areas are assessed in the same manner as the incision. Make sure they are intact and functioning.
- Assess the amount, color, odor, and consistency of any wound drainage.
- Assess the patient's pain, using an objective scale. Incisional pain is usually most severe for the first 2 to 3 days, after which it progressively diminishes. Increased or constant pain, especially an acute change in pain, requires further assessment. It can be a sign of delayed healing, infection, or other complication.
- Assess the patient's general condition for signs and symptoms of infection and hemorrhage.

BOX 8-5 **Preventing Pressure Ulcers**

- In patients at risk, assess the skin daily. Pay particular attention to bony prominences.
- Cleanse the skin routinely and whenever soiling occurs. Use mild cleansing agents and minimal friction, and avoid hot water.
- Maintain higher humidity in the environment. Use skin moisturizers for dry skin.
- Avoid massage over bony prominences.
- Protect skin from moisture associated with incontinence or wound drainage.
- Minimize skin injury from friction and shearing forces by using proper positioning, turning, and transfer techniques.
- Monitor dietary intake of protein and calories. Use nutritional supplements and appropriate interventions to ensure adequate intake.
- Initiate interventions to improve mobility and activity.
- Document measures used to prevent pressure ulcers.

BOX 8-6 **Measurement of a Pressure Ulcer**

- Size: Draw the shape and describe it. Measure the length, width, and diameter.
- Depth: Moisten a sterile swab with saline and insert it gently into the wound at a 90-degree angle with the tip down. Mark the point on the swab that is even with the surrounding skin surface. Remove the swab and measure the depth with a ruler.
- Presence of undermining, tunneling, or sinus tract: Insert a saline-moistened sterile swab under the wound edge. Apply gentle pressure and assess for any abnormal pathways. Do not use force. Measure the location and depth of penetration.

BOX 8-7 Comparison of Stages of Pressure Ulcers

Stage I

An observable pressure-related alteration of intact skin whose indicators as compared to the adjacent or opposite area on the body may include changes in one or more of the following: skin temperature (warmth or coolness), tissue consistency (firm or boggy feel) and/or sensation (pain, itching). The ulcer appears as a defined area of persistent redness in lightly pigmented skin, whereas in darker skin tones, the ulcer may appear with persistent red, blue, or purple hues.

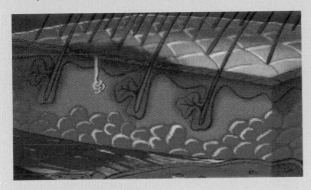

Pressure-relieving measures:
- Frequent turning
- Pressure-relieving devices
- Positioning

Stage II

Partial-thickness skin loss involving epidermis and/or dermis. The ulcer is superficial and presents clinically as an abrasion, blister, or shallow crater.

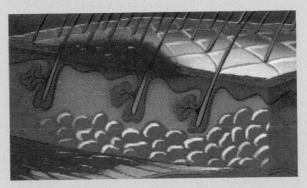

Maintenance of a moist healing environment:
- Saline or
- Occlusive dressing that promotes natural healing but prevents formation of a scar

Stage III

Full-thickness skin loss involving damage or necrosis of subcutaneous tissue that may extend down to, but not through, underlying fascia. The ulcer presents clinically as a deep crater with or without undermining of adjacent tissue.

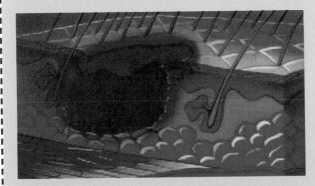

Requires débridement, which can be accomplished by one of the following:
- Wet-to-dry dressings
- Surgical intervention
- Proteolytic enzymes

Stage IV

Full-thickness skin loss with extensive destruction, tissue necrosis, or damage to muscle, bone, or supporting structures (eg, tendon or joint capsule). Sinus tracts may also be associated with stage IV ulcers.

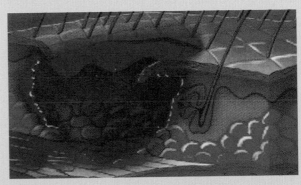

Wounds are treated in the following manner:
- Covered with nonadherent dressing
- Changed every 8–12 hours
- May require skin grafts

From U.S. Department of Health and Human Services. Agency for Health Care Policy and Research. (1992). *Pressure ulcers in adults: Prediction and prevention.* Rockville, MD: DHHS; Porth, C. (1994). *Pathophysiology: Concepts of altered health states.* Philadelphia: JB Lippincott; and National Pressure Ulcer Advisory Panel (NPUAP). http://www.npuap.org.

TABLE 8-1 Examples of Moisture-Retentive Dressings

Type	Purposes	Use
Transparent films Acu-derm Bioclusive BlisterFilm Mefilm Polyskin Uniflex Op-Site Tegaderm	• Allow exchange of oxygen between wound and environment • Are self-adhesive • Protect against contamination • Prevent loss of wound fluid • Maintain a moist wound environment • Allow visualization of wound • May remain in place for 24 to 72 hours, resulting in less interference with healing	• Wounds with minimal drainage • Wounds that are small and superficial, such as stage I and II pressure ulcers and superficial burns
Hydrocolloid dressings DuoDerm Intact Comfeel IntraSite Tegasorb Ultec	• Are occlusive • Absorb drainage • Provide cushioning • Do not allow entry of contaminants • May be left in place for 3 to 5 days, resulting in less interference with healing	• Shallow to moderate-depth skin ulcers • Wounds with drainage • In conjunction with packing for open, deep wounds
Hydrogels Vigilon IntraSite Gel Aquasorb ClearSite Nu-Gel Hypergel	• Maintain a moist wound environment • Do not adhere to wound • Reduce pain	• Partial- and full-thickness wounds • Necrotic wounds • Burns
Alginates Sorban AlgiDerm Curasorb Dermacea Melgisorb	• Absorb some exudate • Are compatible with topical medication • Absorb exudate • Maintain moisture	• Infected wounds
Foams LYOfoam Allevyn	• Maintain moist wound surface • Do not adhere to wound • Insulate wound	• Chronic wounds

Removing Sutures

Skin sutures are used to hold tissue and skin together. Sutures may be black silk, synthetic material, or fine wire. Sutures are removed when enough tensile strength has developed to hold the wound edges together during healing. The time frame varies depending on the patient's age, nutritional status, and wound location. Frequently, after skin sutures are removed, Steri-Strips (small wound-closure strips of adhesive) are applied across the wound to give additional support as it continues to heal. The removal of sutures may be done by the physician or by the nurse with a physician's order.

Equipment	• Sterile suture removal kit or sterile forceps and scissors • Gauze • Wound cleansing agent, according to facility policy • Gloves • Steri-Strips • Tincture of benzoin, if indicated
ASSESSMENT	Inspect the surgical incision and the surrounding tissue. Assess the appearance of the wound for the approximation of wound edges, the color of the wound and surrounding area, and signs of dehiscence. Note the stage of the healing process and characteristics of any drainage. Assess the surrounding skin for color, temperature, and the presence of edema or ecchymosis.
NURSING DIAGNOSIS	Determine the related factors for the nursing diagnoses based on the patient's current status. An appropriate nursing diagnosis is Risk for Infection. Other nursing diagnoses that may be appropriate include: • Anxiety • Pain • Acute Pain • Impaired Skin Integrity • Delayed Surgical Recovery • Risk for Situational Low Self-Esteem
OUTCOME IDENTIFICATION AND PLANNING	The expected outcome to achieve when removing surgical sutures is that the sutures are removed without contaminating the incisional area by maintaining sterile technique, without causing trauma to the wound, and without causing the patient to experience pain or discomfort. In addition, other outcomes that are appropriate include: the patient remains free from exposure to infectious microorganisms; the patient remains free of complications that would delay recovery; and the patient verbalizes positive aspects about self.

IMPLEMENTATION

ACTION	RATIONALE
1. Review the physician's order for suture removal.	Reviewing the order validates the correct patient and correct procedure.
2. Gather the necessary supplies.	Adequate preparation ensures efficient time management.
3. Identify the patient. Explain the procedure to the patient. Describe the sensation as a pulling or slightly uncomfortable experience.	Identification validates the correct patient and correct procedure. Discussion and explanation help allay anxiety and prepare the patient for what to expect.
4. Perform hand hygiene.	Hand hygiene prevents the spread of microorganisms.
5. Close the room door or curtains. Place the bed at an appropriate and comfortable working height.	Closing the door or curtains provides privacy. Placing the bed at an appropriate height helps reduce back strain when performing the procedure.

continues

SKILL 8-1   Removing Sutures (continued)

ACTION	RATIONALE
6. Assist the patient to a comfortable position that provides easy access to the wound area. Use the bath blanket to cover any exposed area other than the wound.	A comfortable patient position helps reduce anxiety. Bath blanket provides for comfort and warmth.
7. Put on gloves. Remove and dispose of any dressings on the surgical incision. Remove gloves and put on a new pair. Inspect the incision area.	Use of gloves and proper removal of dressings help prevent spread of microorganisms. Removal of dressings allows access to the incision.
8. Clean the incision using the wound cleanser and gauze, according to facility policies and procedures.	Incision cleaning prevents the spread of microorganisms and contamination of the wound.
9. **Using the sterile forceps, grasp the knot of the first suture and gently lift the knot up off the skin.**	Raising the suture knot prevents accidental injury to the wound or skin when cutting.
10. Using the sterile scissors, cut one side of the suture below the knot, close to the skin. **Grasp the knot with the forceps and pull the cut suture through the skin. Avoid pulling the visible portion of the suture through the underlying tissue.**	Pulling the cut suture through the skin helps reduce the risk for contamination of the incision area and resulting infection.

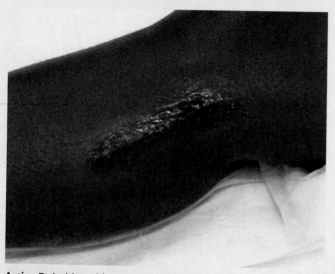

Action 7: Incision with sutures.

Action 10: Using gloved hands to pull up on a suture with forceps and cutting the suture with sterile scissors.

11. Remove every other suture to be sure the wound edges are healed. If they are, remove the remaining sutures as ordered.	Removing every other suture allows for inspection of the wound, while leaving adequate suture in place to promote continued healing if the edges are not totally approximated.
12. Apply Steri-Strips if ordered. If necessary, prepare skin with tincture of benzoin before applying Steri-Strips.	Steri-Strips provide additional support to the wound as it continues to heal. Applying benzoin aids in adherence of Steri-Strips.

continues

ACTION   **RATIONALE**

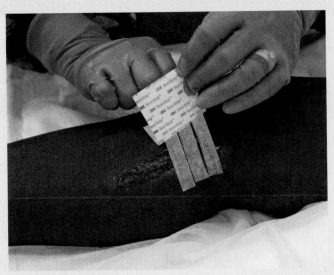

Action 12: Applying Steri-Strips on incision.

13. Reapply the dressing, depending on the physician's orders and facility policy.

A new dressing protects the wound.

14. Remove gloves and perform hand hygiene.

Removing gloves and performing hand hygiene prevent the spread of microorganisms.

15. Document the procedure and assessments.

Documentation promotes continuity of care and communication.

> 3/4/06 1800   Right leg surgical wound appears healed. Incision edges are approximated, without erythema, edema, ecchymosis, or drainage. Skin warm and pink. Sutures removed without difficulty, Steri-Strips applied. Patient instructed in how to care for wound and expectations regarding Steri-Strips; patient and wife verbalized an understanding of information and asked appropriate questions.
> —R. Downs, RN

Action 15: Documentation.

EVALUATION

The expected outcome is met when the patient exhibits an incision area that is clean, dry, and intact without sutures. The incision area is free of trauma and infection, and the patient verbalizes minimal to no complaints of pain or discomfort and positive aspects about self.

Unexpected Situations and Associated Interventions

- *Sutures are crusted with dried blood or secretions, making them difficult to remove:* Moisten sterile gauze with sterile saline and gently loosen crusts prior to removing sutures.
- *Resistance is met when attempting to pull suture through the tissue:* Use a gentle, continuous pulling motion to remove the suture. If the suture still does not come out, do not use excessive force. Report your findings to the physician and document the event in the patient's record.

Special Considerations

- Encourage the patient to splint chest and abdominal wounds during activity, such as changing position, ambulation, coughing, and sneezing. This provides increased support for the underlying tissues and can decrease discomfort.

SKILL 8-2   Removing Surgical Staples

Surgical skin staples are made of stainless steel and are used to hold tissue and skin together. Staples decrease the risk of infection and allow faster wound closure. Surgical staples are removed when enough tensile strength has developed to hold the wound edges together during healing. The time frame varies depending on the patient's age, nutritional status, and wound location. After skin staples are removed, Steri-Strips (small wound-closure strips of adhesive) are applied across the wound to keep the skin edges approximated as it continues to heal. The removal of surgical staples may be done by the physician or by the nurse with a physician's order.

Equipment
- Sterile staple remover
- Gauze
- Wound cleansing agent, according to facility policy
- Gloves
- Steri-Strips
- Tincture of benzoin if indicated

ASSESSMENT

Inspect the surgical incision and the surrounding tissue. Assess the appearance of the wound for the approximation of wound edges, the color of the wound and surrounding area, and signs of dehiscence. Note the stage of the healing process and the characteristics of any drainage. Assess the surrounding skin for color, temperature, and the presence of edema or ecchymosis.

NURSING DIAGNOSIS

Determine the related factors for the nursing diagnoses based on the patient's current status. An appropriate nursing diagnosis is Risk for Infection. Other nursing diagnoses that may be appropriate include:
- Anxiety
- Impaired Comfort
- Acute Pain
- Impaired Skin Integrity
- Delayed Surgical Recovery
- Risk for Situational Low Self-Esteem

OUTCOME IDENTIFICATION AND PLANNING

The expected outcome to achieve when removing surgical staples is that the staples are removed without contaminating the incision area, without causing trauma to the wound, and without causing the patient to experience pain or discomfort. Other outcomes that are appropriate include: the patient remains free from exposure to infectious microorganisms; the patient remains free of complications that would delay recovery; and the patient verbalizes positive aspects about self.

IMPLEMENTATION

ACTION	RATIONALE
1. Review the physician's order for staple removal.	Reviewing the order validates the correct patient and correct procedure.
2. Gather the necessary supplies.	Preparation promotes efficient time management.
3. Identify the patient. Explain the procedure to the patient. Describe the sensation as a pulling or slightly uncomfortable experience.	Patient identification validates the correct patient and correct procedure. Discussion and explanation help allay anxiety and prepare the patient for what to expect.
4. Perform hand hygiene.	Hand hygiene prevents the spread of microorganisms.

continues

Removing Surgical Staples (continued)

ACTION	RATIONALE
5. Close the room door or curtains. Place the bed at an appropriate and comfortable working height.	Closing the door or curtain provides privacy. Raising the bed to an appropriate height helps reduce back strain when performing the procedure.
6. Assist the patient to a comfortable position that provides easy access to the wound area. Use the bath blanket to cover any exposed area other than the wound.	A comfortable position helps reduce the patient's anxiety. Bath blankets provide for comfort and warmth.
7. Put on gloves. Remove and dispose of any dressings on the surgical incision using proper technique. Remove gloves and put on a new pair.	Use of gloves and proper dressing removal prevent the spread of microorganisms. Dressing removal also allows access to the incision.
8. Clean the incision using the wound cleanser and gauze, according to facility policies and procedures.	Wound cleaning prevents the spread of microorganisms and contamination of the wound.
9. **Position the sterile staple remover under the staple to be removed. Firmly close the staple remover. The staple will bend in the middle and the edges will pull up out of the skin.**	Correct use of staple remover prevents accidental injury to the wound and contamination of the incision area and resulting infection.
10. Remove every other staple to be sure the wound edges are healed. If they are, remove the remaining staples as ordered.	Removing every other staple allows for inspection of the wound, while leaving an adequate number of staples in place to promote continued healing if the edges are not totally approximated.
11. Apply Steri-Strips according to facility policy or physician's order. Prepare skin with tincture of benzoin if indicated.	Steri-Strips provide additional support to the wound as it continues to heal. Applying benzoin helps to ensure adherence of Steri-Strips.
12. Reapply the dressing, depending on the physician's orders and facility policy.	A dressing protects the wound.
13. Remove gloves and perform hand hygiene.	Removing gloves and performing hand hygiene prevent the spread of microorganisms.
14. Document the procedure and assessments.	Documentation promotes continuity of care and communication.

10/3/06 0930   Patient reports itching and "new stuff coming from my incision." Leg incision examined. Noted to have serosanguineous drainage from proximal 6 cm of the incision. Proximal 6 to 8 cm with erythema and slight opening of wound edges, rest of incision with approximated edges, no erythema or drainage. Staples removed 10/1/04. Dr. Coles notified. Incision cleansed with normal saline solution, dried, Steri-Strips applied to proximal 6 cm of incision, dressed with dry gauze and wrapped with stretch gauze per order.—S. Hoffman, RN

Action 14: Documentation.

continues

EVALUATION

The expected outcome is met when the patient exhibits a wound that is clean, dry, and intact with the staples removed. Additionally, the patient's wound is free of contamination and trauma. Other outcomes are met when the patient verbalizes little to no pain or discomfort during the removal and states positive aspects about self.

Unexpected Situations and Associated Interventions

- *The wound edges appear approximated prior to staple removal but pull apart afterward:* Report your findings to the physician and document the event in the patient's record. Apply Steri-Strips according to facility policy or physician's order.
- *The staples are stuck to the wound because of dried blood or secretions:* Per facility policy or physician's order, apply moist saline compresses to loosen crusts prior to attempting to remove the staples.

Special Considerations

- Encourage the patient to splint chest and abdominal wounds during activity, such as changing position, ambulation, coughing, and sneezing. This provides increased support for the underlying tissues and can help decrease patient discomfort.

SKILL
8-3   **Caring for a Penrose Drain**

Drains are inserted into or near a wound when it is anticipated that a collection of fluid in a closed area would delay healing. A Penrose drain is a hollow, fat rubber tube. It allows fluid to drain via capillary action into absorbent dressings. Penrose drains are commonly used after the incision and drainage of an abscess, and in abdominal surgery. After a surgical procedure, the surgeon places one end of the drain in or near the area to be drained. The other end passes through the skin, directly through the incision or through a separate incision. A Penrose drain is not sutured. A large safety pin is usually placed in the part outside the wound to prevent the drain from slipping back into the incised area. This type of drain can be advanced or shortened to drain different areas. The patency and placement of the drain are included in the wound assessment.

Equipment

- Sterile cleansing solution and sterile container
- Sterile gloves
- Gauze dressings
- Sterile cotton-tipped applicators, if appropriate
- Drain sponges
- Surgi-pads or ABD pads
- Sterile dressing set or suture set (for the sterile scissors and forceps)
- Sterile cleaning solution as ordered (commonly 0.9% normal saline solution)
- Clean disposable gloves
- Sterile basin (optional)
- Sterile drape (optional)
- Plastic bag or other appropriate waste container for soiled dressings
- Waterproof pad and bath blanket
- Tape or ties
- Additional dressings and supplies needed or as required by the physician's order   *continues*

Caring for a Penrose Drain (continued)

ASSESSMENT

Assess the situation to determine the necessity for wound cleaning and a dressing change. Confirm any physician orders relevant to drain care and any drain care included in the nursing plan of care. Assess the current dressing to determine if it is intact, and assess for the presence of excess drainage or bleeding or saturation of the dressing. Assess the patency of the Penrose drain.

Inspect the wound and the surrounding tissue. Assess the appearance of the wound for the approximation of wound edges, the color of the wound and surrounding area, and signs of dehiscence. Note the stage of the healing process and the characteristics of any drainage. Assess the surrounding skin for color, temperature, and the presence of edema, ecchymosis, or maceration.

NURSING DIAGNOSIS

Determine the related factors for the nursing diagnosis based on the patient's current status. An appropriate nursing diagnosis is Risk for Infection. Other nursing diagnoses may also be appropriate, including:

- Anxiety
- Disturbed Body Image
- Acute Pain
- Deficient Knowledge
- Impaired Skin Integrity
- Delayed Surgical Recovery
- Impaired Tissue Integrity

OUTCOME IDENTIFICATION AND PLANNING

The expected outcome to achieve when performing care for a Penrose drain is that the Penrose drain remains patent and intact. Care is accomplished without contaminating the wound area, without causing trauma to the wound, and without causing the patient to experience pain or discomfort. Other outcomes that are appropriate may include: the wound shows signs of progressive healing without evidence of complications and the patient demonstrates understanding about the need for drain care.

IMPLEMENTATION

ACTION	RATIONALE
1. Review the physician's order for drain and site care or the nursing plan of care related to drain care.	Review of the order or plan of care validates the correct patient and correct procedure.
2. Gather the necessary supplies.	Preparation promotes efficient time management and organized approach to the task.
3. Identify the patient. Explain the procedure to the patient. Inquire about any allergies, specifically related to the products being used for wound care.	Patient identification validates the correct patient and correct procedure. Discussion and explanation help allay anxiety, encourage patient cooperation, and prepare the patient for what to expect.
4. Perform hand hygiene.	Hand hygiene prevents the spread of microorganisms.
5. Close the room door or curtains. Place the bed at an appropriate and comfortable working height.	Closing the door or curtain provides privacy. Placing the bed at an appropriate height helps reduce back strain when providing drain care.
6. Place a waste receptacle at a convenient location for use during the procedure.	Soiled dressing may be discarded easily, without the spread of microorganisms.
7. Assist the patient to a comfortable position that provides easy access to the drain area. Use the bath blanket to cover any exposed area other than the drain. If necessary, place the waterproof pad under the drain site.	Proper patient positioning and use of bath blankets provide for comfort and warmth. Waterproof pad protects underlying surfaces.

continues

SKILL 8-3   Caring for a Penrose Drain (continued)

ACTION

RATIONALE

8. Check the position of the drain or drains before removing the dressing. Put on clean, disposable gloves and loosen tape on the old dressings. Use an adhesive remover to help get the tape off, if necessary.

Checking the position ensures that a drain is not removed accidentally if one is present. Use of gloves protects the nurse from contaminated dressings and prevents the spread of microorganisms. Using adhesive remover helps to reduce patient discomfort during removal of dressing.

9. **Carefully remove the soiled dressings.** If any part of the dressing sticks to the underlying skin, use small amounts of sterile saline to help loosen and remove it. Do not reach over the drain site.

Cautious removal of the dressing is more comfortable for the patient and ensures that any drain present is not inadvertently removed. Sterile saline provides for easier removal of the dressing and prevents tissue damage.

10. After removing the dressing, note the presence, amount, type, color, and odor of any drainage on the dressings. Place soiled dressings in the appropriate waste receptacle. Remove gloves and dispose of them in the appropriate waste receptacle.

The presence of drainage should be documented. Proper use and disposal of gloves prevent the spread of microorganisms.

11. Inspect the drain site for appearance and drainage. Assess if any pain is present. **Closely observe the safety pin in the drain.** Include any problems noted in documentation.

The wound healing process and/or the presence of irritation or infection must be documented.

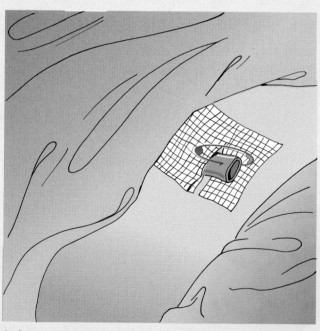

Action 11: Penrose drain in place.

12. If the pin or drain is crusted, replace the pin with a new sterile pin. Take care not to dislodge the drain.

Microorganisms grow more easily in a soiled environment. The safety pin ensures proper placement because the drain is not sutured in place.

13. Using sterile technique, prepare a sterile work area and open the needed supplies.

Supplies are within easy reach and sterility is maintained.

continues

Caring for a Penrose Drain (continued)

ACTION

14. Open the sterile cleaning solution. Pour the cleansing solution into the basin. Add the gauze sponges.

15. Put on sterile gloves.

16. Cleanse the drain site with the cleansing solution. Use the forceps and the moistened gauze or cotton-tipped applicators. **Start at the drain insertion site, moving in a circular motion toward the periphery. Use each gauze sponge or applicator only once. Discard and use new gauze if additional cleansing is needed.**

17. Dry the skin with a new gauze pad. Place the drain sponge under the drain. Place several gauze pads around the drain site. Apply gauze pads over the drain.

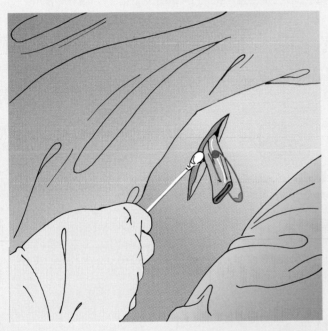

Action 16: Using gloved hands to clean around a Penrose drain with saline-soaked gauze sponge.

18. Apply ABD pads over the gauze. Remove gloves and dispose of them.

19. Tape the ABD pads securely to the patient's skin.

20. After securing the dressing, remove all remaining equipment, place the patient in a position of comfort with side rails up and bed in the lowest position, and perform hand hygiene.

21. Record the procedure, wound assessment, and the patient's reaction to the procedure according to institution's guidelines.

RATIONALE

Sterility of dressings and solution is maintained.

Sterile gloves help to maintain surgical asepsis and sterile technique and prevent the spread of microorganisms.

Using a circular motion ensures that cleaning occurs from the least to most contaminated area and a previously cleaned area is not contaminated again.

Drying prevents skin irritation. The gauze absorbs drainage and prevents the drainage from accumulating on the patient's skin.

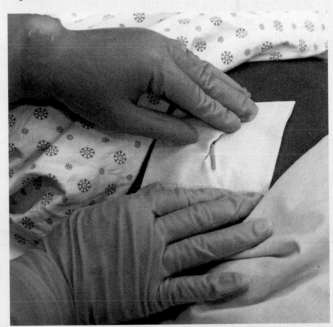

Action 17: Changing the drainage sponge around Penrose drain with gloved hands.

Pads provide extra absorption for excess drainage and provide a moisture barrier. It is easier to handle the tape without gloves.

Taping keeps the dressing secure.

Proper positioning after care maintains patient safety. Hand hygiene prevents the spread of microorganisms.

Documentation promotes continuity of care and communication.

continues

ACTION

RATIONALE

> 3/13/06   1400   Patient medicated with morphine 3 mg IV as ordered prior to dressing change. Dressing to right forearm removed. Dressings noted with small amount of serosanguineous drainage. Forearm with gross edema and erythema. Penrose drain intact. Incision edges approximated, staples intact. Area irrigated with normal saline, dried, and redressed with gauze, ABD pads, and stretch gauze. Reinforced the importance of keeping arm elevated on pillows, with patient verbalizing understanding.—P. Towns, RN

Action 21: Documentation.

22. Check all dressings every shift. More frequent checking may be needed if a wound is more complex or dressings become saturated more frequently.

Frequent checking ensures the assessment of changes in patient condition and timely intervention to prevent complications.

EVALUATION

The expected outcome is met when the patient exhibits a wound that is clean, dry, and intact, with a patent, intact Penrose drain. Other outcomes that are appropriate may include: the patient remains free of wound contamination and trauma; the patient reports minimal to no pain or discomfort; the patient exhibits signs and symptoms of progressive wound healing; and the patient states the reason for drain care.

Unexpected Situations and Associated Interventions

- *Assessment of the drain site reveals significantly increased edema, erythema, and drainage from the site, in addition to drainage via the drain:* Cleanse the site as ordered or per the nursing plan of care. Obtain vital signs, including the patient's temperature. Document care and assessments. Notify the physician of your findings.
- *Assessment of the drain site reveals that the drain has slipped back into the incision:* Follow facility policy and the physician's orders related to advancing Penrose drains. Document assessments and interventions. Notify the physician of your findings and interventions.
- *When preparing to change a dressing on a Penrose drain site, you remove the old dressing and note that the drain is completely out, lying in the dressing when you remove it:* Assess the site and the patient for other symptoms. Provide site care as ordered. Notify the physician. Often, depending on the patient's stage of recovery, the drain is left out. Document your findings and interventions.

Special Considerations

- Depending on facility policy, nurses may be responsible for advancing a Penrose drain as part of their nursing care. To advance a Penrose drain, use sterile forceps to pull the drain out of the incision site the number of centimeters ordered. Reposition the safety pin at the level of the skin. Trim excess tubing, leaving at least 2″ of exposed tubing.
- Wound care is often uncomfortable, and patients may experience significant pain. Assess the patient's comfort level and past experiences with wound care. Offer analgesics as ordered to maintain the patient's level of comfort.

SKILL 8-4

Caring for a T-Tube Drain

A biliary drain or T-tube is sometimes placed in the common bile duct after removal of the gallbladder (cholecystectomy) or a portion of the bile duct (choledochostomy). The tube drains bile while the surgical site is healing. A portion of the tube is inserted into the common bile duct and the remaining portion is anchored to the abdominal wall, passed through the skin, and connected to a closed drainage system. Often, a three-way valve is inserted between the drain tube and the drainage system to allow for clamping and flushing of the tube if necessary. The drainage amount is measured every shift, recorded, and included in output totals.

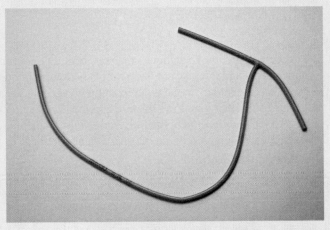

T-tube.

Equipment

- Sterile gloves
- Clean gloves
- Sterile gauze pads
- Sterile drain sponges
- Cleansing solution, usually sterile normal saline
- Sterile cotton-tipped applicators (if appropriate)
- Transparent dressing
- Graduated collection container
- Trash receptacle
- Sterile basin
- Sterile forceps
- Tape
- Skin protectant wipe
- Waterproof pad

ASSESSMENT

Assess the situation to determine the need for wound cleaning, a dressing change, or emptying of the drain. Confirm any physician orders relevant to drain care and any drain care included in the nursing plan of care. Assess the current dressing to determine if it is intact, and assess for evidence of excessive drainage or bleeding or saturation of the dressing. Assess the patency of the T-tube and the drain site.

Inspect the wound and the surrounding tissue. Assess the appearance of the incision for the approximation of wound edges, the color of the wound and surrounding area, and signs of dehiscence. Note the stage of the healing process and characteristics of any drainage. Assess the surrounding skin for color, temperature, and edema, ecchymosis, or maceration.

continues

Caring for a T-Tube Drain (continued)

NURSING DIAGNOSIS	Determine the related factors for the nursing diagnoses based on the patient's current status. An appropriate nursing diagnosis is Risk for Infection. Other nursing diagnoses may also be appropriate, including:

- Anxiety
- Disturbed Body Image
- Impaired Comfort
- Deficient Knowledge
- Impaired Skin Integrity
- Delayed Surgical Recovery
- Impaired Tissue Integrity

OUTCOME IDENTIFICATION AND PLANNING

The expected outcome to achieve when performing care for a T-tube drain is that the drain remains patent and intact. Care is accomplished without contaminating the wound area, without causing trauma to the wound, and without causing the patient to experience pain or discomfort. Other outcomes that are appropriate may include: the wound continues to show signs of progression of healing, and the drainage amounts are measured accurately at the frequency required by facility policy and recorded as part of the intake and output record.

IMPLEMENTATION

ACTION	RATIONALE
1. Review the physician's order for drain and site care or the nursing plan of care related to drain care.	Review validates the correct patient and correct procedure.
2. Gather the necessary supplies.	Preparation promotes efficient time management and organized approach to the task.
3. Identify the patient. Explain the procedure to the patient. Inquire about any allergies, specifically related to the products being used for wound care.	Patient identification validates the correct patient and correct procedure. Discussion and explanation help allay anxiety, encourage patient cooperation, and prepare the patient for what to expect.
4. Perform hand hygiene.	Hand hygiene prevents the spread of microorganisms.
5. Close the room door or curtains. Place the bed at an appropriate and comfortable working height.	Closing the door or curtain provides privacy. Proper bed positioning helps reduce back strain when providing care.
6. Place a waste receptacle at a convenient location for use during the procedure.	Having a waste receptacle handy means that the soiled dressing may be discarded easily, without the spread of microorganisms.
7. Assist the patient to a comfortable position that provides easy access to the drain area. Use the bath blanket to cover any exposed area other than the drain. Place the waterproof pad under the drain site.	Patient positioning and use of a bath blanket provide for comfort and warmth. Waterproof pad protects underlying surfaces.

Emptying Drainage

8. Put on clean gloves.	Gloves help prevent the spread of microorganisms.
9. Using sterile technique, open a gauze pad, making a sterile field with the outer wrapper.	Using sterile technique deters the spread of microorganisms.
10. Place the graduated collection container under the outlet valve of the drainage bag.**Without contaminating the outlet valve, pull the cap off and empty the bag's contents completely into the container; use the gauze to wipe the valve, and reseal the outlet valve.**	Draining contents into container allows for accurate measurement of the drainage. Wiping the valve with gauze prevents contamination of the valve. Wiping the valve and resealing it prevents the spread of microorganisms.

continues

ACTION

RATIONALE

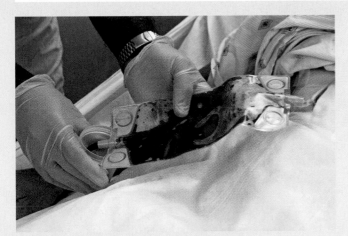

Action 10: Collection container held at the outlet valve.

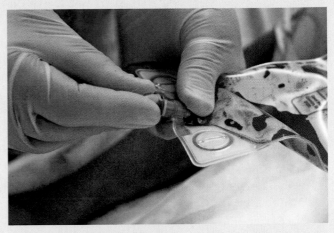

Action 10: Resealing the outlet valve.

11. Carefully measure and record the character, color, and amount of the drainage. Discard the drainage according to facility policy.

Documentation promotes continuity of care and communication. Appropriate disposal of biohazard material reduces the risk for microorganism transmission.

12. Remove gloves and perform hand hygiene.

Proper glove removal and performing hand hygiene prevent spread of microorganisms.

Cleaning the Drain Site

13. Check the position of the drain or drains before removing the dressing. Put on clean, disposable gloves and loosen tape on the old dressings. If necessary, use an adhesive remover to help get the tape off.

Checking position ensures that a drain is not removed accidentally. Gloves protect the nurse from contaminated dressings and prevent the spread of microorganisms. Adhesive tape remover helps to reduce patient discomfort during dressing removal.

14. Carefully remove the soiled dressings. If any part of the dressing sticks to the underlying skin, use small amounts of sterile saline to help loosen and remove. Do not reach over the drain site.

Cautious removal of the dressing is more comfortable for the patient and ensures that any drain present is not removed. Sterile saline provides for easier removal of the dressing and prevents tissue damage. Not reaching over the drain site reduces the risk for contamination.

15. After removing the dressing, note the presence, amount, type, color, and odor of any drainage on the dressings. Place soiled dressings in the appropriate waste receptacle. Remove gloves and dispose of in appropriate waste receptacle.

The presence of drainage should be documented. Proper disposal of gloves prevents spread of microorganisms.

16. Inspect the drain site for appearance and drainage. Assess if any pain is present. Note any problems to include in your documentation.

Wound healing process and/or the presence of irritation or infection should be documented.

17. Using sterile technique, prepare a sterile work area and open the needed supplies.

Preparing a sterile work area ensures that supplies are within easy reach and sterility is maintained.

18. Open the sterile cleaning solution. Pour the cleansing solution into the basin. Add the gauze sponges.

Sterility of dressings and solution is maintained.

19. Put on sterile gloves.

Use of sterile gloves maintains surgical asepsis and sterile technique and reduces the risk of microorganism transmission.

20. Cleanse the drain site with the cleansing solution. Use the forceps and the moistened gauze or cotton-tipped applicators. **Start at the drain insertion site, moving in a circular motion toward the periphery. Use each gauze sponge only once. Discard and use new gauze if additional cleansing is needed.**

Cleaning is done from the least to most contaminated area so that a previously cleaned area is not contaminated again.

continues

ACTION	RATIONALE
21. Allow the area to dry or dry with a new sterile gauze.	Drying deters the growth of microorganisms, which occurs in moist environments.
22. Place the drain sponge under the drain. Place several gauze pads around the drain site. Apply gauze pads over the drain. Alternatively, place the transparent dressing over the tube and dressings.	Dressings absorbs any drainage from the site.
23. Secure the dressings with tape as needed. **Be careful not to kink the tubing.**	Kinked tubing could block drainage.
24. After securing the dressing, remove all remaining equipment, place the patient in a position of comfort with side rails up and bed in the lowest position, and perform hand hygiene.	Proper patient positioning promotes safety. Hand hygiene prevents spread of microorganisms.
25. Record the procedure, your wound assessment, and the patient's reaction to the procedure using your institution's guidelines.	Documentation promotes continuity of care and communication.

> 8/9/06   1500   Dressing removed from
> T-tube site. No drainage noted on dressings.
> Drain site without redness, edema, drainage,
> or ecchymosis. Suture intact. Exit site cleansed
> with normal saline, dried, and redressed with
> dry dressing. Patient denies pain. Emptied col-
> lection bag of 20 cc bile-colored drainage.
> —L. Saunders, RN

Action 25: Documentation.

26. Check all dressings every shift. More frequent checking may be needed if a wound is more complex or dressings become saturated quickly.	Follow-up assessment ensures identification of changes in patient condition and timely intervention to prevent complications.

EVALUATION

The expected outcome is met when the patient exhibits a patent and intact T-tube drain with a wound area that is free of contamination and trauma. The patient verbalizes minimal to no pain or discomfort. Other outcomes that are appropriate may include: the patient exhibits signs and symptoms of progressive wound healing, with drainage being measured accurately at the frequency required by facility policy and amounts recorded as part of the intake and output record; and the patient states the reason for T-tube care.

Unexpected Situations and Associated Interventions

- *A patient's T-tube has been consistently draining 30 to 50 mL a shift, but now there is no output for the current shift. You check the tubing and site and do not observe kinks or other exterior obstructions:* Assess for signs of obstructed bile flow, including chills, fever, tachycardia, nausea, right upper quadrant fullness and pain, jaundice, dark foamy urine, and clay-colored stools. Obtain vital signs. Notify the physician of the situation and your findings and document the event in the patient's record. Flushing of the tube with sterile saline may be ordered as part of the patient's care.
- *Patient had a T-tube placed after surgery. The surgeon has asked that the tube be clamped for 1 hour before and after meals:* This diverts bile into the duodenum to aid in digestion and is accomplished by occluding the tube with a clamp or rubber band. Monitor the patient's response to clamping the tube. If the patient reports new symptoms, such as right upper quadrant pain, nausea, or vomiting, unclamp the tube. Assess for other symptoms and obtain vital signs. Report your findings to the surgeon and document the event in the patient's record.

Caring for a Jackson-Pratt Drain

A Jackson-Pratt (J-P) or grenade drain collects wound drainage in a bulblike device that is compressed to create gentle suction. It consists of perforated tubing connected to a portable vacuum unit. After a surgical procedure, the surgeon places one end of the drain in or near the area to be drained. The other end passes through the skin via a separate incision. These drains are usually sutured in place. The site may be treated as an additional surgical wound, but often these sites are left open to air after the first 24 hours after surgery. They are typically used with breast and abdominal surgery.

As the drainage accumulates in the bulb, the bulb expands and suction is lost, requiring recompression. Typically these drains are emptied every 4 to 8 hours, and when they are half full of drainage or air. However, based on nursing assessment and judgment, the drain could be emptied and recompressed more frequently. The patency, placement of the drain, and the amount and characteristics of the drainage are included in the wound assessment.

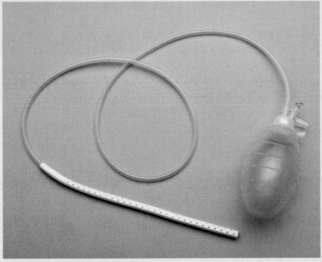

Jackson-Pratt drain.

Equipment

- Graduated container for measuring drainage
- Clean gloves
- Alcohol pad
- Cleansing solution, usually sterile normal saline
- Sterile gauze pads
- Personal protective equipment such as mask or face shield, if indicated

ASSESSMENT

Assess the patency of the Jackson-Pratt drain and the drain site. Confirm any physician orders relevant to drain care and any drain care included in the nursing plan of care.

Assess the situation to determine the need for wound cleaning, a dressing change, or emptying of the drain. Assess the current dressing, if there is one, to determine whether it is intact. Assess for the presence of excess drainage or bleeding or saturation of the dressing.

Inspect the wound and the surrounding tissue. Assess the appearance of the incision for the approximation of wound edges, the color of the wound and surrounding area, and signs of dehiscence. Note the stage of the healing process and characteristics of any drainage. Also assess the surrounding skin for color, temperature, and edema, ecchymosis, or maceration.

continues

NURSING DIAGNOSIS

Determine the related factors for the nursing diagnoses based on the patient's current status. An appropriate nursing diagnosis is Risk for Infection. Many other nursing diagnoses may also be appropriate, including:

- Anxiety
- Disturbed Body Image
- Acute Pain
- Deficient Knowledge
- Impaired Skin Integrity
- Delayed Surgical Recovery
- Impaired Tissue Integrity

OUTCOME IDENTIFICATION AND PLANNING

The expected outcome to achieve when performing care for a Jackson-Pratt drain is that the drain is patent and intact. Care is accomplished without contaminating the wound area, without causing trauma to the wound, and without causing the patient to experience pain or discomfort. Other outcomes that are appropriate may include: drainage amounts are measured accurately at the frequency required by facility policy and amounts are recorded as part of the intake and output record; the patient states positive aspects about self and verbalizes an understanding of the need for drain care.

IMPLEMENTATION

ACTION	RATIONALE
1. Review the physician's order for drain and site care or the nursing plan of care related to drain care.	Reviewing the order and plan of care validates the correct patient and correct procedure.
2. Gather the necessary supplies.	Preparation promotes efficient time management and organized approach to the task.
3. Identify the patient. Explain the procedure to the patient. Inquire about any allergies, specifically related to the products being used for wound care.	Patient identification validates the correct patient and correct procedure. Discussion and explanation help allay anxiety, encourage patient cooperation, and prepare the patient for what to expect.
4. Perform hand hygiene.	Hand hygiene prevents the spread of microorganisms.
5. Close the room door or curtains. Place the bed at an appropriate and comfortable working height.	Closing the door or curtain provides privacy. Placing the bed at the appropriate height helps reduce back strain when providing care.
6. Assist the patient to a comfortable position that provides easy access to the drain area. Use the bath blanket to cover any exposed area other than the drain. Place the waterproof pad under the drain site.	Patient positioning and use of a bath blanket promote comfort and warmth. Waterproof pad protects underlying surfaces.
7. Put on clean gloves; don mask or face shield if indicated.	Gloves prevent the spread of microorganisms; mask reduces the risk of transmission should splashing occur.
8. Place the graduated collection container under the outlet valve of the drain. Without contaminating the outlet valve, pull the cap off. The chamber will expand completely as it draws in air. **Empty the chamber's contents completely into the container. Use the alcohol pad to clean the chamber's spout and cap. Fully compress the chamber with one hand and replace the plug with your other hand.**	Emptying the drainage allows for accurate measurement. Cleaning the spout and cap reduces the risk of contamination and helps prevent the spread of microorganisms. Compressing the chamber reestablishes the vacuum.
9. Check the patency of the equipment. Make sure the tubing is free from twists and kinks.	Patent, untwisted, or unkinked tubing promotes appropriate drainage from wound.

continues

Caring for a Jackson-Pratt Drain (continued)

ACTION

RATIONALE

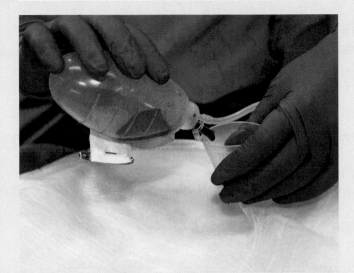

Action 8: Emptying contents of Jackson-Pratt drain into collection device.

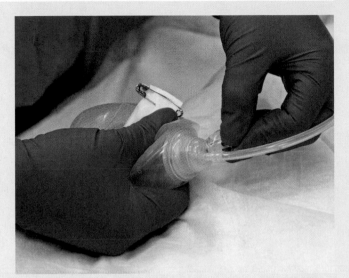

Action 8: With gloved hand, compressing a Jackson-Pratt drain and replacing plug.

10. Secure the Jackson-Pratt drain to the patient's gown below the wound, making sure that there is no tension on the tubing.

11. Carefully measure and record the character, color, and amount of the drainage. Discard the drainage according to facility policy.

12. If the drain site has a dressing, redress the site as outlined in Skill 8-3.

13. If the drain site is open to air, observe the sutures that secure the drain to the skin. Look for signs of pulling, tearing, swelling, or infection of the surrounding skin.

14. Gently clean the sutures with the gauze pad soaked in normal saline. Dry with a new gauze pad.

15. Remove gloves and all remaining equipment, place the patient in a position of comfort with side rails up and bed in the lowest position, and perform hand hygiene.

16. Record the procedure, your wound assessment, and the patient's reaction to the procedure using your institution's guidelines.

Securing the drain prevents injury to the patient and accidental removal of the drain.

Documentation promotes continuity of care and communication. Appropriate disposal of biohazard material reduces the risk for microorganism transmission.

Dressing protects the site.

Early detection of problems leads to prompt intervention and prevents complications.

Gentle cleaning and drying prevent the growth of microorganisms.

Proper patient positioning promotes safety. Proper removal of gloves and hand hygiene prevent spread of microorganisms.

Documentation promotes continuity of care and communication.

> 2/7/06 2400 Right chest incision and drain open to air. Wound edges approximated, slight ecchymosis, no edema, redness, or drainage. Steri-Strips intact. Drain patent and secured with suture. Exit site without edema, drainage, or redness. Drain emptied and recompressed. 40 cc sanguineous drainage recorded.
> —Carol White, RN

Action 16: Documentation.

continues

SKILL 8-5 Caring for a Jackson-Pratt Drain (continued)

EVALUATION

The expected outcome is met when the patient exhibits a patent and intact Jackson-Pratt drain with a wound that is free of contamination and trauma. The patient reports minimal to no pain or discomfort with the care. Other outcomes are met when the patient exhibits signs and symptoms of progressive healing without evidence of complications, with wound drainage being measured accurately at the frequency required by facility policy and recorded as part of the intake and output record.

Unexpected Situations and Associated Interventions

- *A patient has a Jackson-Pratt drain in the right lower quadrant following abdominal surgery. The record indicates it has been draining serosanguineous fluid, 40 to 50 mL every shift. While performing your initial assessment, you note that the dressing around the drain site is saturated with serosanguineous secretions and there is minimal drainage in the collection chamber:* Inspect the tubing for kinks or obstruction. Assess the patient for changes in condition. Remove the dressing and assess the site. Often, if the tubing becomes blocked with a blood clot or drainage particles, the wound drainage will leak around the exit site of the drain. Cleanse the area and redress the site. Notify the physician of your findings and document the event in the patient's record.
- *Your patient calls you to the room and says, "I found this in the bed when I went to get up." He has his Jackson-Pratt drain in his hand. It is completely removed from the patient:* Assess the patient for any new symptoms, and assess the surgical site and drain site. Apply a sterile dressing with gauze and tape to the drain site. Notify the physician of your findings and document the event in the patient's record.

Special Considerations

- Often patients have more than one Jackson-Pratt drain. Number or letter the drains for easy identification. Record the drainage from each drain separately, identified by the number or letter, on the intake and output record.

SKILL 8-6 Caring for a Hemovac Drain

A Hemovac drain is placed into a vascular cavity where blood drainage is expected after surgery, such as with abdominal and orthopedic surgery. The drain consists of perforated tubing connected to a portable vacuum unit. Suction is maintained by compressing a spring-like device in the collection unit. After a surgical procedure, the surgeon places one end of the drain in or near the area to be drained. The other end passes through the skin via a separate incision. These drains are usually sutured in place. The site may be treated as an additional surgical wound, but often these sites are left open to air after the first 24 hours after surgery.

As the drainage accumulates in the collection unit, it expands and suction is lost, requiring recompression. Typically the drain is emptied every 4 or 8 hours and when it is half full of drainage or air. However, based on the physician's orders and nursing assessment and judgment, it could be emptied and recompressed more frequently. The patency, placement of the drain, and the amount and characteristics of the drainage are included in the wound assessment.

continues

Caring for a Hemovac Drain (continued)

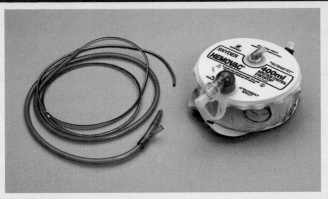

Hemovac drain.

Equipment

- Graduated container for measuring drainage
- Clean gloves
- Alcohol pad
- Cleansing solution, usually sterile normal saline
- Sterile gauze pads
- Personal protective equipment such as mask or face shield, if indicated

ASSESSMENT

Assess the patency of the Hemovac drain and the drain site. Confirm any physician orders relevant to drain care and any drain care included in the nursing plan of care. Also assess the situation to determine the need for wound cleaning, a dressing change, or emptying of the drain. Assess the current dressing, if there is one, to determine if it is intact. Assess for the presence of excess drainage or bleeding or saturation of the dressing. Inspect the wound and the surrounding tissue. Assess the appearance of the incision for the approximation of wound edges, the color of the wound and surrounding area, and signs of dehiscence. Note the stage of the healing process and characteristics of any drainage. Assess the surrounding skin for color, temperature, and edema, ecchymosis, or maceration.

NURSING DIAGNOSIS

Determine the related factors for the nursing diagnoses based on the patient's current status. An appropriate nursing diagnosis is Risk for Infection. Many other nursing diagnoses may also be appropriate, including:

- Anxiety
- Disturbed Body Image
- Impaired Comfort
- Deficient Knowledge
- Impaired Skin Integrity
- Delayed Surgical Recovery
- Impaired Tissue Integrity

OUTCOME IDENTIFICATION AND PLANNING

The expected outcome to achieve when performing care for a Hemovac drain is that the drain is patent and intact. Care is performed without contaminating the wound area, without causing trauma to the wound, and without causing the patient to experience pain or discomfort. Other outcomes that are appropriate may include: drainage amounts are measured accurately at the frequency required by facility policy and recorded as part of the intake and output record; and the patient demonstrates understanding of the need for drain care.

continues

IMPLEMENTATION
ACTION

RATIONALE

1. Review the physician's order for drain and site care or the nursing plan of care related to drain care.

   Review of the order and plan of care validates the correct patient and correct procedure.

2. Gather the necessary supplies.

   Preparation promotes efficient time management and organized approach to the task.

3. Identify the patient. Explain the procedure to the patient. Inquire about any allergies, specifically related to the products being used for wound care.

   Patient identification validates the correct patient and correct procedure. Discussion and explanation help allay anxiety, encourage patient cooperation, and prepare the patient for what to expect.

4. Perform hand hygiene.

   Hand hygiene prevents the spread of microorganisms.

5. Close the room door or curtains. Place the bed at an appropriate and comfortable working height.

   Closing the door or curtain provides privacy. Positioning the bed at the proper height helps reduce back strain when providing care.

6. Assist the patient to a comfortable position that provides easy access to the drain area. Use the bath blanket to cover any exposed area other than the drain. Place the waterproof pad under the drain site.

   Patient positioning and use of a bath blanket provide for comfort and warmth. Waterproof pad protects underlying surfaces.

7. Put on clean gloves and other personal protective equipment, such as mask or face shield, as necessary.

   Gloves prevent the spread of microorganisms. Personal protective equipment such as a face shield prevents transmission should splashing occur.

8. Place the graduated collection container under the pouring spout of the drain. Without contaminating the outlet valve, uncap the valve. The chamber will expand completely as it draws in air. Empty the chamber's contents completely into the container. Use the alcohol pad to clean the chamber's spout and cap. **Fully compress the chamber by pushing the top and bottom together with your hands. Keep the device tightly compressed while you reinsert the plug.**

   Uncapping allows for accurate measurement of the drainage. Cleaning with alcohol prevents contamination of the valve and reduces the risk for microorganism transmission. Compression with both hands helps to reestablish the vacuum.

9. Check the patency of the equipment. Make sure the tubing is free from twists and kinks.

   Free, untwisted, and unkinked tubing promotes drainage from wound.

10. Secure the Hemovac drain to the patient's gown below the wound, making sure that there is no tension on the tubing.

    Securing the drain prevents injury to the patient or accidental removal of the drain.

11. Carefully measure and record the character, color, and amount of the drainage. Discard the drainage according to facility policy.

    Documentation promotes continuity of care and communication. Appropriate disposal of biohazard material prevents transmission of microorganisms.

12. If the drain site has a dressing, redress the site as outlined in Skill 8-3.

    Dressing protects the site.

13. If the drain site is open to air, observe the sutures that secure the drain to the skin. Look for signs of pulling, tearing, swelling, or infection of the surrounding skin.

    Early detection of problems leads to prompt intervention and prevents complications.

14. Gently clean the sutures with the gauze pad soaked in normal saline. Dry with a new gauze pad.

    Cleaning prevents the growth of microorganisms.

15. Remove gloves and all remaining equipment, place the patient in a position of comfort with side rails up and bed in the lowest position, and perform hand hygiene.

    Patient positioning promotes safety. Proper glove removal and hand hygiene prevent spread of microorganisms.

continues

SKILL 8-6 Caring for a Hemovac Drain (continued)

ACTION   **RATIONALE**

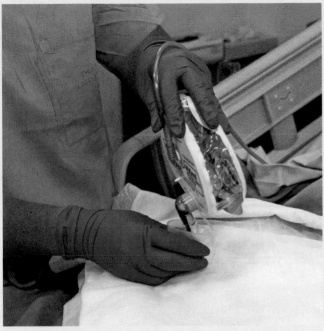

Action 8: Emptying Hemovac drain into collection device.

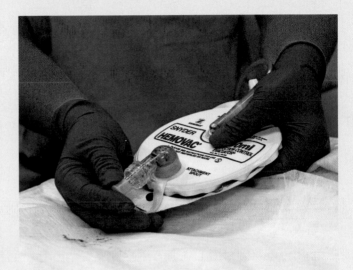

Action 8: Compressing the Hemovac and securing the cap.

16. Record the procedure, your wound assessment, and the patient's reaction to the procedure using your institution's guidelines.

Documentation promotes continuity of care and communication.

> 1/18/06   1000   Hemovac drain in place in left lower extremity, site open to air. Suture intact; exit site slightly pink, without redness, edema, or drainage. Surrounding skin without edema, ecchymosis, or redness. Exit site and suture cleansed with normal saline. Hemovac emptied of 90 cc sanguineous secretions and recompressed.—A. Smith, RN

Action 16: Documentation.

EVALUATION

The expected outcome is met when the patient demonstrates a patent, intact Hemovac drain with a wound that is free of contamination and trauma. The patient verbalizes little to no pain or discomfort. Other outcomes are met when the patient exhibits signs and symptoms of progressive healing without evidence of complications, with wound drainage being measured accurately at the frequency required by facility policy and recorded as part of the intake and output record.

continues

Caring for a Hemovac Drain (continued)

Unexpected Situations and Associated Interventions	• *A patient has a Hemovac drain placed in the left knee following surgery. The record indicates it has been draining serosanguineous secretions, 40 to 50 mL every shift. While performing your initial assessment, you note that the collection chamber is completely expanded. You empty the device and compress to resume suction. A short time later, you observe that the chamber is completely expanded again:* Inspect the tubing for kinks or obstruction. Inspect the device, looking for breaks in the integrity of the chamber. Make sure the cap is in place and closed. Assess the patient for changes in condition. Remove the dressing and assess the site. Make sure the drainage tubing has not advanced out of the wound, exposing any of the perforations in the tubing. If you are not successful in maintaining the vacuum, notify the physician of your findings and interventions and document the event in the patient's record.
Special Considerations	• When the patient with a drain is ready to ambulate, empty and compress the drain prior to activity. Secure the drain to the patient's gown below the wound, making sure there is no tension on the drainage tubing. This removes excess drainage, maintains maximum suction, and avoids strain on the drain's suture line.

Cleaning a Wound and Applying a Sterile Dressing

The goal of wound care is to promote tissue repair and regeneration to restore skin integrity. Many times wound care includes cleaning of the wound and the use of a dressing as a protective covering over the wound. Wound cleansing is performed to remove debris, contaminants, and excess exudate. Sterile normal saline is the preferred cleansing solution.

Dressings can rub or stick to the wound, causing superficial injury. They also can create a warm, damp, dark environment, an environment conducive to the growth of organisms, creating a potential for infection. Dressings are routinely changed to prevent these complications. The frequency of dressing changes depends on the amount of drainage, the physician's order, the nature of the wound, and nursing judgment. One of the most common causes of nosocomial infections is carelessness in practicing asepsis when providing wound care. It is extremely important to use appropriate aseptic technique and follow standard precautions.

Equipment	• Sterile gloves • Gauze dressings • Sterile dressing set or suture set (for the sterile scissors and forceps) • Sterile cleaning solution as ordered (commonly 0.9% normal saline solution) • Clean disposable gloves • Sterile basin (may be optional) • Sterile drape (may be optional) • Plastic bag or other appropriate waste container for soiled dressings • Waterproof pad and bath blanket • Tape or ties • Surgi-pads or ABD pads • Additional dressings and supplies needed or required by the physician's order

continues

Cleaning a Wound and Applying a Sterile Dressing (continued)

ASSESSMENT

Assess the situation to determine the need for wound cleaning and a dressing change. Confirm any physician orders relevant to wound care and any wound care included in the nursing plan of care. Assess the current dressing to determine if it is intact. Assess for excess drainage or bleeding or saturation of the dressing. Inspect the wound and the surrounding tissue. Assess the appearance of the wound for the approximation of wound edges, the color of the wound and surrounding area, and signs of dehiscence. Note the stage of the healing process and characteristics of any drainage. Also assess the surrounding skin for color, temperature, and edema, ecchymosis, or maceration.

NURSING DIAGNOSIS

Determine the related factors for the nursing diagnoses based on the patient's current status. Appropriate nursing diagnoses may include:

- Risk for Infection
- Anxiety
- Disturbed Body Image
- Impaired Comfort
- Deficient Knowledge
- Impaired Skin Integrity
- Delayed Surgical Recovery
- Impaired Tissue Integrity

In addition, many other nursing diagnoses may require the use of this skill.

OUTCOME IDENTIFICATION AND PLANNING

The expected outcome to achieve when cleaning a wound and applying a sterile dressing is that the wound is cleaned and protected with a dressing without contaminating the wound area, without causing trauma to the wound, and without causing the patient to experience pain or discomfort. Other outcomes that are appropriate include: the wound continues to show signs of progression of healing and the patient demonstrates understanding of the need for wound care and dressing change.

IMPLEMENTATION

ACTION	RATIONALE
1. Review the physician's order for wound care or the nursing plan of care related to wound care.	Reviewing the order and plan of care validates the correct patient and correct procedure.
2. Gather the necessary supplies.	Preparation promotes efficient time management and organized approach to the task.
3. Identify the patient. Explain the procedure to the patient. Inquire about any allergies, specifically related to the products being used for wound care.	Patient identification validates the correct patient and correct procedure. Discussion and explanation help allay anxiety, encourage patient cooperation, and prepare the patient for what to expect.
4. Perform hand hygiene.	Hand hygiene prevents the spread of microorganisms.
5. Close the room door or curtains. Place the bed at an appropriate and comfortable working height.	Closing the door or curtain promotes privacy. Proper bed positioning helps reduce back strain while you are performing the procedure.
6. Place a waste receptacle or bag at a convenient location for use during the procedure.	Having a waste container handy means the soiled dressing may be discarded easily, without the spread of microorganisms.
7. Assist the patient to a comfortable position that provides easy access to the wound area. Use the bath blanket to cover any exposed area other than the wound. If necessary, place the waterproof pad under the wound site.	Patient positioning and use of a bath blanket provide for comfort and warmth. Waterproof pad protects underlying surfaces.

continues

Cleaning a Wound and Applying a Sterile Dressing (continued)

ACTION	RATIONALE
8. Check the position of drains, tubes, or other adjuncts before removing the dressing. Put on clean, disposable gloves and loosen tape on the old dressings. If necessary, use an adhesive remover to help get the tape off.	Checking ensures that a drain is not removed accidentally if one is present. Gloves protect the nurse from contaminated dressings and prevent the spread of microorganisms. Adhesive tape remover helps reduce patient discomfort during removal of dressing.

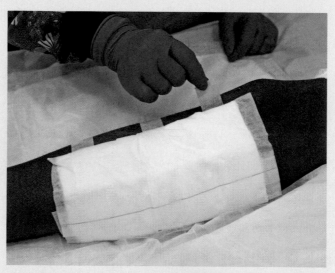

Action 8: Gloved hands loosening dressing tape.

9. Carefully remove the soiled dressings. If any part of the dressing sticks to the underlying skin, use small amounts of sterile saline to help loosen and remove. Do not reach over the wound.	Cautious removal of the dressing is more comfortable for the patient and ensures that any drain present is not removed. Sterile saline provides for easier removal of the dressing and prevents tissue damage.

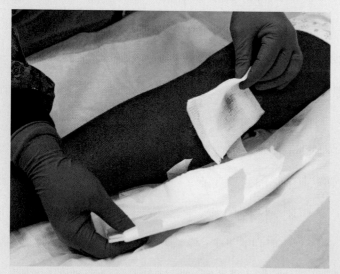

Action 9: Gloved hands removing dressing.

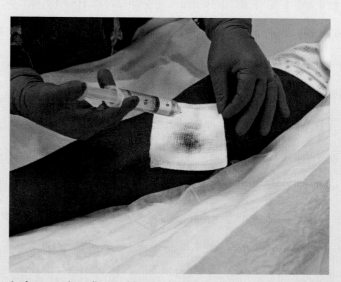

Action 9: Using saline to aid in removing dressing.

continues

Cleaning a Wound and Applying a Sterile Dressing (continued)

ACTION	RATIONALE
10. After removing the dressing, note the presence, amount, type, color, and odor of any drainage on the dressings. Place soiled dressings in the appropriate waste receptacle. Remove your gloves and dispose of them in an appropriate waste receptacle.	The presence of drainage should be documented. Proper disposal of soiled dressings and used gloves prevents spread of microorganisms.

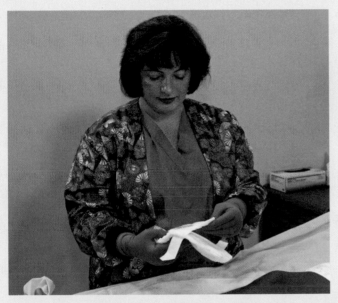

Action 10: Assessing dressing that has been removed.

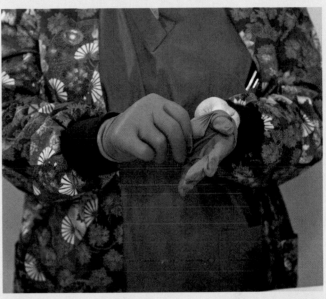

Action 10: Removing gloves.

11. Inspect the wound site for size, appearance, and drainage. Assess if any pain is present. Check the sutures, Steri-Strips, staples, and drains or tubes. Note any problems to include in your documentation.	Wound healing or the presence of irritation or infection should be documented.
12. **Using sterile technique, prepare a sterile work area and open the needed supplies.**	Supplies are within easy reach and sterility is maintained.

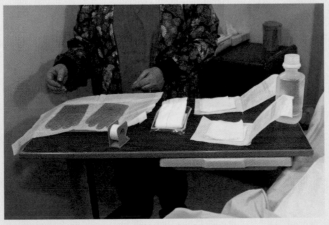

Action 12: Setting up sterile field.

continues

ACTION

RATIONALE

13. Open the sterile cleaning solution. Depending on the amount of cleaning needed, the solution might be poured directly over gauze sponges for small cleaning jobs or into a basin for more complex or larger cleaning.

Sterility of dressings and solution is maintained.

14. Put on sterile gloves.

Use of sterile gloves maintains surgical asepsis and sterile technique and reduces the risk for spreading micro-organisms.

15. Clean the wound. If needed, use sterile forceps to clean the area. **Clean the wound from top to bottom and from the center to the outside. Following this pattern, use gauze for each wipe, placing the used gauze in the waste receptacle. Do not touch any surface with the gloves or forceps.**

Cleaning occurs from the least to most contaminated area. Using a single gauze for each wipe ensures that the previously cleaned area is not contaminated again.

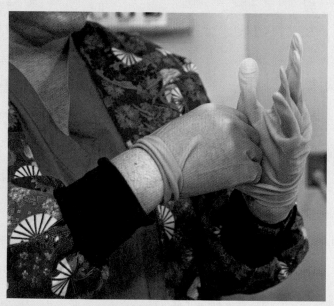

Action 14: Putting on sterile gloves.

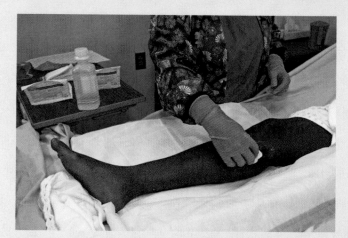

Action 15: Gloved hands cleaning wound with dampened gauze.

16. **If a drain is in use, clean around the drain using a circular motion. Wipe from the center toward the outside. Use the gauze a single time and then dispose of it.**

Cleaning occurs from least to most contaminated area.

18. Once the wound is cleansed, dry the area using a gauze sponge in the same manner. Apply ointment or any other treatments if ordered.

Moisture provides a medium for growth of microorganisms. The growth of microorganisms may be retarded and the healing process improved with the use of ordered ointments or other applications.

19. Apply a layer of dry sterile dressing over the wound. Forceps may be used to apply the dressing.

Primary dressing serves as a wick for drainage. Use of forceps helps ensure that sterile technique is maintained.

20. Place a second layer of gauze over the wound site.

A second layer provides for increased absorption of drainage.

continues

ACTION

RATIONALE

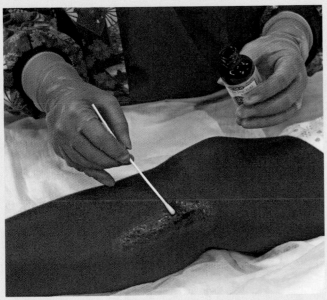

Action 18: Gloved hand applying antiseptic ointment to wound with cotton applicator.

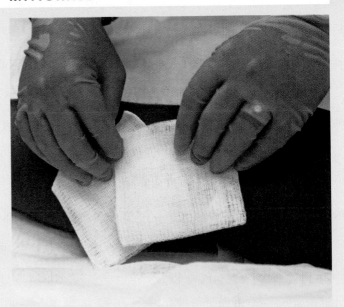

Action 19: Gloved hands applying dry dressing to site.

21. Apply a Surgi-pad or ABD dressing over the gauze at the site as the outermost layer of the dressing.

22. Remove and discard sterile gloves. Apply tape or tie tapes to secure the dressings.

23. After securing the dressing, label dressing with date and time. Remove all remaining equipment, place the patient in a position of comfort with side rails up and bed in the lowest position, and perform hand hygiene.

The dressing acts as additional protection for the wound against microorganisms in the environment.

Tape is easier to apply after gloves have been removed. Proper disposal of gloves prevents the spread of microorganisms.

Recording date and time provides communication and demonstrates adherence to plan of care. Proper patient and bed positioning promotes safety. Hand hygiene prevents spread of microorganisms.

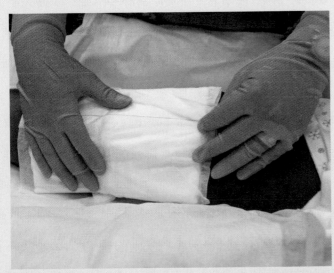

Action 21: Gloved hands applying a Surgi-pad (ABD) over dressing and securing with tape.

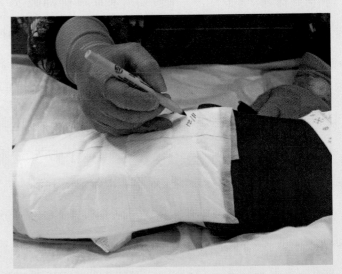

Action 23: Recording date and time of dressing change.

continues

ACTION	RATIONALE
24. Record the procedure, wound assessment, and the patient's reaction to the procedure according to institution's guidelines.	Documentation promotes continuity of care and communication.

> 9/8/06   0600   Dressing removed from leg incision. Scant purulent secretions noted on dressing. Incision edges approximately 1 mm apart, red, with ecchymosis and edema present. Small amount of purulent drainage from wound noted. Area cleansed with normal saline, dried, antibiotic ointment applied per order. Surrounding tissue red and ecchymotic. Redressed with nonadhering dressing, gauze, and wrapped with stretch gauze. Patient reports adequate pain control after preprocedure analgesic.—N. Joiner, RN

Action 24: Documentation.

| 25. Check all wound dressings every shift. More frequent checks may be needed if the wound is more complex or dressings become saturated quickly. | Checking dressings ensures the assessment of changes in patient condition and timely intervention to prevent complications. |

EVALUATION

The expected outcome is met when the patient exhibits a clean, intact wound with a clean sterile dressing in place; the wound is free of contamination and trauma; the patient reports little to no pain or discomfort during care; and the patient demonstrates signs and symptoms of progressive wound healing.

Unexpected Situations and Associated Interventions

- *The previous wound assessment states that the incision was clean and dry and the wound edges were approximated, with the staples and surgical drain intact. The surrounding tissue was without inflammation, edema, or erythema. After the dressing is removed, you note the incision edges are not approximated at the distal end, multiple staples are evident in the old dressing, the surrounding skin tissue is red and swollen, and purulent drainage is on the dressing and leaking from the wound:* Assess the patient for any other signs and symptoms, such as pain, malaise, fever, and paresthesias. Place a dry sterile dressing over the wound site. Report your findings to the physician and document the event in the patient's record. Be prepared to obtain a wound culture and implement any changes in wound care as ordered.
- *After you have put on sterile gloves, the patient moves too close to the edge of the bed and you support her with your hands to prevent her from falling:* If nothing else in the sterile field was touched, remove the contaminated gloves and put on new sterile gloves. If you did not bring a second pair, use the call light to summon a coworker to provide a new pair of gloves.
- *You have set up your supplies, removed the old dressing, and put on sterile gloves to clean the wound. You realize you have forgotten a necessary piece of dressing material:* Ask the patient to press the call bell to summon a coworker to provide the missing supplies.

Special Considerations

- Instruct the patient, if appropriate, and ancillary staff members to observe for excessive drainage that may overwhelm the dressing. They should also report when dressings become soiled or loosened from the skin.

Older Adult Considerations

- The skin of older adults is less elastic and more sensitive, so use paper tape or Montgomery straps to prevent tearing of the skin.

SKILL 8-8

Collecting a Wound Culture

If your assessment of a patient and the patient's wound suggests infection, a wound culture may be ordered to identify the causative organism. Identifying the invading microorganism will provide useful information to select the most appropriate therapy. A nurse or physician can perform a wound culture. Maintaining strict asepsis is crucial so that only the pathogen present in the wound is isolated.

Equipment

- A sterile Culturette kit with swab, or a culture tube with individual sterile swabs
- Sterile gloves
- Clean disposable gloves
- Plastic bag or appropriate waste receptacle
- Patient label for the sample tube
- Biohazard specimen bag
- Bath blanket (if necessary to drape the patient)
- Supplies to clean the wound and reapply a sterile dressing after obtaining the culture

ASSESSMENT

Assess the situation to determine the need for a wound culture. Confirm any physician orders relevant to obtaining a wound culture. Complete an assessment of the wound and the surrounding tissue. Inspect the wound for the approximation of wound edges, the color of the wound and surrounding area, and signs of dehiscence. Note the stage of the healing process and characteristics of any drainage. Assess the surrounding skin for color, temperature, and edema, ecchymosis, or maceration.

NURSING DIAGNOSIS

Determine the related factors for the nursing diagnoses based on the patient's current status. An appropriate nursing diagnosis would be Risk for Infection. Other appropriate diagnoses may include:

- Acute Pain
- Impaired Skin Integrity
- Impaired Tissue Integrity
- Delayed Surgical Recovery
- Disturbed Body Image
- Hyperthermia

OUTCOME IDENTIFICATION AND PLANNING

The expected outcome to achieve when collecting a wound culture is that the culture is obtained without evidence of contamination and without exposing the patient to additional pathogens.

IMPLEMENTATION

ACTION	RATIONALE
1. Review the physician's order for obtaining a wound culture.	Review of the order validates the correct patient and correct procedure.
2. Gather the necessary supplies.	Preparation promotes efficient time management and provides for organized approach to task.
3. Identify the patient, and check the specimen label to make sure the information matches. Explain the procedure to the patient.	Patient identification validates the correct patient and correct procedure. Discussion and explanation help allay anxiety and prepare the patient for what to expect.

continues

SKILL
8-8   **Collecting a Wound Culture** (continued)

ACTION	RATIONALE
4. Perform hand hygiene.	Hand hygiene prevents the spread of microorganisms.
5. Close the room door or curtains. Place the bed at an appropriate and comfortable working height.	Closing the door or curtain promotes privacy. Proper bed positioning helps reduce back strain while you are performing the procedure.
6. Place an appropriate waste receptacle within easy reach for use during the procedure.	Having the waste container handy means that soiled materials may be discarded easily, without the spread of microorganisms.
7. Assist the patient to a comfortable position that provides easy access to the wound. If necessary, drape the patient with the bath blanket to expose only the wound area. Check the culture label again against the patient's identification bracelet.	Patient positioning and use of a bath blanket provide for comfort and warmth. Checking the culture label with the patient's identification ensures the correct patient and the correct procedure.

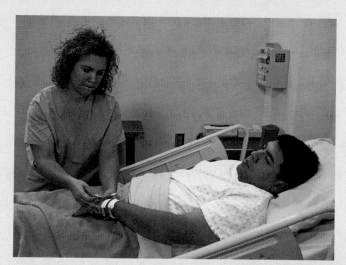

Action 7: Checking culture label with the patient's identification band.

8. Put on the clean, disposable gloves to remove any dressings. Loosen the tape and old dressings. Do not reach over the wound. Remove the dressing and dispose of it in the receptacle. Assess the wound and the characteristics of any drainage. Remove gloves and dispose of them.	Gloves protect the nurse from handling contaminated dressings. Assessment provides information about wound healing or the presence of irritation or infection that should be documented.
9. Set up sterile field with supplies if necessary. Put on sterile gloves and clean the wound according to facility policies and procedures.	A sterile field prevents contamination of the wound. Previous drainage and skin flora, which could contaminate the culture, are removed.

continues

Collecting a Wound Culture (continued)

ACTION	RATIONALE
10. Twist the cap to loosen the swab on the Culturette tube, or open the separate swab and remove the cap from the culture tube. **Keep the swab and inside of the culture tube sterile.**	Supplies are ready to use and within easy reach and aseptic technique is maintained.

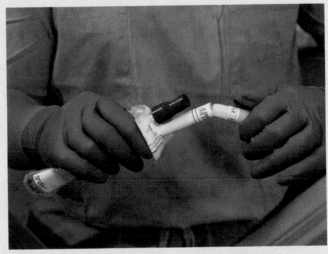

Action 10: Twisting cap on Culturette, keeping swab in the tube.

11. Put on a clean glove or new sterile glove, if necessary.	The use of a Culturette or swab does not require immediate contact with the skin or wound. If contact with the wound is necessary to collect the specimen, wear a sterile glove on that hand.
12. **Carefully insert the swab into the wound and gently roll the swab to obtain a sample. Use another swab if collecting a specimen from another site.**	Cotton tip absorbs wound drainage. Using another swab at a different site prevents cross-contamination of the wound.

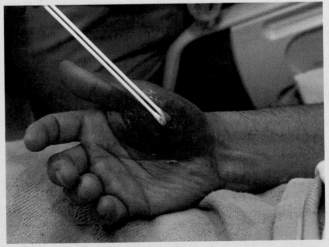

Action 12: Swabbing the wound with cotton applicator from Culturette.

continues

SKILL 8-8

Collecting a Wound Culture (continued)

ACTION

RATIONALE

13. Place the swab back in the culture tube. **Do not touch the outside of the tube with the swab.** Secure the cap. Some Culturette tubes have an ampule of medium at the bottom of the tube. It might be necessary to crush this ampule to activate. Follow the manufacturer's instructions for use.

The outside of the container is protected from contamination with microorganisms and the sample is not contaminated with organisms not in the wound. Surrounding the swab with culture medium is necessary for accurate culture results.

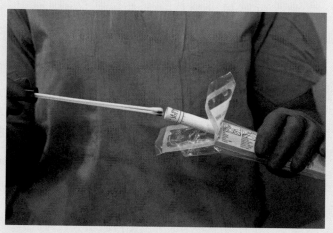

Action 13: Placing applicator swab back in the Culturette.

14. Remove gloves and discard them accordingly. Perform hand hygiene.

Hand hygiene prevents the spread of microorganisms.

15. Don sterile gloves and replace the dressing as needed following the appropriate procedure.

Gloving maintains aseptic technique. Dressings provide for drainage absorption and protect the wound.

16. Remove gloves and perform hand hygiene. Remove any equipment and leave the patient comfortable, with the side rails up and the bed in the lowest position.

Removing gloves and performing hand hygiene prevent the spread of microorganisms. Proper bed positioning promotes patient safety.

17. Label the specimen according to your institution's guidelines and send it to the laboratory in a biohazard bag.

Proper labeling ensures proper identification of the specimen.

18. Document the procedure, the wound assessment, and the patient's reaction to the procedure following your institution's guidelines.

Documentation promotes continuity of care and communication.

continues

SKILL
8-8   **Collecting a Wound Culture** (continued)

ACTION   **RATIONALE**

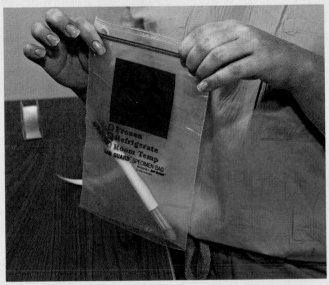

6/22/06   2100   Wound noted on patient's left ankle; 2 cm × 3 cm × 1 cm, red, tender, with purulent drainage present. Edges macerated, without erythema and tenderness. Wound cleaned with normal saline, culture obtained. Skin barrier applied to surrounding area, wound packed with moist saline gauze, dressed with dry gauze and Kling. Left lower extremity elevated. Culture labeled and sent to lab.—J. Wentz, RN

Action 17: Culturette/specimen container in biohazard bag.

Action 18: Documentation.

EVALUATION

The expected outcome is met when the patient's wound is cultured without evidence of contamination and the patient remains free of exposure to additional pathogens.

Unexpected Situations and Associated Interventions

- *You have the culture swab in the patient's wound to obtain the specimen. You realize that you did not clean the wound first:* Discard this swab. Obtain the additional supplies needed to clean the wound according to facility policy and a new culture swab. Clean the wound, then proceed to obtain the culture specimen.
- *As you prepare to insert the culture swab into the wound, you inadvertently touch the swab to the patient's bedclothes:* Discard this swab, obtain a new culture swab, and collect the specimen.

Irrigating a Sterile Wound

An irrigation is a directed flow of solution over tissues. Physicians may order wound irrigations to clean the area of pathogens and other debris and to promote wound healing. Irrigation procedures may also be ordered to apply heat or antiseptics locally. If the wound is closed, clean technique may be used; if the wound is open, sterile equipment and solutions are used for irrigation. Normal saline is often the solution of choice when irrigating wounds.

Equipment

- A sterile irrigation set, including a basin, irrigant container, and irrigation syringe
- Sterile irrigation solution as ordered by the physician, warmed to body temperature
- Waste receptacle to dispose of contaminated materials
- Sterile gloves and a set of clean disposable gloves
- Sterile scissors and forceps
- Waterproof pad and bath blanket
- Sterile supplies for a dressing change
- Sterile packing gauze (if needed)
- Personal protective equipment such as a gown, mask, and eye protection

ASSESSMENT

Assess the situation to determine the need for wound irrigation. Confirm any physician orders relevant to wound care and any wound care included in the nursing plan of care. Assess the current dressing to determine if it is intact. Assess for excess drainage or bleeding or saturation of the dressing. Inspect the wound and the surrounding tissue. Assess the wound for the approximation of wound edges, the color of the wound and surrounding area, and signs of dehiscence. Note the stage of the healing process and characteristics of any drainage. Assess the surrounding skin for color, temperature, and edema, ecchymosis, or maceration. Determine the patient's level of pain and administer analgesics as ordered.

NURSING DIAGNOSIS

Determine the related factors for the nursing diagnoses based on the patient's current status. An appropriate nursing diagnosis would be Risk for Infection. Other nursing diagnoses may include:

- Anxiety
- Acute Pain
- Disturbed Body Image
- Deficient Knowledge
- Impaired Skin Integrity
- Delayed Surgical Recovery
- Impaired Tissue Integrity
- Risk for Trauma

OUTCOME IDENTIFICATION AND PLANNING

The expected outcome to achieve when irrigating a wound is that the wound is cleaned without contamination or trauma and without causing the patient to experience pain or discomfort. Other outcomes that might be appropriate include: the wound continues to show signs of progression of healing, and the patient demonstrates understanding about the need for wound irrigation.

IMPLEMENTATION

ACTION	RATIONALE
1. Review the physician's order for wound care or the nursing plan of care related to wound care.	Reviewing the order and nursing plan of care validates the correct patient and correct procedure.
2. Gather the necessary supplies.	Preparation promotes efficient time management and provides an organized approach to the task.
3. Identify the patient and explain the procedure. Determine if the patient is allergic to any of the materials or solutions needed for the procedure.	Patient identification validates the correct patient and correct procedure. Discussion and explanation help allay anxiety, encourage patient cooperation, and prepare the patient for what to expect.

continues

Irrigating a Sterile Wound (continued)

ACTION

RATIONALE

4. Perform hand hygiene.

5. Close the room door or curtains. Place the bed at a comfortable working height.

6. Assist the patient to a comfortable position that provides easy access to the wound area. **Position the patient so that the irrigation solution will flow from the upper end of the wound toward the lower end.** Expose the area and drape the patient with a bath blanket if needed. Put the waterproof pad under the wound area.

7. Have the disposal bag or waste receptacle within easy reach for use during the irrigation.

8. Put on a gown, mask, and eye protection.

9. Put on clean disposable gloves and remove the soiled dressings.

10. Assess the wound for size, appearance, and drainage. Assess the appearance of the surrounding tissue.

Hand hygiene prevents the spread of microorganisms.

Closing the door or curtains provides privacy. Proper bed positioning helps reduce back strain while you are performing the procedure.

Patient positioning and use of a bath blanket provide for comfort and warmth. Gravity directs the flow of liquid from the least contaminated to the most contaminated area. Waterproof pad protects the patient and the bed linens.

Having the waste container handy means that soiled dressings and supplies may be discarded easily, without the spread of microorganisms.

Using personal protective equipment such as gowns, masks, and eye protection is part of standard precautions. A gown protects clothes from contamination should splashing occur. Goggles protect mucous membranes of eyes from contact with irrigant fluid.

The nurse is protected from handling contaminated dressings.

Assessment provides information about the wound healing process or the presence of infection.

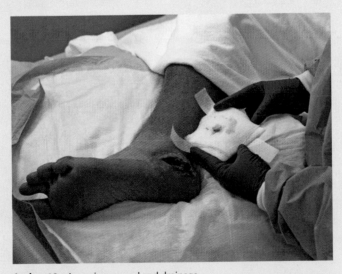

Action 10: Assessing wound and drainage.

11. Discard the dressings in the receptacle. Remove gloves and put them in the receptacle.

12. **Using sterile technique, prepare a sterile field and add all the sterile supplies needed for the procedure to the field. Pour warmed sterile irrigating solution into the sterile container.**

Proper disposal of dressings and gloves prevents the spread of microorganisms.

Supplies are within easy reach and sterile technique is maintained. Using warmed solution prevents chilling of the patient.

continues

ACTION	RATIONALE
13. Put on sterile gloves.	Using sterile gloves maintains surgical asepsis.
14. Position the sterile basin below the wound to collect the irrigation fluid.	Patient and bed linens are protected from contaminated fluid.
15. Fill the irrigation syringe with solution. **Using your non-dominant hand, gently apply pressure to the basin against the skin below the wound to form a seal with the skin.**	The solution will collect in the basin and prevent the irrigant from running down the skin. Patient and bed linens are protected from contaminated fluid.

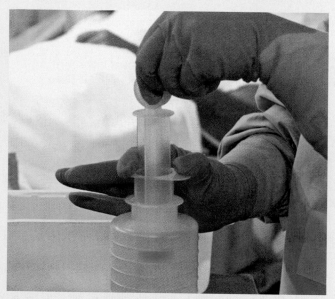

Action 15: Drawing up sterile solution from sterile container into irrigation syringe.

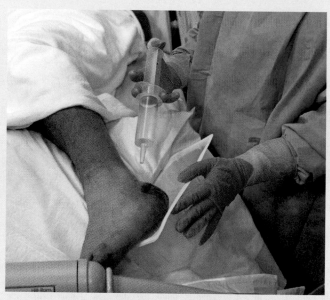

Action 15: Patient lying on side with wound exposed, sterile collection container placed against skin, bed protected with waterproof pad.

ACTION	RATIONALE
16. **Gently direct a stream of solution into the wound. Keep the tip of the syringe at least 1" above the upper tip of the wound. When using a catheter tip, insert it gently into the wound until it meets resistance. Gently flush all wound areas.**	Debris and contaminated solution flow from the least contaminated to most contaminated area. A catheter tip allows the introduction of irrigant into a wound with a small opening or one that is deep.
17. Watch for the solution to flow smoothly and evenly. When the solution from the wound flows out clear, discontinue irrigation.	Irrigation removes exudate and debris.
18. Dry the surrounding skin with a sterile gauze sponge.	Moisture provides a medium for growth of microorganisms.
19. Apply a new sterile dressing to the wound (see Skill 8-7).	Dressings absorb drainage and protect the surrounding skin.
20. Remove gloves and dispose of them properly. Apply tie straps or tape as needed to secure the dressing.	Tape is easier to apply after gloves have been removed.
21. Return the bed to the lowest position while making the patient comfortable and raising the side rails as needed.	Repositioning the bed promotes patient safety.

continues

Irrigating a Sterile Wound (continued)

ACTION   RATIONALE

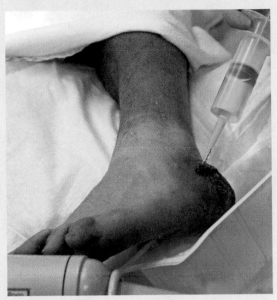

Action 16: Irrigating wound with a gentle stream of solution. Solution drains into collection container.

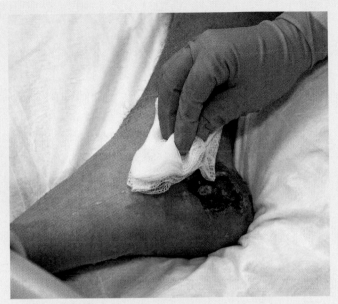

Action 18: Drying around wound, not in wound, with sterile gauze pad.

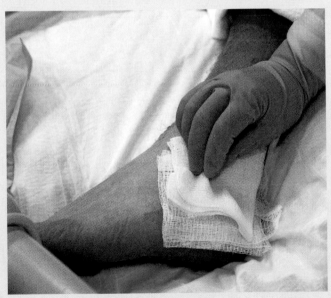

Action 19: Applying sterile dressing to wound.

22. Remove any remaining personal protective equipment. Remove the equipment and dispose of it properly. If any irrigating solution remains in the bottle, recap the bottle and note on the bottle the date and time it was opened.

23. Perform hand hygiene.

Open bottles of solution for wound care are usually good for 24 hours and can be reused. Always follow your facility's guidelines regarding solution storage and disposal.

Hand hygiene prevents spread of microorganisms.

continues

ACTION	RATIONALE
24. Document the procedure, wound assessment, and the patient's reaction to the according to institution's guidelines.	Documentation promotes continuity of care and communication.

3/5/06   1700   Dressing removed from left outer heel area. Minimal serosanguineous drainage noted on dressings. Wound 4 × 5 × 2 cm, pink, with granulation tissue evident. Surrounding skin tone consistent with patient's skin, no edema or redness noted. Irrigated with normal saline, lightly packed with moist saline gauze, and redressed with gauze.—J. Lark, RN

Action 24: Documentation.

25. Check all wound dressings every shift. You might need to check more frequently if a wound is more complex or dressings become saturated more frequently.	Frequent assessment ensures identification of changes in patient condition and timely intervention to prevent complications.

EVALUATION

The expected outcome is met when the patient exhibits a wound that is clean and dry after being irrigated; the wound is free of contamination and trauma; the patient verbalizes little to no pain or discomfort; the patient verbalizes understanding of the need for irrigation; and the wound exhibits signs and symptoms of progressive healing.

Unexpected Situations and Associated Interventions

- *The patient experiences pain when you begin the wound irrigation:* Stop the procedure and administer an analgesic as ordered. Obtain new sterile supplies and begin the procedure after an appropriate amount of time has elapsed to allow the analgesic to begin working. Note the patient's pain on the nursing plan of care so that pain medication can be given prior to future wound treatments.
- *During the wound irrigation, you note bleeding from the wound. This has not happened in the past:* Stop the procedure. Assess the patient for other symptoms. Obtain vital signs. Report your findings to the physician and document the event in the patient's record.

Applying a Wound Vacuum-Assisted Closure

Vacuum-assisted closure (VAC) is a therapy that assists in wound closure by applying localized negative pressure to the wound bed. It is also known as topical negative pressure (TNP). An open-cell foam dressing is applied in the wound. A fenestrated tube is embedded in the foam, allowing the application of the negative pressure. The dressing and distal tubing are covered by a transparent, occlusive, air-permeable dressing that provides a seal, allowing the application of the negative pressure. Excess wound fluid is removed through tubing.

This wound treatment increases blood flow to the wound, promotes granulation tissue formation, removes excess exudate, and reduces wound bacterial counts. Wound VAC dressings are changed every 48 to 72 hours, depending on the manufacturer's specifications and physician's orders.

Vacuum-assisted therapy is indicated for acute and traumatic wounds, pressure ulcers, and chronic open wounds. It should be used cautiously in patients with active bleeding and those taking anticoagulants. It is contraindicated in malignant wounds, untreated osteomyelitis, exposed arteries, or veins and in wounds with large amounts of necrosis or slough.

Equipment

- Vacuum unit
- Evacuation/collection canister
- Reticulated foam
- Fenestrated tubing
- Evacuation tubing
- Transparent occlusive air-permeable dressing
- Skin protectant wipe
- Sterile gauze sponge
- A sterile irrigation set, including a basin, irrigant container, and irrigation syringe
- Sterile irrigation solution as ordered by the physician, warmed to body temperature
- A waste receptacle to dispose of contaminated materials
- Sterile gloves (two pairs) and a set of clean disposable gloves
- Sterile scissors
- Waterproof pad and bath blanket
- Personal protective equipment such as a gown, mask, and eye protection

ASSESSMENT

Confirm the physician's order for the application of wound VAC therapy. Check the patient's chart and question the patient about current treatments that may make the application contraindicated, such as current or recent past anticoagulation therapy, bleeding from the wound, malignant wound, unstable diabetes, untreated osteomyelitis, or the presence of large amounts of necrosis. Assess the equipment to be used, including the condition of cords and plugs.

Complete a wound assessment. Inspect the wound and the surrounding tissue. Assess the wound for the approximation of wound edges, the color of the wound and surrounding area, and signs of dehiscence. Note the stage of the healing process and characteristics of any drainage. Assess the surrounding skin for color, temperature, and edema, ecchymosis, or maceration.

NURSING DIAGNOSIS

Determine the related factors for the nursing diagnoses based on the patient's current status. An appropriate nursing diagnosis is Impaired Skin Integrity. Other nursing diagnoses that may be appropriate or require the use of this skill include:

- Anxiety
- Disturbed Body Image
- Impaired Comfort
- Risk for Infection
- Risk for Injury
- Deficient Knowledge
- Acute Pain
- Impaired Tissue Integrity

continues

SKILL 8-10   Applying a Wound Vacuum-Assisted Closure (continued)

OUTCOME IDENTIFICATION AND PLANNING

The expected outcome to achieve when applying a wound VAC is that the therapy is accomplished without contaminating the wound area, without causing trauma to the wound, and without causing the patient to experience pain or discomfort. Other outcomes that may be appropriate include: the vacuum device functions correctly; the appropriate and ordered pressure is maintained throughout therapy; and the wound exhibits healing.

IMPLEMENTATION

ACTION	RATIONALE
1. Review the physician's order for the application of wound VAC therapy, including the ordered setting for the negative pressure.	Reviewing the order validates the correct patient and correct procedure.
2. Gather the necessary supplies.	Preparation promotes efficient time management and provides an organized approach to the task.
3. Identify the patient and explain the procedure. Determine if the patient is allergic to any of the materials or solutions needed for the procedure.	Patient identification validates the correct patient and correct procedure. Discussion and explanation help allay anxiety, encourage patient cooperation, and prepare the patient for what to expect.
4. Perform hand hygiene.	Hand hygiene prevents the spread of microorganisms.
5. Close the room door or curtains. Place the bed in a comfortable working height.	Closing the door or curtains provides privacy. Proper bed positioning helps reduce back strain while you are performing the procedure.
6. Assist the patient to a comfortable position that provides easy access to the wound area. Position the patient so the irrigation solution will flow from the upper end of the wound toward the lower end. Expose the area and drape the patient with a bath blanket if needed. Put a waterproof pad under the wound area.	Patient positioning and draping provide for comfort and warmth. Gravity directs the flow of liquid from the least contaminated to the most contaminated area. Waterproof pad protects the patient and the bed linens.
7. Have the disposal bag or waste receptacle within easy reach for use during the procedure.	Having the waste container handy means that soiled dressings and supplies may be discarded easily, without the spread of microorganisms.
8. Assemble the VAC device according to the manufacturer's instructions. Set the negative pressure according to the physician's order (25 to 200 mm Hg).	Assembling the equipment promotes efficient time management and provides an organized approach to the task. Setting the pressure ensures appropriate pressure is applied to the wound.
9. Using sterile technique, prepare a sterile field and add all the sterile supplies needed for the procedure to the field. Pour warmed sterile irrigating solution into the sterile container.	Proper preparation ensures that supplies are within easy reach and sterility is maintained.
10. Put on a gown, mask, and eye protection.	Use of personal protective equipment is part of standard precautions. A gown protects your clothes from contamination if splashing should occur. Goggles protect mucous membranes of your eyes from contact with irrigant fluid.
11. Put on clean disposable gloves and remove the soiled dressings.	Gloves provide protection from contaminated dressings.
12. Assess the wound for appearance and drainage. Assess the appearance of the surrounding tissue.	Assessment provides information about the wound healing process or the presence of infection.

continues

Applying a Wound Vacuum-Assisted Closure (continued)

ACTION	RATIONALE
13. Discard the dressings in the receptacle. Remove your gloves and put them in the receptacle.	Proper disposal of dressings and used gloves prevents the spread of microorganisms.
14. Using sterile technique, irrigate the wound (see Skill 8-9).	Irrigation removes exudate and debris.
15. Clean the area around the skin with normal saline. Dry the surrounding skin with a sterile gauze sponge.	Moisture provides a medium for growth of microorganisms.
16. **Wipe intact skin around the wound with a skin protectant wipe and allow it to dry well.**	Skin protectant provides a barrier against irritation and breakdown.
17. Remove gloves if they become contaminated and discard them into the receptacle.	Proper disposal of gloves prevents spread of microorganisms.
18. Put on a new pair of sterile gloves. **Using sterile scissors, cut the foam to the shape and measurement of the wound.** More than one piece of foam may be necessary if the first piece is cut too small. **Carefully place the foam in the wound.**	Aseptic technique maintains sterility of items to come in contact with wound. Foam should fill the wound but not cover intact surrounding skin.
19. **Place the fenestrated tubing into the center of the foam. There should be foam between the tubing and the base of the wound and foam over top of the tubing.**	The fenestrated tubing embedded into the foam delivers negative pressure to the wound.

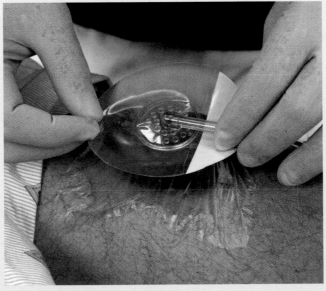

Action 19: Applying fenestrated tubing.

20. **Cover the foam and tubing with the transparent occlusive air-permeable dressing, leaving at least a 2" margin onto the intact skin around the wound.**	The occlusive air-permeable dressing provides a seal, allowing the application of the negative pressure.
21. Connect the free end of the fenestrated tubing to the tubing that is connected to the evacuation canister.	Connection to canister provides a collection chamber for wound drainage and allows measurement of drainage.
22. Remove and discard gloves. Turn on the vacuum unit. **Observe the shrinking of the transparent dressing to the foam** and skin.	Shrinkage confirms good seal, allowing for accurate application of pressure and treatment.

continues

ACTION   RATIONALE

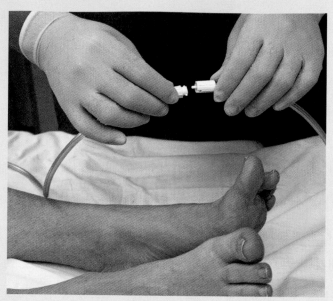

Action 21: Connecting tubing to collection canister.

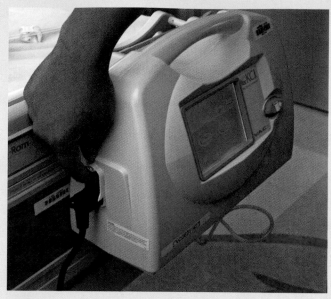

Action 22: Turning on wound VAC.

23. Lower the bed and make sure the patient is comfortable.

24. Perform hand hygiene.

25. Dispose of used supplies and equipment according to facility policy.

26. Document the procedure, the pressure setting, wound assessment, and the patient's reaction according to institution's guidelines.

27. Check all wound dressings every shift.

Repositioning the bed and the patient promotes safety and comfort.

Hand hygiene prevents spread of microorganisms.

Proper disposal of supplies and equipment prevents spread of microorganisms.

Documentation promotes continuity of care and communication.

Assessment ensures identification of changes in patient condition and timely intervention to prevent complications.

4/5/06   0800   Wound VAC dressing intact with good seal maintained, VAC system patent, pressure setting 50 mm Hg. Purulent, sanguineous drainage noted in collection chamber and tubing. Surrounding tissue without edema, redness, ecchymosis, or signs of irritation. Patient verbalizes an understanding of movement limitations related to the system.—B. Clark, RN

Action 26: Documentation.

EVALUATION

The expected outcome is met when the patient exhibits a wound VAC applied without contamination or trauma to the wound. The patient verbalizes little to no pain or discomfort. Other outcomes that may be appropriate include: the patient demonstrates a wound with the appropriate and ordered pressure being maintained; the device functions properly; and the wound shows signs of progressive healing.

continues

SKILL 8-10

Applying a Wound Vacuum-Assisted Closure (continued)

Unexpected Situations and Associated Interventions

- *While assessing the patient, you note that the seal between the transparent dressing and the foam and skin is not tight:* If the seal is broken, the appropriate pressure is not being applied to the wound. Change the dressing, regardless of the length of time it is has been in place.
- *The patient complains of acute pain while the wound VAC is operating:* Assess the patient for other symptoms, obtain vital signs, assess the wound, and assess the vacuum device for proper functioning. Report your findings to the physician and document the event in the patient's record. Administer analgesics as ordered. Continue or change the wound therapy as ordered.

Special Considerations

- Change the wound dressing every 48 to 72 hours, as ordered. Time dressing changes to allow for wound assessment by the other members of the healthcare team.
- Measure and record the amount of drainage each shift as part of the intake and output record.
- Be alert for audible and visual alarms on the vacuum device to alert you to problems, such as tipping of the device greater than 45 degrees, a full collection canister, an air leak in the dressing, or dislodgment of the canister.

SKILL 8-11

Applying an External Heating Device: Aquathermia Pad and Hot Water Bag

Heat dilates peripheral blood vessels, helping to dissipate heat from the body and increasing blood flow to the area. This increases the supply of oxygen and nutrients to the area and reduces venous congestion. Heat applications accelerate the inflammatory response, promoting healing. Heat is also used to reduce muscle tension, relieve muscle spasm, and relieve joint stiffness. Heat also helps relieve pain. It is used to treat infections, surgical wounds, inflammation, arthritis, joint pain, muscle pain, and chronic pain.

Heat is applied by moist and dry methods. The physician's order should include the type of application, the body area to be treated, the frequency of application, and the length of time for the applications. Water used for heat applications needs to be at the appropriate temperature to avoid skin damage: 115° to 125°F for older children and adults and 105° to 110°F for infants, young children, older adults, and patients with diabetes or those who are unconscious.

Two common types of external heating devices are Aquathermia pads and hot water bags. Aquathermia pads are used in healthcare agencies and are safer to use than heating pads. The temperature setting for an Aquathermia pad should not exceed 105° to 109.4°F, depending on facility policy.

Hot water bags are easy and inexpensive to use but have several disadvantages. They may leak and pose a danger from burns related to improper use. They are used most often in the home setting.

Equipment

- Hot water bag with cover
- Water at the appropriate temperature
- Bath thermometer
- Aquathermia pad with electronic unit
- Distilled water
- Cover for the pad, if not part of pad
- Gauze bandage or tape to secure the pad
- Waterproof pad for under the hot water bag

continues

SKILL 8-11 | Applying an External Heating Device: Aquathermia Pad and Hot Water Bag (continued)

ASSESSMENT

Assess the situation to determine the appropriateness for the application of heat. Assess the patient's physical and mental status and the condition of the body area to be treated with heat. Confirm the physician's order for heat therapy, including frequency, type of therapy, body area to be treated, and length of time for the application. Check the equipment to be used, including the condition of cords, plugs, and heating elements. Look for fluid leaks. Once the equipment is turned on, make sure there is a consistent distribution of heat and the temperature is within safe limits.

NURSING DIAGNOSIS

Determine the related factors for the nursing diagnoses based on the patient's current status. Nursing diagnoses that may be appropriate or require the use of this skill include:

- Chronic Pain
- Acute Pain
- Impaired Skin Integrity
- Risk for Impaired Skin Integrity
- Delayed Surgical Recovery
- Impaired Tissue Integrity
- Risk for Injury

Many other nursing diagnoses may require the use of this skill.

OUTCOME IDENTIFICATION AND PLANNING

The expected outcome to achieve when applying an external heat source depends on the patient's nursing diagnosis. Outcomes that may be appropriate include the following: the patient experience increased comfort; the patient experiences decreased muscle spasms; the patient exhibits improved wound healing; the patient demonstrates a reduction in inflammation; and the patient remains free of injury.

IMPLEMENTATION

ACTION	RATIONALE
1. Review the physician's order for the application of heat therapy, including frequency, type of therapy, body area to be treated, and length of time for the application.	Reviewing the order validates the correct patient and correct procedure.
2. Gather the necessary supplies.	Preparation promotes efficient time management and provides an organized approach to the task.
3. Identify the patient and explain the procedure.	Patient identification validates the correct patient and correct procedure. Discussion and explanation help allay anxiety, encourage patient cooperation, and prepare the patient for what to expect.
4. Assess the condition of the skin where the heat is to be applied.	Assessment supplies baseline data for posttreatment comparison and identifies conditions that may contraindicate the application.
5. Perform hand hygiene.	Hand hygiene prevents the spread of microorganisms.
6. Close the room door or curtains. Place the bed at a comfortable working height.	Closing door or curtains provides privacy. Proper bed positioning helps reduce back strain while you are performing the procedure.
7. Assist the patient to a comfortable position that provides easy access to the area to be treated. Expose the area and drape the patient with a bath blanket if needed. Put a waterproof pad under the wound area to protect the bed, if necessary.	Patient positioning and use of a bath blanket provide for comfort and warmth. Waterproof pad protects the patient and the bed linens.

continues

ACTION	RATIONALE
For Aquathermia Pad	
8. Check that the water is at the appropriate level. Fill the control unit two-thirds full with distilled water, or to the fill mark, if necessary. Check the temperature setting on the unit to ensure it is within the safe range.	Tap water leaves mineral deposits in the unit. Checking the temperature setting helps to prevent skin or tissue damage.
9. Check for leaks and tilt the unit in several directions.	This action clears the pad's tubing of air.
10. Plug in the unit and warm the pad before use. Cover the pad with an absorbent cloth. Apply the heat source to the prescribed area. Secure with gauze bandage or tape.	Plugging in the pad readies it for use. Cover protects the skin from direct contact with the bag. Heat travels by conduction from one object to another. Gauze bandage or tape holds the pad in position; do not use pins, as they may puncture and damage the pad.
11. **Assess the condition of the skin and the patient's response to the heat at frequent intervals, according to facility policy. Do not exceed the prescribed length of time for the application of heat.**	Maximum therapeutic effects from the application of heat occur within 20 to 30 minutes. Using heat for more than 45 minutes results in tissue congestion and vasoconstriction, which can result in an increased risk of burns.
12. Remove after the prescribed amount of time. Perform hand hygiene.	Removal reduces risk of injury. Hand hygiene prevents spread of microorganisms.
14. Document the procedure, the patient's response, and your assessment of the area before and after the application.	Documentation promotes continuity of care and communication.

> 9/13/06   2300   Patient complaining of pain, rating it 5 out of 10. Aquathermia pad applied to patient's lower back for 30 minutes; now rating pain as 2 out of 10. Skin without signs of redness or irritation before and after application.—M. Martinez, RN

Action 14: Documentation.

EVALUATION

The expected outcome is met when the patient exhibits increased comfort, decreased muscle spasm, less pain, improved wound healing, or decreased inflammation. In addition, the patient remains free of injury.

Unexpected Situations and Associated Interventions

- *When performing your periodic assessment of the site during the application of heat, you note excessive swelling and redness at the site and the patient complains of pain that was not present prior to applying the heat:* Remove the hot water bag or Aquathermia pad. Assess the patient for other symptoms and obtain vital signs. Report your findings to the physician and document your interventions in the patient's record.
- *When performing your periodic assessment of the site during the application of heat, you note that the hot water bag seems to be significantly cooler:* Refill the hot water bag as necessary to maintain the correct temperature.

continues

Applying an External Heating Device: Aquathermia Pad and Hot Water Bag (continued)

Special Considerations

- Direct heat treatment is contraindicated for patients at risk for bleeding, patients with a sprained limb in the acute stage, or patients with a condition associated with acute inflammation. Use cautiously with children and older adults. Patients with diabetes, stroke, spinal cord injury, and peripheral neuropathy are at risk for thermal injury, as are patients with very thin or damaged skin. Be extremely careful when applying to heat-sensitive areas, such as scar tissue and stomas.
- Instruct the patient not to lean or lie directly on the heating device, as this reduces air space and increases the risk of burns.
- Check the water level in the Aquathermia unit periodically. Evaporation may occur. If the unit runs dry, it could become damaged. Refill with distilled water periodically.

Home Care Considerations

- A hot water bag may be used in the home to apply heat. Fill the hot water bag with hot tap water to warm the bag, then empty it to detect any leaks. Check the temperature of the water with the bath thermometer or test on your inner wrist, adjusting the temperature as ordered (usually 115° to 125°F for adults). Checking the temperature ensures that the heat applied is within the acceptable range of temperatures. Fill the bag one-half to two-thirds full. Partial filling keeps the bag lightweight and flexible so that it can be molded to the treatment area. Squeeze the bag until the water reaches the neck; this expels air, which would make the bag inflexible and would reduce heat conduction. Fasten the top, and cover the bag with an absorbent cloth. The covering protects the skin from direct contact with the bag.

Applying a Warm Sterile Compress to an Open Wound

Sterile warm moist compresses are used on wounds to help promote circulation to the wound, encourage wound healing, decrease edema, promote consolidation of wound exudate, and decrease pain and discomfort at the wound site. Moist heat softens crusted material and is less drying to the skin. Moist heat also penetrates tissues more deeply than dry heat.

The heat of a warm compress dissipates quickly, so the compresses must be changed frequently. Applying a layer of plastic over the compress can help retain the heat longer. If a constant warm temperature is required, a heating device such as an Aquathermia pad is applied over the compress. However, because moisture conducts heat, a low temperature setting is needed on the heating device. Many facilities have warming devices to heat the dressing package to an appropriate temperature for the compress. These devices help reduce the risk of burning or skin damage.

Equipment

- Prescribed solution to moisten the compress material, warmed to 105° to 110°F
- Sterile container for solution
- Sterile gauze dressings or compresses
- Sterile gloves
- Clean disposable gloves
- Waterproof pad and bath blanket
- Dry bath towel
- Tape or ties

continues

- Aquathermia or other external heating device, if ordered or required to maintain the temperature of the compress
- Sterile bath thermometer (if available) to check the solution's temperature
- Sterile supplies to replace the wound dressing after the procedure is completed

ASSESSMENT

Assess for circulatory compromise in the area where compress will be applied, including skin color, pulses distal to the site, evidence of edema, and the presence of sensation. Assess the situation to determine the appropriateness for the application of heat. Confirm the physician's order for the compresses, including the solution to be used, frequency, body area to be treated, and length of time for the application. Assess the equipment to be used, if necessary, including the condition of cords, plugs, and heating elements. Look for fluid leaks. Once the equipment is turned on, make sure there is a consistent distribution of heat and the temperature is within safe limits. Assess the application site frequently during the treatment, as tissue damage can occur.

NURSING DIAGNOSIS

Determine the related factors for the nursing diagnoses based on the patient's current status. An appropriate nursing diagnosis is Risk for Injury. Many other nursing diagnoses may be appropriate, including:

- Anxiety
- Disturbed Body Image
- Acute Pain
- Chronic Pain
- Impaired Skin Integrity
- Risk for Impaired Skin Integrity
- Impaired Tissue Integrity
- Deficient Knowledge

OUTCOME IDENTIFICATION AND PLANNING

The expected outcome to achieve when applying warm sterile compresses is the patient shows signs such as decreased inflammation, decreased muscle spasms, or decreased pain that indicate problems have been relieved. Other outcomes that may be appropriate include: the patient experiences improved wound healing and the patient remains free from injury.

IMPLEMENTATION

ACTION	RATIONALE
1. Review the physician's order.	Reviewing the order validates the correct patient and correct procedure.
2. Gather the necessary supplies.	Preparation promotes efficient time management and provides an organized approach to the task.
3. Identify the patient and explain the procedure. Determine if the patient is allergic to any of the materials or solutions needed for the procedure.	Patient identification validates the correct patient and correct procedure. Discussion and explanation help allay anxiety, encourage patient cooperation, and prepare the patient for what to expect.
4. Perform hand hygiene.	Hand hygiene prevents the spread of microorganisms.
5. Close the room door or curtains. Place the bed at a comfortable working height.	Closing the door or curtain provides privacy. Proper bed positioning helps reduce back strain while you are providing care.
6. Assist the patient to a comfortable position that provides easy access to the wound area. Expose the area and drape the patient with a bath blanket if needed. Put the waterproof pad under the wound area.	Patient positioning and use of a bath blanket provide for comfort and warmth. Waterproof pad protects the patient and the bed linens.

continues

SKILL 8-12   Applying a Warm Sterile Compress to an Open Wound (continued)

ACTION	RATIONALE
7. Have the disposal bag or waste receptacle within easy reach for use during the procedure.	Having a waste container handy means that soiled dressings and supplies may be discarded easily, without the spread of microorganisms.
8. Prepare the external heating pad or Aquathermia pad if one is being used.	Having equipment ready provides for an organized approach to the task. The external heating device allows the compress to retain heat for a longer interval.

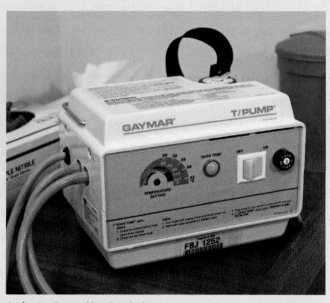

Action 8: External heating device.

ACTION	RATIONALE
9. Using sterile technique, prepare a working field and open all sterile packaging, dressings, and the warmed solution. Pour the solution into the sterile container and drop the sterile gauze for the compress into the solution.	Sterile technique is used for warm moist compresses to an open wound to prevent contamination with microorganisms.
10. Put on clean disposable gloves and remove any old dressing in place. Discard the old dressing in the appropriate receptacle. Remove your gloves and discard them.	Adherence to medical aseptic practices and proper disposal of soiled dressings and supplies prevent the spread of microorganisms.
12. Assess wound site and surrounding tissues. Look for inflammation, drainage, skin color, ecchymosis, and odor.	Assessment provides information about the wound healing process and about the presence of infection and allows for documentation of the condition of the wound before the compress is applied.
13. Put on sterile gloves, following proper procedure.	Use of sterile gloves maintains sterile technique.
14. **Retrieve the sterile compress from the warmed solution, squeezing out any excess moisture. Apply the compress by gently and carefully molding it around the wound site.**	Excess moisture may contaminate the surrounding area and is uncomfortable for the patient. Molding the compress to the skin promotes retention of warmth around the site.
15. **Cover the site with a single layer of gauze and with a dry bath towel;** secure in place if necessary.	Towel provides extra insulation.
16. Place the Aquathermia or heating device, if used, over the towel.	Use of heating device maintains the temperature of the compress and extends the therapeutic effect.

continues

Applying a Warm Sterile Compress to an Open Wound (continued)

ACTION

RATIONALE

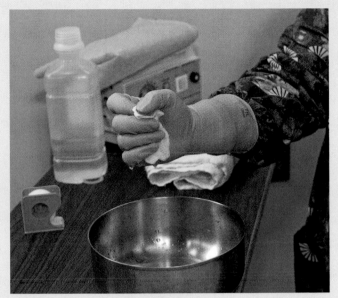

Action 14: With gloves on, squeezing excess solution out of a dressing.

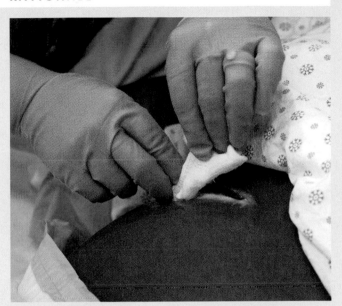

Action 14: Gloved hands molding moist gauze around the wound.

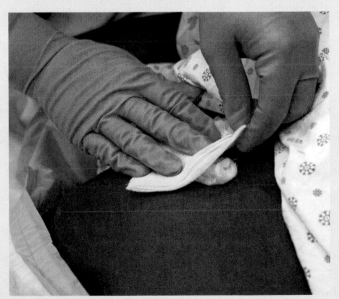

Action 15: Applying single layer of gauze.

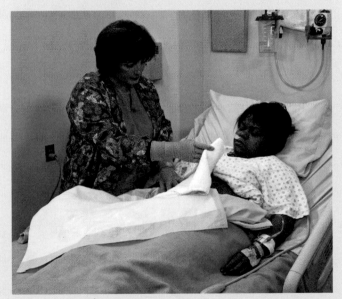

Action 16: Applying external heating device.

17. Remove sterile gloves and discard them appropriately. Perform hand hygiene.

Hand hygiene prevents the spread of microorganisms.

18. **Monitor the time the compress is in place to prevent burns or skin damage. Monitor the condition of the patient's skin and the patient's response at frequent intervals.**

Extended use of heat results in an increased risk for burns from the heat. Impaired circulation may affect the patient's sensitivity to heat.

19. After the prescribed time for the treatment (up to 30 minutes), remove the external heating device (if used) and put on sterile gloves.

Use of sterile gloves helps to maintain sterile technique.

continues

ACTION	RATIONALE
20. Carefully remove the compress while assessing the skin condition around the wound site and observing the patient's response to the heat application. Note any wound changes.	Assessment provides information about the wound healing process; the presence of irritation or infection should be documented.
21. Apply a new sterile dressing to the wound, following proper procedure.	Dressing provides protection for the wound.
23. Remove gloves. Place the patient in a comfortable position. Lower the bed. Dispose of any other supplies appropriately.	Repositioning promotes patient comfort and safety.
24. Perform hand hygiene.	Hand hygiene prevents spread of microorganisms.
26. Document the procedure, the length of time the compress was applied, your assessments of the wound and surrounding tissue, and the patient's response to the procedure.	Documentation promotes continuity of care and communication.

7/6/06   0900   *Left forearm with positive radial pulse, sensation and movement within normal limits, skin pale with brisk capillary refill. Wound dressing removed from left forearm. Wound 2 × 2 × 2 cm on dorsal aspect, red, scant purulent drainage, surrounding area red, with edema, no evidence of maceration. Moist saline compress applied with Aquathermia pad set at 100°F for 30 min. Site assessed every 10 min; no evidence of injury noted. Wound redressed and wrapped with stretch gauze. Left arm elevated on pillows.*—S. Tran, RN

Action 26: Documentation.

EVALUATION

The expected outcome is met when the patient reports relief of symptoms, such as decreased inflammation, pain, or muscle spasms. In addition, the patient remains free of signs and symptoms of injury.

Unexpected Situations and Associated Interventions

- *You are monitoring a patient with a warm compress applied to a wound. Procedure requires that you check the area of application every 5 minutes for tissue tolerance. You note excessive redness and slight maceration of the surrounding skin, and the patient verbalizes increased discomfort:* Stop the heat application. Remove the compress. Apply a new sterile dressing. Assess the patient for other symptoms. Obtain vital signs. Report your findings to the physician and document the event in the patient's record.
- *You are monitoring a patient with a warm compress applied to a wound. Procedure requires that you check the area of application every 5 minutes for tissue tolerance. You note bleeding from the wound and on the compress:* Stop the heat application. Remove the compress. Apply a new sterile dressing. Assess the patient for other symptoms. Obtain vital signs. Report your findings to the physician and document the event in the patient's record.

Special Considerations

- Patients with diabetes, stroke, spinal cord injury, and peripheral neuropathy are at risk for thermal injury, as are patients with very thin or damaged skin.
- Be extremely careful when applying to heat-sensitive areas, such as scar tissue and stomas.

Using a Cooling Blanket

A cooling blanket, or hypothermia pad, is a blanket-sized Aquathermia pad that conducts a cooled solution, usually distilled water, through coils in a rubber or plastic blanket or pad. Placing a patient on a hypothermia blanket or pad helps to lower body temperature. The nurse monitors the patient's body temperature and can reset the blanket setting accordingly. The blanket also may be preset to maintain a specific body temperature; the device continually monitors the patient's body temperature using a temperature probe (which is inserted rectally or in the esophagus, or placed on the skin) and adjusts the temperature of the circulating liquid accordingly.

Equipment

- Disposable cooling blanket or pad
- Control panel
- Distilled water to fill the device, if necessary
- Thermometer, if needed to monitor the patient's temperature
- Sphygmomanometer
- Stethoscope
- Temperature probe, if needed
- Thin blanket or sheet
- Towels
- Clean gloves

ASSESSMENT

Assess the patient's condition, including current body temperature, to determine the need for the cooling blanket. Consider alternative measures to help lower the patient's body temperature before implementing the blanket. Also verify the physician's order for the application of a hypothermia blanket. Assess the patient's vital signs, neurologic status, mental status, peripheral circulation, and skin integrity. Assess the equipment to be used, including the condition of cords, plugs, and cooling elements. Look for fluid leaks. Once the equipment is turned on, make sure there is a consistent distribution of cooling.

NURSING DIAGNOSIS

Determine the related factors for the nursing diagnoses based on the patient's current status. Appropriated nursing diagnoses may include:

- Hyperthermia
- Risk for Injury
- Deficient Knowledge
- Risk for Impaired Skin Integrity
- Ineffective Thermoregulation
- Acute Pain

OUTCOME IDENTIFICATION AND PLANNING

The expected outcome to achieve when using a hypothermia blanket is that the patient maintains a normal body temperature. Other outcomes that may be appropriate include: the patient does not experience shivering; the patient's vital signs are within normal limits; and the patient does not experience alterations in skin integrity.

IMPLEMENTATION

ACTION	RATIONALE
1. Review the physician's order for the application of the hypothermia blanket. Obtain consent for the therapy per facility policy.	Reviewing the order validates the correct patient and correct procedure.
2. Gather the necessary supplies.	Preparation promotes efficient time management and provides an organized approach to the task.

continues

Using a Cooling Blanket (continued)

ACTION	RATIONALE

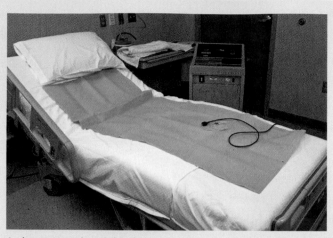

Action 2: Hypothermia blanket.

ACTION	RATIONALE
3. Identify the patient and explain the procedure.	Patient identification validates the correct patient and correct procedure. Discussion and explanation help allay anxiety, encourage cooperation, and prepare the patient for what to expect.
4. Assess the patient's vital signs, neurologic status, mental status, peripheral circulation, and skin integrity.	Assessment supplies baseline data for comparison during therapy and identifies conditions that may contraindicate the application.
5. Perform hand hygiene.	Hand hygiene prevents the spread of microorganisms.
6. Close the room door or curtains. Place the bed at a comfortable working height.	Closing the room or curtains provides privacy. Proper bed positioning helps reduce back strain while you are performing the procedure.
7. Make sure the patient's gown has cloth ties, not snaps or pins.	Cloth ties minimize the risk of cold injury.
8. Apply lanolin or a mixture of lanolin and cold cream to the patient's skin where it will be in contact with the blanket.	These agents help protect the skin from cold.
9. Turn on the blanket and make sure the cooling light is on. Verify that the temperature limits are set within the desired safety range.	Turning on the blanket prepares it for use. Keeping temperature within the safety range prevents excessive cooling.
10. Cover the hypothermia blanket with a thin sheet or bath blanket.	A sheet or blanket protects the patient's skin from direct contact with the cooling surface, reducing the risk for injury.
11. Position the blanket under the patient so that the top edge of the pad is aligned with the patient's neck.	The blanket's rigid surface may be uncomfortable. The cold may lead to tissue breakdown.
12. Put on gloves. Lubricate the rectal probe and insert it into the patient's rectum unless contraindicated. Or tuck the skin probe deep into the patient's axilla and tape it in place. For patients who are comatose or anesthetized, use an esophageal probe. Attach the probe to the control panel for the blanket.	The probe allows continuous monitoring of the patient's core body temperature. Rectal insertion may be contraindicated in patients with a low white blood cell count or platelet count.

continues

SKILL 8-13 Using a Cooling Blanket (continued)

ACTION	RATIONALE

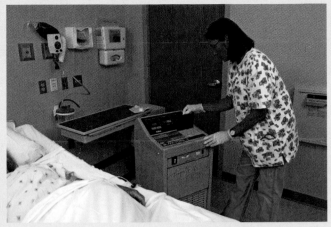

Action 9: Checking the settings on the cooling blanket control unit and turning it on.

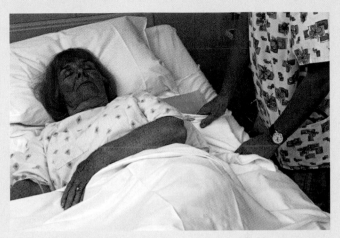

Action 11: Cooling blanket on bed.

13. Wrap the patient's hands and feet in gauze if ordered, or if the patient desires. **For male patients, elevate the scrotum off the cooling blanket with towels.**

These actions minimize chilling, promote comfort, and protect sensitive tissues from direct contact with cold.

14. Recheck the thermometer and settings on the control panel.

Rechecking verifies that the blanket temperature is maintained at a safe level.

15. Remove gloves and perform hand hygiene.

Hand hygiene prevents spread of microorganisms.

16. **Turn and position the patient regularly (every 30 minutes to 1 hour).** Keep linens free from condensation. Reapply cream as needed. Observe the patient's skin for change in color, changes in lips and nail beds, edema, pain, and sensory impairment.

Turning and repositioning prevent alterations in skin integrity and provide for assessment of potential skin injuries.

17. **Monitor vital signs and perform a neurologic assessment per facility policy, usually every 15 minutes, until the body temperature is stable.**

Continuous monitoring provides evaluation of the patient's response to the therapy and permits early identification and intervention if adverse effects occur.

18. Observe for signs of shivering, including verbalized sensations, facial muscle twitching, hyperventilation, or twitching of extremities.

Shivering increases heat production.

19. Assess the patient's level of comfort.

Hypothermia therapy can cause discomfort. Prompt assessment and action can prevent injuries.

20. Turn off blanket according to facility policy, usually when the patient's body temperature reaches 1° above the desired temperature. Continue to monitor the patient's temperature until it stabilizes.

Body temperature can continue to fall after this therapy.

21. Document assessments, vital signs, and time of initiation of therapy. Document the control settings, the duration of treatment, and the patient's response.

Documentation promotes continuity of care and communication.

continues

ACTION	RATIONALE

> 11/10/06   1800   Patient's temp 106°F, pulse
> 122, respirations 24, BP 118/72. Dr. Fenter noti-
> fied. Order received for application of cooling
> blanket. Procedure explained to patient. Lano-
> lin applied to skin, bath sheet applied between
> blanket and patient, axillary probe applied,
> cooling blanket setting 99°F per order. Vital
> signs and skin assessment every 30 min; see
> flow sheet.—J. Lee, RN
>
> 11/10/06   1930   Patient reports chills and
> shivering. Temperature 100°F, pulse 104, respi-
> rations 20, BP 114/68. Dr. Fenter notified. Cool-
> ing blanket discontinued per order.—J. Lee, RN

Action 21: Documentation.

EVALUATION

The expected outcome is met when the patient exhibits a stable, body temperature and other vital signs within acceptable parameters. In addition, the patient remains free from shivering and the patient's skin is pink, clean, warm, and dry, without evidence of injury.

Unexpected Situations and Associated Interventions

- *The patient states he is cold and has chills. You observe shivering of his extremities:* Obtain vital signs. Assess for other symptoms. Increase the blanket temperature to a more comfortable range. Administer tranquilizers as ordered. If shivering persists or is excessive, discontinue the therapy. Notify the physician of your findings and document the event in the patient's record.
- *When performing a skin assessment during therapy, you note increased pallor on pressure points and sluggish capillary refill. The patient reports alterations in sensation on these points:* Discontinue therapy, obtain vital signs, assess for other symptoms, notify the physician, and document the event in the patient's record.

Special Considerations

- The patient may experience a secondary defense reaction, vasodilation, that causes body temperature to rebound, defeating the purpose of the therapy.

Older Adult Considerations

- Older adults are more at risk for skin and tissue damage because of their thin skin, loss of cold sensation, decreased subcutaneous tissue, and changes in the body's ability to regulate temperature. Check these patients more frequently during therapy.

Applying Cold Therapy

Cold constricts the peripheral blood vessels, reducing blood flow to the tissues and decreasing the local release of pain-producing substances. Cold reduces the formation of edema and inflammation, reduces muscle spasm, and promotes comfort by slowing the transmission of pain stimuli. The application of cold therapy reduces bleeding and hematoma formation. The application of cold, using ice, is appropriate after direct trauma, for dental pain, for muscle spasms, after muscle sprains, and for the treatment of chronic pain. Ice can be used to apply cold therapy, usually in the form of an ice bag or ice collar, or in a glove. Commercially prepared cold packs are also available.

Equipment

- Ice
- Ice bag, ice collar, glove
- Small towel or washcloth
- Clean gloves
- Disposable waterproof pad
- Gauze wrap or tape

ASSESSMENT

Assess the situation to determine the appropriateness for the application of cold therapy. Assess the patient's physical and mental status and the condition of the body area to be treated with the cold therapy. Confirm the physician's order, including frequency, type of therapy, body area to be treated, and length of time for the application. Assess the equipment to be used to make sure it will function properly.

NURSING DIAGNOSIS

Determine the related factors for the nursing diagnoses based on the patient's current status. An appropriate nursing diagnosis is Acute Pain. Other nursing diagnoses that may be appropriate or require the use of this skill include:

- Impaired Skin Integrity
- Chronic Pain
- Ineffective Tissue Perfusion
- Delayed Surgical Recovery

OUTCOME IDENTIFICATION AND PLANNING

The expected outcome to achieve when applying an external cold source depends on the patient's nursing diagnosis. Outcomes that may be appropriate include the following: the patient experiences increased comfort; the patient experiences decreased muscle spasms; the patient experiences decreased inflammation; and the patient does not show signs of bleeding or hematoma at the treatment site.

IMPLEMENTATION

ACTION	RATIONALE
1. Review the physician's order for the application of cold therapy, including frequency, type of therapy, body area to be treated, and length of time for the application.	Reviewing the order validates the correct patient and correct procedure.
2. Gather the necessary supplies.	Preparation promotes efficient time management and provides an organized approach to the task.
3. Identify the patient and explain the procedure.	Patient identification validates the correct patient and correct procedure. Discussion and explanation help allay anxiety, encourage cooperation, and prepare the patient for what to expect.
4. Assess the condition of the skin where the ice is to be applied.	Assessment supplies baseline data for posttreatment comparison and identifies any conditions that may contraindicate the application.

continues

Applying Cold Therapy (continued)

ACTION	RATIONALE
5. Perform hand hygiene.	Hand hygiene prevents the spread of microorganisms.
6. Close the room door or curtains. Place the bed at a comfortable working height.	Closing the door or curtain provides privacy. Proper bed positioning helps reduce back strain while you perform the procedure.
7. Assist the patient to a comfortable position that provides easy access to the area to be treated. Expose the area and drape the patient with a bath blanket if needed. Put the waterproof pad under the wound area, if necessary.	Patient positioning and use of a bath blanket provide for comfort and warmth. Waterproof pad protects the patient and the bed linens.
8. Fill the bag, collar, or glove about three-fourths full with ice. **Remove any excess air from the device.** Securely fasten the end of the bag or collar; tie the glove closed.	Ice provides a cold surface. Excess air interferes with cold conduction. Fastening the end prevents leaks.
9. **Cover the device with a towel or washcloth.** (If the device has a cloth exterior, this is not necessary.)	The cover protects the skin and absorbs condensation.

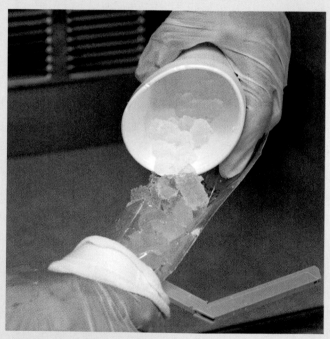

Action 8: Filling ice bag with ice.

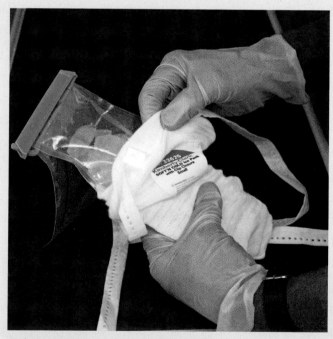

Action 9: Wrapping ice bag with cloth.

10. Put on gloves. Remove and dispose of any dressings at the site, if present.	Use of gloves prevents spread of microorganisms. Dressing removal allows access to the treatment site.
11. Place the device lightly against the area. **Remove the ice and assess the site for redness after 30 seconds. Ask the patient about the presence of burning sensations.**	These actions prevent burn injury.
12. Replace the device snugly against the site if no problems are evident. Secure it in place with gauze wrap or tape.	Wrapping or taping stabilizes the device in the proper location.

continues

Applying Cold Therapy (continued)

ACTION   **RATIONALE**

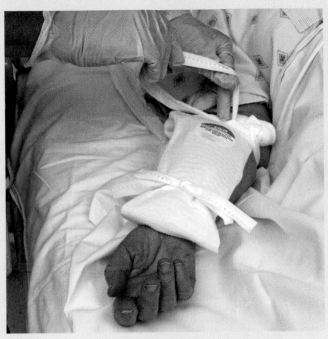

Action 12: Applying cloth-wrapped bag and securing with gauze.

13. Reassess the treatment area every 5 minutes or according to facility policy.

Assessment of the patient's skin is necessary for early detection of adverse effects, thereby allowing prompt intervention to avoid complications.

14. **After 20 minutes or the prescribed amount of time, remove the ice and dry the skin.**

Limiting the time of application prevents injury due to overexposure to cold. Prolonged application of cold may result in decreased blood flow with resulting tissue ischemia. A compensatory vasodilation may occur as a means to provide warmth to the area.

15. Apply a new dressing to site, if necessary.

Dressing provides protection to the skin.

16. Perform hand hygiene.

Hand hygiene prevents spread of microorganisms.

17. Document the procedure, the patient's response, and your assessment of the area before and after the application.

Documentation promotes continuity of care and communication.

11/1/06   1430   Swelling noted on right lower extremity from mid-calf to foot. Toes warm, pink, positive sensation and movement, negative for numbness, tingling, and pain. Ice bags wrapped in cloth applied to right ankle and lower calf. Patient instructed to communicate any changes in sensation or pain; verbalizes an understanding of information.
—L. Semet, RN

Action 17: Documentation.

continues

SKILL 8-14   Applying Cold Therapy (continued)

EVALUATION   The expected outcome is met when the patient reports a relief of pain and increased comfort. Other outcomes that may be appropriate include: the patient verbalizes a decrease in muscle spasms; the patient exhibits a reduction in inflammation; and the patient remains free of any injury, including signs of bleeding or hematoma at the treatment site.

Unexpected Situations and Associated Interventions
- *When performing a skin assessment during therapy, you note increased pallor at the treatment site and sluggish capillary refill, and the patient reports alterations in sensation at the application site:* Discontinue therapy, obtain vital signs, assess for other symptoms, notify the physician, and document the event in the patient's record.

Special Considerations
- The patient may experience a secondary defense reaction, vasodilation, that causes body temperature to rebound, defeating the purpose of the therapy.

Older Adult Considerations
- Older adults are more at risk for skin and tissue damage because of their thin skin, loss of cold sensation, decreased subcutaneous tissue, and changes in the body's ability to regulate temperature. Check these patients more frequently during therapy.

SKILL 8-15   Applying Montgomery Straps

Montgomery straps are recommended to secure dressings on wounds that require frequent dressing changes, such as wounds with increased drainage. These straps allow the nurse to perform wound care without the need to remove adhesive strips, such as tape, with each dressing change, thus decreasing the risk of skin irritation and injury.

Montgomery straps are prepared strips of nonallergenic tape with ties inserted through holes at one end. One set of straps is placed on either side of a wound and the straps are tied like shoelaces to secure the dressings. When it is time to change the dressing, the straps are untied, the wound is cared for, and then the straps are retied to hold the new dressing. Often a skin barrier is applied before the straps to protect the skin. The straps or ties need to be changed only if they become loose or soiled.

Equipment
- Gloves
- Dressings for wound care as ordered
- Commercially available Montgomery straps or 2″ to 3″ hypoallergenic tape and strings for ties
- Cleansing solution, usually normal saline
- Gauze pads
- Skin protectant wipe
- Skin barrier sheet (hydrocolloidal or non-hydrocolloidal)

ASSESSMENT   Assess the wound for amount of drainage and the frequency of dressing changes. Assess the integrity of any straps currently in use. Loose or soiled straps or ties should be replaced. Assess the wound and surrounding skin (see Skill 8-7).

continues

| NURSING DIAGNOSIS | Determine the related factors for the nursing diagnoses based on the patient's current status. An appropriate nursing diagnosis is Risk for Impaired Skin Integrity. Other nursing diagnoses that may be appropriate include: |

- Impaired Tissue Integrity
- Risk for Infection
- Risk for Injury
- Anxiety
- Disturbed Body Image
- Deficient Knowledge
- Impaired Skin Integrity
- Delayed Surgical Recovery

OUTCOME IDENTIFICATION AND PLANNING   The expected outcome to achieve when applying Montgomery straps is that the patient's skin is free from irritation and injury. Other outcomes that may be appropriate include that the care is accomplished without contaminating the wound area, without causing trauma to the wound, and without causing the patient to experience pain or discomfort, and the wound continues to show signs of progression of healing.

IMPLEMENTATION

ACTION	RATIONALE
1. Review the physician's order for wound care or the nursing care plan related to wound care.	Reviewing the order validates the correct patient and correct procedure.
2. Gather the necessary supplies.	Preparation promotes efficient time management and an organized approach to the task.
3. Identify the patient. Explain the procedure to the patient. Inquire about any allergies, specifically those related to the products being used for wound care.	Patient identification validates the correct patient and correct procedure. Discussion and explanation help allay anxiety, encourage patient cooperation, and prepare the patient for what to expect.
4. Perform hand hygiene.	Hand hygiene prevents the spread of microorganisms.
5. Close the room door or curtains. Place the bed at an appropriate and comfortable working height.	Closing the door or curtains provides privacy. Proper bed positioning helps reduce back strain while you are performing the procedure.
6. Place a waste receptacle at a convenient location for use during the procedure.	Having a waster container handy means that the soiled dressing may be discarded easily, without the spread of microorganisms.
7. Assist the patient to a comfortable position that provides easy access to the wound area. Use a bath blanket to cover any exposed area other than the wound. If necessary, place a waterproof pad under the wound site.	Patient positioning and use of a bath blanket provide for comfort and warmth. Waterproof pad protects underlying surfaces.
8. Perform wound care and a dressing change as outlined in Skill 8-7, as ordered.	Wound care aids in healing and provides protection for the wound.
9. If ready-made straps are not available, cut four to six strips of tape long enough to extend about 6″ beyond the wound. The number of strips will depend on the size of the wound and dressing.	Proper sizing is necessary to allow enough tape to secure to the patient's skin and hold the dressing in place.

continues

SKILL 8-15   Applying Montgomery Straps (continued)

ACTION

RATIONALE

10. Fold one end of each strip 2″ to 3″ back on itself, sticky sides together, to form a nonadhesive tab. Cut a small hole in the folded tab's center, close to the top edge. Make as many pairs of straps as necessary to secure the dressing.

Straps should be long enough to allow removal and replacement of the dressing multiple times.

11. Put on clean gloves. Clean the skin on either side of the wound with the gauze, moistened with normal saline. Dry the skin.

Gloves prevent the spread of microorganisms. Cleaning and drying the skin prevents irritation and injury.

12. **Apply a skin protectant to the skin where the straps will be placed.**

Skin protectant minimizes the risk for skin breakdown.

13. Remove gloves.

Tape is easier to handle without gloves. Wound is covered with the dressing.

14. Apply the sticky side of each tape or strap to a skin barrier sheet. Apply the sheet directly to the skin near the dressing. Repeat for the other side.

Skin barrier prevents skin irritation and breakdown.

15. Thread a separate string through each pair of holes in the straps. Tie one end of the string in the hole. Fasten the other end with the opposing tie, like a shoelace. **Do not secure too tightly.** Repeat according to the number of straps needed. If commercially prepared straps are used, tie strings like a shoelace. Note date and time of application on strap.

Ties hold the dressing in place. However, tying the ties too tightly puts additional stress on the surrounding skin. Recording date and time provides a baseline for changing straps.

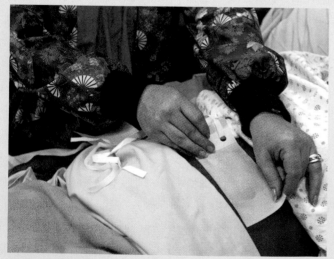

Action 14: Applying Montgomery straps (on a skin barrier sheet) to the patient's abdomen.

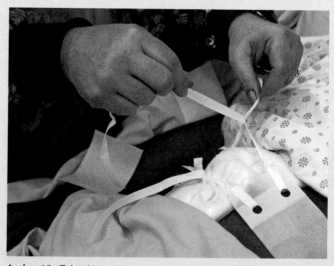

Action 15: Tying Montgomery straps.

16. Return the bed to the lowest position while making the patient comfortable and raising the side rails as needed.

Repositioning the bed and patient promotes safety.

17. Perform hand hygiene.

Hand hygiene prevents spread of microorganisms.

18. Document the procedure, the patient's response, and your assessment of the area before and after application.

Documentation promotes continuity of care and communication.

19. Replace the ties and straps whenever they are soiled, or every 2 to 3 days.

Replacing soiled ties and straps prevents the growth of pathogens.

continues

SKILL 8-15 Applying Montgomery Straps (continued)

ACTION   **RATIONALE**

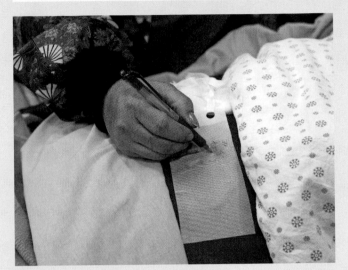

Action 15: Labeling Montgomery straps in place.

10/20/06 1930   Patient's abdominal
wound has large amounts of serosanguineous
drainage, saturating multiple layers of gauze
and ABDs, requiring dressing changes at least
q 3 hours. Surrounding skin cleansed, skin
protectant applied, and Montgomery straps
applied to secure wound dressings.
—D. Rightner, RN

Action 18: Documentation.

EVALUATION

The expected outcome when applying Montgomery straps is met when the patient's skin is clean, dry, intact, and free from irritation and injury. Other outcomes are met when the patient exhibits a clean wound area free of contamination and trauma. In addition, the patient verbalizes minimal to no pain or discomfort, and the patient exhibits signs and symptoms indicative of progressive wound healing.

Unexpected Situations and Associated Interventions

- *Your patient has had an abdominal wound for several weeks. Despite careful wound and skin care, you observe signs of redness and irritation where the tape for the dressings has been repeatedly placed:* Obtain the supplies listed in this skill. Apply Montgomery straps, being sure to move the skin barrier sheet at least 1″ away from the area of irritation.

Applying a Saline-Moistened Dressing

A dressing is a protective covering placed on a wound. Gauze dressings are easy to use and adapt to many applications. Gauze can be moistened with saline to keep the surface of open wounds moist. This type of dressing promotes moist wound healing and protects the wound from contamination and trauma. A moist wound surface enhances the cellular migration necessary for tissue repair and healing. This dressing is often used with chronic wounds and pressure wounds. It is important that the dressing material be moist, not wet, when placed in open wounds. Dressing materials are soaked in normal saline solution and squeezed to remove excess saline so that the dressing is only slightly moist. The dressing is applied loosely in the wound bed, then covered with a secondary dressing to absorb drainage.

Equipment

- Clean gloves
- Sterile gloves
- Sterile dressing instrument set, including forceps and scissors
- Sterile thin-mesh gauze dressing
- Sterile gauze dressings
- Absorbent secondary dressing, such as an ABD
- Skin protectant wipe
- Sterile basin
- Prescribed sterile solution, usually normal saline, for wetting dressings
- Sterile saline
- Tape or ties
- Waterproof waste receptacle
- Sterile cotton-tipped applicators
- Supplies for wound cleansing or irrigation, as necessary
- Waterproof pad and bath blanket
- Personal protective equipment, such as a gown, mask, and eye protection

ASSESSMENT

Assess the situation to determine the need for a dressing change. Confirm any physician orders relevant to wound care and any wound care included in the nursing care plan. Assess the current dressing, if there is one, to see if it is intact and if there is excess drainage or bleeding or saturation of the dressing. Assess the patient's level of comfort and the need for analgesics before wound care. Assess the location, stage, drainage, and types of tissue present in the wound. Measure the wound. Assess the surrounding skin for color, temperature, edema, ecchymosis, or maceration.

**NURSING
DIAGNOSIS**

Determine the related factors for the nursing diagnoses based on the patient's current status. An appropriate nursing diagnosis is Impaired Skin Integrity. Other nursing diagnoses that may be appropriate include:

- Anxiety
- Disturbed Body Image
- Impaired Comfort
- Risk for Infection
- Acute Pain
- Chronic Pain
- Impaired Tissue Integrity

**OUTCOME
IDENTIFICATION
AND PLANNING**

The expected outcome to achieve when applying a saline-moistened dressing is that the procedure is accomplished without contaminating the wound area, without causing trauma to the wound, and without causing the patient to experience pain or discomfort. Other outcomes that are appropriate include sterile technique is maintained (if appropriate); wound healing is promoted; the surrounding skin is without signs of irritation, infection, and maceration; and the wound continues to show signs of progression of healing.

continues

Applying a Saline-Moistened Dressing (continued)

IMPLEMENTATION

ACTION	RATIONALE
1. Review the physician's order and/or nursing care plan for the application of a saline-moistened dressing.	This action validates the correct patient and correct procedure.
2. Gather the necessary supplies.	This action promotes efficient time management and provides an organized approach to the task.
3. Identify the patient and explain the procedure. Determine if the patient is allergic to any of the materials or solutions needed for the procedure.	Identifying the patient validates the correct patient and correct procedure. Discussion and explanation help allay anxiety, encourage patient cooperation, and prepare the patient for what to expect.
4. Perform hand hygiene.	Hand hygiene prevents the spread of microorganisms.
5. Close the room door or curtains. Place the bed at a comfortable working height.	Closing the door or curtains provides privacy. Having the bed at a comfortable height helps reduce back strain while you are performing the procedure.
6. Assist the patient to a comfortable position that provides easy access to the wound area. Position the patient so the irrigation solution will flow from the upper end of the wound toward the lower end, if wound irrigation is necessary. Expose the area and drape the patient with the bath blanket if needed. Put the waterproof pad under the wound area to protect the bed.	A comfortable position and bath blanket provide comfort and warmth for the patient. Gravity directs the flow of liquid from the least contaminated to the most contaminated area. The waterproof pad protects the patient and the bed linens.
7. Have the disposal bag or waste receptacle within easy reach.	Having the waste receptacle handy means that soiled dressings and supplies may be discarded easily, without the spread of microorganisms.
8. Put on personal protective equipment as appropriate.	Using personal protective equipment prevents contamination from microorganisms and the spread of infection.
9. Put on clean disposable gloves and gently remove the soiled dressings. If the dressing adheres to the underlying tissues, moisten it with saline to loosen.	Gloves protect the nurse from handling contaminated dressings. Moistening the dressing prevents disruption of healing tissue.
10. After removing the dressing, note the presence, amount, type, color, and odor of any drainage on the dressings. Place soiled dressings in the appropriate waste receptacle.	The presence of drainage should be documented. Discarding dressings appropriately prevents the spread of microorganisms.
11. Assess the wound for appearance, stage, the presence of eschar, granulation tissue, epithelialization, undermining, tunneling, necrosis, sinus tract, and drainage. Assess the appearance of the surrounding tissue. Measure the wound.	This information provides evidence about the wound healing process and/or the presence of infection.
12. Remove your gloves and put them in they receptacle.	Discarding gloves prevents the spread of microorganisms.
13. Using sterile technique, open the supplies and dressings. Place the fine-mesh gauze into the basin and pour the ordered solution over the mesh to saturate it.	Gauze touching the wound surface must be moistened to increase the absorptive ability and promote healing.
14. Put on the sterile gloves.	Sterile gloves maintain surgical asepsis.
15. Cleanse or irrigate the wound as prescribed or with normal saline. (See Skills 8-7 and 8-9.)	Cleaning removes debris, contaminants, and excess exudate.

continues

ACTION	RATIONALE
16. Apply a skin protectant to the skin surrounding the wound.	A skin protectant prevents skin irritation and breakdown.
17. Squeeze excess fluid from the gauze dressing. Unfold and fluff the dressing.	The gauze provides a thin, moist layer to contact all the wound surfaces.
18. Gently press the moistened gauze into the wound. If necessary, use the forceps or cotton-tipped applicators to press the gauze into all wound surfaces.	The dressing provides a moist environment for all wound surfaces.
19. Apply several dry, sterile gauze pads over the wet gauze.	Dry gauze absorbs excess moisture and drainage.
20. Place the ABD pad over the gauze.	The ABD pad prevents contamination.
21. Remove and discard your sterile gloves. Apply tape or tie tapes to secure the dressings.	Discarding gloves prevents the spread of microorganisms. Tape is easier to apply after gloves have been removed.
22. After securing the dressing, remove all remaining equipment, place the patient in a position of comfort with side rails up and the bed in the lowest position, and perform hand hygiene.	These actions ensure safety. Hand hygiene prevents the spread of microorganisms.
23. Record the procedure, your wound assessment, and the patient's reaction to the procedure using your institution's guidelines.	Documentation promotes continuity of care and communication.
24. Check all wound dressings every shift. You might need to check more frequently if a wound is more complex or dressings become saturated more frequently.	Frequent checks ensure that changes in patient condition are noted and timely intervention is performed to prevent complications.

EVALUATION

The expected outcome when applying a saline-moistened dressing is met when the procedure is accomplished without contaminating the wound area, without causing trauma to the wound, and without causing the patient to experience pain or discomfort. Other outcomes are met when sterile technique is maintained (if appropriate); wound healing is promoted; the surrounding skin is without signs of irritation, infection, and maceration; and the wound continues to show signs of progression of healing.

Unexpected Situations and Related Interventions

- *When removing a patient's dressing, you note eschar in the wound:* The presence of eschar in a wound precludes the staging of the wound. The eschar must be removed for adequate pressure ulcer staging to be done.
- *You note several depressions or crater-like areas on inspection of a wound:* Notify the physician, who may order the wound to be packed. Pack wound cavities loosely with dressing material. Overpacking may increase pressure and interfere with tissue healing.
- *You note that the wound dressing is dry upon removal:* Reduce the time interval between changes to prevent drying of the materials, which may disrupt healing tissue.

Special Considerations

- Make sure ancillary staff understand the importance of reporting excessive drainage from the dressing, and any soiled or loose dressings.
- Many products are available to treat chronic and pressure ulcers. Treatment varies based on facility policy, nursing protocol, clinical specialist referrals, and physician orders.

SKILL 8-17   **Applying a Hydrocolloid Dressing**

Hydrocolloid dressings are wafer-shaped dressings that come in many shapes and thicknesses. An adhesive backing provides adherence to the wound and surrounding skin. They absorb drainage, maintain a moist wound surface, and decrease the risk for infection by covering the wound surface. They are used for shallow to moderate-depth wounds with minimal drainage and stay in place for 3 to 7 days. Polyurethane dressings are nonadhesive hydrocolloid dressings that must be secured to prevent wound contamination, as they do not adhere to the wound or surrounding skin. Application can be done using clean or sterile technique, depending on facility policy (see Special Considerations).

Equipment

- Hydrocolloid dressing
- Clean gloves
- Sterile gloves
- Sterile dressing instrument set, for the scissors
- Skin protectant wipe
- Supplies needed for wound cleansing, as necessary
- Sterile cotton-tipped applicator
- Waterproof waste receptacle
- Bath blanket
- Personal protective equipment such as gown, mask, and eye protection

ASSESSMENT

Assess the situation to determine the need for a dressing change. Check the date when the current dressing (if present) was placed. Confirm any physician orders relevant to wound care and any wound care included in the nursing care plan. Assess the current dressing, if there is one, to determine if it is intact. Assess the patient's level of comfort and the need for analgesics before wound care. Assess the location, stage, drainage, and types of tissue present in the wound. Measure the wound. Assess the surrounding skin for color, temperature, edema, ecchymosis, or maceration.

NURSING DIAGNOSES

Determine the related factors for the nursing diagnoses based on the patient's current status. An appropriate nursing diagnosis is Impaired Skin Integrity. Other nursing diagnoses that may be appropriate include:

- Anxiety
- Disturbed Body Image
- Impaired Comfort
- Risk for Infection
- Acute Pain
- Chronic Pain
- Impaired Tissue Integrity

OUTCOME IDENTIFICATION AND PLANNING

The expected outcome to achieve when applying a hydrocolloid dressing is that the procedure is accomplished without contaminating the wound area, without causing trauma to the wound, and without causing the patient to experience pain or discomfort. Other outcomes that are appropriate include sterile technique is maintained (if appropriate); wound healing is promoted; the surrounding skin is without signs of irritation, infection, and maceration; and the wound continues to show signs of progression of healing.

IMPLEMENTATION

ACTION	RATIONALE
1. Review the physician's order and/or nursing care plan for the application of a hydrocolloid dressing.	Checking the order validates the correct patient and correct procedure.
2. Gather the necessary supplies.	Having supplies at hand promotes efficient time management and provides an organized approach to the task.

continues

ACTION	RATIONALE
3. Identify the patient and explain the procedure. Determine if the patient is allergic to any of the materials or solutions needed for the procedure.	Identifying the patient validates the correct patient and correct procedure. Discussion and explanation help allay anxiety, encourage patient cooperation, and prepare the patient for what to expect.
4. Perform hand hygiene.	Hand hygiene prevents the spread of microorganisms.
5. Close the room door or curtains. Place the bed at a comfortable working height.	Closing the door or curtains provides privacy. Having the bed at a comfortable height helps reduce back strain while you are performing the procedure.
6. Assist the patient to a comfortable position that provides easy access to the wound area. Position the patient so the irrigation solution will flow from the upper end of the wound toward the lower end, if necessary. Expose the area and drape the patient with the bath blanket if needed. Put the waterproof pad under the wound area to protect the bed.	A comfortable position and the bath blanket provide for comfort and warmth. Gravity directs the flow of liquid from the least contaminated to the most contaminated area. The waterproof pad protects the patient and the bed linens.
7. Have the disposal bag or waste receptacle within easy reach.	Having the waste receptacle handy means that dressings and supplies may be discarded easily, without the spread of microorganisms.
8. Put on personal protective equipment as appropriate.	Using personal protective equipment prevents contamination from microorganisms and the spread of infection.
9. Put on clean disposable gloves and gently remove the soiled dressing. Discard it in the receptacle.	The nurse is protected from handling a contaminated dressing.
10. Assess the wound for appearance, stage, granulation tissue, epithelialization, undermining, tunneling, necrosis, sinus tract, and drainage. Assess the appearance of the surrounding tissue. Measure the wound.	This information provides evidence about the wound healing process and/or the presence of infection.
11. Remove your gloves and put them in the receptacle.	Discarding gloves prevents the spread of microorganisms.
12. Set up a sterile field and put on the sterile gloves if indicated.	Using sterile gloves prevents contamination of the wound or supplies and prevents the spread of microorganisms.
13. Cleanse or irrigate the wound as prescribed or with normal saline. (See Skills 8-7 and 8-9.)	Cleansing removes debris, contaminants, and excess exudate.
14. Apply a skin protectant to the skin surrounding the wound.	Using a skin protectant prevents skin irritation and breakdown.
15. Choose a clean, dry, presized dressing or cut one to size using sterile scissors. The dressing must be sized generously, allowing at least a 1″ margin of healthy skin around the wound to be covered with the dressing.	These actions ensure proper adherence, coverage of the wound, and wear of the dressing.
16. Remove the release paper from the adherent side of the dressing. Apply the dressing to the wound without stretching the dressing. Smooth wrinkles as it is applied.	Proper application prevents shearing force on the wound and minimizes irritation.
17. If necessary, secure the dressing edges with tape. Dressings that are near the anus need to have the edges taped. Apply additional skin barrier to the areas to be covered with tape, if necessary.	Taping helps keep the dressing intact. Taping the edges of dressings near the anus prevents wound contamination from fecal material.

continues

Applying a Hydrocolloid Dressing (continued)

ACTION	RATIONALE
18. Remove and discard your sterile gloves.	Discarding gloves prevents the spread of microorganisms.
19. Remove all remaining equipment, place the patient in a position of comfort with side rails up and the bed in the lowest position, and perform hand hygiene.	These actions ensure safety. Hand hygiene prevents the spread of microorganisms.
20. Record the procedure, your wound assessment, and the patient's reaction to the procedure using your institution's guidelines. Note the date for the next dressing change, based on facility policy (normally 3 to 7 days).	Documentation promotes continuity of care and communication.
21. Check all wound dressings every shift to validate that they are intact.	Frequent checks ensure that changes in patient condition are noted and timely intervention is performed to prevent complications.

EVALUATION   The expected outcome when applying a hydrocolloid dressing is met when the procedure is accomplished without contaminating the wound area, without causing trauma to the wound, and without causing the patient to experience pain or discomfort. Other outcomes are met when sterile technique is maintained (if appropriate); wound healing is promoted; surrounding skin is without signs of irritation, infection, and maceration; and the wound continues to show signs of progression of healing.

Unexpected Situations and Related Interventions

- *When performing wound care, you observe adherent necrotic material in the wound:* Notify the wound care specialist and/or the physician, as further débridement may be necessary.

Special Considerations

- Guidelines from the Agency for Health Care Policy and Research state that clean gloves and clean dressings may be used to treat pressure ulcers as long as the agency infection control procedures are followed. The *no-touch technique* may be used within these guidelines. Clean gloves are used to handle dressing material. Irrigants and dressings are sterile. The wound is redressed by picking up dressing materials by the corner and placing the untouched side over the pressure ulcer.
- Many products are available to treat chronic and pressure ulcers. Treatment varies based on facility policy, nursing protocol, clinical specialist referrals, and physician orders.

■ Developing Critical Thinking Skills

1. While providing wound care for Lori Downs' foot ulcer, you note that the drainage, which was scant and yellow yesterday, is now green and has saturated the old dressing. Should you continue with the prescribed wound care?
2. Three days ago Tran Nguyen underwent a modified radical mastectomy. She has three Jackson-Pratt drains at her surgical site. She has started asking questions about her surgery and anticipated discharge home. Until this morning, she has avoided looking at her surgical site. You are helping her with her bathing and dressing. As you help her remove her gown, she becomes visibly upset and anxious and exclaims, "Oh no! What's wrong? I'm bleeding from the cuts!" You realize she is looking at her drains. How should you respond?

3. Arthur Lowes has come to his surgeon's office today for a follow-up examination after a colon resection. After he sees the physician, you, the treatment nurse, will remove the surgical staples from the incision. As you prepare to remove the staples, Mr. Lowes comments, "I hope my stomach doesn't pop out now!" What should you tell him?

Bibliography

Atkinson, A. (2002). Body image considerations in patients with wounds. *Journal of Community Nursing, 16*(10), 32–36.

Centers for Disease Control and Prevention (2000). Monitoring hospital-acquired infections to promote patient safety, US, 1990–1999. *Morbidity and Mortality Weekly Report, 49*(08), 149–153.

Centers for Disease Control and Prevention. (Oct. 25, 2002). Guideline for hand hygiene in health-care settings. *Morbidity and Mortality Weekly Report, 51*(RR-16), 1–45.

Clinical Skills. (Jan. 21–27, 2003). Wound VACs. *Nursing Times, 99*(3), 29.

Craven, R., & Hirnle, C. (2003). *Fundamentals of nursing. Human health and function* (4th ed.). Philadelphia: Lippincott Williams & Wilkins.

Davidson, M. (2002). Sharpen your wound assessment skills. *Nursing, 32*(10), 32hn1.

McConnell, E. A. (July 2001). Clinical do's & don'ts: Emptying a closed wound drainage device. *Nursing, 31*(7), 17.

Ovington, L., & Schaum, K. (2001). Wound care products: How to choose. *Home Healthcare Nurse, 19*(4), 224–240.

Pieper, B., Templin, T., et al. (2002). Home care nurses' ratings of appropriateness of wound treatments and wound healing. *Journal of WOCN, 29*(1), 20–28.

Pullen, R. L., Jr. (October 2003). Clinical do's & don'ts: Removing sutures and staples. *Nursing, 33*(10), 18.

Stotts, N. (1999). Evidence-based practice: What is it and how is it used in wound care? *Nursing Clinics of North America, 34*(4), 955–963.

Taylor, C., Lillis, C., & LeMone, P. (2004). *Fundamentals of nursing. The art & science of nursing care* (5th ed.). Philadelphia: Lippincott Williams & Wilkins.

U.S. Department of Health and Human Services, Agency for Health Care Policy and Research. (1994). *Treatment of pressure ulcers.* Rockville, MD: Author.

Vincent, J. (June 14, 2003). Nosocomial infections in adult intensive care units. *Lancet, 361*(9374), 2068–2077.

Winslow, E. H. (September 1992). Hospital extra. Working smart. Warm up the cooling blanket. *American Journal of Nursing, 92*(9), 24J.

Activity

Focusing on Patient Care

This chapter will help you develop some of the skills related to activity necessary to care for the following patients:

Bobby Rowden was knocked down during soccer practice and has come to the emergency room with pain, swelling, and deformity of his right forearm. He is diagnosed with a fracture.

Esther Levitz has been admitted to the hospital with nausea, anorexia, debilitating fatigue, and weight loss. Her underlying diagnosis of lymphoma and inactivity put her at risk for thrombus formation.

Manuel Esposito is scheduled for surgery tomorrow to repair a fractured hip. His physician has ordered skin traction to immobilize the injury prior to surgery.

Learning Outcomes

After studying this chapter, the student should be able to:

1. Assist a patient with turning in bed
2. Provide range-of-motion exercises
3. Move a patient up in bed with the assistance of another nurse
4. Transfer a patient from the bed to a stretcher
5. Transfer a patient from the bed to a chair
6. Transfer a patient from the bed to a chair with the assistance of another nurse
7. Transfer a patient using a hydraulic lift
8. Assist a patient with ambulation
9. Assist a patient with ambulation using a walker
10. Assist a patient with ambulation using crutches
11. Assist a patient with ambulation using a cane
12. Apply pneumatic compression devices
13. Apply a continuous passive motion device
14. Apply a sling
15. Apply a figure-eight bandage
16. Assist with a cast application
17. Care for a patient with a cast
18. Care for a patient in skin traction, including application
19. Care for patient in skeletal traction
20. Care for a patient with an external fixation device
21. Care for patient in halo traction

Key Terms

abduction: movement away from the center or median line of the body

adduction: movement toward the center or median line of the body

anorexia: loss of appetite

arthroplasty: surgical formation or reformation of a joint

compartment syndrome: occurs when there is increased tissue pressure within a limited space; leads to compromises in the circulation and the function of the involved tissue

contracture: permanent shortening or tightening of a muscle due to spasm or paralysis

contusion: an injury in which the skin is not broken; a bruise

deep vein thrombosis: a blood clot in a blood vessel originating in the large veins of the legs

diabetes mellitus: a group of metabolic diseases characterized by elevated blood glucose levels resulting from defects in insulin secretion, insulin action, or both

extension: the return movement from flexion; the joint angle is increased

flexion: bending of a joint so that the angle of the joint diminishes

fracture: a break in the continuity of the bone

goniometer: an apparatus to measure joint movement and angles

Homans' sign: pain in the calf when the toe is passively dorsiflexed; an early sign in venous thrombosis of the deep veins of the calf

hyperextension: extreme or abnormal extension

orthostatic hypotension: an abnormal drop in blood pressure that occurs as a person changes from a supine to a standing position

peripheral vascular disease: pathologic conditions of the vascular system characterized by reduced blood flow through the peripheral blood vessels

pronation: the act of lying face downward; the act of turning the hand so the palm faces downward or backward

pulmonary embolism: obstruction of the pulmonary artery or one of its branches by a blood clot

rotation: process of turning on an axis; twisting or revolving

shearing force: force created by the interplay of gravity and friction on the skin and underlying tissues; shear causes tissue layers to slide over one another and blood vessels to stretch and twist and disrupts the microcirculation of the skin and subcutaneous tissue

supination: turning of the palm or foot upward

thrombophlebitis: a blood clot that accompanies vein inflammation

thrombosis: the formation or development of a blood clot

venous stasis: decrease in blood flow in the venous system related to dysfunctional valves or inactivity of the muscles of the affected extremity

Most healthy individuals take the ability to move and be active for granted. People simply expect our amazingly complex musculoskeletal and nervous systems to work together smoothly and on command to enable us to stand upright, walk, and reach for and grasp what we want. People usually give little thought to caring for the systems that promote and coordinate healthy movement until disuse, trauma, or illness interferes with some aspect of movement or activity. The ability to move is closely related to the fulfillment of other basic human needs. Although breathing continues during rest, movement facilitates pulmonary functioning and increases peripheral blood flow. Because regular exercise contributes to the healthy functioning of each body system and, conversely, immobility negatively affects each body system, nurses actively encourage exercise to promote wellness, prevent illness, and restore health.

The human body was designed for motion, and regular activity and exercise are necessary for its healthy functioning. Individuals who choose inactive lifestyles or who are forced into inactivity by illness or injury place themselves at high risk for serious health problems. Complications resulting from inactivity and immobility differ in their occurrence and severity according to the patient's age and overall health state. Promoting exercise and emphasizing wellness behaviors are challenging opportunities for nurses. Nurses must recognize cues that indicate both potential and actual problems related to a patient's activity and mobility status. Nursing interventions are directed to preventing these problems whenever possible. Strategies designed to promote correct body alignment, mobility, and fitness are important parts of nursing care.

This chapter will cover skills to assist the nurse in providing care related to activity, inactivity, and healthcare problems related to the musculoskeletal system. Please look over the summary boxes at the beginning of this chapter for a quick review of critical knowledge to assist you in understanding the skills related to these topics.

BOX 9-1 Principles of Body Mechanics

- Correct body alignment is important to prevent undue strain on joints, muscles, tendons, and ligaments while maintaining balance.
- Maintaining balance involves keeping the spine in vertical alignment, body weight close to the center of gravity, and feet spread for a broad base of support.
- Using the body's major muscle groups and natural levers and fulcrums allows for coordinated movement to avoid musculoskeletal strain and injury.
- Assess the situation before acting so that you can plan to use good body mechanics.
- Use the large muscle groups in the legs to provide force for movement. Keep the back straight, with hips and knees bent. Slide, roll, push, or pull rather than lift an object.
- Perform work at the appropriate height for your body position, close to your center of gravity.
- Use mechanical lifts and/or assistance to ease the movement.

BOX 9-2 Effects of Immobility on the Body

- Decreased muscle strength and tone, decreased muscle size
- Decreased joint mobility and flexibility
- Limited endurance and activity intolerance
- Bone demineralization
- Lack of coordination and altered gait
- Decreased ventilatory effort and increased respiratory secretions, atelectasis, respiratory congestion
- Increased cardiac workload, orthostatic hypotension, venous thrombosis
- Impaired circulation and skin breakdown
- Decreased appetite, constipation
- Urinary stasis, infection
- Altered sleep patterns, pain, depression, anger, anxiety

BOX 9-3 Principles of Effective Traction

- Countertraction must be applied for effective traction.
- Traction must be continuous to be effective.
- Skeletal traction is never interrupted unless a life-threatening emergency occurs.
- Weights are not removed unless intermittent traction is prescribed.
- The patient must maintain good body alignment in the center of the bed.
- Ropes must be unobstructed.
- Weights must hang free.

SKILL 9-1   Assisting a Patient With Turning in Bed

Individuals who are forced into inactivity by illness or injury are at high risk for serious health complications. One of the most common skills that you may use involves helping patients who cannot turn themselves in bed without assistance. You need to use your knowledge of correct body mechanics and correct body alignment to turn the patient in bed. Mastering and using these techniques will help you maintain a turn schedule to prevent complications for an immobile patient. If patient requires logrolling, please refer to Skill 17-4.

Equipment

No special equipment is required for this skill. Pillows or other supports may be used to help the patient maintain the desired position after turning and to maintain correct body alignment for the patient. If indicated, clean gloves may be worn.

ASSESSMENT

Before moving a patient, check the medical record for any conditions or orders that will limit mobility. Perform a pain assessment prior to the time for the activity. If the patient reports pain, administer the prescribed medication in sufficient time to allow for the full effect of the analgesic. Assess the patient's ability to assist with moving and the need for a second individual to assist with the activity.

NURSING DIAGNOSIS

Determine the related factors for the nursing diagnoses based on the patient's current status. Appropriate nursing diagnoses may include:

- Activity Intolerance
- Risk for Activity Intolerance
- Anxiety
- Impaired Comfort
- Risk for Falls
- Fatigue
- Risk for Injury
- Impaired Bed Mobility
- Acute Pain
- Chronic Pain
- Risk for Impaired Skin Integrity
- Impaired Skin Integrity

OUTCOME IDENTIFICATION AND PLANNING

The expected outcome to achieve when assisting a patient with turning in bed is that the activity takes place without injury to patient or nurse. An additional outcome is that the patient is comfortable and in proper body alignment.

IMPLEMENTATION

ACTION	RATIONALE
1. Review the physician's orders and nursing plan of care for patient activity. Identify any movement limitations and the ability of the patient to assist with turning.	Checking the physician's order and plan of care validates the correct patient and correct procedure. Identification of limitations and ability helps to prevent injury.
2. Gather any positioning aids, if necessary.	Having aids readily available promotes efficient time management.
3. Identify the patient. Explain the procedure to the patient.	Patient identification validates the correct patient and correct procedure. Discussion and explanation help allay anxiety and prepare the patient for what to expect.
4. Perform hand hygiene and put on gloves, if necessary.	Hand hygiene and gloving prevent the spread of micro-organisms.
5. Close the room door or curtains. Place the bed at an appropriate and comfortable working height.	Closing the door or curtain provides privacy. Proper bed height helps reduce back strain while performing the procedure.

continues

Assisting a Patient With Turning in Bed (continued)

ACTION	RATIONALE
6. Adjust the head of the bed to a flat position or as low as the patient can tolerate. Place pillows, wedges, or any other supports to be used for positioning within easy reach.	This position facilitates the turning maneuver and minimizes strain on the nurse. Having supports readily available promotes efficient care.
7. Using the drawsheet, move the patient to the edge of the bed, opposite the side to which he or she will be turned.	With this placement, the patient will be on the center of the bed after turning is accomplished.
8. Stand on the side of the bed toward which the patient is turning. Make sure the side rail on the opposite side of the bed from where you are standing is raised. Lower the side rail nearest you.	This positions the nurse opposite the center of the body mass; raising the opposite side rail prevents the patient from possible injury; lowering the near side rail prevents strain on the nurse.
9. **Place the patient's arms across his or her chest and cross his or her far leg over the leg nearest you.**	This facilitates the turning motion and protects the patient's arms during the turn.
10. Stand opposite the patient's center with your feet spread about shoulder width and with one foot ahead of the other. **Tighten your gluteal and abdominal muscles and flex your knees. Use your leg muscles to do the pulling.**	This helps avoid straining the nurse's lower back. The nurse is in a stable position with good body alignment and prepared to use large muscle masses to turn the patient.

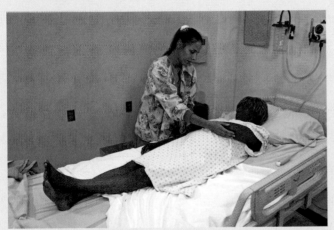

Action 9: Placing patient's arms across chest and patient's far leg crossed over the leg nearest the nurse.

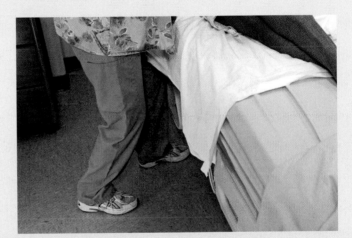

Action 10: Standing opposite the patient's center, with feet spread about shoulder width and with one foot ahead of the other.

11. Position your hands on the patient's far shoulder and hip, and roll the patient toward you. Or, you may use the draw sheet to gently pull the patient over on his or her side.	This maneuver supports the patient's body and makes use of the nurse's weight to assist with turning.
12. Use a pillow or other support behind the patient's back. Pull the shoulder blade forward and out from under the patient.	Pillow will provide support and help the patient maintain the desired position. Positioning the shoulder blade removes pressure from the bony prominence.
13. Make the patient comfortable and position him or her in proper alignment, using pillows or other supports under the leg and arm as needed. Readjust the pillow under the patient's head. Elevate the head of the bed as needed for comfort.	Positioning in proper alignment with supports ensures that the patient will be able to maintain the desired position and will be comfortable.

continues

ACTION	RATIONALE

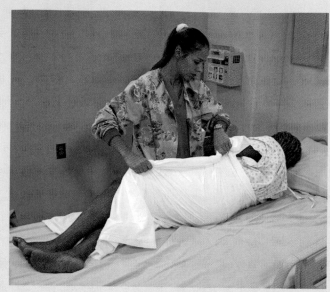

Action 11: Using drawsheet to pull patient over on her side.

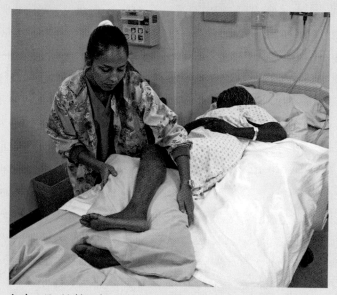

Action 13: Making the patient comfortable.

14. Place the bed in the lowest position, with the side rails up. Make sure the call bell and other necessary items are within easy reach.

Adjusting the bed height ensures patient safety.

15. Perform hand hygiene and document the position change per your facility's policy.

Hand hygiene prevents the spread of microorganisms. Documentation promotes continuity of care and communication.

EVALUATION

The expected outcome is met when the patient is turned and repositioned without injury to patient or nurse. The patient demonstrates proper body alignment and verbalizes comfort.

Unexpected Situations and Associated Interventions

- *You are turning a patient by yourself, but you realize that the patient cannot help as much as you thought and is heavier than you anticipated:* Use the call bell to summon assistance from a coworker. Alternatively, cover the patient, make sure all rails are up, lower the bed to the lowest position, and get someone to assist you.

SKILL 9-2   Providing Range-of-Motion Exercises

Range of motion is the complete extent of movement of which a joint is normally capable. Taking part in routine activities of daily living helps to use muscle groups that keep many joints in an effective range of motion. When all or some of the normal activities are impossible, attention is given to the joints not being used or to those that have limited use. When the patient does the exercise for himself or herself, it is referred to as active range of motion. Exercises performed by the nurse without participation by the patient are referred to as passive range of motion. Exercises should be as active as the patient's physical condition permits. Allow the patient to do as much individual activity as his or her condition permits. Range-of-motion exercises should be initiated as soon as possible because body changes can occur after only 3 days of impaired mobility.

Equipment

No special equipment or supplies are necessary to perform range-of-motion exercises. If appropriate, clean gloves may be worn.

ASSESSMENT

Review the medical record and nursing plan of care for any conditions or orders that will limit mobility. Perform a pain assessment prior to the time for the exercises. If the patient reports pain, administer the prescribed medication in sufficient time to allow for the full effect of the analgesic. Assess the patient's ability to perform range-of-motion exercises. Inspect and palpate joints for redness, tenderness, pain, swelling, or deformities.

NURSING DIAGNOSIS

Determine the related factors for the nursing diagnoses based on the patient's current status. An appropriate nursing diagnosis is Impaired Physical Mobility. Other appropriate nursing diagnoses could include:

- Impaired Bed Mobility
- Activity Intolerance
- Anxiety
- Fatigue
- Risk for Injury
- Deficient Knowledge
- Acute Pain
- Chronic Pain
- Impaired Skin Integrity

OUTCOME IDENTIFICATION AND PLANNING

The expected outcome to achieve when performing range-of-motion exercises is that the patient maintains joint mobility. Other outcomes include improving or maintaining muscle strength, and preventing muscle atrophy and contractures.

IMPLEMENTATION

ACTION	RATIONALE
1. Review the physician's orders and nursing plan of care for patient activity. Identify any movement limitations.	Reviewing the order and plan of care validates the correct patient and correct procedure. Identification of limitations prevents injury.
2. Identify the patient. Explain the procedure to the patient.	Patient identification validates the correct patient and correct procedure. Discussion and explanation help allay anxiety and prepare the patient for what to expect.
3. Perform hand hygiene and put on gloves, if necessary.	Hand hygiene and gloving prevent the spread of microorganisms.
4. Close the room door or curtains. Place the bed at an appropriate and comfortable working height. Adjust the head of the bed to a flat position or as low as the patient can tolerate.	Closing the door or curtains provides privacy. Proper bed height helps reduce back strain while performing the procedure.

continues

SKILL 9-2   Providing Range-of-Motion Exercises (continued)

ACTION

5. Stand on the side of the bed where the joints are to be exercised. Uncover only the limb to be used during the exercise.

6. Perform the exercises slowly and gently, providing support by holding the areas proximal and distal to the joint. Repeat each exercise two to five times, moving each joint in a smooth and rhythmic manner. **Stop movement if the patient complains of pain or if you meet resistance.**

7. **While performing the exercises, begin at the head and move down one side of the body at a time.**

8. Move the chin down to rest on the chest. Return the head to a normal upright position. Tilt the head as far as possible toward each shoulder.

9. Move the head from side to side, bringing the chin toward each shoulder.

RATIONALE

Standing on the side to be exercised prevents strain on the nurse's back. Proper draping provides for privacy and warmth.

Slow, gentle movements with support prevent discomfort and muscle spasms resulting from jerky movements. Repeated movement of muscles and joints improves flexibility and increases circulation to the body part. Pain may indicate the exercises are causing damage.

Proceeding from head to toe one side at a time promotes efficient time management and an organized approach to the task.

These movements provide for flexion, extension, and lateral flexion of the head and neck.

These movements provide for rotation of neck.

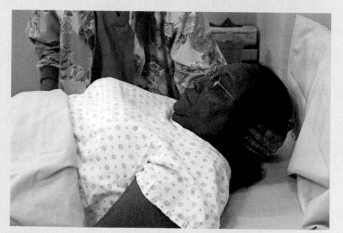

Action 8: Moving patient's chin down to rest on chest.

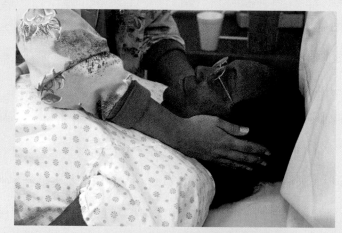

Action 8: Holding patient's head upright and centered.

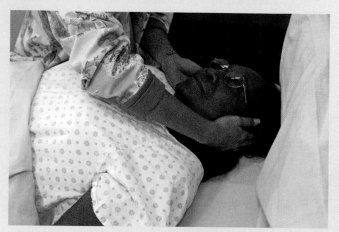

Action 8: Moving patient's head to one shoulder.

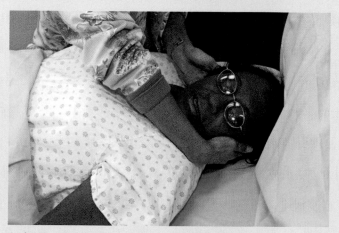

Action 9: Moving patient's chin toward one shoulder.

continues

SKILL 9-2 Providing Range-of-Motion Exercises (continued)

ACTION	RATIONALE
10. Start with the arm at the patient's side and lift the arm forward to above the head. Return the arm to the starting position at the side of the body.	These movements provide for flexion and extension of the shoulder.
11. With the arm back at the patient's side, move the arm laterally to an upright position above the head, and then return to the original position. Move the arm across the body as far as possible.	These movements provide for abduction and adduction of the shoulder.

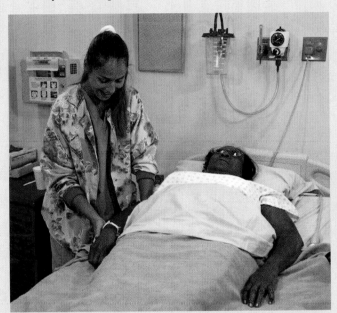

Action 10: Holding patient's arm at side.

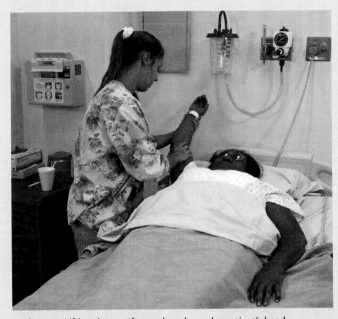

Action 10: Lifting the arm forward to above the patient's head.

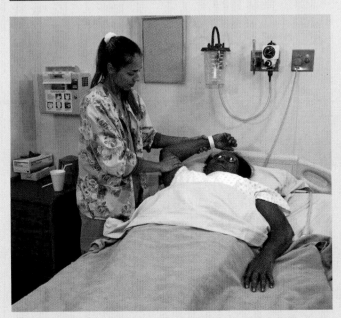

Action 11: Moving the patient's arm laterally to an upright position above the patient's head.

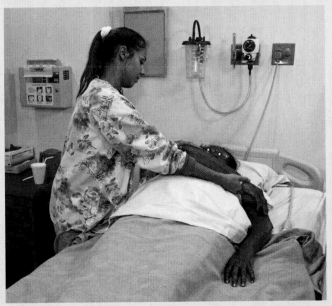

Action 11: Moving the arm across the patient's body as far as possible.

continues

Providing Range-of-Motion Exercises (continued)

ACTION	RATIONALE
12. Raise the arm at the side until the upper arm is in line with the shoulder. Bend the elbow at a 90-degree angle and move the forearm upward and downward, then return the arm to the side.	These movements provide for internal and external rotation of the shoulder.
13. Bend the elbow and move the lower arm and hand upward toward the shoulder. Return the lower arm and hand to the original position while straightening the elbow.	These movements provide for flexion and extension of the elbow.

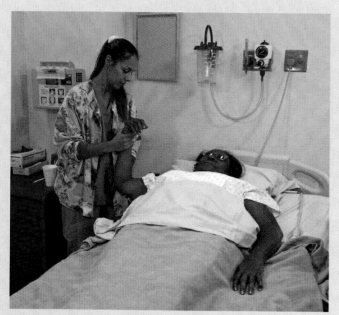

Action 12: Raising the patient's arm until the upper arm is in line with the patient's shoulder, with elbow bent.

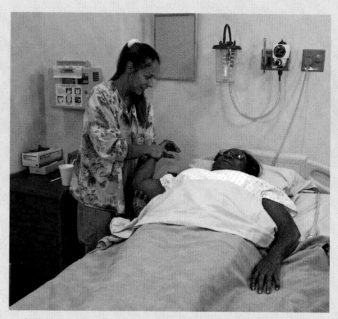

Action 13: Bending the patient's elbow and move the lower arm and hand upward toward the shoulder.

14. Rotate the lower arm and hand so the palm is up. Rotate the lower arm and hand so the palm of the hand is down.	These movements provide for supination and pronation of the forearm.
15. Move the hand downward toward the inner aspect of the forearm. Return the hand to a neutral position even with the forearm. Then move the dorsal portion of the hand backward as far as possible.	These movements provide for flexion, extension, and hyperextension of the wrist.
16. Bend the fingers to make a fist, then straighten them out. Spread the fingers apart and return them back together. Touch the thumb to each finger on the hand.	These movements provide for flexion, extension, abduction, and adduction of the fingers.
17. Extend the leg and lift it upward. Return the leg to the original position beside the other leg.	These movements provide for flexion and extension of the hip.
18. Lift the leg laterally away from the patient's body. Return the leg back toward the other leg and try to extend it beyond the midline.	These movements provide for abduction and adduction of the hip.

continues

Providing Range-of-Motion Exercises (continued)

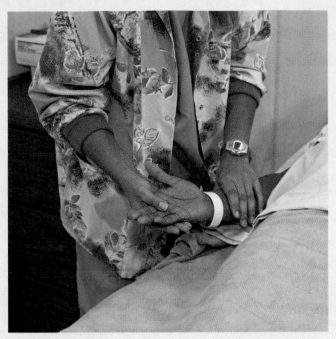

Action 14: Rotating the patient's lower arm and hand so palm is up.

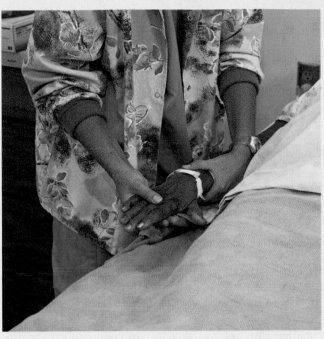

Action 14: Rotating the patient's lower arm and hand so palm is down.

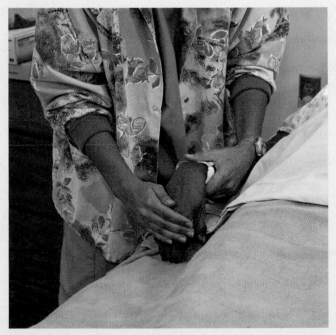

Action 15: Moving the patient's hand downward toward the inner aspect of forearm.

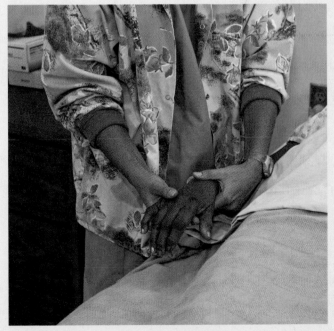

Action 15: Returning hand to the neutral position.

continues

Providing Range-of-Motion Exercises (continued)

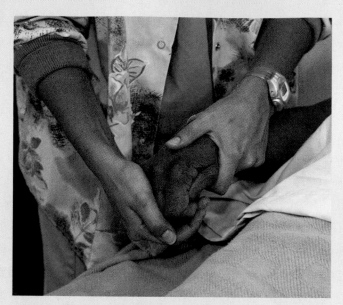

Action 16: Bending patient's fingers to make a fist.

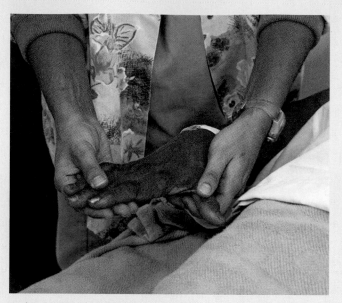

Action 16: Straightening out patient's fingers.

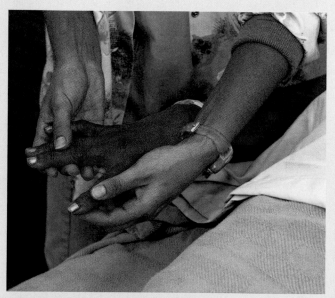

Action 16: Spreading the patient's fingers apart.

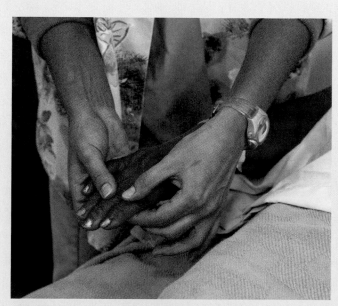

Action 16: Returning the patient's fingers back together.

continues

Providing Range-of-Motion Exercises (continued)

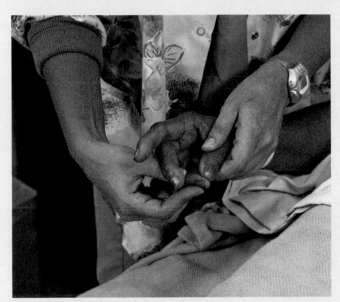

Action 16: Assisting patient to touch thumb to each finger.

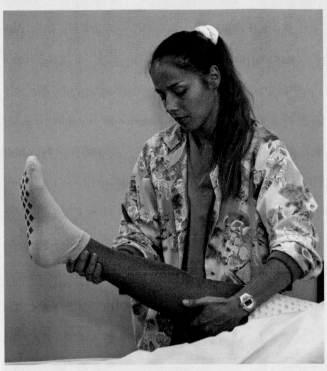

Action 17: Extending and lifting the patient's leg.

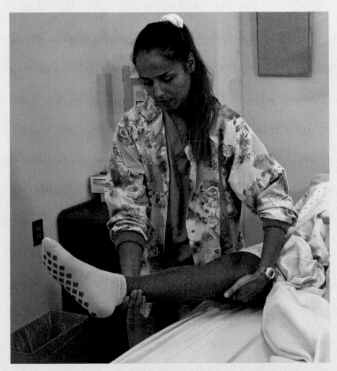

Action 18: Lifting the patient's leg laterally away from the body (abduction).

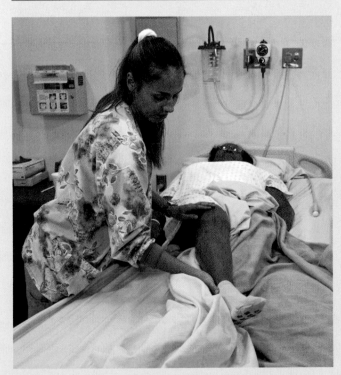

Action 18: Returning the leg back toward the other leg and trying to extend it beyond the midline if possible.

continues

ACTION	RATIONALE
19. Turn the foot and leg toward the other leg to rotate it internally. Turn the foot and leg outward away from the other leg to rotate it externally.	These movements provide for internal and external rotation of the hip.
20. Bend the leg and bring the heel toward the back of the leg; then return the leg to a straight position.	These movements provide for flexion and extension of the knee.

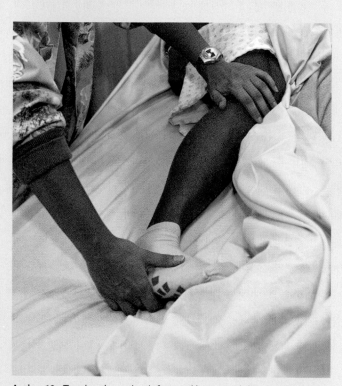

Action 19: Turning the patient's foot and leg toward the opposite leg to rotate it internally.

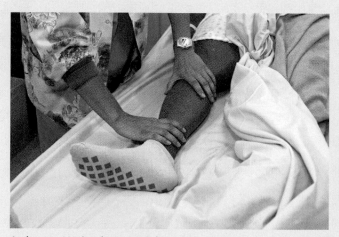

Action 19: Moving the patient's foot and leg outward away from the opposite leg to rotate it externally.

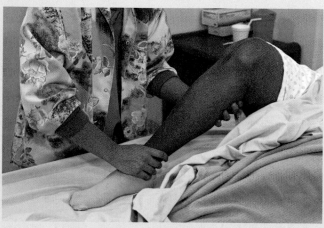

Action 20: Bending the patient's leg and bringing the heel toward the back of the leg.

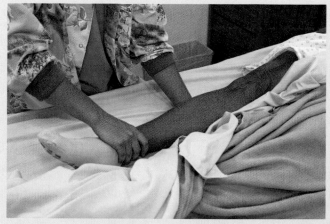

Action 20: Returning the leg to a straight position.

continues

ACTION	**RATIONALE**
21. Move the foot up and back until the toes are upright. Move the foot with the toes pointing downward.	These movements provide for dorsiflexion and plantarflexion of the ankle.
22. Turn the sole of the foot toward the midline. Turn the sole of the foot outward.	These movements provide for inversion and eversion of the ankle.

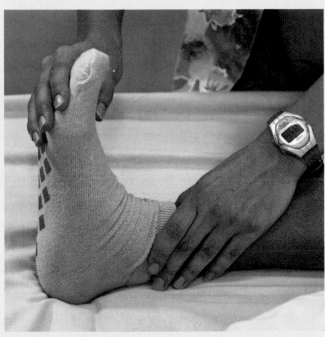

Action 21: At the ankle, moving the patient's foot up and back until the toes are upright.

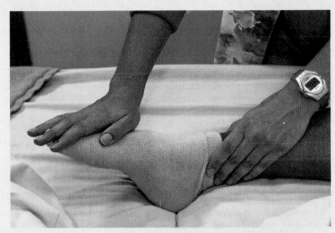

Action 21: Moving the patient's foot with the toes pointing down.

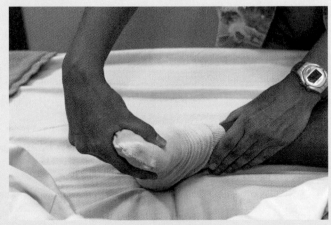

Action 22: Turning the sole toward the midline.

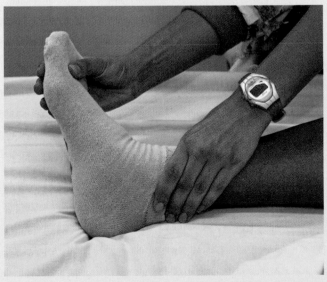

Action 22: Turning the sole outward.

continues

SKILL 9-2   Providing Range-of-Motion Exercises (continued)

ACTION	RATIONALE
23. Curl the toes downward, then straighten them out. Spread the toes apart and bring them together.	These movements provide for flexion, extension, abduction, and adduction of the toes.
24. Repeat these exercises on the other side of the body. Encourage the patient to do as many of these exercises by himself or herself as possible.	Repeating motions on the other side provides exercise for the entire body.
25. When finished, make sure the patient is comfortable, with the side rails up and the bed in the lowest position.	Proper positioning with raised side rails and proper bed height provides for patient comfort and safety.

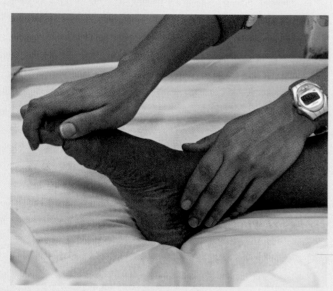

Action 23: Curling the patient's toes down.

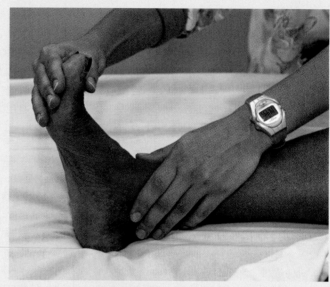

Action 23: Straightening the patient's toes.

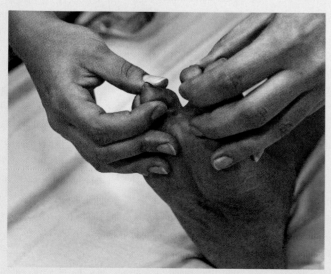

Action 23: Spreading the patient's toes apart.

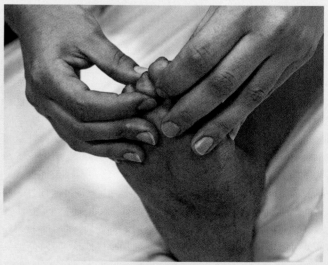

Action 23: Bringing the patient's toes together.

continues

Providing Range-of-Motion Exercises (continued)

ACTION	RATIONALE
26. Remove gloves if used and perform hand hygiene. Document the exercises performed, any observations, and the patient's reaction to the activities.	Proper glove removal and hand hygiene prevent the spread of microorganisms. Documentation promotes continuity of care and communication.

> 5/1/06   0945   Range-of-motion exercises performed to all joints. Patient able to perform active range of motion of head, neck, shoulders, and arms. Required moderate assistance with ROM to lower extremities. Denied any complaints of pain during exercises. Patient tolerated exercise session well. Sitting in semi-Fowler's position with side rails up, watching television.—J. Chrisp, RN

Action 26: Documentation.

EVALUATION

The expected outcome is met when the patient maintains or improves joint mobility and muscle strength, and muscle atrophy and contractures are prevented.

Unexpected Situations and Associated Interventions

- *While you are performing range-of-motion exercises, the patient complains of feeling tired:* Stop the activity for that time. Reevaluate the nursing plan of care. Space the exercises out at different times of the day. Schedule exercise times for the parts of the day the patient is typically feeling more rested.
- *While exercising your patient's leg, he complains of sudden, sharp pain:* Stop the exercises. Assess the patient for other symptoms. Notify the physician of the event and your findings. Joints should be moved until there is resistance but not pain. Uncomfortable reactions should be reported and exercises halted. The activity plan may have to be revised.

Special Considerations

- Many of these exercises can be incorporated into daily activities, such as during bathing.
- A physician's order and specific instructions should be obtained to perform range-of-motion exercises for patients with acute arthritis, fractures, torn ligaments, joint dislocation, acute myocardial infarction, and bone tumors or metastases.

Older Adult Considerations

- Avoid neck hyperextension and attempts to achieve full range of motion in all joints with older patients.

Moving a Patient Up in Bed With the Assistance of Another Nurse

When a patient needs to be moved up in bed, it is important to avoid injuring yourself and the patient. The patient is at risk for injuries from shearing forces while being moved. Evaluate the patient's condition, any activity restrictions, the patient's ability to assist with positioning and ability to understand directions, the patient's body weight, and your strength to decide if additional assistance is needed. When the patient cannot assist with movement or weighs more than one person can safely move, you need to enlist the assistance of another staff person. Using assistance, good body mechanics, and correct technique is important to avoid injuries to yourself and the patient.

Equipment

No special equipment is needed for this skill, but a drawsheet should be present on the bed. If appropriate, clean gloves may be worn.

ASSESSMENT

Assess the situation to determine the need to move the patient up in the bed. Review the medical record and nursing plan of care for conditions that may influence the patient's ability to move or to be positioned. Assess for tubes, intravenous lines, incisions, or equipment that may alter the positioning procedure. Assess the patient's level of consciousness, ability to understand and follow directions, and ability to assist with moving. Assess the patient's weight and your strength to determine if additional assistance is needed.

NURSING DIAGNOSIS

Determine the related factors for the nursing diagnoses based on the patient's current status. Appropriate nursing diagnosis may include:

- Activity Intolerance
- Risk for Injury
- Acute Pain
- Chronic Pain
- Impaired Tissue Integrity
- Ineffective Tissue Perfusion
- Impaired Skin Integrity
- Impaired Gas Exchange
- Risk for Impaired Skin Integrity
- Impaired Bed Mobility

OUTCOME IDENTIFICATION AND PLANNING

The expected outcome to achieve when moving a patient up in bed with the assistance of another nurse is that the patient remains free from injury and maintains proper body alignment. Additional outcomes may include: the patient reports improved comfort; the patient demonstrates maximal ventilation and lung expansion; and the patient's skin is clean, dry, and intact without any redness, irritation, or breakdown.

IMPLEMENTATION

ACTION	RATIONALE
1. Review the medical record and nursing plan of care for conditions that may influence the patient's ability to move or to be positioned. Assess for tubes, intravenous lines, incisions, or equipment that may alter the positioning procedure. Identify any movement limitations.	Reviewing the order and plan of care validates the correct patient and correct procedure. Identifying limitations or interfering equipment helps to minimize the risk for injury.
2. Identify the patient. Explain the procedure to the patient.	Patient identification validates the correct patient and correct procedure. Discussion and explanation help allay anxiety and prepare the patient for what to expect.
3. Perform hand hygiene and put on gloves, if necessary.	Hand hygiene and gloving prevent the spread of microorganisms.

continues

Moving a Patient Up in Bed With the Assistance of Another Nurse (continued)

ACTION	RATIONALE
4. Close the room door or curtains. Place the bed at an appropriate and comfortable working height. Adjust the head of the bed to a flat position or as low as the patient can tolerate.	Closing the door or curtain provides for privacy. Proper bed height helps reduce back strain while you are performing the procedure. Flat positioning helps to decrease the gravitational pull of the upper body.
5. Remove all pillows from under the patient. Leave one at the head of the bed, leaning upright against the headboard.	Removing pillows from under the patient facilitates movement; placing a pillow at the head of the bed prevents accidental head injury against the top of the bed.
6. Position one nurse on either side of the bed, and lower both side rails.	Proper positioning and lowering the side rails facilitate moving the patient and minimize strain on the nurses.
7. If a drawsheet is not in place under the patient, place one under the patient's midsection.	A drawsheet supports the patient's weight and reduces friction during the lift.
8. Ask the patient (if able) to bend his or her legs and put his or her feet flat on the bed to assist with the movement.	Patient can use major muscle groups to push. Even if the patient is too weak to push on the bed, placing the legs in this fashion will assist with movement and prevent shearing of the skin on the heels.
9. **Have the patient fold the arms across the chest. Have the patient (if able) lift the head with chin on chest.**	Positioning in this manner provides assistance, reduces friction, and prevents hyperextension of the neck.

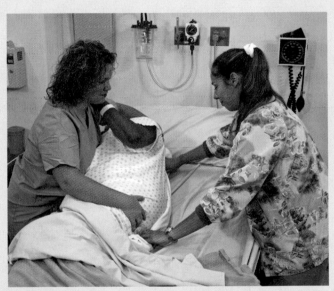

Action 7: Placing drawsheet under the patient.

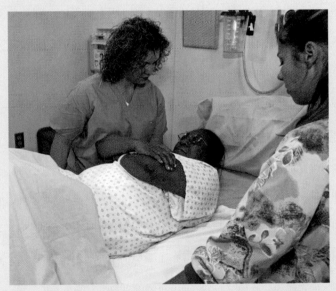

Action 9: Assisting the patient to flex the neck with chin on chest.

10. Position yourself at the patient's midsection with your feet spread shoulder width apart and one foot slightly in front of the other.	Doing so positions each nurse opposite the center of the body mass, lowers the center of gravity, and reduces the risk for injury.
11. **Fold or bunch the drawsheet close to the patient before grasping it securely and preparing to move the patient.**	Having the drawsheet close to the body brings the patient's center of gravity closer to each nurse and provides for a secure hold.
12. Flex your knees and hips. Tighten your abdominal and gluteal muscles and keep your back straight.	Using the legs' large muscle groups and tightening muscles during transfer prevent back injury.

continues

ACTION	RATIONALE

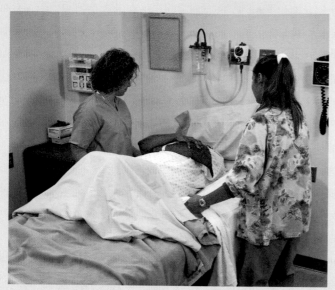

Action 10: Nurses positioned at the patient's midsection.

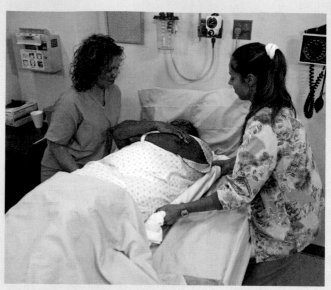

Action 11: Folding drawsheet close to the patient.

13. **Shift your weight back and forth from your back leg to your front leg and count to three. On the count of three, move the patient up in bed. If possible, the patient can assist with the move by pushing with the legs.** Repeat the process if necessary to get the patient to the right position.

The rocking motion uses the nurses' weight to counteract the patient's weight. Rocking develops momentum, which provides a smooth lift with minimal exertion by the nurses. If the patient assists, less effort is required by the nurses.

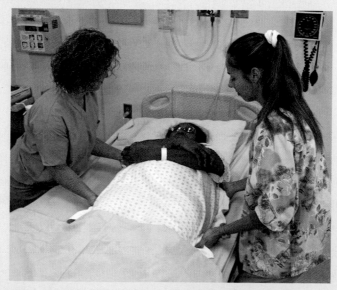

Action 14: Moving the patient up in bed to a comfortable position.

14. Assist the patient to a comfortable position and readjust the pillows and supports as needed. Raise the side rails. Place the bed in the lowest position.

Readjusting the bed with supports and side rails ensures patient safety and comfort.

15. Perform hand hygiene.

Hand hygiene prevents the spread of microorganisms.

continues

SKILL 9-3 Moving a Patient Up in Bed With the Assistance of Another Nurse (continued)

EVALUATION

The expected outcome is met when the patient is moved up in bed without injury and maintains proper body alignment, is comfortable and in the optimal position for ventilation and lung expansion, and demonstrates intact skin without evidence of any breakdown.

Unexpected Outcomes and Associated Interventions

- *You are attempting to move a patient up in the bed with another nurse. Your first attempt is unsuccessful, and you realize the patient is too heavy for only two people to transfer:* Obtain the assistance of at least two other coworkers. Position opposing pairs at the patient's shoulders and buttocks to distribute the weight. If necessary, have a fifth person lift the patient's legs or heels. The transfer of very large patients is aided by putting the bed in a slight Trendelenburg position temporarily, provided the patient can tolerate it.

Special Considerations

- When moving a patient with a leg or foot problem, such as a cast, wound, or fracture, one assistant should be assigned to lift and move that extremity.

SKILL 9-4 Transferring a Patient From the Bed to a Stretcher

While in the hospital, patients are often transported by stretcher to other areas for tests or procedures. Considerable care must be taken when moving someone from a bed to a stretcher or from a stretcher to a bed to prevent injury to the patient or staff. If the patient has an altered mental status or is unable to help, additional personnel will be required to perform this activity. When transferring patients from a bed to a stretcher, using a transfer board or roller board may help reduce strain on your back.

Equipment

- Transport stretcher
- Drawsheet
- Bath blanket
- Regular blanket
- At least two assistants, depending on the patient's condition
- Clean gloves (optional)

ASSESSMENT

Review the medical record and nursing plan of care for conditions that may influence the patient's ability to move or to be transferred. Assess for tubes, intravenous lines, incisions, or equipment that may alter the transfer process. Assess the patient's level of consciousness, ability to understand and follow directions, and ability to assist with the transfer. Assess the patient's weight and your strength to determine if additional assistance is needed. Assess the patient's comfort level; if needed, medicate as ordered with analgesics.

NURSING DIAGNOSIS

Determine the related factors for the nursing diagnoses based on the patient's current status. An appropriate nursing diagnosis is Risk for Injury. Other appropriate nursing diagnoses may include:

- Activity Intolerance
- Anxiety
- Risk for Falls
- Fear
- Acute Pain
- Risk for Impaired Skin Integrity
- Impaired Transfer Ability

continues

OUTCOME IDENTIFICATION AND PLANNING

The expected outcome to achieve when transferring a patient from the bed to a stretcher is that the patient is transferred without injury to patient or nurse.

IMPLEMENTATION

ACTION	RATIONALE
1. Review the medical record and nursing plan of care for conditions that may influence the patient's ability to move or to be positioned. Assess for tubes, intravenous lines, incisions, or equipment that may alter the positioning procedure. Identify any movement limitations.	Reviewing the medical record and plan of care validates the correct patient and correct procedure. Checking for interfering equipment helps reduce the risk for injury.
2. Identify the patient. Explain the procedure to the patient.	Patient identification validates the correct patient and correct procedure. Discussion and explanation help allay anxiety and prepare the patient for what to expect.
3. Perform hand hygiene and put on gloves, if necessary.	Hand hygiene and gloving prevent the spread of microorganisms.
4. Close the room door or curtains. Adjust the head of the bed to a flat position or as low as the patient can tolerate. Raise the bed to the same height as the transport stretcher. Lower the side rails.	Closing the door or curtain provides privacy. Proper bed height and lowering side rails makes transfer easier and decreases the risk for injury.
5. Place a drawsheet under the patient if one is not already there. Have patient fold arms against chest and move chin to chest. Use the drawsheet to move the patient to the side of the bed where the stretcher will be placed.	A drawsheet supports the patient's weight, reduces friction during the lift, and provides for a secure hold.

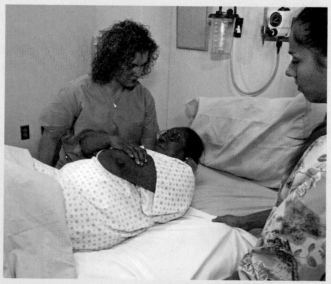

Action 5: Using the drawsheet to move the patient to the side of the bed where the stretcher will be placed.

6. Place the bath blanket over the patient and remove the top covers from underneath.	Bath blanket provides privacy and warmth.
7. Position the stretcher next to and parallel to the bed. **Lock the wheels on the stretcher and the bed.**	Positioning equipment makes the transfer easier and decreases the risk for injury. Locking the wheels keeps the bed and stretcher from moving.

continues

Transferring a Patient From the Bed to a Stretcher (continued)

ACTION

8. Remove the pillow from the bed and place it on the stretcher. The two nurses should stand on the stretcher side of the bed. The third nurse should stand on the side of the bed without the stretcher.

9. Have the nurse on the side of the bed without the stretcher kneel on the bed, with his or her knee at the upper torso closer to the patient than the other knee. Fold or bunch the drawsheet close to the patient before grasping it securely in preparation for the transfer. Use a transfer board if one is available.

RATIONALE

Team coordination provides for patient safety during transfer.

The nurse uses major muscle groups to assist in moving the patient. A transfer board makes it easier to move the patient and minimizes the risk for injury to the patient and nurses.

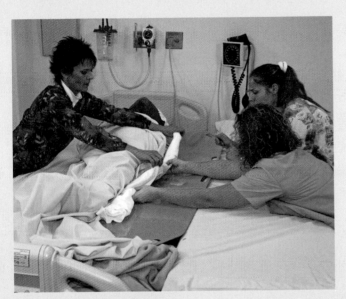

Action 9: Using a transfer board.

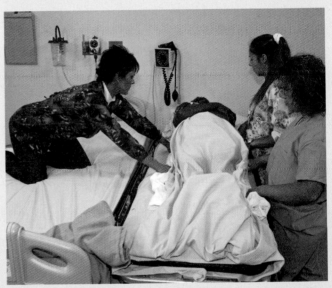

Action 12: One nurse kneeling on the bed as patient is moved to the stretcher.

10. Have one of the nurses on the stretcher side of the bed reach across the stretcher and grasp the drawsheet at the head and chest areas of the patient.

11. Have the other nurse reach across the stretcher and grasp the drawsheet at the patient's waist and thigh area.

12. **At a signal given by one of the nurses, have the nurses standing on the stretcher side of the bed pull the sheet. At the same time, the nurse kneeling on the bed should lift the patient from the bed to the stretcher.**

Doing so supports the patient's head and upper body.

Doing so supports the lower part of the patient's body.

Working in unison distributes the work of moving the patient and facilitates the transfer.

continues

SKILL
9-4   Transferring a Patient From the Bed to a Stretcher (continued)

ACTION

13. Once the patient is transferred to the stretcher, secure the patient until the side rails are raised. Raise the side rails. Ensure the patient's comfort. Cover the patient with a blanket. Leave the drawsheet in place for the return transfer.

14. Perform hand hygiene and document the time and patient's destination, according to facility policy.

RATIONALE

Side rails promote safety; blanket promotes comfort.

Hand hygiene prevents the spread of microorganisms. Documentation promotes continuity of care and communication.

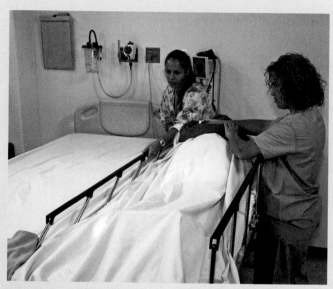

Action 13: Securing the patient.

5/12/06   1005   Patient transferred to stretcher via two-person assistance. Transported to radiology for chest x-ray.—M. Joliet, RN

Action 14: Documentation.

EVALUATION

The expected outcome is met when the patient is transferred to the stretcher without injury to patient or nurse.

Unexpected Situations and Associated Interventions

- *Your patient needs to be transported to another department by stretcher. The patient is very heavy and somewhat confused, so you are concerned about his ability to cooperate with the transfer:* Obtain the assistance of three additional coworkers. Use a transfer board to move the patient. To place the transfer board, turn the patient on his side using the drawsheet, with his back toward the stretcher. Position the transfer board lengthwise and midway between the bed and the stretcher. Return the patient to his back with the drawsheet between the patient and the board. Using the drawsheet, slide the patient across the transfer board and onto the stretcher. Reposition the patient on the stretcher, remove the board, and secure the patient on the stretcher.

Special Considerations

- The transfer of patients is often delegated to unlicensed personnel. Before moving patients, all personnel need to complete instruction about this skill and must be able to provide return demonstrations of transfer skills. When a patient is being transferred, communicate clearly any mobility restrictions or special care needs.

SKILL 9-5   Transferring a Patient From the Bed to a Chair

Often, moving a patient from the bed to a chair helps him or her begin engaging in physical activity. Also, changing a patient's position will help prevent complications related to immobility. Safety and comfort are key concerns when assisting the patient out of bed. Assessing the patient's response to activity is a major nursing responsibility. Before performing the transfer, identify any restrictions related to the patient's condition and determine how activity levels may be affected.

Equipment
- Chair or wheelchair
- Blanket to cover the patient in the chair
- Clean gloves (optional)

ASSESSMENT

Assess the situation to determine the need to get the patient out of bed. Review the medical record and nursing plan of care for conditions that may influence the patient's ability to move or to be transferred. Check for tubes, intravenous lines, incisions, or equipment that may require modifying the transfer procedure. Assess the patient's level of consciousness, ability to understand and follow directions, and ability to assist with the transfer. Assess the patient's weight and your strength to determine if additional assistance is needed. Assess the patient's comfort level; if needed, medicate as ordered with analgesics.

NURSING DIAGNOSIS

Determine the related factors for the nursing diagnoses based on the patient's current status. Appropriate nursing diagnoses may include:
- Activity Intolerance
- Risk for Activity Intolerance
- Anxiety
- Fear
- Risk for Falls
- Impaired Transfer Ability
- Acute Pain
- Chronic Pain
- Impaired Physical Mobility
- Risk for Injury

OUTCOME IDENTIFICATION AND PLANNING

The expected outcome to achieve when transferring a patient from the bed to a chair is that the transfer is accomplished without injury to patient or nurse and the patient remains free of any complications of immobility.

IMPLEMENTATION

ACTION	RATIONALE
1. Review the medical record and nursing plan of care for conditions that may influence the patient's ability to move or to be positioned. Assess for tubes, intravenous lines, incisions, or equipment that may alter the positioning procedure. Identify any movement limitations.	Reviewing the medical record and plan of care validates the correct patient and correct procedure. Identification of equipment or limitations helps reduce the risk for injury.
2. Identify the patient. Explain the procedure to the patient.	Patient identification validates the correct patient and correct procedure. Discussion and explanation help allay anxiety and prepare the patient for what to expect.
3. Perform hand hygiene and put on gloves, if necessary.	Hand hygiene and gloving prevent the spread of microorganisms.
4. If needed, move equipment to make room for the chair. Close the door or draw the curtains.	A clear pathway from the bed to the chair facilitates the transfer. Closing the door or curtain provides for privacy.

continues

ACTION

5. Place the bed in the lowest position. Raise the head of the bed to a sitting position, or as high as the patient can tolerate.

6. **Make sure the bed brakes are locked. Put the chair next to the bed, facing the foot of the bed. If available, lock the brakes of the chair. If the chair does not have brakes, brace the chair against a secure object.**

7. Assist the patient to a side-lying position, facing the side of the bed the patient will sit on. Lower the side rail if necessary and stand near the patient's hips. Stand with your legs shoulder width apart with one foot near the head of the bed, slightly in front of the other foot.

8. Ask the patient to swing his or her legs over the side of the bed. At the same time, pivot on your back leg to lift the patient's trunk and shoulders. **Keep your back straight; avoid twisting.**

RATIONALE

Proper bed height and positioning facilitate the transfer. The amount of energy needed to move from a sitting position or elevated position to a sitting position is decreased.

Locking brakes or bracing the chair prevents movement during transfer and increases stability and patient safety.

The nurse's center of gravity is placed near the patient's greatest weight to safely assist the patient to a sitting position.

Gravity lowers the patient's legs over the bed. The nurse transfers weight in the direction of motion and protects his or her back from injury.

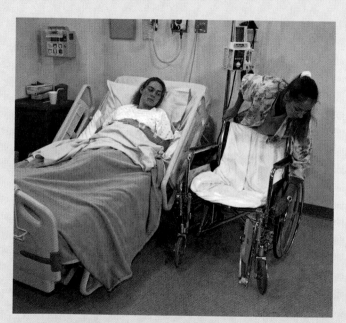

Action 6: Putting the chair next to the bed, facing the foot of the bed, and locking the brakes.

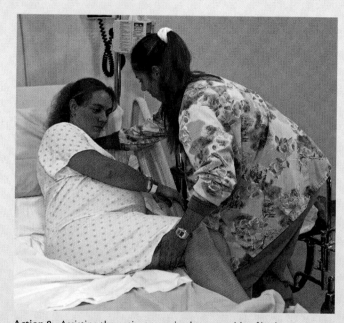

Action 8: Assisting the patient to swing legs over side of bed.

9. **Stand in front of the patient, and assess for any balance problems or complaints of dizziness. Allow legs to dangle a few minutes before continuing.**

10. Assist the patient to put on a robe and nonskid footwear.

11. Stand facing the patient. Spread your feet about shoulder width apart and flex your hips and knees.

Standing in front of the patient prevents falls or injuries from orthostatic hypotension. The sitting position facilitates transfer to the chair and allows the circulatory system to adjust to a change in position.

Robe provides warmth and privacy. Nonskid soles reduce the risk for falling.

This position provides stability and allows for smooth movement using the legs' large muscle groups.

continues

Transferring a Patient From the Bed to a Chair (continued)

ACTION

12. Place your hands around the patient's waist while the patient holds on to you with one hand on your shoulder and the other hand on your waist. Apply a transfer belt if necessary.

13. Ask the patient to slide his or her buttocks to the edge of the bed until the feet touch the floor. Position yourself as close as possible to the patient, with your foot positioned on the outside of the patient's foot.

14. Rock back and forth while counting to three. **On the count of three, use your legs (not your back) to help raise the patient to a standing position. If indicated, brace your front knee against the patient's weak extremity as he or she stands.**

15. Pivot on your back foot until the patient feels the chair against his or her legs.

16. Ask the patient to use an arm to steady himself or herself on the arm of the chair while slowly lowering to a sitting position. **Continue to brace the patient's knees with your knees. Flex your hips and knees when helping the patient sit in the chair.**

RATIONALE

This positioning avoids injury to the nurse if the patient should fall and grasp the nurse around the neck.

Doing so provides balance and support.

Rocking prevents muscle strain by providing momentum and requiring less of the nurse's energy to lift. Bracing your knee against a weak extremity prevents a weak knee from buckling and the patient from falling.

This action ensures proper positioning before sitting.

The patient uses his or her own arm for support and stability. Flexing hips and knees uses major muscle groups to aid in movement and reduce strain on the nurse's back.

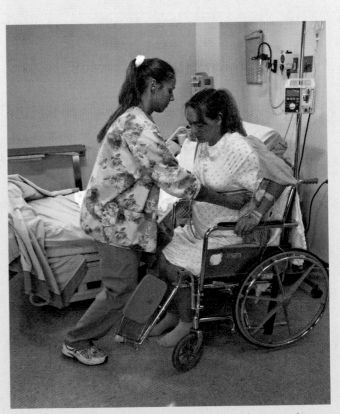

Action 14: Nurse using her own legs to help raise the patient to a standing position.

Action 16: Patient using her own arms to remain steady. Nurse using good body mechanics.

continues

Transferring a Patient From the Bed to a Chair (continued)

ACTION	RATIONALE
17. Assess the patient's alignment in the chair. Cover with a blanket if needed. Place the call bell close.	Assessment promotes comfort; blanket provides warmth and privacy; having the call bell readily available helps promote safety.
18. Perform hand hygiene. Document the activity, including the length of time the patient sat in the chair, any observations, and the patient's tolerance of and reaction to the activity.	Hand hygiene prevents the spread of microorganisms. Documentation promotes continuity of care and communication.

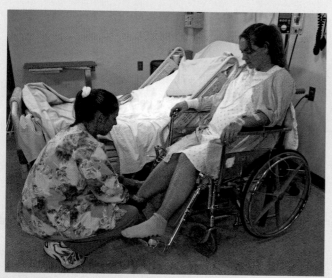

Action 17: Assessing the patient's alignment in the chair.

> 5/13/06 1135   Patient dangled at side of bed for 5 minutes without complaints of dizziness or lightheadedness. Patient assisted out of bed to chair with minimal difficulty; tolerated sitting in chair for 30 minutes. Assisted back to bed, in semi-Fowler's position. Both side rails up.—J. Minkins, RN

Action 18: Documentation.

EVALUATION

The expected outcome is met when the patient transfers from the bed to the chair without injury and exhibits no signs and symptoms of problems or complications related to immobility. In addition, the nurse remains free of injury during the transfer.

Unexpected Situations and Associated Interventions

- *You are assisting a patient out of bed. The previous times the patient has gotten up, you have not had any difficulty helping him by yourself, so you are working alone this time. The patient is positioned on the side of the bed. You flex your hips and knees to help him stand. As you move to pivot to the chair, the patient becomes very lightheaded and weak and his knees buckle. The patient is too heavy for you to lift to the chair:* Do not continue the move to the chair. Lower the patient back to the side of the bed. Pivot him back into bed, cover him, and raise the side rails. Check vital signs and assess for any other symptoms. After his symptoms have subsided and you are ready to get him up again, arrange for the assistance of another staff member. Have the patient dangle his legs for a longer period of time before standing. Assess for lightheadedness or dizziness before helping him stand up. Notify the physician if there are any significant findings or if his symptoms persist.

Special Considerations

- The transfer of patients is often delegated to unlicensed personnel. Before moving patients, all personnel need to complete instruction and must be able to provide return demonstrations of transfer skills. Before the transfer, communicate clearly any mobility restrictions or special care needs.

Transferring a Patient From the Bed to a Chair With the Assistance of Another Nurse

Depending on the patient's ability to assist with a transfer, it is often safer and simpler to have two nurses assist with the activity. Good body mechanics and teamwork during this transfer will help prevent injury to you, your coworker, and the patient. If the bed and chair seat are not the same height, more than one person should be involved in transferring the patient.

Equipment

- Chair or wheelchair
- Blanket to cover the patient
- Coworker to assist
- Chair transfer board, if indicated
- Clean gloves (optional)

ASSESSMENT

Assess the situation to determine the need to get the patient out of bed. Review the medical record and nursing plan of care for conditions that may influence the patient's ability to move or to be transferred. Assess for tubes, intravenous lines, incisions, or equipment that may alter the transfer procedure. Assess the patient's level of consciousness, ability to understand and follow directions, and ability to assist with the transfer. Assess the patient's weight and your strength to determine if additional assistance is needed. Assess the patient's comfort level; if needed, medicate as ordered with analgesics.

NURSING DIAGNOSIS

Determine the related factors for the nursing diagnoses based on the patient's current status. Appropriate nursing diagnoses may include:

- Activity Intolerance
- Risk for Activity Intolerance
- Anxiety
- Fear
- Risk for Falls
- Impaired Transfer Ability
- Acute Pain
- Chronic Pain
- Impaired Physical Mobility
- Risk for Injury

OUTCOME IDENTIFICATION AND PLANNING

The expected outcome to achieve when transferring a patient from the bed to a chair is that the transfer is accomplished without injury to patient or nurse and complications of immobility are prevented.

IMPLEMENTATION

ACTION	RATIONALE
1. Review the medical record and nursing plan of care for conditions that may influence the patient's ability to move or to be positioned. Assess for tubes, intravenous lines, incisions, or equipment that may alter the positioning procedure. Identify any movement limitations.	Review of medical record and plan of care validates the correct patient and correct procedure. Checking for equipment and limitations helps minimize the risk for injury.
2. Identify the patient. Explain the procedure to the patient.	Patient identification validates the correct patient and correct procedure. Discussion and explanation help allay anxiety and prepare the patient for what to expect.
3. Perform hand hygiene and put on gloves, if necessary.	Hand hygiene and gloving prevent the spread of microorganisms.

continues

ACTION	RATIONALE
4. If needed, move the equipment to make room for the chair. Close the door or draw the curtains.	Moving equipment out of the way provides a clear path and facilitates the transfer. Closing the door or curtain provides for privacy.
5. **Make sure the bed brakes are locked.** Adjust the height of the bed to a comfortable working height, or to the level of the armrest (if one is present) on the chair.	Locking bed brakes increases stability and patient safety. Having the bed at the proper height facilitates the transfer with minimal muscle strain on the nurses.
6. Move the patient to the near side of the bed and have patient cross his or her arms on the chest if possible. Position the chair next to the bed near the upper end, with the back of the chair parallel to the head of the bed. If possible, remove the armrest closest to the bed. Lock the chair wheels, if available. Use a chair transfer board if appropriate.	Moving the patient to the near side of the bed allows the nurses to expend less effort when moving the patient. A transfer board makes it easier to move the patient and minimizes the risk of injury to the patient and nurses.
7. Prepare to lift the patient from the bed to the chair. Have the lead nurse stand behind the chair and slip his or her arms under the patient's axillae and grasp the patient's wrists securely. The second nurse faces the wheelchair and supports the patient's knees by placing his or her arms under the patient's knees.	Positioning in this manner minimizes muscle strain on the nurses.
8. On a predetermined signal, flex your hips and knees, keeping your back straight, and simultaneously lift the patient and gently lower the patient into the chair.	Having two people lift the patient distributes the weight and decreases the effort needed for the transfer.

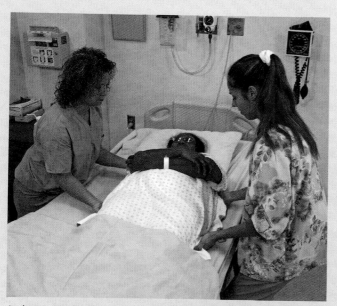

Action 6: Moving the patient to the edge of the bed.

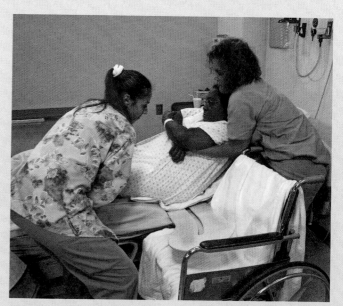

Action 7: Preparing to lift the patient using a chair transfer board.

continues

ACTION   **RATIONALE**

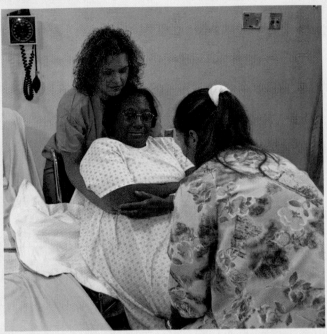

Action 8: Lifting patient into chair.

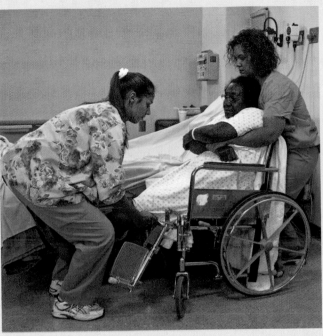

Action 8: Lowering the patient gently into the chair.

9. Adjust the patient's position using pillows if necessary. Check the patient's alignment in the chair. Cover him or her with a blanket if necessary. Place the call bell within reach.

These actions provide for patient safety and comfort.

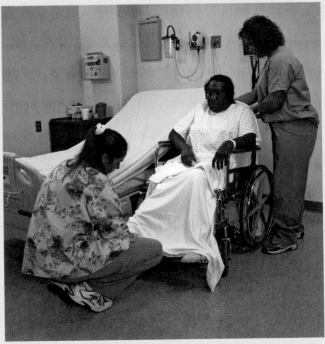

Action 9: Adjusting the patient's position, using pillows if necessary, and checking the patient's alignment in the chair.

continues

ACTION	RATIONALE
10. Perform hand hygiene. Document the activity, transfer, any observations, the patient's tolerance of the procedure, and the length of time in the chair.	Hand hygiene prevents the spread of microorganisms. Documentation promotes continuity of care and communication.

5/10/06   1310   Patient transferred with two-person assistance via chair transfer board to wheelchair. Patient out of bed to chair for 10 minutes. Patient complained of dizziness; skin pale and slightly moist. Pulse increased 15 beats from baseline; blood pressure decreased to 100/50 mm Hg from baseline of 112/60 mm Hg. Transferred back to bed. Lying with head of bed elevated 15 degrees and side rails up. Pulse rate and blood pressure returned to baseline after 5 minutes of returning to bed.
—P. Collins, RN

Action 10: Documentation.

EVALUATION

The expected outcome is met when the transfer is accomplished without injury to patient or nurse and complications of immobility are prevented.

Unexpected Situations and Associated Interventions

- *You and a coworker are attempting to get a patient out of bed using the previously described transfer method for two nurses. You cannot lift the patient high enough to get him out of the bed, over the armrest, and into the chair:* Stop trying: you, your coworker, or the patient could be injured. Use a hydraulic lift to transfer the patient into the chair.

Special Considerations

- The transfer of patients is often delegated to unlicensed personnel. Before moving patients, all personnel need to complete instruction and must be able to provide return demonstrations of transfer skills. Before the transfer, communicate clearly any mobility restrictions or special care needs.

SKILL 9-7   Transferring a Patient Using a Hydraulic Lift

A hydraulic device such as the Hoyer lift is a mechanical device that permits a patient to be transferred from the bed to a chair. It is used when transferring a patient poses a risk for injury to the nurses or the patient. The patient is positioned in a sling that is attached to the device by straps or chains. The lift raises the patient up off the bed, moves the patient clear of the bed, and lowers the patient into the chair. Each manufacturer's device is slightly different, so review the instructions for your particular device.

Equipment
- Hydraulic lift
- Sheet or pad to cover the sling
- Chair or wheelchair
- Clean gloves (optional)

ASSESSMENT

Assess the situation to determine the need to use the hydraulic lift. Review the medical record and nursing plan of care for conditions that may influence the patient's ability to move or to be transferred. Assess for tubes, intravenous lines, incisions, or equipment that may alter the transfer procedure. Assess the patient's level of consciousness and ability to understand and follow directions. Assess the patient's comfort level; if needed, medicate as ordered with analgesics. Assess the condition of the equipment.

NURSING DIAGNOSIS

Determine the related factors for the nursing diagnoses based on the patient's current status. Nursing diagnoses that may be appropriate include:
- Activity Intolerance
- Anxiety
- Fear
- Risk for Injury
- Acute Pain
- Chronic Pain
- Impaired Transfer Ability
- Risk for Falls

OUTCOME IDENTIFICATION AND PLANNING

The expected outcome to achieve when transferring a patient from the bed to a chair using a hydraulic lift is that the transfer is accomplished without injury to patient or nurse and the patient is free of any complications of immobility.

IMPLEMENTATION

ACTION	RATIONALE
1. Review the medical record and nursing plan of care for conditions that may influence the patient's ability to move or to be positioned. Assess for tubes, intravenous lines, incisions, or equipment that may alter the positioning procedure. Identify any movement limitations.	Reviewing the medical record and plan of care validates the correct patient and correct procedure. Checking for equipment and limitations reduces the risk for injury during the transfer.
2. Identify the patient. Explain the procedure to the patient.	Patient identification validates the correct patient and correct procedure. Discussion and explanation allay anxiety and prepare the patient for what to expect.
3. Perform hand hygiene and put on gloves, if necessary.	Hand hygiene and gloving prevent the spread of microorganisms.
4. If needed, move the equipment to make room for the chair. Close the door or draw the curtains.	Moving equipment out of the way provides a clear path and facilitates the transfer. Closing the door or curtain provides for privacy.

continues

Transferring a Patient Using a Hydraulic Lift (continued)

ACTION

RATIONALE

5. Bring the chair to the side of the bed. **Lock the wheels, if present.**

Bringing the chair close to the bed minimizes the distance needed for transfer. Locking the wheels prevents chair movement and ensures patient safety.

6. Adjust the bed to a comfortable working height. **Lock the bed brakes.**

Having the bed at the proper height prevents back and muscle strain. Locking the brakes prevents bed movement and ensures patient safety.

7. Place the sling evenly under the patient. Roll the patient to one side and place half of the sling with the sheet or pad on it under the patient from shoulders to midthigh. Roll the patient to the other side and pull the sling under the patient.

Rolling the patient positions the patient on the sling with minimal movement. Even distribution of the patient's weight in the sling provides for patient comfort and safety.

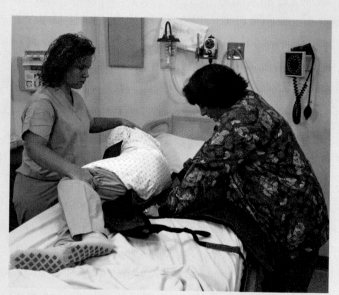

Action 7: Rolling the patient to one side and placing the rolled sling underneath the patient.

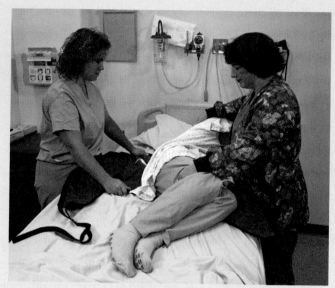

Action 7: Rolling the patient to the opposite side and flattening out sling under the patient.

8. **Roll the base of the lift under the side of the bed nearest to the chair. Center the frame over the patient. Lock the wheels of the lift.**

Doing so reduces the distance necessary for transfer. Centering the frame helps maintain the balance of the lift. Locking the lift's wheels prevents the lift from rolling.

9. Using the base-adjustment lever, widen the stance of the base.

A wider stance provides greater stability and prevents tipping.

10. Lower the arms close enough to attach the sling to the frame.

Lowering the arms is necessary to allow for the attachment of the sling's hooks.

11. Place the strap or chain hooks through the holes of the sling. Short straps attach behind the patient's back and long straps at the other end. Check the patient to make sure the hooks are not pressing into the skin. Some lifts have straps on the sling that attach to hooks on the frame. Check the manufacturer's instructions for each lift.

Connecting the straps or chains permits attachment of the sling to the lift. Checking the patient's skin for pressure from the hooks prevents injury.

continues

ACTION   **RATIONALE**

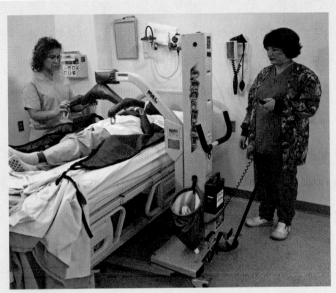

Action 9: Spreading the base of the Hoyer lift.

Action 10: Lowering the arms of the Hoyer lift.

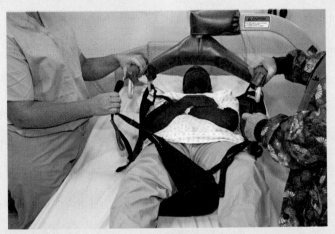

Action 11: Connecting the straps to the lift.

12. Check all equipment, lines, and drains attached to the patient so that they are not interfering with the device. Have the patient fold his or her arms across the chest.

Ensuring that equipment and lines are free of the device prevents dislodgement and possible injury.

13. With a person standing on each side of the lift, tell the patient that he or she will be lifted from the bed. Support injured limbs as necessary. Engage the pump to raise the patient about 6″ above the bed.

Having the necessary persons available provides for safety. Supporting injured limbs helps maintain stability. Informing the patient about what will occur reassures the patient and reduces fear.

14. Unlock the wheels of the lift. **Carefully wheel the patient straight back and away from the bed.** Support the patient's limbs as needed.

Moving in this manner promotes stability and safety.

15. Position the patient over the chair with the base of the lift straddling the chair. Lock the wheels of the lift.

Proper positioning of the patient and device promotes stability and safety.

continues

ACTION   **RATIONALE**

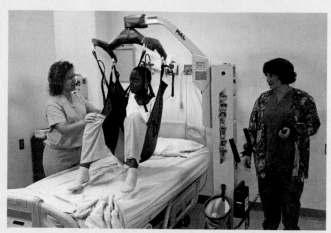

Action 13: Raising the patient 6" above the bed.

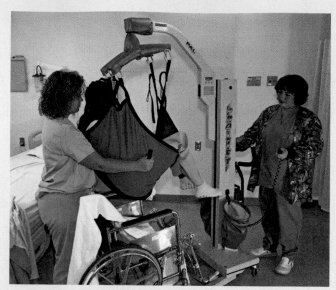

Action 15: Positioning the patient in the sling over the chair.

16. Gently lower the patient to the chair until the hooks or straps are slightly loosened from the sling or frame. Guide the patient into the chair with your hands as the sling lowers.

Gently lowering the patient in this manner places the patient fully in the chair and reduces the risk for injury.

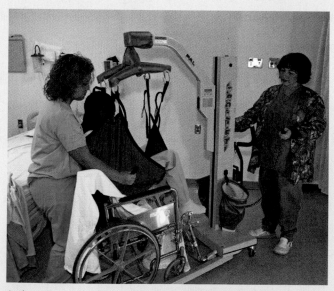

Action 16: Lowering the patient in the sling into the chair.

17. Disconnect the hooks or strap from the frame. Keep the sling in place under the patient.

Disconnecting the hooks or straps allows the patient to be supported by the chair and promotes comfort. The sling will need to be reattached to the lift to move the patient back to bed.

continues

ACTION	RATIONALE
18. Adjust the patient's position using pillows if necessary. Check the patient's alignment in the chair. Cover the patient with a blanket if necessary. Place the call bell within reach. When it is time for the patient to return to bed, reattach the hooks or straps and reverse the steps.	Pillows and proper alignment provide for patient safety and comfort. Reattaching the hooks or straps allows the lift to support the patient for transfer back to bed.
19. Perform hand hygiene. Document the activity, transfer, any observations, the patient's tolerance of the procedure, and the length of time in the chair.	Hand hygiene prevents the spread of microorganisms. Documentation promotes continuity of care and communication.

> 5/13/06   1430   Patient transferred out of bed to chair using hydraulic lift. Tolerated sitting in chair for 25 minutes without complaints of dizziness or pain. Assisted back to bed via hydraulic lift. Left sitting in semi-Fowler's position with all four side rails up.—P. Jefferson, RN

Action 19: Documentation.

EVALUATION   The expected outcome is met when the transfer is accomplished without injury to patient or nurse and the patient exhibits no evidence of complications of immobility.

Unexpected Situations and Associated Interventions

- *You are preparing to move a patient using a hydraulic lift. After you apply the sling and attach it to the frame, the patient becomes anxious and tells you she is afraid:* Acknowledge the patient's feelings and explain the procedure again. Reassure the patient about the safety of the device. Obtain an additional person to support the patient during the move by holding her hand or supporting her head. If possible, plan the transfer when a family member or friend is present to offer support.

Special Considerations

- The transfer of patients is often delegated to unlicensed personnel. Before moving patients, all personnel need to complete instruction and must be able to provide return demonstrations of transfer skills. Before the transfer, communicate clearly any mobility restrictions or special care needs.

SKILL 9-8   Assisting a Patient With Ambulation

Walking exercises most of the body's muscles and increases joint flexibility. It improves respiratory and gastrointestinal function. Ambulating also reduces the risk for complications of immobility. However, even a short period of immobility can decrease a person's tolerance for ambulating.

Equipment

- Transfer belt (optional, based on patient status and facility policy)
- Nonskid shoes or slippers
- Additional staff for assistance as needed

ASSESSMENT

Assess the patient's ability to walk and the need for assistance. Review the patient's record for conditions that may affect ambulation. Perform a pain assessment prior to the time for the activity. If the patient reports pain, administer the prescribed medication in sufficient time to allow for the full effect of the analgesic. Take vital signs and assess the patient for dizziness or lightheadedness with position changes.

NURSING DIAGNOSIS

Determine the related factors for the nursing diagnoses based on the patient's current status. An appropriate nursing diagnosis is Impaired Physical Mobility. Other nursing diagnoses that may be appropriate include:

- Risk for Injury
- Activity Intolerance
- Impaired Comfort
- Risk for Falls
- Fatigue
- Acute Pain
- Chronic Pain
- Impaired Walking

OUTCOME IDENTIFICATION AND PLANNING

The expected outcome to achieve when assisting a patient with ambulation is that the patient ambulates safely, without falls or injury. Additional appropriate outcomes include the patient demonstrates improved muscle strength and joint mobility; the patient's level of independence increases; and the patient remains free of complications of immobility.

IMPLEMENTATION

ACTION	RATIONALE
1. Review the medical record and nursing plan of care for conditions that may influence the patient's ability to move and ambulate. Assess for tubes, intravenous lines, incisions, or equipment that may alter the procedure for ambulation. Identify any movement limitations.	Reviewing the medical record and plan of care validates the correct patient and correct procedure. Checking for equipment and limitations reduces the risk for patient injury.
2. Identify the patient. Explain the procedure to the patient. Ask the patient to report any feelings of dizziness, weakness, or shortness of breath while walking. Decide how far to walk.	Patient identification validates the correct patient and correct procedure. Discussion and explanation help allay anxiety and prepare the patient for what to expect.
3. Perform hand hygiene.	Hand hygiene prevents the spread of microorganisms.
4. Place the bed in the lowest position.	Proper bed height ensures safety when getting the patient out of bed.
5. Assist the patient to the side of the bed. Have the patient sit on the side of the bed for several minutes and assess for dizziness or lightheadedness. Have the patient stay sitting until he or she feels secure.	Having the patient sit at the side of the bed minimizes the risk for blood pressure changes (orthostatic hypotension) that can occur with position change. Allowing the patient to sit until he or she feels secure reduces anxiety and helps prevent injury.

continues

Assisting a Patient With Ambulation (continued)

ACTION

6. Assist the patient to don footwear and a robe, if desired.

7. Wrap the transfer belt around the patient's waist, based on assessed need and facility policy.

8. Assist the patient to stand. Have the patient hold your waist or shoulders for support when standing, if needed. Assess the patient's balance and leg strength. If the patient is weak or unsteady, return the patient to bed or assist to a chair.

9. If you are the only nurse assisting, position yourself to the side and slightly behind the patient. Support the patient by the waist or transfer belt.

   a. When two nurses assist, position yourself to the side and slightly behind the patient, supporting the patient by the waist or transfer belt. Have the other nurse carry or manage equipment or provide additional support from the other side.

   b. Alternatively, when two nurses assist, stand at the patient's sides (one nurse on each side) with near hands grasping the inferior aspect of the patient's near upper arm and far hands holding the patient's lower arm or hand.

RATIONALE

Doing so ensures safety and patient warmth.

Transfer belt provides for a safe, firm hold and minimizes the risk for injury.

Holding at the waist or shoulders prevents injury to the nurse. Assessing balance and strength helps to identify need for additional assistance to prevent falling.

Positioning to the side and slightly behind the patient encourages the patient to stand and walk erect. It also places the nurse in a safe position if the patient should lose his or her balance or begin to fall. With two nurses, grasping the patient's arms as described provides additional support to the patient and distributes the patient's weight equally.

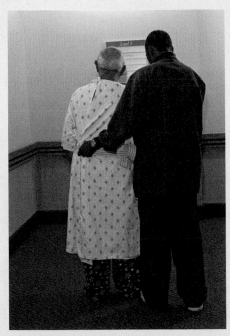

Action 9: Nurse positioned to the side and slightly behind the patient while walking, supporting the patient by the waist or transfer belt.

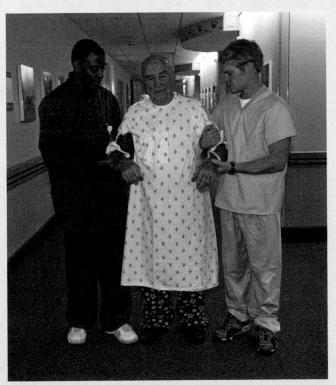

Action 9b: Two nurses holding the patient's upper arms and supporting lower arms or hands.

continues

ACTION	RATIONALE

c. Alternatively, when two nurses assist, stand at the patient's sides (one nurse on each side) and slip near arms under the patient's arms and around his or her back, grasping each other's arms. Have the patient stretch his or her arms over the nurses' shoulders and then grasp your far hands.

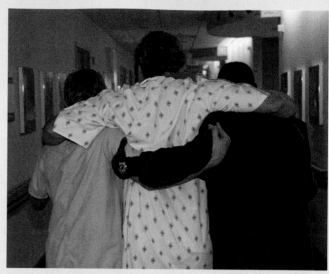

Action 9c: Two nurses grasping each other's arms behind the patient's back, with the patient's arms stretched over the nurses' shoulders.

10. Take several steps forward with the patient. **Continue to assess the patient's strength and balance.** Remind patient to stand erect.

Taking several steps with the patient and standing erect promote good balance and stability. Continued assessment helps maintain patient safety.

11. Continue with ambulation for the planned distance and time. Return the patient to the bed or chair based on the patient's tolerance and condition.

Ambulation as prescribed promotes activity and prevents fatigue.

12. Perform hand hygiene. Document the activity, any observations, the patient's tolerance of the procedure, and the distance walked.

Hand hygiene prevents the spread of microorganisms. Documentation promotes continuity of care and communication.

> 5/14/06   1720   Patient ambulated with as-
> sistance in hallway for a distance of approxi-
> mately 15 feet. Patient tolerated ambulation
> well; denied any complaints of dizziness, pain,
> or fatigue. Ambulated back to room and sitting
> in chair listening to music.—J. Minkins, RN

Action 12: Documentation.

EVALUATION

The expected outcome is met when the patient ambulates safely for the prescribed distance and time and remains free from falls or injury. Additional outcomes are met when the patient exhibits increasing muscle strength, joint mobility, and independence and the patient remains free of any signs and symptoms of immobility.

continues

SKILL 9-8 Assisting a Patient With Ambulation (continued)

Unexpected Situations and Associated Interventions

- *You are walking with a postoperative patient in the hallway. She tells you she feels faint and begins to lean over as if she is going to fall:* Place your feet wide apart, with one foot in front. Rock your pelvis out on the side nearest the patient. This widens and stabilizes the base of support. Put your arms under the patient's axillae and encircle the patient. This ensures a safe hold on the patient. Support the patient by pulling her weight backward against your body. Gently slide her down your body to the floor, protecting her head. This enables you to support the patient's weight with large muscle groups and protects you from back strain. Stay with the patient. Call for help. If another staff member was assisting you with ambulation, each of you should use one hand to support the patient under the axillae and grasp the patient's hand or wrist with your other hands. Slowly lower her to the floor. If a transfer belt is in place, grasp the belt to steady and lower the patient.

Special Considerations

- All equipment, such as indwelling urinary catheters, drains, or intravenous infusions, should be secured to a pole for ambulation. Do not carry equipment while helping the patient. Your hands should be free to provide support.

SKILL 9-9 Assisting a Patient With Ambulation Using a Walker

A walker is a lightweight metal frame with four legs. Nonskid caps cover the end of the legs to prevent slipping. Walkers provide stability and security for patients with insufficient strength and balance to use other ambulatory aids. There are several kinds of walkers; the choice of which to use is based on the patient's arm strength and balance. Sometimes two of the leg caps are replaced with slides or wheels so the patient can push the walker instead of picking it up to move forward. The walker should extend from the floor to the patient's hip joint. The patient's elbows should be flexed about 30 degrees. Usually, the legs of the walker can be adjusted to the appropriate height.

Equipment

- Walker adjusted to the appropriate height
- Nonskid shoes or slippers
- Additional staff for assistance as needed

ASSESSMENT

Assess the patient's ability to walk and the need for assistance. Review the patient's record for conditions that may affect ambulation. Perform a pain assessment prior to the time for the activity. If the patient reports pain, administer the prescribed medication in sufficient time to allow for the full effect of the analgesic. Take vital signs and assess the patient for dizziness or lightheadedness with position changes. Assess the patient's knowledge regarding the use of a walker.

NURSING DIAGNOSIS

Determine the related factors for the nursing diagnoses based on the patient's current status. An appropriate nursing diagnosis is Risk for Falls. Other nursing diagnoses that may be appropriate include:

- Deficient Knowledge
- Risk for Injury
- Activity Intolerance
- Impaired Comfort
- Fatigue
- Acute Pain
- Chronic Pain
- Impaired Walking

continues

SKILL 9-9   Assisting a Patient With Ambulation Using a Walker (continued)

OUTCOME IDENTIFICATION AND PLANNING

The expected outcome to achieve when assisting a patient with ambulation using a walker is that the patient ambulates safely with the walker and is free from falls or injury. Additional appropriate outcomes include: the patient demonstrates proper use of the walker and states the need for the walker; the patient demonstrates increasing muscle strength, joint mobility, and independence; and the patient remains free of complications of immobility.

IMPLEMENTATION

ACTION	RATIONALE
1. Review the medical record and nursing plan of care for conditions that may influence the patient's ability to move and ambulate and for specific instructions for ambulation such as distance. Assess for tubes, intravenous lines, incisions, or equipment that may alter the procedure for ambulation. Assess the patient's knowledge and previous experience regarding the use of a walker. Identify any movement limitations.	Reviewing the medical record and plan of care validates the correct patient and correct procedure. Checking for equipment and limitations helps minimize the risk for injury.
2. Identify the patient. Explain the procedure to the patient. Tell the patient to report any feelings of dizziness, weakness, or shortness of breath while walking. Decide how far to walk.	Patient identification validates the correct patient and correct procedure. Discussion and explanation help allay anxiety and prepare the patient for what to expect.
3. Perform hand hygiene.	Hand hygiene prevents the spread of microorganisms.
4. Place the bed in the lowest position.	Proper bed height ensures safety when getting the patient out of bed.
5. Assist the patient to the side of the bed. Have the patient sit on the side of the bed. Assess for dizziness or light-headedness. Have the patient stay sitting until he or she feels secure. Alternatively, assist the patient to a chair.	Having the patient sit on the side of the bed minimizes the risk for blood pressure changes (orthostatic hypotension) that can occur with position change. Assessing patient complaints helps prevent injury.
6. Assist the patient to don footwear and a robe, if desired.	Doing so ensures safety and warmth.
7. **Place the walker directly in front of the patient.** Ask the patient to push himself or herself off the bed, or assist the patient to stand if seated in a chair. Assist the patient to stand within the walker, if necessary. Once the patient is standing, have him or her hold the walker's hand grips firmly and equally. The nurse should stand slightly behind the patient, on one side.	Proper positioning with the walker ensures balance. Standing within the walker and holding the hand grips firmly provide stability when moving the walker and helps ensure safety.
8. Have the patient move the walker forward 6″ to 8″ and set it down, making sure all four feet of the walker stay on the floor. Then, tell the patient to step forward with either foot into the walker, supporting himself or herself on his or her arms. Follow through with the other leg. **If one leg is weaker or impaired, have the patient step forward with the involved leg and follow with the uninvolved leg, again supporting himself or herself on his or her arms.**	Having all four feet of the walker on the floor provides a broad base of support. Moving the walker and stepping forward moves the center of gravity toward the walker, ensuring balance and preventing tipping of the walker.
9. Move the walker forward again, and continue the same pattern. Continue with ambulation for the planned distance and time. Return the patient to the bed or chair based on the patient's tolerance and condition.	Moving the walker promotes activity. Continuing for the planned distance and time prevents the patient from becoming fatigued.
10. Perform hand hygiene. Document the activity, any observations, the patient's ability to use the walker, the patient's tolerance of the procedure, and the distance walked.	Hand hygiene prevents the spread of microorganisms. Documentation promotes continuity of care and communication.

continues

Assisting a Patient With Ambulation Using a Walker (continued)

ACTION   **RATIONALE**

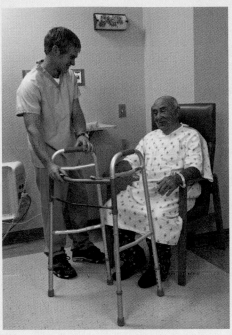

Action 7: Setting the walker in front of a seated patient.

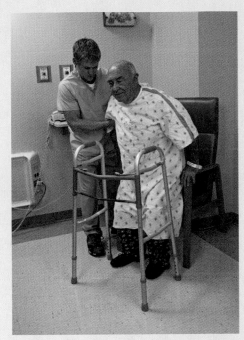

Action 7: Assisting the patient to stand with the walker.

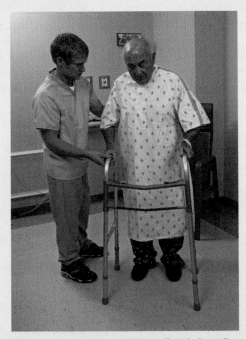

Action 8: Assisting the patient to walk with the walker.

5/15/06   0900   Patient ambulated with walker from bed to bathroom for morning care with minimal assistance; demonstrated proper steps in using walker. Able to ambulate back to bed using walker independently.
—P. Collins, RN

Action 10: Documentation.

continues

EVALUATION

The expected outcome is met when the patient uses the walker to ambulate safely and remains free of injury. Other outcomes are met when the patient exhibits increased muscle strength, joint mobility, and independence; demonstrates independent walker use; and exhibits no evidence of complications of immobility.

Unexpected Situations and Associated Special Considerations

- *You are assisting a patient ambulating in the hallway using a walker. She becomes extremely tired and says she can't pick up the walker anymore ("it's too heavy"). However, she cannot walk without the walker:* Call for assistance. Have a coworker obtain a wheelchair to transport the patient back to her room. Assess the patient for other symptoms, if necessary. In the future, plan to ambulate for shorter distances to prevent her from becoming fatigued.

Interventions

- Never use a walker on the stairs.
- Advise the patient to check the walker before use for signs of damage, deformity of the frame, or loose or missing parts.
- Teach patients to use the arms of the chair for leverage when getting up from a chair. Patients should not pull on the walker to get up; the walker could tip or become unbalanced.

**SKILL
9-10   Assisting a Patient With Ambulation Using Crutches**

Crutches can be used for the short or long term. Crutches enable a patient to walk and remove weight from one or both legs. Crutches are often used when the patient has a sprain, fracture, or nonwalking cast. The patient uses the arms to support the body weight. A short-term crutch, known as an underarm or axillary crutch, is a wooden or metal staff that extends from the floor to below the axilla. Crutches used for the long term provide additional support for weak or paralyzed legs. Long-term crutches, known as forearm support crutches, are metal and extend from the floor to the forearm, with metal bands encircling the forearms. This section will discuss short-term crutch use.

There are five crutch gaits, or patterns, for walking. The four-point gait is used by patients who can bear weight on both legs. It is the safest but requires good coordination. The two-point gait is used for patients with leg weakness but with good coordination and arm strength. The three-point gait is used with patients who can bear only partial or no weight on one leg. The swing-to and swing-through gaits are used by patients with paralysis of the hips and legs.

Equipment

- Crutches with axillary pads, hand grips, and rubber suction tips
- Nonskid shoes or slippers

ASSESSMENT

Review the patient's record and nursing plan of care to determine the reason for using crutches and instructions for weight bearing. Check for specific instructions from physical therapy. Perform a pain assessment prior to the time for the activity. If the patient reports pain, administer the prescribed medication in sufficient time to allow for the full effect of the analgesic. Determine the patient's knowledge regarding the use of crutches and assess the patient's ability to balance on the crutches. Assess for muscle strength in the legs and arms. Determine the appropriate gait for the patient to use.

continues

SKILL 9-10

Assisting a Patient With Ambulation Using Crutches (continued)

NURSING DIAGNOSIS

Determine the related factors for the nursing diagnoses based on the patient's current status. An appropriate nursing diagnosis is Risk for Injury. Other nursing diagnoses that may be appropriate include:

- Deficient Knowledge
- Risk for Falls
- Activity Intolerance
- Impaired Comfort
- Fatigue
- Acute Pain
- Chronic Pain
- Impaired Walking

OUTCOME IDENTIFICATION AND PLANNING

The expected outcome to achieve when assisting a patient with ambulation using crutches is that the patient ambulates safely without experiencing falls or injury. Additional appropriate outcomes include: the patient demonstrates proper crutch-walking technique; demonstrates increased muscle strength and joint mobility; and exhibits no evidence of injury related to crutch use.

IMPLEMENTATION

ACTION	RATIONALE
1. Review the medical record and nursing plan of care for conditions that may influence the patient's ability to move and ambulate. Assess for tubes, intravenous lines, incisions, or equipment that may alter the procedure for ambulation. Assess the patient's knowledge and previous experience regarding the use of crutches. Determine that the appropriate size crutch has been obtained.	Reviewing the medical record and plan of care validates the correct patient and correct procedure. Assessment helps identify problem areas to minimize the risk for injury.
2. Identify the patient. Explain the procedure to the patient. Tell the patient to report any feelings of dizziness, weakness, or shortness of breath while walking. Decide how far to walk.	Patient identification validates the correct patient and correct procedure. Discussion and explanation help allay anxiety and prepare the patient for what to expect.
3. Perform hand hygiene.	Hand hygiene prevents the spread of microorganisms.
4. Assist the patient to stand erect, face forward in the tripod position. This means the patient holds the crutches 6″ in front of and 6″ to the side of each foot.	Positioning the crutches in this manner provides a wide base of support to increase stability and balance
5. For the four-point gait:	This movement ensures stability and safety.
a. Have the patient move the right crutch forward 6″ and then move the left foot forward to the level of the right crutch.	
b. Then have the patient move the left crutch forward 6″ and then move the right foot forward to the level of the left crutch.	
6. For the three-point gait:	Patient continues to bears weight on the stronger leg.
a. Have the patient move the affected leg and both crutches forward about 6″.	
b. Have the patient move the stronger leg forward to the level of the crutches.	

continues

ACTION   **RATIONALE**

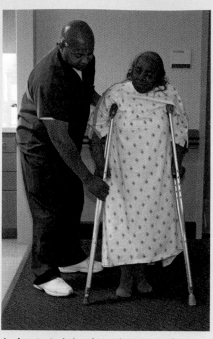

Action 4: Assisting the patient to stand erect, facing forward in the tripod position.

7. For the two-point gait:

   a. Have the patient move the left crutch and the right foot forward about 6″ at the same time.

   b. Have the patient move the right crutch and left leg forward to the level of the left crutch at the same time.

8. For the swing-to gait:

   a. Have the patient move both crutches forward about 6″.

   b. Have the patient lift the legs and swing them to the crutches, supporting his or her body weight on the crutches.

9. For the swing-through gait:

   a. Have the patient move both crutches forward about 6″.

   b. Have the patient lift the legs and swing through and ahead of the crutches, supporting his or her weight on the crutches.

10. **Continue with ambulation for the planned distance and time. Return the patient to the bed or chair based on the patient's tolerance and condition.**

11. Perform hand hygiene. Document the activity, any observations, the patient's ability to use the crutches, the patient's tolerance of the procedure, and the distance walked.

Patient bears partial weight on both feet.

Swing-to gait provides mobility for patients with weakness or paralysis of the hips or legs.

The swing-through gait provides mobility for patients with weakness or paralysis of the hips or legs.

Continued ambulation promotes activity. Adhering to the planned distance and time prevents the patient from becoming fatigued.

Hand hygiene prevents the spread of microorganisms. Documentation promotes continuity of care and communication.

continues

Assisting a Patient With Ambulation Using Crutches (continued)

ACTION	RATIONALE

> 5/10/06   1830   Patient instructed in crutch
> walking using four-point gait. Patient return-
> demonstrated gait, ambulating for approxi-
> mately 15 feet in hallway, without difficulty.
> —H. Pointer, RN

Action 11: Documentation.

EVALUATION

The expected outcome is met when the patient demonstrates correct use of crutches to ambulate safely and without injury. Additional outcomes are met when the patient demonstrates increased muscle strength and joint mobility and exhibits no evidence of injury related to crutch use.

Unexpected Situations and Associated Interventions

- *You are assisting a patient ambulating in the hallway using crutches when the patient reports fatigue. You notice that the patient is bearing weight on the axillary area:* Call for assistance and have a coworker obtain a wheelchair to transport the patient back to the room. Once the patient is back in bed, reinforce instructions about avoiding pressure on the axillary area. In the future, plan for a shorter distance to prevent the patient from becoming fatigued. Talk with the multidisciplinary healthcare team about possible exercises for upper extremity strengthening.

Special Considerations

- Crutches can be used when climbing stairs. The patient grasps both crutches as one on one side of the body and uses the stair railing. Have the patient stand in the tripod position facing the stairs. The patient transfers his or her weight to the crutches and holds the railing. The patient places the unaffected leg on the first stair tread. The patient then transfers his or her weight to the unaffected leg, moving up onto the stair tread. The patient moves the crutches and affected leg up to the stair tread and continues to the top of the stairs. Using this process, the crutches always support the affected leg.
- The crutch is appropriately sized when about three finger-widths remain between the axilla and the top of the crutch when the crutch is placed in a tripod position.
- Long-term use of the swing-to and swing-through gaits can lead to atrophy of the hips and legs. Appropriate exercises need to be included in the patient's plan of care to avoid this complication.
- Patients should not lean on the crutches. Prolonged pressure on the axillae can damage the brachial nerves, causing brachial nerve palsy, with resulting loss of sensation and inability to move the upper extremities.
- Patients using crutches should perform arm and shoulder strengthening exercises to aid with crutch walking.

Canes are useful for patients who can bear weight but need support for balance. Canes are also useful for patients who have decreased strength in one leg. Canes are made of wood or metal. The cane should rise from the floor to the height of the person's waist, and the elbow should be flexed about 30 degrees when holding the cane. Canes provide an additional point of support during ambulation. The patient holds the cane in the hand opposite the weak or injured leg.

Equipment
- Cane of appropriate size with rubber tip
- Nonskid shoes or slippers

ASSESSMENT

Assess the patient's upper body strength, ability to bear weight, ability to walk, and the need for assistance. Review the patient's record for conditions that may affect ambulation. Perform a pain assessment prior to the time for the activity. If the patient reports pain, administer the prescribed medication in sufficient time to allow for the full effect of the analgesic. Take vital signs and assess the patient for dizziness or lightheadedness with position changes. Assess the patient's knowledge regarding the use of a cane.

NURSING DIAGNOSIS

Determine the related factors for the nursing diagnoses based on the patient's current status. An appropriate nursing diagnosis is Risk for Falls. Other nursing diagnoses that may be appropriate include:
- Deficient Knowledge
- Risk for Injury
- Activity Intolerance
- Fatigue
- Acute Pain
- Chronic Pain
- Impaired Walking

OUTCOME IDENTIFICATION AND PLANNING

The expected outcome to achieve when assisting a patient with ambulation using a cane is that the patient ambulates safely without falls or injury. Additional appropriate outcomes include: the patient demonstrates proper use of the cane; the patient demonstrates increased muscle strength, joint mobility, and independence; the patient exhibits no evidence of injury from use of the cane.

IMPLEMENTATION

ACTION	RATIONALE
1. Review the medical record and nursing plan of care for conditions that may influence the patient's ability to move and ambulate. Assess for tubes, intravenous lines, incisions, or equipment that may alter the procedure for ambulation. Assess the patient's knowledge and previous experience regarding the use of a cane. Identify any movement limitations.	Review of the medical record and plan of care validates the correct patient and correct procedure. Identification of equipment and limitations helps reduce the risk for injury.
2. Identify the patient. Explain the procedure to the patient. Tell the patient to report any feelings of dizziness, weakness, or shortness of breath while walking. Decide how far to walk.	Patient identification validates the correct patient and correct procedure. Discussion and explanation help allay anxiety and prepare the patient for what to expect.
3. Perform hand hygiene.	Hand hygiene prevents the spread of microorganisms.

continues

ACTION	RATIONALE
4. Assist the patient to stand with weight evenly distributed between the feet and the cane.	This position provides a broad base of support and balance.
5. Have the patient hold the cane on his or her stronger side, close to the body.	Holding the cane on the stronger side helps to distribute the patient's weight away from the involved side and prevents leaning.
6. Tell the patient to advance the cane 4″ to 12″ (10 to 30 cm) and then, while supporting his or her weight on the stronger leg and the cane, advance the weaker foot forward, parallel with the cane.	Moving in this manner provides support and balance.
7. While supporting his or her weight on the weaker leg and the cane, have the patient advance the stronger leg forward ahead of the cane (heel slightly beyond the tip of the cane).	Moving in this manner provides support and balance.
8. Tell the patient to move the weaker leg forward until it is even with the stronger leg, and then advance the cane again.	This motion provides support and balance.
9. Continue with ambulation for the planned distance and time. Return the patient to the bed or chair based on the patient's tolerance and condition.	Continued ambulation promotes activity. Adhering to the planned distance and patient's tolerance prevents the patient from becoming fatigued.
10. Perform hand hygiene. Document the activity, any observations, the patient's ability to use the cane, the patient's tolerance of the procedure, and the distance walked.	Hand hygiene prevents the spread of microorganisms. Documentation promotes continuity of care and communication.

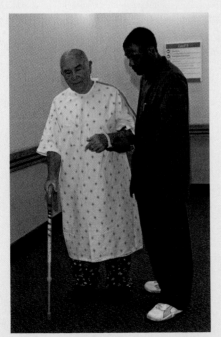

Action 5: Standing with the patient with the cane held on the patient's stronger side, close to the body.

5/14/06   1330   Patient instructed in cane use. Patient return-demonstrated gait, ambulating approximately 10 feet in room. Patient needed continued reminders about leaning to one side. Requires continued instruction in cane use. Another teaching session planned for early evening.—J. Phelps, RN

Action 10: Documentation.

continues

EVALUATION

The expected outcome is met when the patient uses the cane to ambulate safely and is free from falls or injury. Additional outcomes are met when the patient demonstrates proper use of the cane; exhibits increased muscle strength, joint mobility, and independence; and experiences no injury related to cane use.

Unexpected Situations and Associated Interventions

- *You are assisting a patient ambulating in the hallway using a cane when the patient says she can't walk any more:* Call for assistance. Have a coworker obtain a wheelchair to transport the patient back to her room. Assess the patient for possible causes, such as anxiety, fatigue, or a change in her condition. In the future, plan shorter distances to prevent her from becoming fatigued. Anticipate the need for referral to physical therapy for muscle strengthening.

Special Considerations

- Patients with bilateral weakness should not use a cane. Crutches or a walker would be more appropriate.
- To climb stairs, the patient should advance the stronger leg up the stair first, followed by the cane and with weaker leg. To descend, reverse the process.
- When less support is required from the cane, the patient can advance the cane and weaker leg forward simultaneously while the stronger leg supports the patient's weight.
- Patients should be taught to position their canes within easy reach when they sit down so that they can rise easily.

**SKILL
9-12   Applying Pneumatic Compression Devices**

Pneumatic compression devices (PCDs) consist of fabric sleeves containing air bladders that apply brief pressure to the legs. Intermittent compression pushes blood from the smaller blood vessels into the deeper vessels and into the femoral veins. This action enhances blood flow and venous return and promotes fibrinolysis, deterring venous thrombosis. The sleeves are attached by tubing to an air pump. The sleeve may cover the entire leg or may extend from the foot to the knee. PCDs may be used in combination with antiembolism stockings and anticoagulant therapy to prevent thrombosis formation. They can be used preoperatively and postoperatively with patients at risk for blood clot formation. They are also prescribed for patients with other risk factors for clot formation, including inactivity or immobilization, chronic venous disease, and malignancies.

Equipment

- Compression sleeves of appropriate size based on the manufacturer's guidelines
- Inflation pump with connection tubing

ASSESSMENT

Assess the patient's history, medical record, and current condition and status to identify patients at risk for development of deep vein thrombosis. Assess the skin integrity of the lower extremities. Identify any leg conditions that would be exacerbated by the use of the compression device or would contraindicate its use. Review the patient's record and nursing plan of care to verify the physician's order for use.

continues

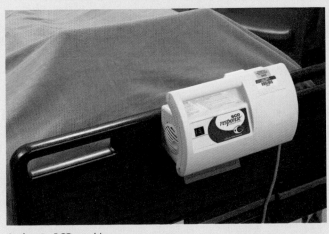

SKILL 9-12 Applying Pneumatic Compression Devices (continued)

NURSING DIAGNOSIS

Determine the related factors for the nursing diagnoses based on the patient's current status. An appropriate nursing diagnosis is Risk for Peripheral Neurovascular Dysfunction. Other nursing diagnoses that may be appropriate include:

- Impaired Physical Mobility
- Fatigue
- Delayed Surgical Recovery
- Risk for Injury

OUTCOME IDENTIFICATION AND PLANNING

The expected outcome to achieve when applying PCDs is that the patient maintains adequate circulation in extremities and is free from symptoms of neurovascular compromise.

IMPLEMENTATION

ACTION	RATIONALE
1. Review the medical record and nursing plan of care for conditions that may contraindicate the use of the PCD.	Reviewing the medical record and plan of care validates the correct patient and correct procedure and minimizes the risk for injury.
2. Identify the patient. Explain the procedure to the patient.	Patient identification validates the correct patient and correct procedure. Discussion and explanation help allay anxiety and prepare the patient for what to expect.
3. Perform hand hygiene.	Hand hygiene prevents the spread of microorganisms.
4. Close the room door or curtains. Place the bed at an appropriate and comfortable working height.	Closing the door or curtains provides privacy. Proper bed height helps reduce back strain.
5. Hang the compression pump on the foot of the bed and plug it into an electrical outlet. Attach the connecting tubing to the pump.	Equipment preparation promotes efficient time management and provides an organized approach to the task.

Action 5: PCD machine.

6. Remove the compression sleeves from the package and unfold them. Lay the unfolded sleeves on the bed with the cotton lining facing up. Take note of the markings indicating the correct placement for the ankle and popliteal areas.	Proper placement of the sleeves prevents injury.

continues

ACTION

RATIONALE

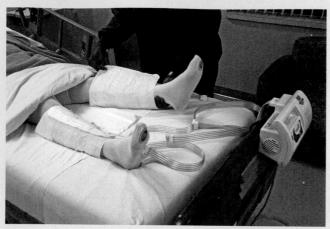

Action 7: Placing PCD sleeves under the patient's legs with the tubing toward the heel.

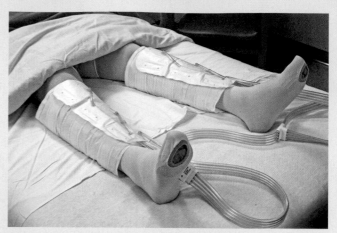

Action 8: PCD sleeves snugly around the patient's legs.

7. Apply antiembolism stockings if ordered. Place a sleeve under the patient's leg with the tubing toward the heel. Each one fits either leg. For total leg sleeves, place the behind-the-knee opening at the popliteal space to prevent pressure there. For knee-high sleeves, make sure the back of the ankle is over the ankle marking.

Proper placement prevents injury.

8. Wrap the sleeve snugly around the patient's leg so that two fingers fit between the leg and the sleeve. Secure the sleeve with the Velcro fasteners. Repeat for the second leg, if bilateral therapy is ordered. Connect each sleeve to the tubing for the pump. Follow the manufacturer's recommendations.

Correct placement ensures appropriate, but not excessive, compression of the extremity.

9. Set the pump to the prescribed maximum pressure (usually 35 to 55 mm Hg). Make sure the tubing is free from kinks. Check that the patient can move about without interrupting the airflow. Turn on the pump.

Proper pressure setting ensures patient safety and prevents injury.

10. Observe the patient and the device during the first cycle. Check the audible alarms. Check the sleeves and pump at least once per shift or per facility policy.

Observation and frequent checking ensure proper fit and inflation and reduce the risk for injury from the device

11. Place the bed in the lowest position, with the side rails up. Make sure the call bell and other necessary items are within easy reach.

Returning the bed to the lowest position and having the call bell and other items readily available promote patient safety.

12. Assess the extremities for peripheral pulses, edema, changes in sensation, and movement. Remove the sleeves and assess and document skin integrity every 8 hours.

Assessment provides for early detection and prompt intervention for possible complications, including skin irritation.

13. Perform hand hygiene. Document the time and date of application of the PCD, the patient's response to the therapy, and the patient's understanding of the therapy. Document the status of the alarms and the cooling settings.

Hand hygiene prevents the spread of microorganisms. Documentation promotes continuity of care and communication.

continues

SKILL
9-12

Applying Pneumatic Compression Devices (continued)

ACTION	RATIONALE

4/27/06 1615   Patient instructed in reason for pneumatic compression device therapy; verbalizes understanding of therapy. Knee-high PCDs applied to both lower extremities; pressure set at 45 mm Hg as ordered. Patient denies any complaints of numbness or tingling. Feet and toes warm and pink; quick capillary refill; bilateral pedal pulses present and equal. Alarms and cooling settings as ordered.—J. Trotter, RN

Action 13: Documentation.

EVALUATION

The expected outcome is met when the patient exhibits adequate circulation in extremities without symptoms of neurovascular compromise.

Unexpected Situations and Associated Interventions

- *Your postoperative patient is wearing PCDs on both legs. While you are performing a routine assessment, he tells you that he has started to have pain in his left leg, along with tingling and numbness:* Remove the PCDs and assess both lower extremities. Perform a skin and neurovascular assessment. Assess the extremities for peripheral pulses, edema, changes in sensation, and movement. Report the patient's symptoms and assessment to the physician.

Special Considerations

- PCDs are contraindicated in patients with suspected or existing deep vein thrombosis. They should not be used for patients with arterial occlusive disease, severe edema, cellulitis, phlebitis, a skin graft, or an infection of the extremity.
- Use the cooling setting, if the unit has one. The skin under the sleeve can become wet with diaphoresis, which can increase the risk for impaired skin integrity.
- Generally, the PCDs should be worn continuously. They may be removed for bathing, walking, and physical therapy. Use is usually discontinued when the patient is ambulating consistently.
- The risk for deep vein thrombosis formation and injury is greater if the sleeves are not applied correctly.

SKILL 9-13   Applying a Continuous Passive Motion Device

A continuous passive motion (CPM) device promotes range of motion, circulation, and healing of a joint. It is frequently used after arthroplasty surgery, especially after total knee arthroplasty. The amount of flexion and extension of the joint and the cycle rate (the number of revolutions per minute) are determined by the physician, but nurses place the patient in and out of the device and monitor the patient's response to the therapy.

Equipment

- CPM device
- Single-patient-use soft goods kit
- Tape measure
- Goniometer

ASSESSMENT

Review the medical record and nursing plan of care for orders for degrees of flexion and extension. Assess the neurovascular status of the involved extremity. Perform a pain assessment. Administer the prescribed medication in sufficient time to allow for the full effect of the analgesic before starting the device. Assess for proper alignment of the joint in the CPM device. Assess the patient's ability to tolerate the prescribed treatment.

NURSING DIAGNOSIS

Determine the related factors for the nursing diagnoses based on the patient's current status. An appropriate nursing diagnosis is Impaired Physical Mobility. Other appropriate nursing diagnoses may include:

- Activity Intolerance
- Anxiety
- Fatigue
- Risk for Injury
- Acute Pain
- Risk for Impaired Skin Integrity
- Delayed Surgical Recovery
- Risk for Peripheral Neurovascular Dysfunction

OUTCOME IDENTIFICATION AND PLANNING

The expected outcome to achieve when applying a CPM device is that the patient experiences increased joint mobility. Other outcomes include: the patient displays improved or maintained muscle strength, muscle atrophy and contractures are prevented, circulation is promoted in the affected extremity, effects of immobility are decreased, and healing is stimulated.

IMPLEMENTATION

ACTION	RATIONALE
1. Review the medical record and nursing plan of care for the appropriate degrees of flexion and extension, the cycle rate, and the length of time the CPM is to be used.	Reviewing the medical record and plan of care validates the correct patient and correct procedure and reduces the risk for injury.
2. Identify the patient. Explain the procedure to the patient.	Patient identification validates the correct patient and correct procedure. Discussion and explanation help allay anxiety and prepare the patient for what to expect.
3. Obtain equipment. Apply the soft goods to the CPM device.	Equipment preparation promotes efficient time management and provides an organized approach to the task. The soft goods help to prevent friction to the extremity during motion.
4. Perform hand hygiene.	Hand hygiene prevents the spread of microorganisms.

continues

Applying a Continuous Passive Motion Device (continued)

ACTION

5. Close the room door or curtains. Place the bed at an appropriate and comfortable working height.

6. Using the tape measure, determine the distance between the gluteal crease and the popliteal space.

7. Measure the leg from the knee to one quarter inch beyond the bottom of the foot.

8. Position the patient in the middle of the bed. The affected extremity should be in a slightly abducted position.

9. Support the affected extremity and elevate it, placing it in the padded CPM device.

10. Make sure the knee is at the hinged joint of the CPM device.

11. Adjust the footplate to maintain the patient's foot in a neutral position. Make sure the leg is not internally or externally rotated.

RATIONALE

Closing the door or curtains provides privacy. Proper bed height helps reduce back strain.

The thigh length on the CPM device is adjusted based on this measurement.

The position of the footplate is adjusted based on this measurement.

Proper positioning promotes correct body alignment and prevents pressure on the unaffected extremity.

Support and elevation assist in movement of the affected extremity without injury.

Proper positioning in the device prevents injury.

Adjustment helps ensure proper positioning and prevent injury.

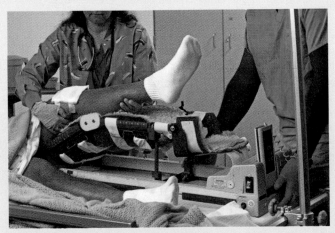

Action 9: Placing the patient's leg into the CPM machine.

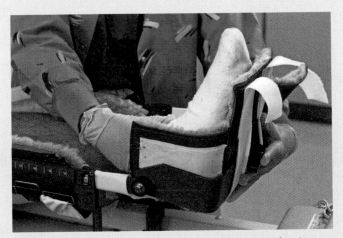

Action 11: Adjusting the footplate to maintain the patient's foot in a neutral position.

12. Apply the restraining straps under the CPM device and around the leg. **Check that two fingers fit between the strap and the leg.**

13. Explain the use of the STOP/GO button to the patient. Set the controls to the levels ordered by the physician. Turn on the power to the CPM.

14. Set the device to ON and start the therapy by pressing the GO button. Observe the patient and the device during the first cycle. Determine the angle of flexion when the device reaches its greatest height using the goniometer.

15. Check the patient's level of comfort and perform skin and neurovascular assessment at least every 8 hours or per facility policy.

Restraining straps maintain the leg in position. Leaving a space between the strap and leg prevents injury from excessive pressure from the strap.

Explanation decreases anxiety by allowing the patient to participate in care.

Observation ensures that the device is working properly, thereby ensuring patient safety. Measuring with a goniometer ensures the device is set to the prescribed parameters.

Frequent assessments provide for early detection and prompt intervention should problems arise.

continues

ACTION   **RATIONALE**

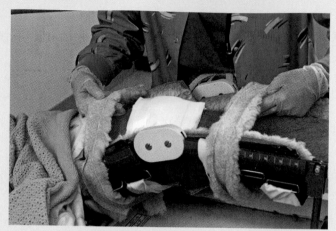

Action 12: Using two fingers to check the fit between the straps and the leg.

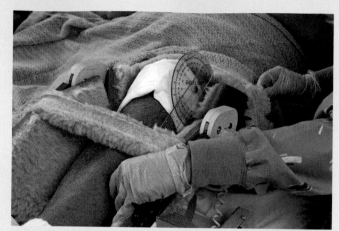

Action 14: Using the goniometer, determining the angle of joint flexion when the device reaches its greatest height.

16. Place the bed in the lowest position, with the side rails up. Make sure the call bell and other necessary items are within easy reach.

Having the bed at the proper height and having the call bell and other items handy ensure patient safety.

17. Perform hand hygiene. Document the time and date of application of the CPM, the extension and flexion settings, the speed of the device, the patient's response to the therapy, and your assessment of the extremity.

Hand hygiene prevents the spread of microorganisms. Documentation promotes continuity of care and communication.

> 5/03/06   1430   Right knee incision clean and dry; dressing intact. Right toes pink and warm with brisk capillary refill; equal to left. Pedal pulses present and equal bilaterally. CPM device applied with range of motion at 30 degrees of knee flexion for 5 cycles per minute for 30 minutes. Patient complains of slight increase in pain from a rating of 4 out of 10 to 5 out of 10 but states, "I don't want anything for the pain right now." Will reassess in 15 minutes and offer analgesic as ordered.
> —K. Dugas, RN

Action 17: Documentation.

EVALUATION

The expected outcome is met when the patient demonstrates increased joint mobility. In addition, the patient exhibits improved muscle strength without evidence of atrophy or contractures.

Unexpected Situations and Associated Interventions

- *A patient is prescribed therapy with a CPM device. After you initiate the prescribed flexion and extension of the joint, the patient complains of sudden pain in the joint:* Stop the CPM device. Check the settings to make sure the device is set correctly for the prescribed therapy. Assess the patient for other signs and symptoms and obtain vital signs. Perform a neurovascular assessment of the affected extremity. Notify the physician of the patient's pain and any other findings. When therapy is resumed, evaluate the need for premedication with analgesics. Continue pain intervention with analgesics as prescribed.

SKILL 9-14   Applying a Sling

A sling is a bandage that can provide support for an arm or immobilize an injured arm, wrist, or hand. Slings can be used to restrict movement of a fracture or dislocation and to support a muscle sprain. They may also be used to support a splint or secure dressings. Healthcare agencies usually use commercial slings. The sling should distribute the supported weight over a large area, not the back of the neck, to prevent pressure on the cervical spinal nerves.

Equipment
- Commercial arm sling
- ABD gauze pad

ASSESSMENT

Assess the situation to determine the need for a sling. Assess the affected limb for pain and edema. Perform a neurovascular assessment of the affected extremity. Assess body parts distal to the site for cyanosis, pallor, coolness, numbness, tingling, swelling, and absent or diminished pulses.

NURSING DIAGNOSIS

Determine the related factors for the nursing diagnoses based on the patient's current status. An appropriate nursing diagnosis is Impaired Physical Mobility. Other nursing diagnoses that may be appropriate include:

- Risk for Injury
- Acute Pain
- Risk for Peripheral Neurovascular Dysfunction
- Risk for Impaired Skin integrity
- Dressing or Grooming Self-Care Deficit

OUTCOME IDENTIFICATION AND PLANNING

The expected outcome to achieve when applying a sling is that the arm is immobilized, and the patient maintains muscle strength and joint range of motion. In addition, the patient shows no evidence of contractures, venous stasis, thrombus formation, or skin breakdown.

IMPLEMENTATION

ACTION	RATIONALE
1. Review the medical record and nursing plan of care to determine the need for the use of a sling.	Reviewing the medical record and plan of care validates the correct patient and correct procedure and prevents injury.
2. Identify the patient. Explain the procedure to the patient.	Patient identification validates the correct patient and correct procedure. Discussion and explanation help allay anxiety and prepare the patient for what to expect.
3. Perform hand hygiene.	Hand hygiene prevents the spread of microorganisms.
4. Close the room door or curtains. Place the bed at an appropriate and comfortable working height, if necessary.	Closing the door or curtain provides privacy. Proper bed height helps reduce back strain.
5. Assist the patient to a sitting position. Place the patient's forearm across the chest with the elbow flexed and the palm against the chest. Measure the sleeve length, if indicated.	Proper positioning facilitates sling application. Measurement ensures proper sizing of the sling and proper placement of the arm.
6. Enclose the arm in the sling, making sure the elbow fits into the corner of the fabric. Run the strap up the patient's back and across the shoulder opposite the injury, then down the chest to the fastener on the end of the sling.	This position ensures adequate support and keeps the arm out of a dependent position, preventing edema.
7. Place the ABD pad under the strap, between the strap and the patient's neck. Ensure that the sling and forearm are slightly elevated and at a right angle to the body.	Padding prevents skin irritation and reduces pressure on the neck. Proper positioning ensures alignment, provides support, and prevents edema.

continues

SKILL 9-14 Applying a Sling (continued)

ACTION

RATIONALE

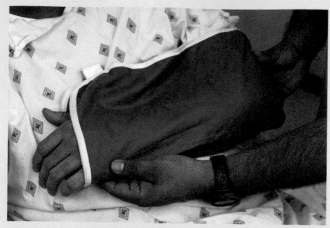

Action 6: Placing the patient's arm into the canvas sling with the elbow flush in the corner of the sling.

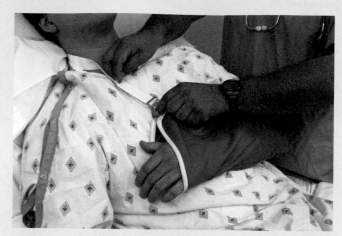

Action 6: Placing the strap around the patient's neck.

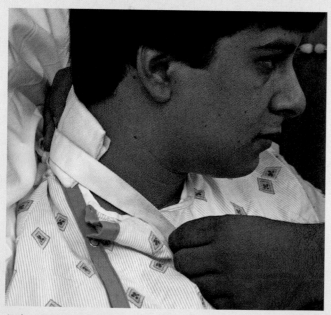

Action 7: Placing padding between the strap and the patient's neck.

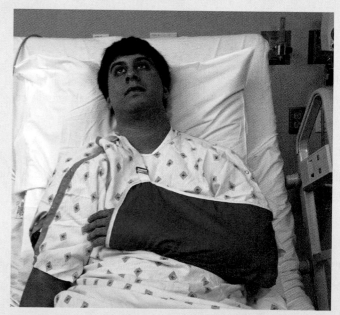

Action 7: Patient with sling in place.

8. Place the bed in the lowest position, with the side rails up. Make sure the call bell and other necessary items are within easy reach.

9. Check the patient's level of comfort, arm positioning, and neurovascular status of the affected limb every 4 hours or according to facility policy. Assess the axillary and cervical skin frequently for irritation or breakdown.

10. Perform hand hygiene. Document the time and date the sling was applied. Document the patient's response to the sling and the neurovascular status of the extremity.

Having the bed at proper height and leaving the call bell and other items within reach ensure patient safety.

Frequent assessment ensures patient safety, prevents injury, and provides early intervention for skin irritation and other complications.

Hand hygiene prevents the spread of microorganisms. Documentation promotes continuity of care and communication.

continues

SKILL 9-14   Applying a Sling (continued)

ACTION	RATIONALE

> 5/22/06   2015   Sling applied to left arm as ordered. Left hand and fingers warm to touch and pink. Brisk capillary refill. Left radial pulse present and equal to right. Patient denies any complaints of numbness, pain, or tingling of left upper extremity.—P. Peterson, RN

Action 10: Documentation.

EVALUATION

The expected outcome is met when the patient demonstrates extremity in proper alignment with adequate muscle strength and joint range of motion. In addition, the patient demonstrates proper use of sling and remains free of complications, including contractures, venous stasis, thrombus formation, or skin breakdown.

Unexpected Situations and Associated Interventions

- *Your patient needs a sling to support a wrist fracture, but you cannot obtain a commercially prepared sling:* Make a sling using a triangular bandage or cloth. Place the cloth or bandage on the chest with a corner of the cloth at the elbow. Place the affected arm across the chest with the elbow flexed and the palm on the chest. Wrap the end closest to the head around the neck, on the opposite side from the injured arm. Bring the end of the cloth that is farthest from the head up over the injured arm and tie it at the side of the neck. The sling and forearm should be slightly elevated and at a right angle to the body. Fold the material at the elbow and secure the sling with a safety pin above and behind the elbow.

Special Considerations

- The patient's wrist should be enclosed in the sling. Do not allow it to hang out and down over the edge. This prevents pressure on nerves and blood vessels and prevents muscle contractures, deformity, and discomfort.
- Assess circulation and comfort at regular intervals.

SKILL 9-15   Applying a Figure-Eight Bandage

Bandages are used to apply pressure over an area, immobilize a body part, prevent or reduce edema, and secure splints and dressings. Bandages can be elasticized or made of gauze, flannel, or muslin. In general, narrow bandages are used to wrap feet, the lower legs, hands, and arms, and wider bandages are used for the thighs and trunk. A roller bandage is a continuous strip of material wound on itself to form a roll. The free end is anchored and the roll is passed or rolled around the body part, taking care to exert equal tension in all turns. Unwind the bandage gradually and only as needed. The bandage should overlap itself evenly and by one-half to two-thirds the width the bandage. The figure-eight turn consists of oblique overlapping turns that ascend and descend alternately. It is used around the knee, elbow, ankle, and wrist.

Equipment

- Elastic or other bandage of the appropriate width
- Tape, pins, or self-closures
- Gauze pads
- Clean gloves, if indicated

continues

Applying a Figure-Eight Bandage (continued)

ASSESSMENT

Review the medical record, physician's orders, and nursing plan of care and assess the situation to determine the need for a bandage. Assess the affected limb for pain and edema. Perform a neurovascular assessment of the affected extremity. Assess body parts distal to the site for evidence of cyanosis, pallor, coolness, numbness, tingling, and swelling and absent or diminished pulses. Assess the distal circulation of the extremity after the bandage is in place and at least every 4 hours.

NURSING DIAGNOSIS

Determine the related factors for the nursing diagnoses based on the patient's current status. Appropriate nursing diagnoses may include:

- Impaired Physical Mobility
- Risk for Injury
- Acute Pain
- Risk for Peripheral Neurovascular Dysfunction
- Risk for Impaired Skin Integrity
- Ineffective Tissue Perfusion
- Dressing or Grooming Self-Care Deficit

OUTCOME IDENTIFICATION AND PLANNING

The expected outcome to achieve when applying a figure-eight bandage is that the bandage is applied correctly without injury or complications. Other outcomes that may be appropriate include: patient maintains circulation to the affected part and remains free of neurovascular complications.

IMPLEMENTATION

ACTION	RATIONALE
1. Review the medical record and nursing plan of care to determine the need for a figure-eight bandage.	Reviewing the medical record and plan of care validates the correct patient and correct procedure and reduces risk for injury.
2. Identify the patient. Explain the procedure to the patient.	Patient identification validates the correct patient and correct procedure. Discussion and explanation help allay anxiety and prepare the patient for what to expect.
3. Perform hand hygiene and put on gloves if contact with drainage is possible.	Hand hygiene and gloving prevent the spread of microorganisms.
4. Close the room door or curtains. Place the bed at an appropriate and comfortable working height.	Closing the door or curtains provides privacy. Proper bed height helps reduce back strain.
5. Assist the patient to a comfortable position, with the affected body part in a normal functioning position.	Keeping the body part in a normal functioning position promotes circulation and prevents deformity and discomfort.
6. Hold the bandage roll with the roll facing upward in one hand. Hold the free end of the roll in the other hand. Hold the bandage so it is close to the affected body part.	Proper handling of the bandage allows application of even tension and pressure.
7. Wrap the bandage around the limb twice, below the joint, to anchor it.	Anchoring the bandage ensures that it will stay in place.
8. Use alternating ascending and descending turns to form a figure eight. Overlap each turn of the bandage by one-half to two-thirds the width of the strip.	Making alternating ascending and descending turns helps to ensures the bandage will stay in place on a moving body part.
9. **Unroll the bandage as you wrap, not before wrapping.**	Unrolling the bandage with wrapping prevents uneven pressure, which could interfere with blood circulation.

continues

SKILL 9-15   Applying a Figure-Eight Bandage (continued)

ACTION	RATIONALE

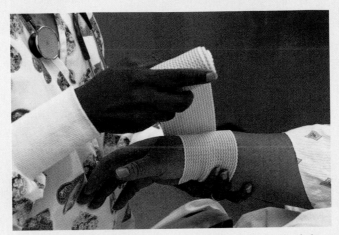

Action 7: Wrapping the bandage around the patient's limb twice, below the joint, to anchor it.

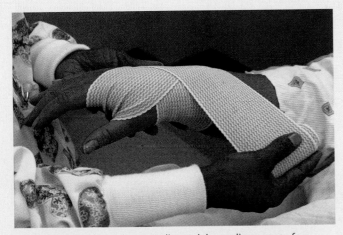

Action 8: Using alternating ascending and descending turns to form a figure eight.

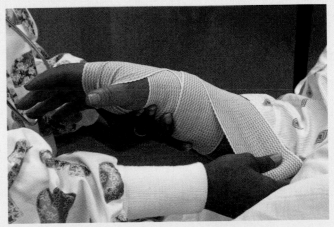

Action 8: Overlapping each turn of the bandage by one-half to two-thirds the width of the strip.

10. **Wrap firmly, but not tightly.** Assess the patient's comfort as you wrap. If the patient reports tingling, itching, numbness, or pain, loosen the bandage.

Firm wrapping is necessary to provide support and prevent injury, but wrapping too tightly interferes with circulation. Patient complaints are helpful indicators of possible circulatory compromise.

11. After the area is covered, wrap the bandage around the limb twice, above the joint, to anchor it. Secure the end of the bandage with tape, pins, or self-closures. Avoid metal clips.

Anchoring at the end ensures the bandage will stay in place. Metal clips can cause injury.

12. Remove your gloves, if worn, and discard them. Place the bed in the lowest position, with the side rails up. Make sure the call bell and other necessary items are within easy reach.

Repositioning the bed and having items nearby ensure patient safety.

13. Assess the distal circulation after the bandage is in place.

Elastic may tighten as it is wrapped. Frequent assessment of distal circulation ensures patient safety and prevents injury.

continues

SKILL 9-15
Applying a Figure-Eight Bandage (continued)

ACTION   **RATIONALE**

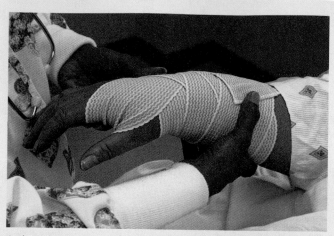

Action 11: Wrapping the bandage around the patient's limb twice, above the joint, to anchor it, and secure the end of the bandage with tape, pins, or self-closures.

14. **Elevate the wrapped extremity for 15 to 30 minutes after application of the bandage.**

    Elevation promotes venous return and reduces edema.

15. Lift the distal end of the bandage and assess the skin for color, temperature, and integrity. Assess for pain and perform a neurovascular assessment of the affected extremity at least every 4 hours, or per facility policy.

    Assessment aids in prompt detection of compromised circulation and allows for early intervention for skin irritation and other complications.

16. Remove and change the bandage at least once a day, or per physician order or facility policy. Cleanse the skin and dry thoroughly before applying a new bandage. Assess the skin for irritation and breakdown.

    Changing bandage as ordered prevents skin irritation and allows for close inspection of the skin to detect changes. Cleaning and drying the skin before application reduces the risk for skin irritation and breakdown.

17. Perform hand hygiene. Document the time, date, and site that the bandage was applied and the size bandage used. Include the skin assessment and care provided before application. Document the patient's response to the bandage and the neurovascular status of the extremity.

    Hand hygiene prevents the spread of microorganisms. Documentation promotes continuity of care and communication.

> 5/27/06 1615   Three-inch bandage applied to right knee using figure-eight technique. Skin pink, warm, and dry with quick capillary refill; pedal and dorsalis pedis pulses present and equal bilaterally. Patient denies any complaints of pain, numbness, or tingling. Patient instructed to report any complaints immediately. Right lower extremity resting on two pillows at present.—J. Wilkins, RN

Action 17: Documentation.

continues

Applying a Figure-Eight Bandage (continued)

EVALUATION

The expected outcome is achieved when the patient exhibits a bandage that is applied correctly, without causing injury or neurovascular compromise. In addition, the patient demonstrates proper alignment of the bandaged body part; the patient remains free of evidence of complications; and the patient demonstrates understanding of signs and symptoms to report immediately.

Unexpected Situations and Associated Interventions

- *After you have applied a figure-eight bandage to a patient's elbow to hold dressings in place, the patient reports tingling, numbness, and pain in his hand during a routine assessment:* Remove the bandage, wait 30 minutes, and reapply the bandage with less tension. Continue to monitor the neurovascular status of the extremity. Symptoms should subside fairly quickly. If symptoms persist, notify the physician.
- *You remove the bandage on a patient's ankle and note the bandage is limp and less elastic than when it was applied:* Obtain a new bandage and apply it to the ankle. Launder the old bandage to restore its elasticity. Keep two bandages at the bedside: one can be applied while the other is laundered.

Special Considerations

- A figure-eight bandage may be contraindicated if skin breakdown or lesions are present on the area to be wrapped.
- When wrapping an extremity, elevate it for 15 to 30 minutes before applying the bandage, if possible. This promotes venous return and prevents edema. Avoid applying the bandage to a dependent extremity.
- Place gauze pads or cotton between skin surfaces, such as toes and fingers, to prevent skin irritation. Skin surfaces should not touch after the bandage is applied.
- Include the heel when wrapping the foot, but do not wrap the toes or fingers unless necessary. Assess distal body parts to detect impaired circulation.
- Avoid leaving gaps in bandage layers or leaving skin exposed, as this may result in uneven pressure on the body part.

SKILL 9-16   Assisting With Cast Application

A cast is a rigid external immobilizing device that encases a body part. Casts are used to immobilize a body part in a specific position and to apply uniform pressure on the encased soft tissue. They may be used to treat injuries, correct a deformity, stabilize weakened joints, or promote healing after surgery. Casts generally allow the patient mobility while restricting movement of the affected body part. Casts may be made of plaster or synthetic materials, such as fiberglass. Each material has advantages and disadvantages. Non-plaster casts set in 15 minutes and can sustain weight bearing or pressure in 15 to 30 minutes. Plaster casts can take 24 to 72 hours to dry, with no weight bearing or pressure being applied during this period. Patient safety is of utmost importance during the application of a cast. Typically, a physician applies the cast. Nursing responsibilities include preparing the patient and equipment and assisting during the application. The nurse provides skin care to the affected area before, during, and after the cast is applied. In some settings, nurses with special preparation may apply or change casts.

Equipment

- Casting materials, such as plaster rolls or fiberglass, depending on the type of cast being applied
- Padding material, such as stockinette, sheet wadding, or Webril, depending on the type of cast being applied
- Plastic bucket or basin filled with warm water
- Disposable gloves and aprons
- Scissors
- Waterproof disposable pads

ASSESSMENT

Assess the skin condition in the affected area, noting redness, contusions, or open wounds. Assess the neurovascular status of the affected extremity, including distal pulses, color, temperature, presence of edema, capillary refill to fingers or toes, and sensation and motion. Perform a pain assessment. If the patient reports pain, administer the prescribed analgesic in sufficient time to allow for the full effect of the medication. Assess for muscle spasms and administer the prescribed muscle relaxant in sufficient time to allow for the full effect of the medication. Assess for the presence of disease processes that may contraindicate the use of a cast or interfere with wound healing, including skin diseases, peripheral vascular disease, diabetes mellitus, and open or draining wounds.

NURSING DIAGNOSIS

Determine the related factors for the nursing diagnoses based on the patient's current status. An appropriate nursing diagnosis is Risk for Peripheral Neurovascular Dysfunction. Other nursing diagnoses that may be appropriate include:

- Acute Pain
- Impaired Physical Mobility
- Risk for Injury
- Anxiety
- Fear
- Disturbed Body Image
- Risk for Impaired Skin Integrity
- Ineffective Tissue Perfusion
- Deficient Knowledge

OUTCOME IDENTIFICATION AND PLANNING

The expected outcome to achieve when assisting with a cast application is that the cast is applied without interfering with neurovascular function and that healing occurs. Other outcomes that may be appropriate include that the patient is free from complications, has knowledge of the treatment regimen, and experiences increased comfort.

continues

SKILL 9-16 Assisting With Cast Application (continued)

IMPLEMENTATION

ACTION	RATIONALE
1. Review the medical record and physician's orders to determine the need for the cast.	Reviewing the medical record and order validates the correct patient and correct procedure.
2. Identify the patient. Explain the procedure to the patient and verify area to be casted.	Patient identification validates the correct patient and correct procedure. Discussion and explanation help allay anxiety and prepare the patient for what to expect.
3. Perform a pain assessment and assess for muscle spasm. Administer prescribed medications in sufficient time to allow for the full effect of the analgesic and/or muscle relaxant.	Assessment of pain and analgesic administration ensure patient comfort and enhance cooperation.
4. Perform hand hygiene and put on gloves, if necessary.	Hand hygiene and gloving prevent the spread of micro-organisms; gloving also protects the nurse from residual casting materials collecting on hands.
5. Close the room door or curtains. Place the bed at an appropriate and comfortable working height, if necessary.	Closing the door or curtains provides privacy. Proper bed height helps reduce back strain while you are performing the procedure.
6. Position the patient as needed, depending on the type of cast being applied and the location of the injury. Support the extremity or body part to be casted.	Proper positioning minimizes movement, maintains alignment, and increases patient comfort.
7. Drape the patient with the waterproof pads.	Draping provides warmth and privacy and helps protect other body parts from contact with casting materials.
8. Cleanse and dry the affected body part.	Skin care before cast application helps prevent skin breakdown.
9. Position and maintain the affected body part in the position indicated by the physician as the stockinette, sheet wadding, and padding is applied. The stockinette should extend beyond the ends of the cast. As the wadding is applied, check for wrinkles.	Stockinette and other materials protect skin from casting materials and create a smooth, padded edge, protecting the skin from abrasion. Padding protects the skin, tissues, and nerves from the pressure of the cast.

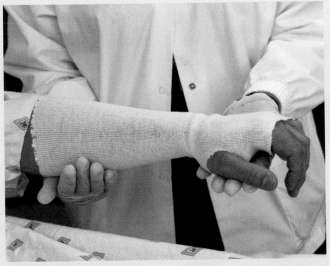

Action 9: Stockinette in place.

continues

SKILL 9-16　Assisting With Cast Application (continued)

ACTION

RATIONALE

10. Position and maintain the affected body part in the position indicated by the physician as the casting material is applied. Assist with finishing by folding the stockinette or other padding down over the outer edge of the cast.

Smooth edges lessen the risk for skin irritation and abrasion.

11. **Support the cast during hardening.** Handle hardening plaster casts with the palms of hands, not fingers. Support the cast on a firm, smooth surface. Do not rest it on a hard surface or sharp edges. Avoid placing pressure on the cast.

Proper handling avoids denting of the cast and development of pressure areas.

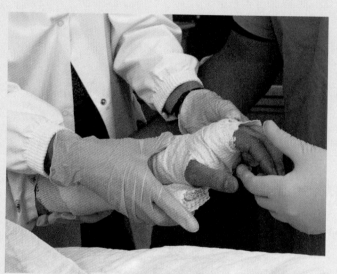

Action 10: Casting material being applied.

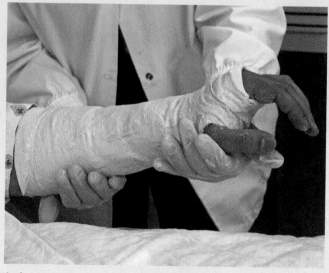

Action 11: Using palms to move the casted limb.

12. **Elevate the injured limb above heart level with pillow or bath blankets as ordered, making sure pressure is evenly distributed under the cast.**

Elevation promotes venous return. Evenly distributed pressure prevents molding and denting of the cast and development of pressure areas.

13. Remove gloves and dispose of them properly; place the bed in the lowest position, if necessary.

Removing gloves properly reduces the risk for infection transmission and contamination of other items. Repositioning the bed promotes safety.

14. Obtain x-rays as ordered.

X-rays identify that the affected area is positioned properly.

15. **Instruct the patient to report pain, odor, drainage, changes in sensation, abnormal sensation, or the inability to move fingers or toes of the affected extremity.**

Pressure within a cast may increase with edema and lead to compartment syndrome. Patient complaints allow for early detection of and prompt intervention for complications such as skin irritation or impaired tissue perfusion.

16. Leave the cast uncovered and exposed to the air. Reposition the patient every 2 hours. Depending on facility policy, a fan may be used to dry the cast.

Keeping the cast uncovered promotes drying. Repositioning prevents development of pressure areas. Using a fan helps increase airflow and speeds drying.

17. Perform hand hygiene. Document the time, date, and site that the cast was applied. Include the skin assessment and care provided before application. Document the patient's response to the cast and the neurovascular status of the extremity.

Hand hygiene prevents the spread of microorganisms. Documentation promotes continuity of care and communication.

continues

ACTION	RATIONALE

6/1/06   1245   Fiberglass cast applied to right forearm from mid-upper arm to middle of hand. Cast clean and dry; edges padded. No signs of irritation noted. Patient able to move fingers freely. Fingers pale pink, warm, and dry. Capillary refill less than 2 seconds. Patient denies any numbness, tingling, or pain. Right forearm resting on two pillows. Patient instructed to report any complaints of pain, pressure, numbness, tingling, or decreased ability to move fingers.—P. Collins, RN

Action 17: Documentation.

EVALUATION

The expected outcome is achieved when neurovascular function is maintained and healing occurs. In addition, the patient is free from complications, has knowledge of the treatment regimen, and experiences increased comfort.

Unexpected Situations and Associated Interventions

• *Your patient, who has a cast on his hand and forearm, has been experiencing pain relief in the extremity with ice application and oral analgesics. He now reports pain unrelieved by the analgesic and a feeling of tightness in his arm. In addition, his fingers are cool, with sluggish capillary refill:* Compartment syndrome may be developing. Adjust the arm so that it is no higher than heart level. This enhances arterial perfusion and controls edema. Notify the physician of the situation immediately. Prepare for bivalving of the cast (cutting of the cast in half longitudinally) to relieve pressure.

Special Considerations

• Perform frequent, regular assessment of neurovascular status. Early recognition of diminished circulation and nerve function is essential to prevent loss of function. Be alert for the presence of compartment syndrome.
• Fiberglass casts dry quickly, usually within 5 to 15 minutes.
• If a fiberglass cast was applied, remove any fiberglass resin residue on the skin with alcohol or acetone.

SKILL 9-17   Caring for a Cast

A cast is a rigid external immobilizing device that encases a body part. Casts are used to immobilize a body part in a specific position and to apply uniform pressure on the encased soft tissue. They may be used to treat injuries, correct a deformity, stabilize weakened joints, or promote healing after surgery. Casts generally allow the patient mobility while restricting movement of the affected body part. Casts may be made of plaster or synthetic materials, such as fiberglass. Each material has advantages and disadvantages. Non-plaster casts set in 15 minutes and can sustain weight bearing or pressure in 15 to 30 minutes. Plaster casts can take 24 to 72 hours to dry, with no weight bearing or pressure application during this period. Nursing responsibilities after the cast is in place include maintaining the cast, preventing complications, and providing patient teaching related to cast care.

Equipment

- Washcloth
- Towel
- Skin cleanser
- Basin of warm water
- Waterproof pads
- Tape
- Pillows
- Clean gloves, if indicated

ASSESSMENT

Review the patient's medical record and nursing plan of care to determine the need for cast care and care of the affected area. Perform a pain assessment and administer the prescribed medication in sufficient time to allow for the full effect of the analgesic prior to starting care. Assess the neurovascular status of the affected extremity, including distal pulses, color, temperature, presence of edema, capillary refill to fingers or toes, and sensation and motion. Assess the skin distal to the cast. Note any indications of infection, including any foul odor from the cast, pain, fever, edema, and extreme warmth over an area of the cast. Assess for complications of immobility, including alterations in skin integrity, reduced joint movement, decreased peristalsis, constipation, alterations in respiratory function, and signs of thrombophlebitis. Inspect the condition of the cast. Be alert for cracks, dents, or the presence of drainage from the cast. Assess the patient's knowledge of cast care.

NURSING DIAGNOSIS

Determine the related factors for the nursing diagnoses based on the patient's current status. An appropriate nursing diagnosis is Risk for Peripheral Neurovascular Dysfunction. Other nursing diagnoses that may be appropriate include:

- Anxiety
- Disturbed Body Image
- Risk for Disuse Syndrome
- Risk for Falls
- Risk for Infection
- Risk for Injury
- Deficient Knowledge
- Impaired Physical Mobility
- Acute Pain
- Self-Care Deficit (bathing/hygiene, feeding, dressing or grooming, or toileting)
- Risk for Impaired Skin Integrity
- Delayed Surgical Recovery
- Impaired Tissue Perfusion
- Impaired Home Maintenance

continues

Caring for a Cast (continued)

OUTCOME IDENTIFICATION AND PLANNING

The expected outcome to achieve when caring for a patient with a cast is that the cast remains intact and the patient does not experience neurovascular compromise. Other outcomes include that the patient is free from infection, the patient experiences only mild pain and slight edema or soreness, the patient experiences only slight limitations of range of joint motion, the skin around the cast edges remains intact, the patient participates in activities of daily living, and the patient demonstrates appropriate cast-care techniques.

IMPLEMENTATION

ACTION	RATIONALE
1. Review the medical record and the nursing plan of care to determine the need for cast care and care for the affected body part.	Reviewing the medical record and plan of care validates the correct patient and correct procedure.
2. Identify the patient. Explain the procedure to the patient.	Patient identification validates the correct patient and correct procedure. Discussion and explanation help allay anxiety and prepare the patient for what to expect.
3. Perform hand hygiene and put on gloves, if necessary.	Hand hygiene and gloving prevent the spread of micro-organisms. Gloves protect the nurse from residual casting materials collecting on hands.
4. Close the room door or curtains. Place the bed at an appropriate and comfortable working height, if necessary.	Closing the door or curtains provides privacy. Proper bed height helps reduce back strain while you are performing the procedure.
5. If a plaster cast was applied, handle the casted extremity or body area with the palms of your hands for the first 24 to 36 hours, until the cast is fully dry.	Proper handling of a plaster cast prevents dents in the cast, which may create pressure areas on the inside of the cast.
6. If the cast is on an extremity, elevate the affected area on pillows covered with waterproof pads. **Maintain the normal curvatures and angles of the cast.**	Elevation helps reduce edema and enhances venous return. Use of a waterproof pad prevents soiling of linen. Maintaining curvatures and angles maintains proper joint alignment, helps prevent flattened areas on the cast as it dries, and prevents pressure areas.

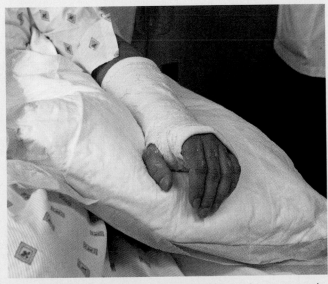

Action 6: Elevating casted limb, maintaining the normal curvatures and angles of the cast.

continues

ACTION

RATIONALE

7. Keep cast (plaster) uncovered until fully dry.

Keeping the cast uncovered allows heat and moisture to dissipate and air to circulate to speed drying.

8. Wash excess antiseptic or antimicrobial agents, such as povidone–iodine (Betadine), or residual casting material from the exposed skin. Dry thoroughly.

Washing the area permits a clear area for inspection and reduces the risk for irritation and breakdown from the agent.

9. Assess the condition of the cast. Be alert for cracks, dents, or the presence of drainage from the cast. Perform skin and neurovascular assessment according to facility policy, as often as every 1 to 2 hours. **Check for pain, edema, inability to move body parts distal to the cast, pallor, pulses, and abnormal sensations. If the cast is on an extremity, compare it to the uncasted extremity.**

Assessment helps detect abnormal neurovascular function or infection and allows for prompt intervention. Assessing the neurovascular status determines the circulation and oxygenation of tissues. Pressure within a cast may increase with edema and lead to compartment syndrome.

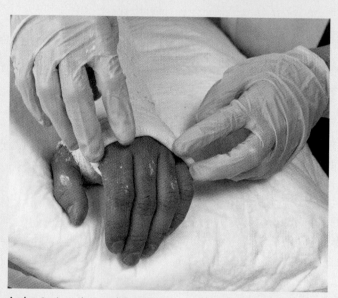

Action 9: Assessing condition of cast.

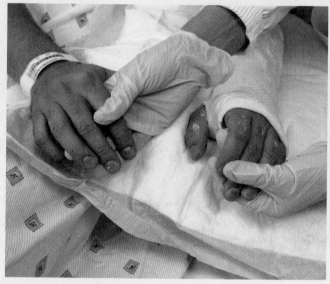

Action 9: Assessing skin and neurovascular function; comparing with the uncasted extremity.

10. **If breakthrough bleeding or drainage is noted on the cast, mark the area on the cast. Indicate the date and time next to the area.** Follow physician orders or facility policy regarding the amount of drainage that needs to be reported to the physician.

Marking the area provides a baseline for monitoring the amount of bleeding or drainage.

11. Assess for signs of infection. Monitor the patient's temperature. Assess for a foul odor from the cast, increased pain, or extreme warmth over an area of the cast.

Infection deters healing. Assessment allows for early detection and prompt intervention.

12. Reposition the patient every 2 hours. Provide back and skin care frequently. Encourage range of motion for unaffected joints. Encourage the patient to cough and deep breathe.

Repositioning promotes even drying of the cast and reduces the risk for the development of pressure areas under the cast. Frequent skin and back care prevents patient discomfort and skin breakdown. Range of motion maintains joint function of unaffected areas. Coughing and deep breathing reduce the risk for respiratory complications associated with immobility.

continues

Caring for a Cast (continued)

ACTION	RATIONALE

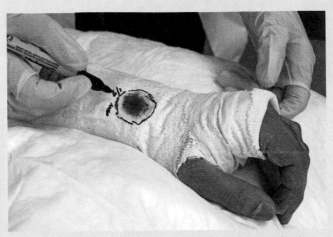

Action 10: Marking any breakthrough bleeding on the cast, indicating the date and time.

13. Instruct the patient to report pain, odor, drainage, changes in sensation, abnormal sensation, or the inability to move fingers or toes of the affected extremity.	Pressure within a cast may increase with edema and lead to compartment syndrome. Patient understanding of signs and symptoms allows for early detection and prompt intervention.
14. Remove gloves and dispose of them appropriately; place the bed in the lowest position, if necessary.	Proper glove removal and disposal reduce the risk for transmission of organisms; bed repositioning promotes safety.
15. Perform hand hygiene. Document all assessments and care provided. Document the patient's response to the cast, repositioning, and any teaching.	Hand hygiene prevents the spread of microorganisms. Documentation promotes continuity of care and communication.

EVALUATION

The expected outcome is achieved when the patient exhibits a cast that is intact without evidence of neurovascular compromise to the affected body part. Other expected outcomes include: the patient remains free from infection, the patient verbalizes only mild pain and slight edema or soreness, the patient maintains range of joint motion, the patient demonstrates intact skin at cast edges, the patient is able to perform activities of daily living, and the patient demonstrates appropriate cast-care techniques.

Unexpected Situations and Associated Interventions

- *Your patient, who has a cast on his hand and forearm, has been experiencing pain relief in the extremity with ice application and oral analgesics. He now reports pain unrelieved by the analgesic and a feeling of tightness in his arm. In addition, his fingers are cool, with sluggish capillary refill:* Compartment syndrome may be developing. Adjust the arm so that it is no higher than heart level. This enhances arterial perfusion and controls edema. Notify the physician of the situation immediately. Prepare for bivalving of the cast (cutting of the cast in half longitudinally) to relieve pressure.

continues

SKILL 9-17   Caring for a Cast (continued)

Special Considerations

- Explain that itching under the cast is normal, but the patient should not stick objects down or in the cast to scratch.
- Begin patient teaching immediately after the cast is applied and continue until the patient or a significant other can provide care.
- If a cast is applied after surgery or trauma, monitor vital signs (the most accurate way to assess for bleeding).

Older Adult Considerations

- Older adults may experience changes in circulation related to their age. They may have slow or poor capillary refill related to peripheral vascular disease. Obtain baseline information for comparison after the cast is applied. Use more than one neurovascular assessment to assess circulation. Compare extremities or sides of the body for symmetry.

SKILL 9-18   Applying Skin Traction and Caring for a Patient in Skin Traction

Traction is the application of a pulling force to a part of the body. It is used to reduce fractures, treat dislocations, correct or prevent deformities, improve or correct contractures, or decrease muscle spasms. It must be applied in the correct direction and magnitude to obtain the therapeutic effects desired.

With traction, the affected body part is immobilized by pulling with equal force on each end of the injured area, mixing traction and countertraction. Weights provide the pulling force or traction. The use of additional weights or positioning the patient's body weight against the traction pull provides the countertraction. Skin traction is applied directly to the skin, exerting indirect pull on the bone. The force may be applied using adhesive or nonadhesive traction tape or a boot, belt, or halter. Skin traction immobilizes a body part intermittently.

Types of skin traction for adults include Buck's extension traction (lower leg), a cervical head halter, and the pelvic belt. Nursing care for skin traction includes setting the traction up, applying the traction, monitoring the application and patient response, and preventing complications from the therapy and immobility.

Equipment

- Bed with traction frame and trapeze
- Weights
- Velcro straps or other straps
- Rope and pulleys
- Boot with footplate
- Elastic hose
- Gloves
- Skin cleansing supplies

ASSESSMENT

Assess the patient's medical record, physician's orders, and the nursing plan of care to determine the type of traction, traction weight, and line of pull. Assess the traction equipment to ensure proper function, including inspecting the ropes for fraying and proper positioning. Assess the patient's body alignment. Perform a skin assessment and neurovascular assessment. Assess for complications of immobility, including alterations in respiratory function, skin integrity, urinary and bowel elimination, and muscle weakness, contractures, thrombophlebitis, pulmonary embolism, and fatigue.

continues

SKILL 9-18

Applying Skin Traction and Caring for a Patient in Skin Traction (continued)

NURSING DIAGNOSIS

Determine the related factors for the nursing diagnoses based on the patient's current status. Appropriate nursing diagnoses may include:

- Risk for Injury
- Ineffective Airway Clearance
- Anxiety
- Risk for Constipation
- Impaired Gas Exchange
- Deficient Knowledge
- Impaired Bed Mobility
- Acute Pain
- Impaired Physical Mobility
- Toileting Self-Care Deficit
- Bathing or Hygiene Self-Care Deficit
- Dressing or Grooming Self-Care Deficit
- Risk for Impaired Skin Integrity

OUTCOME IDENTIFICATION AND PLANNING

The expected outcome to achieve when applying and caring for a patient in skin traction is that the traction is maintained with the appropriate counterbalance and the patient is free from complications of immobility. Other outcomes that may be appropriate include that the patient maintains proper body alignment, the patient reports an increased level of comfort, and the patient is free from injury.

IMPLEMENTATION

ACTION	RATIONALE
1. Review the medical record and the nursing plan of care to determine the type of traction being used and care for the affected body part.	Reviewing the medical record and plan of care validates the correct patient and correct procedure.
2. Identify the patient. Explain the procedure to the patient, emphasizing the importance of maintaining counterbalance, alignment, and position.	Patient identification validates the correct patient and correct procedure. Discussion and explanation help allay anxiety and prepare the patient for what to expect.
3. Perform a pain assessment and assess for muscle spasm. Administer prescribed medications in sufficient time to allow for the full effect of the analgesic and/or muscle relaxant.	Assessing pain and administering analgesics promote patient comfort.
4. Perform hand hygiene.	Hand hygiene prevents the spread of microorganisms.
5. Close the room door or curtains. Place the bed at an appropriate and comfortable working height.	Closing the door or curtains provides for privacy. Proper bed height prevents back and muscle strain.
6. Ensure the traction apparatus is attached securely to the bed. Assess the traction setup. Apply the ordered amount of weight. **The weights should hang freely, not touching the bed or floor.**	Assessment of traction set-up and weights promotes safety. Properly hanging weights and correct patient positioning ensure accurate counterbalance and function of the traction.
7. Check that the ropes move freely through the pulleys. Check that all knots are tight and are positioned away from the pulleys. Pulleys should be free from the linens.	Checking ropes and pulleys ensures that weight is being applied correctly, promoting accurate counterbalance and function of the traction.
8. Place the patient in a supine position with the foot of the bed elevated slightly. The patient's head should be near the head of the bed and in alignment.	Proper patient positioning maintains proper counterbalance and promotes safety.

continues

ACTION

9. Cleanse the affected area. Place the elastic hose on the affected limb.

10. Place the traction boot over the patient's leg. Be sure the patient's heel is in the heel of the boot. Secure the boot with the straps.

11. Attach the traction cord to the footplate of the boot. Pass the rope over the pulley fastened at the end of the bed. Attach the weight to the hook on the rope, usually 5 to 10 pounds for an adult. Gently let go of the weight.

RATIONALE

Skin care aids in preventing skin breakdown. Use of elastic hose prevents edema and neurovascular complications.

The boot provides a means for attaching traction; proper application ensures proper pull.

Attachment of weight applies the pull for the traction. Gently releasing the weight prevents a quick pull on the extremity and possible injury and pain.

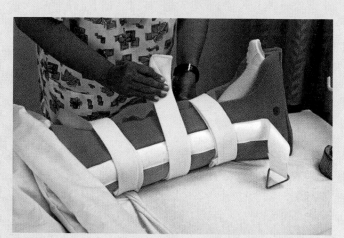

Action 10: Applying the traction boot with an elastic stocking in place on the leg.

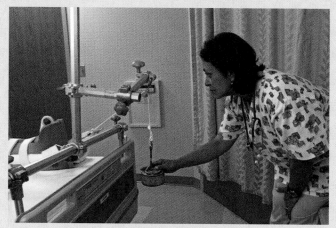

Action 11: Applying the weight for the skin traction.

12. Check the patient's alignment with the traction.

13. Perform a skin traction assessment per facility policy. This assessment includes checking the traction equipment, examining the affected body part, maintaining proper body alignment, and performing a skin assessment and a neurovascular assessment.

14. Check the boot for placement and alignment. **Make sure the line of pull is parallel to the bed and not angled downward.**

15. Remove the straps every 4 hours per the physician's order or facility policy. Check bony prominences for skin breakdown, abrasions, and pressure areas. Remove the boot per physician's order or facility policy every 8 hours. Put on gloves and wash, rinse, and thoroughly dry the skin.

Proper alignment is necessary for proper counterbalance and ensures patient safety.

Assessment provides information to determine proper application and alignment, thereby reducing the risk for injury. Misalignment causes ineffective traction and may interfere with healing.

Misalignment causes ineffective traction and may interfere with healing. A properly positioned boot prevents pressure on the heel.

Removing the straps provides assessment information for early detection and prompt intervention of potential complications should they arise. Washing the area enhances circulation to skin; thorough drying prevents skin breakdown. Using gloves prevents transfer of microorganisms.

continues

Applying Skin Traction and Caring for a Patient in Skin Traction (continued)

ACTION	RATIONALE
16. Assess the extremity distal to the traction for edema, and assess peripheral pulses. Assess the temperature, color, and capillary refill, and compare with the unaffected limb. Check for pain, inability to move body parts distal to the traction, pallor, and abnormal sensations. Assess for indicators of deep vein thrombosis, including calf tenderness, swelling, and a positive Homans' sign.	Doing so helps detect signs of abnormal neurovascular function and allows for prompt intervention. Assessing neurovascular status determines the circulation and oxygenation of tissues. Pressure within the traction boot may increase with edema.

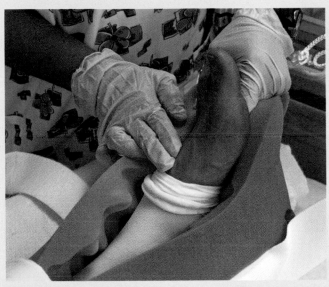

Action 16: Assessing distal pulses.

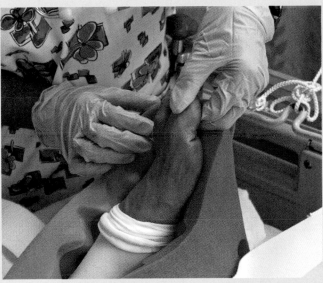

Action 16: Assessing capillary refill.

17. Replace the traction and remove gloves and dispose of them appropriately.	Replacing traction is necessary to provide immobilization and facilitate healing. Proper disposal of gloves prevents the transmission of microorganisms.
18. **Ensure the patient is positioned in the center of the bed, with the affected leg aligned with the trunk of the patient's body.**	Misalignment interferes with the effectiveness of traction and may lead to complications.

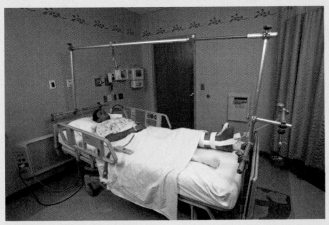

Action 18: Skin traction in place.

continues

SKILL
9-18

Applying Skin Traction and Caring for a Patient in Skin Traction (continued)

ACTION	RATIONALE
19. Examine the weights and pulley system. **Weights should hang freely, off the floor and bed. Knots should be secure. Ropes should move freely through the pulleys. The pulleys should not be constrained by knots.**	Checking the weights and pulley system ensures proper application and reduces the risk for patient injury from traction application.
20. Perform range-of-motion exercises on all joint areas, unless contraindicated. Encourage the patient to cough and deep breathe every 2 hours.	Range of motion maintains joint function. Coughing and deep breathing help to reduce the risk for respiratory complications related to immobility.
21. Raise the side rails. Place the bed in the lowest position that still allows the weight to hang freely.	Raising the side rails promotes patient safety. Proper bed positioning ensures effective application of traction without patient injury.
22. Perform hand hygiene. Document the time, date, type, amount of weight used, and the site where the traction was applied. Include the skin assessment and care provided before application. Document the patient's response to the traction and the neurovascular status of the extremity.	Hand hygiene prevents the spread of microorganisms. Documentation promotes continuity of care and communication.

6/3/06 1500   Patient complaining of pain in left hip due to fracture, rating it 7 out of 10. Administered oxycodone 2 tabs as ordered. Pain rated 3 out of 10, 30 minutes later. Buck's extension traction with 5 lb of weight applied to left extremity. Skin intact. Pedal pulses present and equal, feet pale pink, warm, and dry, with brisk capillary refill bilaterally. Patient able to wiggle toes freely. Denies numbness or tingling. Patient lying flat in bed with head of bed elevated approximately 15 degrees. Surgery planned for tomorrow.—L. James, RN

Action 22: Documentation.

EVALUATION

The expected outcome is met when the patient demonstrates proper body alignment with traction applied and maintained with appropriate counterbalance. Other outcomes include: the patient verbalizes pain relief, with pain rated at lower numbers and the patient remains free of injury.

Unexpected Situations and Associated Interventions

• *Your patient is in Buck's traction and reports pain in the heel of the affected leg:* Remove traction and perform a skin and neurovascular assessment. Reapply the traction and reassess the neurovascular status in 15 to 20 minutes. Notify the physician.

SKILL 9-18   Applying Skin Traction and Caring for a Patient in Skin Traction (continued)

Special Considerations
- Unless contraindicated, encourage the patient to do active flexion–extension ankle exercise and calf pumping exercises at regular intervals to decrease venous stasis.
- Be alert for pressure on peripheral nerves with skin traction. Take care with Buck's traction to avoid pressure on the peroneal nerve at the point where it passes around the neck of the fibula just below the knee.
- Patients in traction for extended periods of time are at risk for developing helplessness, isolation, confinement, and loss of control. Diversional activities, therapeutic communication, and frequent visits by staff and significant others are an important part of care.

Older Adult Considerations
- Be extra vigilant with older adults in skin traction. Elderly patients are prone to alterations in skin integrity due to a decreased amount of subcutaneous fat and thinner, drier, more fragile skin.

SKILL 9-19   Caring for a Patient in Skeletal Traction

Skeletal traction provides pull to a body part by attaching weight directly to the bone using pins, screws, wires, or tongs. It is used to immobilize a body part for prolonged periods. This method of traction is used to treat fractures of the femur, tibia, and cervical spine. Nursing responsibilities related to skeletal traction include maintaining the traction, maintaining body alignment, monitoring neurovascular status, promoting exercise, preventing complications from the therapy and immobility, and preventing infection by providing pin site care.

Equipment
- Sterile gloves
- Sterile applicators
- Cleansing agent for pin care, usually sterile normal saline, per physician order or facility policy
- Sterile container
- Antimicrobial ointment, if ordered
- Foam or gauze dressing, per physician order or facility policy

ASSESSMENT

Review the patient's medical record, physician's orders, and nursing plan of care to determine the type of traction, traction weight, and line of pull. Assess the traction equipment to ensure proper function, including inspecting the ropes for fraying and proper positioning. Assess the patient's body alignment. Perform a skin assessment and neurovascular assessment. Inspect the pin insertion sites for inflammation and infection. Assess for complications of immobility, including alterations in respiratory function, constipation, alterations in skin integrity, alterations in urinary elimination, and muscle weakness, contractures, thrombophlebitis, pulmonary embolism, and fatigue.

NURSING DIAGNOSIS

Determine the related factors for the nursing diagnoses based on the patient's current status. An appropriate nursing diagnosis is Impaired Skin Integrity. Other nursing diagnoses that may be appropriate include:
- Risk for Injury
- Ineffective Airway Clearance
- Anxiety
- Risk for Constipation

continues

- Deficient Knowledge
- Impaired Bed Mobility
- Acute Pain
- Impaired Physical Mobility
- Self-Care Deficit (toileting, bathing or hygiene, or dressing or grooming)
- Risk for Infection
- Impaired Gas Exchange

OUTCOME IDENTIFICATION AND PLANNING

The expected outcome to achieve when caring for a patient in skeletal traction is that the traction is maintained appropriately and that the patient is free from complications of immobility and infection. Other outcomes that may be appropriate include: the patient maintains proper body alignment, the patient reports an increased level of comfort, and the patient is free from injury.

IMPLEMENTATION

ACTION	RATIONALE
1. Review the medical record and the nursing plan of care to determine the type of traction being used and the prescribed care.	Reviewing the medical record and plan of care validates the correct patient and correct procedure.
2. Identify the patient. Explain the procedure to the patient, emphasizing the importance of maintaining counterbalance, alignment, and position.	Patient identification validates the correct patient and correct procedure. Discussion and explanation help allay anxiety and prepare the patient for what to expect.
3. Perform a pain assessment and assess for muscle spasm. Administer prescribed medications in sufficient time to allow for the full effect of the analgesic and/or muscle relaxant.	Assessing for pain and administering analgesics promote patient comfort.
4. Perform hand hygiene.	Hand hygiene prevents the spread of microorganisms.
5. Close the room door or curtains. Place the bed at an appropriate and comfortable working height.	Closing the door or curtains provides for privacy. Proper bed height prevents back and muscle strain.
6. Ensure the traction apparatus is attached securely to the bed. Assess the traction setup, including application of the ordered amount of weight. **Be sure that the weights hang freely, not touching the bed or the floor.**	Proper traction application reduces the risk of injury by promoting accurate counterbalance and function of the traction.
7. Check that the ropes move freely through the pulleys. Check that all knots are tight and are positioned away from the pulleys. Pulleys should be free from the linens.	Free ropes and pulleys ensure accurate counterbalance and function of the traction.
8. Check the alignment of the patient's body as prescribed.	Proper alignment maintains an effective line of pull and prevents injury.
9. Perform a skin assessment. Pay attention to pressure points, including the ischial tuberosity, popliteal space, Achilles tendon, sacrum, and heel.	Skin assessment provides early intervention for skin irritation, impaired tissue perfusion, and other complications.
10. Perform a neurovascular assessment. Assess the extremity distal to the traction for edema and peripheral pulses. Assess the temperature and color and compare with the unaffected limb. Check for pain, inability to move body parts distal to the traction, pallor, and abnormal sensations. Assess for indicators of deep vein thrombosis, including calf tenderness, swelling, and a positive Homans' sign.	Neurovascular assessment aids in early identification and allows for prompt intervention should compromised circulation and oxygenation of tissues develop.

continues

Caring for a Patient in Skeletal Traction (continued)

ACTION	RATIONALE
11. Assess the site at and around the pins for redness, edema, and odor. Assess for skin tenting, prolonged or purulent drainage, elevated body temperature, elevated pin site temperature, and bowing or bending of the pins.	Pin sites provide a possible entry for microorganisms. Skin inspection allows for early detection and prompt intervention should complications develop.

12. Provide pin site care.
  a. Using sterile technique, open the applicator package and pour the cleansing agent into the sterile container.
  b. Put on the sterile gloves.
  c. Place the applicators into the solution.
  d. **Clean the pin site starting at the insertion area and working outward, away from the pin site.**
  e. **Use each applicator once. Use a new applicator for each pin site.**
	Pin site care helps prevent infection and subsequent osteomyelitis. Using sterile technique with sterile gloves reduces the risk for infection transmission. Using sterile applicators ensures adherence to sterile technique, reducing the risk of contamination of pin sites. Cleaning from the center outward ensures movement from the least to most contaminated area. Using an applicator once reduces the risk of microorganism transmission.

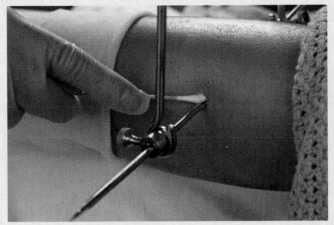

Action 12: Cleaning around pin sites with normal saline on an applicator.

13. Depending on physician order and facility policy, apply the antimicrobial ointment to pin sites and apply a dressing.	Antimicrobial ointment helps reduce the risk of infection. A dressing aids in protecting the pin sites from contamination and contains any drainage.
14. Perform range-of-motion exercises on all joint areas, unless contraindicated. Encourage the patient to cough and deep breathe every 2 hours.	Range-of-motion exercises promote joint mobility. Coughing and deep breathing reduce the risk of respiratory complications related to immobility.
15. Remove gloves. Perform hand hygiene. Document the time, date, type of traction, and the amount of weight used. Include the skin assessment, pin site assessment, and pin site care. Document the patient's response to the traction and the neurovascular status of the extremity.	Gloves and hand hygiene prevent the spread of microorganisms. Documentation promotes continuity of care and communication.

continues

ACTION   **RATIONALE**

> 6/5/06   1020   *Pin site care performed. Pin sites cleaned with normal saline and open to the air. Sites slightly red with serosanguineous crusting noted. Neurovascular status intact. Balanced suspension skeletal traction maintained as ordered.*—M. Leroux, RN

Action 15: Documentation.

EVALUATION

The expected outcome is met when the patient demonstrates maintenance of skeletal traction with pin sites free of infection. In addition, the patient maintains proper body alignment and joint function, patient verbalizes pain relief, patient states signs and symptoms to report, and patient remains free of injury.

Unexpected Situations and Associated Interventions

- *While performing a pin site assessment for your patient with skeletal traction, you note that several of the pins move and slide in the pin tract:* Assess the patient for other symptoms, including signs of infection at the pin sites, pain, and fever. Assess for neurovascular changes. Notify the physician of the findings.

Special Considerations

- Assess the patient for chronic conditions, such as diabetes mellitus, peripheral vascular disease, and chronic obstructive pulmonary disease, which can significantly increase a patient's risk for complications when skeletal traction is in use.
- Never remove the weights from skeletal traction unless a life-threatening situation occurs. Removal of the weights interferes with therapy and can result in injury to the patient.
- Inspect the pin sites for inflammation and evidence of infection at least every 8 hours. Prevention of osteomyelitis is of utmost importance.

SKILL
9-20

Caring for a Patient With an External Fixation Device

External fixators are used to manage open fractures with soft tissue damage. They consist of one of a variety of frames to hold pins that are drilled into or through bones. External fixators provide stable support for severe crushed or splintered fractures and access to and treatment for soft tissue injuries. The use of these devices allows treatment of the fracture and damaged soft tissues while promoting patient comfort, early mobility, and active exercise of adjacent uninvolved joints. Complications related to disuse and immobility are minimized. Nursing responsibilities include reassuring the patient, maintaining the device, monitoring neurovascular status, promoting exercise, preventing complications from the therapy, preventing infection by providing pin site care, and providing teaching to ensure compliance and self-care. Nurses play a major role in preparing the patient psychologically for the application of an external fixator. The devices appear clumsy and large. In addition, the nurse needs to clarify misconceptions regarding pain and discomfort associated with the device.

Equipment

Equipment varies with the type of fixator and the type and location of the fracture but may include:

- Sterile applicators
- Cleansing solution, usually sterile normal saline, per physician order or facility policy
- Ice bag
- Sterile gauze
- Analgesic, per physician order
- Antimicrobial ointment, per physician's order or facility policy

ASSESSMENT

Review the patient's medical record, physician's orders, and the nursing plan of care to determine the type of device being used and prescribed care. Assess the external fixator to ensure proper function and position. Perform a skin assessment and neurovascular assessment. Inspect the pin insertion sites for signs of inflammation and infection. Assess the patient's knowledge regarding the device and self-care activities and responsibilities.

NURSING DIAGNOSIS

Determine the related factors for the nursing diagnoses based on the patient's current status. An appropriate nursing diagnosis is Risk for Infection. Other nursing diagnoses that may be appropriate include:

- Impaired Skin Integrity
- Risk for Injury
- Anxiety
- Deficient Knowledge
- Acute Pain
- Impaired Physical Mobility

OUTCOME IDENTIFICATION AND PLANNING

The expected outcome to achieve when caring for a patient with an external fixator device is that the patient shows no evidence of complication such as infection, contractures, venous stasis, thrombus formation, or skin breakdown. Additional outcomes that may be appropriate include that the patient shows signs of healing, experiences relief from pain, and is free from injury.

IMPLEMENTATION

ACTION	RATIONALE
1. Review the medical record and the nursing plan of care to determine the type of device being used and prescribed care.	Reviewing the medical record and plan of care validates the correct patient and correct procedure.

continues

SKILL 9-20   **Caring for a Patient With an External Fixation Device** (continued)

ACTION	RATIONALE
2. Identify the patient. Explain the procedure to the patient. Assure the patient that there will be little pain after the fixation device is in place. Reinforce that the patient will be able to adjust to the device and will be able to move about with the device, allowing him or her to resume normal activities more quickly.	Patient identification validates the correct patient and correct procedure. Discussion and explanation allay anxiety and prepare the patient psychologically for the application of the device.
3. After the fixation device is in place, **apply ice to the surgical site as ordered or per facility policy. Elevate the affected body part if appropriate.**	Ice and elevation help reduce swelling, relieve pain, and reduce bleeding.
4. Perform a pain assessment and assess for muscle spasm. Administer prescribed medications in sufficient time to allow for the full effect of the analgesic and/or muscle relaxant.	Pain assessment and analgesic administration help promote patient comfort.
5. Administer analgesics as ordered before exercising or mobilizing the affected body part.	Administration of analgesics promotes patient comfort and facilitates movement.
6. Perform neurovascular assessments per facility policy or physician's order, usually every 2 to 4 hours for 24 hours, then every 4 to 8 hours. Assess the affected body part for color, motion, sensation, edema, capillary refill, and pulses. If appropriate, compare with the unaffected side. Assess for pain not relieved by analgesics, burning, tingling, and numbness.	Assessment promotes early detection and prompt intervention of abnormal neurovascular function, nerve damage, or circulatory impairment. Assessment of neurovascular status determines the circulation and oxygenation of tissues.
7. Perform hand hygiene.	Hand hygiene prevents the spread of microorganisms.
8. Close the room door or curtains. Place the bed at an appropriate and comfortable working height.	Closing the door or curtains provides for privacy. Proper bed height prevents back and muscle strain.

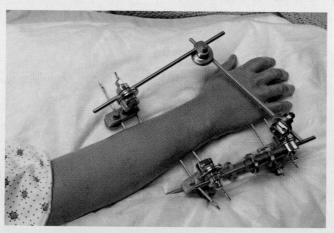

Action 8: External fixator device in place.

9. Assess the pin site for redness, tenting of the skin, prolonged or purulent drainage, swelling, and bowing, bending, or loosening of the pins. Monitor body temperature.	Assessing pin sites aids in early detection of infection and stress on the skin and allows for appropriate intervention.

continues

ACTION

RATIONALE

10. Perform pin site care.
    a. Using sterile technique, open the applicator package and pour the cleansing agent into the sterile container.
    b. Put on the sterile gloves.
    c. Place the applicators into the solution.
    d. **Clean the pin site starting at the insertion area and working outward, away from the pin site.**
    e. **Use each applicator once. Use a new applicator for each pin site.**

Performing pin site care using sterile technique prevents crusting at the site, which could lead to fluid buildup, infection, and osteomyelitis. Cleaning from the center outward promotes movement from the least to most contaminated area. Using each applicator only once prevents transfer of microorganisms.

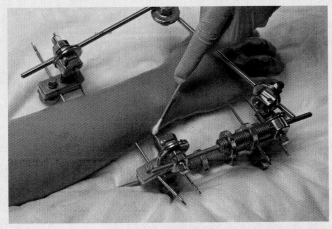

Action 10: Cleaning around pin sites with normal saline on an applicator.

11. Depending on physician order and facility policy, apply the antimicrobial ointment to pin sites and apply a dressing.

Antimicrobial ointment prevents infection; applying a dressing helps contain drainage.

12. Remove gloves. Perform hand hygiene. Document the time, date, and type of device in place. Include the skin assessment, pin site assessment, and pin site care. Document the patient's response to the device and the neurovascular status of the affected area.

Hand hygiene prevents the spread of microorganisms. Documentation promotes continuity of care and communication.

EVALUATION

The expected outcome is met when the patient exhibits an external fixation device in place with pin sites that are clean, dry, and intact, without evidence of infection. The patient remains free of complication such as contractures, venous stasis, thrombus formation, or skin breakdown; the patient verbalizes pain relief; the patient remains free of injury, and the patient demonstrates knowledge of pin site care.

Special Considerations

- Teach the patient and significant others how to provide pin site care and how to recognize the signs of pin site infection. External fixator devices are in place for prolonged periods of time. Clean technique can be used at home.
- Reinforce the importance of keeping the affected body part elevated when sitting or lying down to prevent edema.
- Do not adjust the clamps on the external fixator frame. It is the physician's responsibility to adjust the clamps.
- Fractures often require additional treatment and stabilization with a cast or molded splint after the fixator device is removed.

Caring for a Patient in Halo Traction

Halo traction provides immobilization to patients with spinal cord injury. Halo traction consists of a metal ring that fits over the patient's head, connected with skull pins into the skull, and metal bars that connect the ring to a vest that distributes the weight of the device around the chest. It immobilizes the head and neck after traumatic injury to the cervical vertebrae and allows early mobility. Although most injuries are treated with surgical intervention followed by halo application to stabilize the spinal cord while healing takes place, halo traction can be used alone. Halo traction has less risk of infection than other immobilization techniques because it does not require skin incisions and drill holes to position the skull pins.

Nursing responsibilities include reassuring the patient, maintaining the device, monitoring neurovascular status, monitoring respiratory status, promoting exercise, preventing complications from the therapy, preventing infection by providing pin site care, and providing teaching to ensure compliance and self-care. Nurses play a major role in preparing the patient psychologically for the application of the device. Patients are often unsettled by the appearance of the device and may have feelings of claustrophobia. Misconceptions regarding pain and discomfort associated with the device also must be addressed.

Equipment

- Basin of warm water
- Bath towels
- Medicated skin powder or cornstarch, per physician order or facility policy
- Sterile applicators
- Cleansing solution, per physician order or facility policy
- Sterile gauze
- Antimicrobial ointment, per physician's order or facility policy
- Analgesic, per physician's order
- Sterile gloves

ASSESSMENT

Review the patient's medical record, physician's orders, and nursing plan of care to determine the type of device being used and prescribed care. Assess the halo traction device to ensure proper function and position. Perform a respiratory, neurologic, and skin assessment. Inspect the pin insertion sites for inflammation and infection. Assess the patient's knowledge regarding the device and self-care activities and responsibilities, and his or her feelings related to treatment.

NURSING DIAGNOSIS

Determine the related factors for the nursing diagnoses based on the patient's current status. An appropriate nursing diagnosis is Fear. Other nursing diagnoses that may be appropriate include:

- Anxiety
- Disturbed Body Image
- Risk for Falls
- Ineffective Coping
- Deficient Knowledge
- Impaired Gas Exchange
- Risk for Infection
- Risk for Injury
- Impaired Physical Mobility
- Acute Pain
- Bathing or Hygiene Self-Care Deficit
- Dressing or Grooming Self-Care Deficit
- Toileting Self-Care Deficit
- Impaired Skin Integrity
- Disturbed Sleep Pattern

continues

Caring for a Patient in Halo Traction (continued)

**OUTCOME
IDENTIFICATION
AND PLANNING**

The expected outcome to achieve when caring for a patient with halo traction is that the patient maintains cervical alignment. Additional outcomes that may be appropriate include that the patient shows no evidence of infection; the patient is free from complications such as respiratory impairment, orthostatic hypotension, and skin breakdown; the patient experiences relief from pain; and the patient is free from injury.

IMPLEMENTATION
ACTION

RATIONALE

1. Review the medical record and the nursing plan of care to determine the type of device being used and prescribed care.

Reviewing the medical record and plan of care validate the correct patient and correct procedure.

2. Identify the patient. Explain the procedure to the patient.

Patient identification validates the correct patient and correct procedure. Discussion and explanation help allay anxiety and prepare the patient for what to expect.

3. Perform hand hygiene.

Hand hygiene prevents the spread of microorganisms.

4. Close the room door or curtains. Place the bed at a comfortable working height or have the patient sit up if appropriate.

Closing the door or curtains promotes privacy. Proper bed height helps prevent muscle strain.

5. Monitor vital signs and perform a neurologic assessment, including level of consciousness, motor function, and sensation, per facility policy. This is usually at least every 2 hours for 24 hours, or possibly every hour for 48 hours.

Changes in the neurologic assessment could indicate spinal cord trauma, which would require immediate intervention.

6. Examine the halo vest unit every 8 hours for stability, secure connections, and positioning. Make sure the patient's head is centered in the halo without neck flexion or extension. Check each bolt for loosening.

Assessment ensures correct function of the device and patient safety.

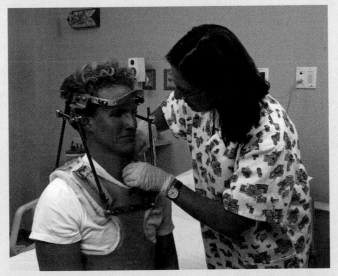

Action 6: Examining the halo vest unit for stability, secure connections, and positioning.

continues

7. Check the fit of the vest. With the patient in a supine position, you should be able to insert one or two fingers under the jacket at the shoulder and chest.

Checking the fit prevents compression on the chest, which could interfere with respiratory status.

8. Wash the patient's chest and back daily. Place the patient on his or her back or sitting up if appropriate. Loosen the bottom Velcro straps.

Daily cleaning prevents skin breakdown and allows assessment. Loosening the straps allows access to the chest and back.

9. Wring out a bath towel soaked in warm water. Pull the towel back and forth in a drying motion beneath the front. Do not use soap or lotion under the vest.

Using an overly wet towel could lead to skin maceration and breakdown. Soaps and lotions can cause skin irritation.

10. Thoroughly dry the skin in the same manner with a dry towel. Inspect the skin for tender, reddened areas or pressure spots. Lightly dust the skin with a prescribed medicated powder or cornstarch.

Drying and using powder or cornstarch, which helps absorb moisture, prevent skin breakdown.

11. Turn the patient on his or her side, less than 45 degrees if lying supine, and repeat the process on the back. Close the Velcro straps. Assist the patient with changing the shirt.

Doing so prevents skin breakdown. Soaps and lotions can cause skin irritation.

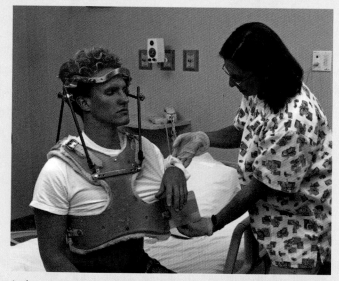

Action 11: Assisting patient to change shirt.

12. Perform a respiratory assessment. Check for respiratory impairment, such as absence of breath sounds, the presence of adventitious sounds, reduced inspiratory effort, or shortness of breath.

The halo vest limits chest expansion, which could lead to alterations in respiratory function. Pulmonary embolus is a common complication associated with spinal cord injury.

13. Assess the pin site for redness, tenting of the skin, prolonged or purulent drainage, swelling, and bowing, bending, or loosening of the pins. Monitor body temperature.

Pin sites provide an entry for microorganisms. Assessment allows for early detection and prompt intervention should problems arise.

14. Perform pin site care. (See Skills 9-19 and 9-20.)

Pin site care reduces the risk of infection and subsequent osteomyelitis.

15. Depending on physician order and facility policy, apply the antimicrobial ointment to pin sites and apply a dressing.

Antimicrobial ointment helps prevent infection. Dressing provides protection and helps contain any drainage.

continues

Caring for a Patient in Halo Traction (continued)

ACTION   **RATIONALE**

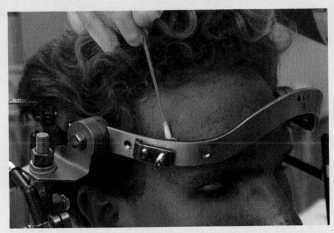

Action 14: Cleaning around pin sites with normal saline on an applicator.

16. Remove gloves and dispose of them appropriately. Place the bed in the lowest position.

Disposing of gloves reduces the risk of microorganism transmission. Proper bed height ensures patient safety.

17. Perform hand hygiene. Document the time, date, and type of device in place. Include the skin assessment, pin site assessment, and pin site care. Document the patient's response to the device and the neurologic assessment and respiratory assessment.

Hand hygiene prevents the spread of microorganisms. Documentation promotes continuity of care and communication.

EVALUATION

The expected outcome is met when the patient maintains cervical alignment. Additional outcomes are met when the patient shows no evidence of infection; the patient is free from complications such as respiratory impairment, orthostatic hypotension, and skin breakdown; the patient experiences relief from pain; and the patient is free from injury.

Unexpected Situations and Associated Interventions

- *Your patient, being treated with halo traction, complains of a headache after the physician has tightened the skull pins:* This is a common complaint; obtain an order for and administer an analgesic. However, if the pain is associated with jaw movement, notify the physician immediately, as the pins may have slipped onto the temporal plate.

Special Considerations

- Wrenches specific for the vest should always be kept at the bedside for emergency removal of the anterior portion of the vest should it be necessary to perform CPR.
- Patient teaching to prevent injury is very important. Patients need to learn to turn slowly and refrain from bending forward to avoid falls.
- Stress to the frame could cause misalignment of the spine and straining or tearing of the skin.

■ Developing Critical Thinking Skills

1. You are preparing to discharge Bobby Rowden from the emergency room. Discuss the teaching you should include for Bobby and his parents related to his injury and his plaster cast.

2. A pneumatic compression device has been ordered as part of the admission orders for Esther Levitz. You bring the pump and sleeves into the room, and she asks, "What is that? It looks like a torture machine!" How will you respond?

3. You are caring for Manuel Esposito the evening before his surgery. Your assessment of his affected extremity reveals skin that is warm to the touch, rapid capillary refill, and positive sensation and movement. What other assessments should you perform as part of your care for Mr. Esposito?

Bibliography

Beaupre, L. (April 1, 2001). Exercise combined with continuous passive motion or slider board therapy compared with exercise only: a randomized controlled trial of patients following total knee arthroplasty. *Physical Therapy, 81*(4), 1029–1037.

Breuninger, C., Follin, S., Munden, J., et al. (eds.) (2001). *Handbook of nursing procedures.* Springhouse, PA: Springhouse Corp.

Craven, R., & Hirnle, C. (2003). *Fundamentals of nursing. Human health and function* (4th ed.). Philadelphia: Lippincott Williams & Wilkins.

Fort, C. W. (September 2002). Get pumped to prevent DVT. *Nursing, 32*(9), 50–52.

Gulanick, M., & Myers, J. (2003). *Nursing plans of care: Nursing diagnosis.* Philadelphia: Mosby.

McConnell, E. A. (December 1997). Clinical do's & don'ts: Assisting with cast application. *Nursing, 27*(12), 28.

Mollabashy, A. (September 1997). Immobilization techniques for the cervical spine: cervical orthoses, skeletal traction, and halo devices. *Topics in Emergency Medicine, 19*(3), 26–33.

Pifer, G. (September 2000). Casting and splinting: prevention of complications. *Topics in Emergency Medicine, 22*(3), 48–54.

Sims, M., & Whiting, J. (Nov. 30, 2000). Pin-site care. *Nursing Times, 96*(48), 46.

Smeltzer, S., & Bare, B. (2004). *Brunner & Suddarth's textbook of medical-surgical nursing* (10th ed.). Philadelphia: Lippincott Williams & Wilkins.

Taylor, C., Lillis, C., & LeMone, P. (2004). *Fundamentals of nursing. The art & science of nursing care* (5th ed.). Philadelphia: Lippincott Williams & Wilkins.

Wood, M. (June 14, 2001). A protocol for care of skeletal pin sites. *Nursing Times, 97*(24), 66–68.

Comfort

Focusing on Patient Care

This chapter will help you develop the skills needed to meet the comfort needs of the following patients:

Mildred Simpson is a 75-year-old woman recovering from a total hip replacement.

Joseph Watkins comes to the emergency department because of acute pain in his lower back that started when he was moving furniture.

Jerome Batiste, age 60, has been diagnosed with bone cancer and is being discharged with an order for patient-controlled analgesia (PCA) at home.

Learning Outcomes

After studying this chapter, the reader should be able to:

1. Give a back massage
2. Apply a TENS unit
3. Care for a patient receiving PCA
4. Care for a patient receiving epidural analgesia

Key Terms

acute pain: pain that is generally rapid in onset, varies in intensity from mild to severe, and may last from a brief period up to 6 months

allodynia: pain that occurs after a normally weak or non-painful stimulus, such as a light touch or a cold drink; a characteristic feature of neuropathic pain

breakthrough pain: a temporary flare-up of moderate to severe pain that occurs even when the patient is taking around-the-clock medication for persistent pain

chronic pain: pain that may be limited, intermittent, or persistent but lasts for 6 months or longer and interferes with normal functioning

cutaneous pain: superficial pain usually involving the skin or subcutaneous tissue

dynorphin: endorphin with the most potent analgesic effect

endorphins: opioid neuromodulators; powerful pain-blocking chemicals that have prolonged analgesic effects and produce euphoria

enkephalins: opioid neuromodulators widespread throughout the brain and dorsal horn of the spinal cord; considered less potent than endorphins

gate control theory: theory that states that certain nerve fibers, those of small diameter, conduct excitatory pain stimuli toward the brain while nerve fibers of a large diameter appear to inhibit the transmission of pain impulses from the spinal cord to the brain

intractable pain: pain that is resistant to therapy and persists despite a variety of interventions

neuromodulators: endogenous opioid compounds; naturally present, morphine-like chemical regulators in the spinal cord and brain

neuropathic pain: pain that results from an injury to or abnormal functioning of peripheral nerves or the central nervous system

continues

Key Terms (continued)

neurotransmitters: substances that either excite or inhibit target nerve cells

nociceptive: pain that is usually acute and transmitted after normal processing of noxious stimuli

pain threshold: the lowest intensity of a stimulus that causes the subject to recognize pain

pain tolerance: point beyond which a person is no longer willing to endure pain

psychogenic pain: pain with a psychogenic origin; one for which a physical cause cannot be identified

referred pain: pain that is perceived in an area distant from its point of origin

somatic pain: diffuse or scattered pain that originates in tendons, ligaments, bones, blood vessels, and nerves

visceral pain: poorly localized pain that originates in body organs in the thorax, cranium, and abdomen

Comfort is an important need, and providing comfort is a major nursing responsibility. Providing comfort can be as simple as straightening the patient's bed linens, offering to hold the patient's hand, or assisting with hygiene needs. However, most often, providing comfort means providing pain relief.

A person in pain often experiences it as an all-consuming reality and wants only one intervention: pain relief. If pain relief were as simple as rubbing a back or administering a prescribed analgesic, nursing's task would be easy. However, no two people experience pain exactly the same way. Differences in individual pain perception and response to pain, as well as the multiple and diverse causes of pain, require the use of highly specialized abilities to promote comfort and relieve pain. The most important of these are the nurse's belief that the patient's pain is real, willingness to become involved in the patient's pain experience, and competence in developing effective pain management regimens.

Pain is an elusive and complex phenomenon, and despite its universality, its exact nature remains a mystery. It is one of the human body's defense mechanisms that indicates the person is experiencing a problem. The definition of pain that is probably of greatest benefit to nurses and patients is that offered by Margo McCaffery (1979, p. 11): "Pain is whatever the experiencing person says it is, existing whenever he (or she) says it does." This definition rests on the belief that the only one who can be a real authority on whether, and how, an individual is experiencing pain is that individual.

Pain is present whenever a person says it is, even when no specific cause of the pain can be found. Healthcare practitioners must rely on the patient's description of the pain because it is a subjective symptom that only the patient can identify and describe.

This chapter will cover the skills to assist the nurse in providing comfort, including pain relief. Please look over the summary tables, boxes, and figure at the beginning of this chapter for a quick review of critical knowledge to assist you in understanding the skills related to comfort and pain relief.

TABLE 10-1 Additional Terms Used by Patients to Describe Pain

Quality

Sharp	Pain that is sticking in nature and that is intense
Dull	Pain that is not as intense or acute as sharp pain, possibly more annoying than painful. It is usually more diffuse than sharp pain.
Diffuse	Pain that covers a large area. Usually, the patient is unable to point to a specific area without moving the hand over a large surface, such as the entire abdomen.
Shifting	Pain that moves from one area to another, such as from the lower abdomen to the area over the stomach.

Other terms used to describe the quality of pain include sore, stinging, pinching, cramping, gnawing, cutting, throbbing, shooting, viselike pressure.

Severity

Severe or excruciating	These terms depend on the patient's interpretation of pain. Behavioral and physiologic signs help assess the severity of pain. On a scale of 1 to 10, slight pain could be described as being between about 1 and 3; moderate pain, between about 4 and 7; and severe pain, between about 8 and 10.
Moderate	
Slight or mild	

Periodicity

Continuous	Pain that does not stop
Intermittent	Pain that stops and starts again
Brief or transient	Pain that passes quickly

TABLE 10-2 Pain Assessment

Factors to Assess	Questions and Approaches
Characteristics of the pain Location	"Where is your pain? Is it external or internal?" (Asking the patient with acute pain to point to the painful area with one finger may help to localize the pain. Patients with chronic pain may have difficulty trying to localize their pain, however.)
Duration	"How long have you been experiencing pain? How long does a pain episode last? How often does a pain episode occur?"
Quantity	Ask the patient to indicate the degree (amount) of pain currently experienced on the scale below: 0 1 2 3 4 5 6 7 8 9 10 No pain Mild Moderate Severe Pain as bad as it can be It is also helpful to ask how much pain the patient has (on the same scale) when the pain is at its least and at its worst: Least _____ Worst _____
Quality	"What words would you use to describe your pain?"
Chronology	"How does the pain develop and progress?" (If pattern can be identified, interventions early in a pain sequence will often be far more effective than those used after the pain is well established.) "Has the pain changed since it first began? If so, how?"
Aggravating factors	"What makes the pain occur or increase in intensity?"
Alleviating factors	"What makes the pain go away or lessen? What methods of relief have you tried in the past? How long were they used? How effective were they?" (Methods of relief currently in effect for hospitalized patients should be apparent from the chart. It is important to verify the use of current orders and their effectiveness with the patient. Outpatients may need to be asked to record a medication profile, a thorough and accurate account of all medications they are taking.)

continues

TABLE 10-2 continued

Factors to Assess	Questions and Approaches
Associated phenomena	"Are there any other factors that seem to relate consistently to your pain? Any other symptoms that occur just before, during, or after your pain?"
Physiologic responses Vital signs (blood pressure, pulse, respirations) Skin color Perspiration Pupil size Nausea	Signs of sympathetic stimulation commonly occur with acute pain. Signs of parasympathetic stimulation (decreased blood pressure and pulse, rapid and irregular respirations, pupil constriction, nausea and vomiting, and warm, dry skin) may be present, especially in prolonged, severe pain, visceral, or deep pain.
Muscle tension	Observe. Ask the patient whether he or she is aware of any tight, tense muscles.
Anxiety	Are signs of anxiety evident? (May include decreased attention span or ability to follow directions, frequent asking of questions, shifting of topics of conversation, avoidance of discussion of feelings, acting out, somatizing.)
Behavioral responses Posture, gross motor activities	Does patient rub or support a particular area? Make frequent position changes? Walk, pace, kneel, or assume a rolled-up position? Does patient rest a particular body part? Protect an area from stimulation? Lie quietly? (In acute pain, postural and gross motor activities are often altered; in chronic pain, the only signs of change may be postures characteristic of withdrawal.)
Facial features	Does the patient have a pinched look? Are there facial grimaces? Knotted brow? Overall taut, anxious appearance? (A look of fatigue is more characteristic of chronic pain.)
Verbal expressions	Does the patient sigh, moan, scream, cry, repetitively use the same words?
Affective responses Anxiety	"Do you feel anxious? Are you afraid? If so, how bad are these feelings?"
Depression	"Do you feel depressed, down, or low? If so, how bad are these feelings? Are your feelings about yourself mostly good or bad? Do you have feelings of failure? Do you see yourself or your illness as a burden to those you care about?"
Interactions with others	How does the patient act when he or she is in pain in the presence of others? How does the patient respond to others when he or she is not in pain? How do significant others and caregivers respond to the patient when the patient is in pain? When the patient is not in pain?
Degree to which pain interferes with patient's life (use past performance as baseline)	"Does the pain interfere with sleep? If so, to what extent? Is fatigue a major factor in the pain experience? Is the conduct of intimate or peer relationships affected by the pain? Is work function affected? Participation in recreational–diversional activities?" (An activity diary is often helpful—sometimes crucial. One to several weeks of hourly activity recorded by the patient may be necessary. Levels of pain, intake of food, and sleep–rest periods are noted along with activities performed. Separate diaries for inpatient and outpatient episodes may be necessary because hospitalization markedly affects the nature and type of activities performed.)
Perception of pain and meaning to patient	"Are you worried about your illness? Do you see any connection between your pain and the nature or course of illness? If so, how do you see them as related? Do you find any meaning in your pain? If so, is this beneficial or detrimental to you? Are you struggling to find some meaning for your pain?"
Adaptive mechanisms used to cope with pain	"What do you usually do to relieve stress? How well do these things work? What techniques do you use at home to help cope with the pain? How well have they worked? Do you use these in the hospital? If not, why not?"
Outcomes	"What would you like to be doing right now, this week, this month, if the pain were better controlled? How much would the pain have to decrease (on the 0 to 10 scale) for you to begin to accomplish these goals?"

BOX 10-1 Common Responses to Pain

Behavioral (Voluntary) Responses
Moving away from painful stimuli
Grimacing, moaning, and crying
Restlessness
Protecting the painful area and refusing to move

Physiologic (Involuntary) Responses
Typical Sympathetic Responses When Pain
Is Moderate and Superficial
Increased blood pressure
Increased pulse and respiratory rates
Pupil dilation
Muscle tension and rigidity
Pallor (peripheral vasoconstriction)
Increased adrenaline output
Increased blood glucose
Typical Parasympathetic Responses When Pain
Is Severe and Deep
Nausea and vomiting
Fainting or unconsciousness

Decreased blood pressure
Decreased pulse rate
Prostration
Rapid and irregular breathing

Affective (Psychological) Responses
Exaggerated weeping and restlessness
Withdrawal
Stoicism
Anxiety
Depression
Fear
Anger
Anorexia
Fatigue
Hopelessness
Powerlessness

BOX 10-2 Selected Nonpharmacologic Pain Relief Methods

Whether used alone or in combination with analgesics, non-pharmacologic methods can be effective in promoting comfort and relieving pain. No one method is more effective than another. Typically the method chosen is based on patient preference.

Distraction
- Patient recalls a pleasant experience or focuses attention on an enjoyable activity.
- Music often is used for distraction: the patient concentrates on listening to the music, raising or lowering the volume based on the amount of pain.
- This method is effective primarily for pain episodes that are brief, typically lasting 5 minutes or less.

Guided Imagery
- Patient concentrates on a peaceful, pleasant image.
- The focus is on the details of the image, such as sights, sounds, smells, tastes, and touches as appropriate.

- Audio tapes of sounds can be helpful with this method.
- Pain relief results from the positive emotions evoked by the image.

Deep Breathing
- Patient stares at an object and then slowly inhales and exhales while counting aloud to maintain a comfortable rate and rhythm.
- The patient concentrates on the rising and falling of the abdomen.
- With each breath, the patient concentrates on feeling more and more weightless.

Muscle Relaxation
- The patient focuses on a particular muscle group and then tenses the muscles and notes the sensation.
- After about 5 to 7 seconds, the patient relaxes the muscle group and concentrates on the relaxation sensation.
- The patient continues this process with another muscle group until he or she has covered the entire body.

Date _____

Patient's name _____ Age _____ Room _____

Diagnosis _____ Physician _____

Nurse _____

1. LOCATION: Patient or nurse marks drawing.

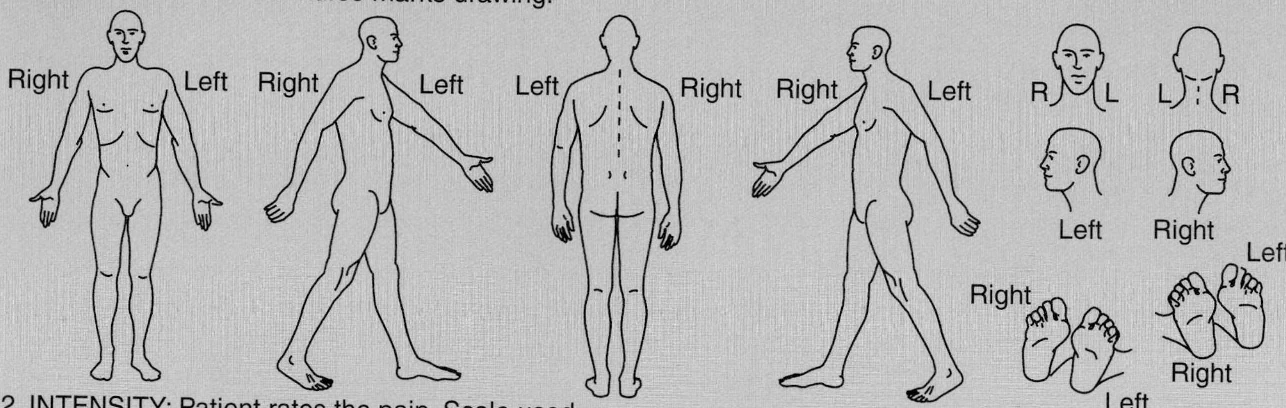

2. INTENSITY: Patient rates the pain. Scale used _____
Present: _____
Worst pain gets: _____
Best pain gets: _____
Acceptable level of pain: _____

3. QUALITY: (Use patient's own words, e.g., prick, ache, burn, throb, pull, sharp)
_____

4. ONSET, DURATION, VARIATION, RHYTHMS: _____
_____

5. MANNER OF EXPRESSING PAIN: _____
6. WHAT RELIEVES THE PAIN? _____
7. WHAT CAUSES OR INCREASES THE PAIN? _____
8. EFFECTS OF PAIN: (Note decreased function, decreased quality of life.)

    Accompanying symptoms (e.g., nausea) _____
    Sleep _____
    Appetite _____
    Physical activity _____
    Relationship with others (e.g., irritability) _____
    Emotions (e.g., anger, suicidal, crying) _____
    Concentration _____
    Other _____

9. OTHER COMMENTS: _____
_____

10. PLAN: _____
_____

May be duplicated for use in clinical practice. Adapted from McCaffery M, Pasero C: *Pain: Clinical manual*, p. 60. Copyright © 1999, Mosby, Inc.

FIGURE 10-1 Pain assessment tool.

Giving a Back Massage

A back massage generally follows the patient's bath. A massage acts as a general body conditioner and can be used to relieve muscle tension and promote relaxation. Some nurses do not always give back massages to patients because they don't think they have enough time. However, giving a back massage provides an opportunity for the nurse to observe the skin for signs of breakdown. It improves circulation; can decrease pain, symptom distress, and anxiety; and improve sleep quality; it also provides a means of communicating with the patient through the use of touch. A back massage also provides cutaneous stimulation as a method of pain relief.

Because some patients consider the back massage a luxury and may be reluctant to accept it, communicate its importance and value to the patient. An effective back massage should take 4 to 6 minutes to complete. A lotion is usually used; warm it before applying it to the back. Be aware of the patient's medical diagnosis when considering giving a back massage. A back massage is contraindicated, for example, when the patient has had back surgery or has fractured ribs. Position the patient on the abdomen or, if this is contraindicated, on the side for a back massage.

Equipment

- Massage lubricant or lotion
- Powder, if not contraindicated
- Bath blanket
- Towel
- Clean gloves, if the patient has lesions or contact with drainage is likely

ASSESSMENT

Review the patient's medical record and plan of care for information about the patient's status and contraindications to back massage. Question the patient about any conditions that might require modifications or that might contraindicate a massage. Inquire about any allergies, such as to lotions or scents. Ask if the patient has any preferences for lotion or has his or her own lotion. Assess the patient's level of pain, asking him or her to rate the pain on a scale of 1 to 10. Check the patient's medication administration record for the time an analgesic was last administered. If appropriate, administering an analgesic early enough so that it has time to take effect.

**NURSING
DIAGNOSIS**

Determine the related factors for the nursing diagnoses based on the patient's current status. An appropriate nursing diagnosis is Acute Pain. Other nursing diagnoses that may be appropriate include:

- Chronic Pain
- Disturbed Sleep Pattern
- Risk for Skin Integrity
- Anxiety
- Ineffective Coping
- Activity Intolerance
- Deficient Knowledge
- Ineffective Tissue Perfusion
- Self-Care Deficit

In addition, many other nursing diagnoses may require the use of this skill.

**OUTCOME
IDENTIFICATION
AND PLANNING**

The expected outcome to achieve when performing a back massage is that the patient states pain is relieved and the patient is relaxed. Other outcomes that may be appropriate include: the patient experiences control of chronic pain; the patient displays decreased anxiety and improved relaxation; skin breakdown is absent; the patient understands the reasons for back massage; and tissue perfusion is improved.

continues

SKILL 10-1   Giving a Back Massage (continued)

IMPLEMENTATION
ACTION

1. Offer a back massage to the patient and explain the procedure.

2. Perform hand hygiene.
3. Close the curtain or door.

4. Assist the patient to the prone or side-lying position with the back exposed from the shoulders to the sacral area. Use the bath blanket to drape the patient. Raise the bed to the high position and lower the side rail closest to you.

5. **Warm the lubricant or lotion in the palm of your hand, or place the container in warm water.**

6. Using light gliding strokes (*effleurage*), apply lotion to patient's shoulders, back, and sacral area.

7. Place your hands beside each other at the base of the patient's spine and stroke upward to the shoulders and back downward to the buttocks in slow, continuous strokes. Continue for several minutes.

RATIONALE

Back massage can facilitate circulation and promote relaxation. Explanation aids in decreasing anxiety and prepares the patient for what is to come.

Hand hygiene deters the spread of microorganisms.

Closing the door or curtain ensures privacy and promotes relaxation.

This position exposes an adequate area for massage. Draping the patient provides privacy and warmth. Having the bed in the high position reduces back strain for the nurse.

Cold lotion causes chilling and discomfort.

Effleurage relaxes the patient and lessens tension.

Continuous contact is soothing and stimulates circulation and muscle relaxation.

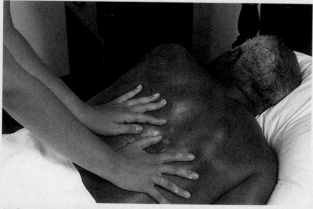
Action 6: Using effleurage on a patient's back.

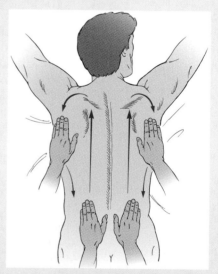
Action 7: Stroking upward to the shoulders.

8. Massage the patient's shoulder, entire back, areas over iliac crests, and sacrum with circular stroking motions. **Keep your hands in contact with the patient's skin.** Continue for several minutes, applying additional lotion as necessary.

9. Knead the patient's skin by gently alternating grasping and compression motions (*pétrissage*).

10. Complete the massage with additional long stroking movements that eventually become lighter in pressure.

A firm stroke with continuous contact promotes relaxation.

Kneading increases blood circulation.

Long stroking motions are soothing and promote relaxation; continued stroking with gradual lightening of pressure helps extend the feeling of relaxation.

continues

Giving a Back Massage (continued)

ACTION	RATIONALE

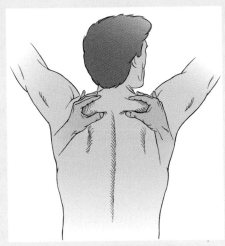

Action 9: Using pétrissage.

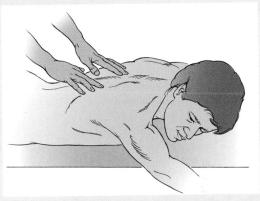

Action 10: Use light stroking with lessening pressure.

11. During massage, observe the patient's skin for reddened or open areas. **Pay particular attention to the skin over bony prominences.**

Pressure may interfere with circulation and lead to pressure ulcers. Back massage stimulates circulation to these areas.

12. Use the towel to pat the patient dry and to remove excess lotion. Apply powder if the patient requests it.

Drying provides comfort and reduces the feeling of moisture on the back.

13. Perform hand hygiene.

Hand hygiene deters the spread of microorganisms.

14. Assess the patient's response and record your observations on the patient's medical record.

Documentation provides communication about the procedure and the condition of the patient's skin and promotes continuity of care.

EVALUATION   The expected outcome is achieved when the patient reports a decrease in pain or control of pain as evidenced by a lower numerical rating. In addition, the patient verbalizes increased comfort and decreased anxiety. The patient exhibits pink, dry, intact skin and verbalizes an understanding of the reasons for and benefits of back massage.

Unexpected Situations and Associated Interventions

- *Your patient cannot lie prone, so you are giving him a back massage while he is lying on his side. However, as you begin to massage the back, the patient cannot maintain the side-lying position:* If possible, have the patient hold onto the side rail on the side to which he is facing. If this is not possible or the patient cannot assist, use pillows and bath blankets to prevent the patient from rolling. If necessary, enlist the help of another person to maintain the patient's position.
- *While massaging the patient's back, you notice a 2″ reddened area on the patient's sacrum:* Note this observation in the patient's medical record and report it to the physician. Do not massage the area. When the back massage is completed, position the patient off the sacral area, using pillows to maintain the patient's position, and institute a turning schedule.

continues

Giving a Back Massage (continued)

Special Considerations

- Before giving a back massage, assess the patient's body structure and skin condition, and tailor the duration and intensity of the massage accordingly. If you are giving a back massage at bedtime, have the patient ready for bed beforehand so the massage can help him or her fall asleep.
- Use a separate bottle of lotion for each patient to prevent cross-contamination. If the patient has oily skin, substitute a talcum powder or lotion of the patient's choice. However, to avoid aspiration, do not use powder if the patient has an endotracheal or tracheal tube in place. Avoid using powder and lotion together because this may lead to skin maceration.
- When massaging the patient's back, stand with one foot slightly forward and your knees slightly bent to allow effective use of your arm and shoulder muscles.
- Give special attention to bony prominences, because these areas are disposed to the formation of pressure ulcers. Develop a turning schedule and give a back massage with each position change.

Applying a TENS Unit

Transcutaneous electrical nerve stimulation (TENS) is a noninvasive technique for providing pain relief that involves the electrical stimulation of large-diameter fibers to inhibit the transmission of painful impulses carried over small-diameter fibers. The TENS unit consists of a battery-powered portable unit, lead wires, and cutaneous electrode pads that are applied to the painful area. It requires a physician's order. TENS therapy has reportedly been effective in reducing postoperative pain and improving mobility after surgery. Positive results have also been noted when it is used as an adjunct with physical therapy and for patients with low back pain. The TENS unit may be applied intermittently throughout the day or worn for extended periods of time, depending on the physician's order.

Equipment

- TENS unit
- Electrodes
- Electrode gel (if electrodes are not pregelled)
- Tape (if electrodes are not self-adhesive)
- Alcohol wipes

ASSESSMENT

Review the patient's medical record and plan of care for specific instructions related to TENS therapy, including the physician's order and conditions indicating the need for therapy. Review the patient's history for conditions that might contraindicate therapy such as pacemaker insertion, cardiac monitoring, or electrocardiography. Determine the location of electrode placement based on consultation with the physician and on the patient's report of pain. Inspect the skin of the area designated for electrode placement for irritation, redness, or breakdown. Assess the patient's pain using a pain rating scale. Check to ensure proper functioning of the unit. Assess the patient's understanding of TENS therapy and the rationale for its use. Check manufacturer's instructions for use.

**NURSING
DIAGNOSIS**

Determine the related factors for the nursing diagnoses based on the patient's current status. Appropriate nursing diagnoses include Acute Pain and Chronic Pain. Other appropriate nursing diagnoses may include:

- Anxiety
- Fear

continues

Applying a TENS Unit (continued)

- Ineffective Coping
- Deficient Knowledge
- Risk for Injury
- Risk for Impaired Skin Integrity

Many other nursing diagnoses may require the use of this skill.

**OUTCOME
IDENTIFICATION
AND PLANNING**

The expected outcome to achieve when applying a TENS unit is that the patient will verbalize a decrease in pain, as evidenced by a lower numerical rating, without experiencing any injury or skin irritation or breakdown. Other appropriate outcomes may include: patient displays decreased anxiety, improved coping skills, and an understanding of the therapy and the reason for its use.

IMPLEMENTATION

ACTION

RATIONALE

1. Identify the patient, show the patient the device, and explain the function of the device and the reason for its use.

Patient identification ensures that the correct patient will receive the therapy. Explanation helps reduce anxiety and prepare the patient for what is to come.

2. Perform hand hygiene.

Hand hygiene deters the spread of microorganisms.

3. Inspect the area where the electrodes are to be placed. Clean and dry it with an alcohol wipe.

Inspection ensures that the electrodes will be applied to intact skin. Cleaning and drying help ensure that electrodes will adhere.

4. Remove the adhesive backing from the electrodes and apply them to the specified location. **If the electrodes are not pregelled, apply a small amount of electrode gel to the bottom of each electrode.** If the electrodes are not self-adhering, tape them in place.

Application to the proper location enhances the success of the therapy. Gel is necessary to promote conduction of the electrical current.

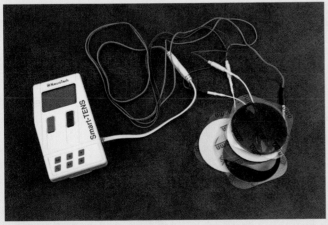

Action 1: TENS unit.

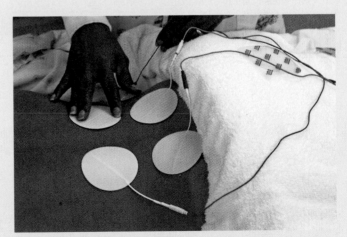

Action 4: Apply the TENS electrodes.

5. **Check the placement of the electrodes; leave at least a 2″ (5 cm) space (about the width of one electrode) between them.**

Proper spacing is necessary to reduce the risk of burns due to the proximity of the electrodes.

6. **Note the controls on the TENS unit to make sure that they are off.** Connect the wires to the electrodes (if not already attached) and plug them into the unit.

This connection completes the electrical circuit necessary to stimulate the nerve fibers.

continues

ACTION

7. Turn on the unit and adjust the intensity setting to the lowest intensity and determine if the patient can feel a tingling, burning, or buzzing sensation. Then adjust the intensity to the prescribed amount or the setting most comfortable for the patient. Secure the unit to the patient.

8. Set the pulse width (duration of the each pulsation) as indicated or recommended.

9. Assess the patient's pain level during therapy.
   a. If intermittent use is ordered, turn the unit off after the specified duration of treatment and remove the electrodes. Provide skin care to the area.
   b. If continuous therapy is ordered, periodically remove the electrodes from the skin (after turning the unit off) to inspect the area and clean the skin. Reapply electrodes and continue therapy.

10. When therapy is discontinued, turn the unit off and remove the electrodes. Clean the patient's skin. Clean the unit and replace the batteries.

11. Perform hand hygiene and document the date and time of application; patient's initial pain assessment; electrode placement location; intensity and pulse width; duration of therapy; pain assessments during therapy and patient's response; and time of removal or discontinuation of therapy.

RATIONALE

Using the lowest setting at first introduces the patient to the sensations. Adjusting the intensity is necessary to provide the proper amount of stimulation

The pulse width determines the depth and width of the stimulation

Pain assessment helps evaluate the effectiveness of therapy.
a. TENS therapy can be ordered for intermittent or continuous use. Skin care reduces the risk for irritation and breakdown.
b. Periodic removal of electrodes allows for skin assessment. Skin care reduces the risk for irritation and breakdown. Reapplication ensures continued therapy.

Turning the unit off and removing electrodes when therapy is discontinued reduces the risk of injury to the patient. Cleaning the unit and replacing the batteries ensures that the unit is ready for use.

Action 7: Turn on the unit.

5/28/06   1105   Patient complaining of severe lower back pain, rating it as 9 out of 10 on pain rating scale. Identified lower sacral area as site of pain. TENS therapy ordered for 30 to 45 minutes. Electrodes applied to right and left sides of sacral area. Intensity initially set at 80 pulses per second with pulse width of 80 microseconds. Pain rating at 7 out of 10 after 15 minutes of therapy. Intensity increased to 100 pulses per second with a pulse width increased to 100 microseconds. Pain rating at 5 out of 10 after 15 minutes at increased settings. Therapy continued for an additional 15 minutes and discontinued. Patient rated pain at 3 out of 10 at end of session. Skin on lower sacral area clean, dry, and intact without evidence of irritation or breakdown. Patient instructed to report increasing pain.
—K. Lewin, RN

Action 11: Documentation.

continues

SKILL 10-2   Applying a TENS Unit (continued)

EVALUATION

The expected outcome is achieved when the patient verbalizes pain relief. In addition, the patient remains free of signs and symptoms of skin irritation and breakdown and injury. The patient reports decreased anxiety and increased ability to cope with pain. The patient verbalizes information related to the functioning of the unit and reasons for its use.

Unexpected Situations and Associated Interventions

- *While receiving TENS therapy, the patient reports pain and intolerable paresthesia:* Check the settings, connections, and placement of the electrodes. Adjust the settings and reposition the electrodes as necessary.
- *During a TENS therapy session, the patient reports muscle twitching:* Assess the patient and check the intensity setting. Readjust the intensity to a lower setting, because the patient is most likely experiencing overstimulation.
- *While assessing the skin where the electrodes are placed for a patient receiving continuous TENS therapy, you notice some irritation and redness:* Clean and dry the area thoroughly. Reposition the electrodes in the same area, but avoid the irritated and reddened area.

Special Considerations

- Never place electrodes over the carotid sinus nerves or over laryngeal or pharyngeal muscles, over the eyes, or over the uterus of a pregnant woman.
- TENS is not used when the etiology of the pain is unknown because it may mask a new pathology.
- Whenever electrodes are being repositioned or removed, turn the unit off first.
- For acute pain, a pulse width of 60 to 100 microseconds is recommended; for chronic or intense pain, a pulse width of 220 to 250 microseconds may be needed.
- A conventional intensity setting ranges from 80 to 125 pulses per second.

SKILL 10-3   Caring for a Patient Receiving PCA

Patient-controlled analgesia (PCA) provides effective individualized analgesia and comfort. This drug delivery system may be used to manage acute and chronic pain in a healthcare facility or the home. PCA relieves pain associated with operative procedures, labor and delivery, trauma, and cancer. This device is most commonly used to deliver analgesics intravenously, but the subcutaneous route is also an option. The most frequently prescribed drug for PCA administration is morphine.

The PCA system consists of a portable infusion pump containing a reservoir or chamber for a syringe that is prefilled with the prescribed opioid. When pain occurs, the patient pushes a button that activates the PCA device to deliver a small preset bolus dose of the analgesic. A lockout interval that is programmed into the PCA unit (usually 5 to 10 minutes) prevents reactivation of the pump and administration of another dose during that period of time. The pump mechanism can also be programmed to deliver only a specified amount of analgesic within a given time interval (most commonly every hour or, occasionally, every 4 hours). These safeguards limit the risk for overmedication and allow the patient to evaluate the effect of the previous dose. PCA pumps also have a locked safety system that prohibits tampering with the device.

Patients need instruction preoperatively if they are expected to use the PCA device postoperatively. Suitable candidates for this type of delivery system include patients who are alert and capable of controlling the unit. Setting up the PCA system and ensuring that it is functioning properly are additional nursing activities.

continues

SKILL 10-3   Caring for a Patient Receiving PCA (continued)

Equipment	• PCA system • Syringe filled with mediation • PCA system tubing • Alcohol wipes (if indicated) • Clean gloves
ASSESSMENT	Review the patient's medical record and plan of care for specific instructions related to PCA therapy, including the physician's order and conditions indicating the need for therapy. Check the physician's order for the prescribed drug, initial loading dose, dose for self-administration, and lockout interval. Review the patient's history for conditions that might contraindicate therapy, such as respiratory limitations, history of substance abuse, or psychiatric disorder. Determine the route for administration, such as intravenously or via a subcutaneous infusion port. Inspect the site to be used for the infusion for signs of infiltration or infection. Assess the intravenous infusion (if this is the route) to ensure that the line is patent and the current solution is compatible with the drug ordered. Assess the patient's pain using a pain rating scale. Check to ensure proper functioning of the unit. Assess the patient's level of consciousness and understanding of PCA therapy and the rationale for its use.
NURSING DIAGNOSIS	Determine the related factors for the nursing diagnoses based on the patient's current status. Appropriate nursing diagnoses include Acute Pain and Chronic Pain. Other appropriate nursing diagnoses may include: • Anxiety • Fear • Ineffective Coping • Deficient Knowledge • Risk for Injury Many other nursing diagnoses may require the use of this skill.
OUTCOME IDENTIFICATION AND PLANNING	The expected outcome to achieve when caring for a patient receiving PCA is that the patient verbalizes a decrease in pain, as evidenced by a lower numerical rating, without experiencing injury. Other appropriate outcomes may include: the patient displays decreased anxiety, improved coping skills, and an understanding of the therapy and the reason for its use.

IMPLEMENTATION

ACTION	RATIONALE
1. Identify the patient, show the patient the device, and explain the function of the device and reason for use.	Patient identification ensures that the correct patient will receive the therapy. Explanation helps reduce anxiety and prepare the patient for what is to come.
2. Plug the PCA device into the electrical outlet.	The PCA devices requires a power source (electricity or battery) to run.
3. Perform hand hygiene and put on gloves.	Hand hygiene and gloving deter the spread of microorganisms.
4. **Check the label on the prefilled drug syringe with the medication record and patient identification.**	This action verifies that the correct drug and dosage will be administered to the correct patient.
5. Connect tubing to prefilled syringe and place the syringe into the PCA device. **Prime the tubing.**	Doing so prepares the device to deliver the drug. Priming the tubing purges air from the tubing and reduces the risk for air embolism.
6. Connect the PCA tubing to the patient's intravenous infusion line or subcutaneous infusion port; tape the connection site.	Connection is necessary to allow drug delivery to the patient. Taping ensures that the tubing will not become dislodged or disconnected.

continues

Caring for a Patient Receiving PCA (continued)

ACTION   **RATIONALE**

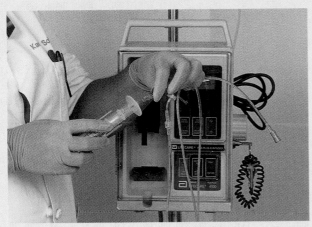

Action 5: Connect the tubing to the prefilled syringe. (Photo © B. Proud.)

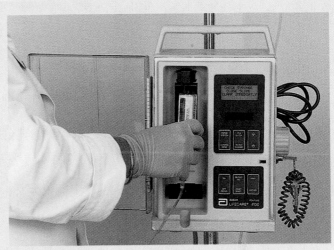

Action 5: Load the syringe into the PCA device. (Photo © B. Proud.)

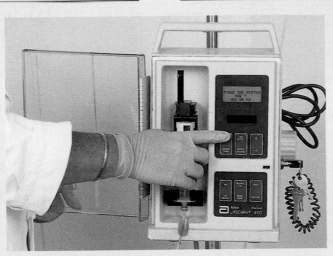

Action 5: Priming the tubing. (Photo © B. Proud.)

7. Set the PCA device to administer the loading dose, and then program the device based on the physician's order for infusion dosage and lockout interval.

These actions ensure that the appropriate drug dosage will be administered.

8. Instruct the patient to press the button each time he or she needs relief from pain.

Instruction promotes correct use of the device.

9. Assess the patient's pain at least every 1 to 2 hours and monitor vital signs, especially respiratory status. Inspect the site and rate of the infusion periodically. Replace the drug syringe when it is empty.

Continued assessment at frequent intervals helps evaluate the effectiveness of the drug and reduce the risk for complications. Respiratory depression may occur with the use of narcotic analgesics. Replacing the syringe ensures continued drug delivery.

10. Remove gloves and dispose of them appropriately, and perform hand hygiene. Document the date and time PCA therapy was initiated, initial pain assessment, drug and loading dose administered, individual dosing and time interval, continued pain assessments, and patient's response to therapy.

Hand hygiene and proper disposal of gloves deter the spread of infection. Documentation promotes communication and continuity of care.

continues

ACTION

RATIONALE

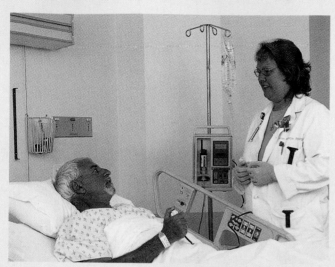

Action 8: Teach the patient how to use the device.   (Photo © B. Proud.)

6/1/06   0645   Patient returned from surgery with PCA therapy with morphine sulfate 1 mg/mL in place via IV infusion. Device programmed to deliver 0.1 mg at 10-minute lockout intervals. Patient complaining of moderate to severe abdominal pain, rating pain as 6 to 8 out of 10 on a pain rating scale. Patient instructed to press PCA button for pain relief. Vital signs within acceptable parameters. Respiratory rate 16 breaths per minute. IV of 1,000 cc D5LR infusing at 100 cc/minute; site clean and dry without evidence of infiltration or infection. —P. Joyner, RN

6/1/06   0700   Patient rates pain at 5. Respirations 16 breaths per minute. Encouraged patient to take deep breaths and cough. Lying on right side with the support of two pillows and head of bed elevated 30 degrees. —P. Joyner, RN

Action 10: Documentation.

EVALUATION

The expected outcome is achieved when the patient verbalizes pain relief. In addition, the patient remains free of signs and symptoms of injury; the patient reports decreased anxiety and increased ability to cope with pain; and the patient verbalizes information related to the functioning of the unit and the reasons for its use.

Unexpected Situations and Associated Interventions

- *While receiving PCA therapy, your patient's respiratory rate drops to 10 breaths per minute and he becomes very lethargic and slow to respond:* Stop the PCA infusion immediately and notify the physician. In the meantime, attempt to arouse the patient by talking to him and shaking him. Encourage the patient to take deep slow breaths if possible. Prepare to administer oxygen and a narcotic antagonist such as naloxone (Narcan).
- *The patient's intravenous infusion line becomes infiltrated:* Stop the PCA infusion and IV infusion. Remove the IV catheter and restart the IV line in another site. Once the site is established, resume the IV and PCA infusion.

Special Considerations

- Check the manufacturer's instructions before using the device because a wide variety of PCA devices are available.
- If using a device that provides continuous and bolus doses, remember that the cumulative doses per hour should not exceed the total hourly dose ordered by the physician.
- Monitor the patient's vital signs, especially when initiating therapy. Encourage the patient to practice coughing and deep breathing to promote ventilation and prevent pooling of secretions.
- Have a narcotic antagonist such as naloxone (Narcan) readily available in case the patient develops respiratory complications related to drug therapy.

continues

SKILL 10-3   Caring for a Patient Receiving PCA (continued)

Infant and Child Considerations

- PCA can be an effective method of pain control for a child. When determining the appropriateness of this therapy for a child, consider the child's chronological age and developmental level, ability to understand (cognitive level), and motor skills.
- PCA has been shown to be very effective for adolescents because it gives them an increased feeling of control over the situation.

Home Care Considerations

- Be sure that the patient understands how to use the PCA device properly. Teach the patient how the device works, when to contact the physician, signs and symptoms of adverse reactions, and signs and symptoms of drug tolerance.
- Advise the patient to change positions gradually to prevent orthostatic hypotension, which may result from use of a narcotic analgesic.
- Ensure that there is a reliable adult who can provide backup assistance should the patient have difficulty.
- Consider a referral to a home healthcare agency to continue teaching and provide assessment of the therapy.

SKILL 10-4   Caring for a Patient Receiving Epidural Analgesia

Epidural analgesia is being used more commonly to provide pain relief during the immediate postoperative phase (particularly after thoracic, abdominal, orthopedic, and vascular surgery) and for chronic pain situations. Epidural pain management is also being used in children with terminal cancer and children undergoing hip, spinal, or lower extremity surgery. The anesthesiologist usually inserts the catheter in the mid-lumbar region into the epidural space that exists between the walls of the vertebral canal and the dura mater or outermost connective tissue membrane surrounding the spinal cord. For temporary therapy, the catheter exits directly over the spine, and the tubing is positioned over the patient's shoulder with the end of the catheter taped to the chest. For long-term therapy, the catheter is usually tunneled subcutaneously and exits on the side of the body or on the abdomen.

The narcotic or opioid acts directly on the opiate receptors in the spinal cord, and pain relief is achieved with smaller doses and less severe side effects. The epidural analgesia can be administered as a bolus dose (either one-time or intermittent), via a continuous infusion pump, or by a patient-controlled epidural analgesia (PCEA) pump (Pasero, 2003b). The drug of choice is usually preservative-free morphine or fentanyl (Sublimaze). Since the epidural space contains blood vessels, nerves, and fat, lipid-soluble fentanyl is readily dissolved; it has a rapid onset of action (5 minutes) but a short duration of action (approximately 2 hours). Morphine is a hydrophilic opioid, meaning that it has a high affinity for water. It has a slower onset of action but may exert its analgesic effect for as long as 24 hours because it remains longer in the cerebrospinal fluid (CSF) and spinal tissue (Pasero, 2003b). Epidural catheters used for the management of acute pain are typically removed 36 to 72 hours after surgery, when oral medication can be substituted for relief of pain.

continues

SKILL 10-4   Caring for a Patient Receiving Epidural Analgesia (continued)

Equipment

- Volume infusion device
- Epidural infusion tubing
- Prescribed epidural analgesic solutions
- Transparent dressing or gauze pads
- Labels for epidural infusion line
- Tape
- Emergency drugs and equipment such as naloxone, oxygen, endotracheal intubation set, handheld resuscitation bag

ASSESSMENT

Review the patient's medical record and plan of care for specific instructions related to epidural analgesia therapy, including the physician's order for the drug and conditions indicating the need for therapy. Review the patient's history for conditions that might contraindicate therapy, such as local or systemic infections, neurologic disease, coagulopathy or use of anticoagulant therapy, spinal arthritis or spinal deformity, hypotension, marked hypertension, allergy to the prescribed medication, or psychiatric disorder. Assess the patient's pain using a pain rating scale. Check to ensure proper functioning of the unit. Assess the patient's level of consciousness and understanding of epidural analgesia therapy and the rationale for its use.

NURSING DIAGNOSIS

Determine the related factors for the nursing diagnoses based on the patient's current status. Appropriate nursing diagnoses include Acute Pain and Chronic Pain. Other appropriate nursing diagnoses may include:

- Anxiety
- Fear
- Ineffective Coping
- Deficient Knowledge
- Risk for Injury
- Risk for Infection

Many other nursing diagnoses may require the use of this skill.

OUTCOME IDENTIFICATION AND PLANNING

The expected outcome to achieve when caring for a patient receiving epidural analgesia is that the patient verbalizes a decrease in pain, as evidenced by a lower numerical rating, without experiencing injury. Other appropriate outcomes may include: the patient displays decreased anxiety and improved coping skills; the patient remains free from infection; and the patient verbalizes understanding of the therapy and the reason for its use.

IMPLEMENTATION

ACTION	RATIONALE
1. Verify the physician's order for analgesia, drug preparation, and rate of infusion with another nurse. Perform hand hygiene and put on gloves if indicated.	Verification provides for safe administration of the correct dose at the correct rate. Hand hygiene and gloving deter the spread of microorganisms.
2. **Have an ampule of 0.4 mg naloxone (Narcan) and a syringe at the bedside.**	Naloxone reverses the respiratory depressant effect of opioids.
3. After the catheter has been inserted, check the infusion bag and ensure that the infusion tubing has been primed and connected to the epidural catheter and the rate of infusion is correct.	Doing so ensures that the drug will be administered correctly as prescribed.
4. Tape all connection sites. Label the bag, tubing, and pump apparatus "For Epidural Infusion Only." **Do not administer any other narcotics or adjuvant drugs without the approval of the clinician responsible for the epidural injection.**	Taping prevents accidental dislodgement. Labeling prevents inadvertent administration of other intravenous medications through this setup. Additional medication may potentiate the action of the opioid, increasing the risk for respiratory depression.

continues

Caring for a Patient Receiving Epidural Analgesia (continued)

ACTION

RATIONALE

5. Assess the exit site and apply a transparent dressing over the catheter insertion site. Monitor the infusion rate.

The transparent dressing protects the site while still allowing assessment. Monitoring the infusion rate prevents incorrect administration of the medication.

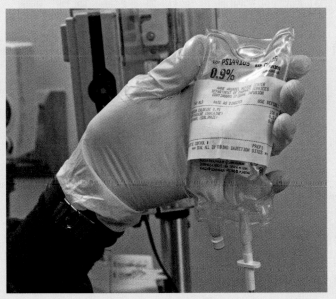

Action 4: Epidural bag.

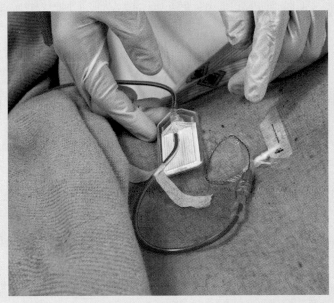

Action 5: Assessing exit site.

6. Assess and record sedation level (using a sedation scale) and respiratory status every hour for the first 24 hours, then at 4-hour intervals (or according to agency policy). **Notify the physician if the sedation rating is 3, the respiratory depth decreases, or the respiratory rate falls below 8 breaths per minute.**

Opioids can depress the respiratory center in the medulla. A change in the level of consciousness is usually the first sign of altered respiratory function.

7. Keep the head of bed elevated 30 degrees unless contraindicated.

Elevation of the patient's head minimizes upward migration of the opioid in the spinal cord, thus decreasing the risk for respiratory depression.

8. Record the patient's level of pain and the effectiveness of pain relief.

This information helps in determining the need for subsequent "breakthrough" pain medication.

9. Monitor urinary output and assess for bladder distention.

Opioids can cause urinary retention.

10. Assess motor strength every 4 hours.

The catheter may migrate into the intrathecal space and allow opioids to block the transmission of nerve impulses completely through the spinal cord to the brain.

11. Monitor for adverse effects (pruritus, nausea, and vomiting).

Opioids may spread into the trigeminal nerve, causing itching, or resulting in nausea and vomiting due to slowed gastrointestinal function or stimulation of a chemoreceptor trigger zone in the brain. Medications are available to treat these adverse effects.

continues

ACTION	RATIONALE
12. Assess for signs of infection at the insertion site.	Inflammation or local infection may develop at the catheter insertion site. Strict aseptic technique and sterile dressing and tubing changes according to agency policy can prevent this complication.
13. Change the dressing over the catheter exit site every 24 to 48 hours or as needed per agency policy. Change the infusion tubing every 48 hours or as specified by agency policy.	Dressing and tubing changes reduce the risk for infection.
14. After providing care, remove and dispose of gloves and perform hand hygiene.	Proper disposal of gloves and hand hygiene deter the spread of microorganisms.
15. Document catheter patency, the condition of the insertion site and dressing, vital signs and assessment information, any change in infusion rate, solution, or tubing, analgesics administered, and the patient's response.	Documentation promotes communication and continuity of care.

6/3/06 0935   Continuous morphine infusion via epidural catheter in place. Exit site clean and slightly moist. Transparent dressing in place. Patient rates pain at 3 out of 10. Temperature 98.2°F; pulse, 76 beats per minute; respirations 16 breaths per minute and effortless; blood pressure, 110/70 mm Hg. Patient alert and quickly responds to verbal stimuli. Bladder nonpalpable; urine output of 100 cc over the last 2 hours. Denies nausea, vomiting, or itching. Able to detect sensation of cold in lower extremities bilaterally. Able to wiggle toes and flex and dorsiflex feet bilaterally. Lower extremity muscle strength equal and moderately strong bilaterally.—T. James, RN

Action 15: Documentation.

EVALUATION

The expected outcome is achieved when the patient verbalizes pain relief. In addition, the patient exhibits a dry, intact dressing and the catheter exit site is free of signs and symptoms of complications, injury, or infection. The patient reports a decrease in anxiety and increased ability to cope with pain. The patient verbalizes information related to the functioning of the epidural catheter and the reasons for its use.

Unexpected Situations and Associated Interventions

- *While receiving epidural analgesia, the patient's respiratory rate drops to 10 breaths per minute and he becomes very lethargic and slow to respond:* Stop the epidural infusion immediately and notify the physician. In the meantime, attempt to arouse the patient by talking to him and shaking him. Encourage the patient to take deep slow breaths if possible. Prepare to administer oxygen and a narcotic antagonist such as naloxone (Narcan) via a peripheral IV site.
- *The patient demonstrates weakness and loss of sensation in the lower extremities while receiving epidural analgesia:* Reassess the patient's lower extremities for motor and sensory function. If positive for sensorimotor loss, notify the physician and expect to decrease the epidural infusion.

continues

- *While receiving epidural analgesia, the patient suddenly develops a severe headache. Inspection of the catheter site reveals clear drainage on the dressing:* Stop the epidural infusion and notify the physician immediately. The catheter may have migrated and entered the dura.

Special Considerations

- The patient receiving epidural analgesia should always have a peripheral IV line in place, either as a continuous IV infusion or as an intermittent infusion device, to allow immediate administration of emergency drugs if warranted.
- Drugs given epidurally diffuse slowly and may cause adverse reactions, including excessive sedation, for up to 12 hours after the infusion has been discontinued.
- Typically an anesthesiologist orders analgesics and removes the catheter. However, facility policy may allow a specially trained nurse to remove the catheter.
- No resistance should be felt during the removal of an epidural catheter.
- Assess the patient's respiratory rate and blood pressure every 2 hours for the first 8 hours and then every 4 hours for the next 8 hours during the first 24 hours after starting the infusion. After this time, assessments can occur every 8 hours, depending on the patient's condition (unless ordered otherwise).

■ Developing Critical Thinking Skills

1. Since her surgery, Mildred Simpson has been spending most of her time in bed. A special pillow is placed between her legs to keep her hips in abduction. The nurse offers to give Mrs. Simpson a back massage. What areas would be most important for the nurse to address when performing this skill?
2. The physician decides to admit Joseph Watkins to the hospital for evaluation of his back. Intermittent TENS therapy is ordered and is to be started in the emergency department. How would the nurse initiate this therapy?
3. Jerome Batiste and his wife are concerned about using the PCA device at home. What information would the nurse provide to help alleviate their concerns?

Bibliography

Acello, B. (2000). Meeting JCAHO standards for pain control. *Nursing, 30*(3), 52–54.

Arnstein, P. (2002). Optimizing perioperative pain management. *AORN, 76*(5), 812–818.

Beyer, J., et al. (1992). The creation, validation, and continuing development of the Oucher: A measure of pain intensity in children. *Journal of Pediatric Nursing, 7*(5), 335.

Clinical Update: New standards for assessment and treatment of pain instituted by JCAHO. (2001). *American Journal for Nurse Practitioners, 5*(1), 43–44.

Criste, A. (2003). AANA Journal course update for nurse anesthetists. *AANA Journal Course, 70*(6), 475–480.

Donovan, H., & Ward, S. (2001). A representational approach to patient education. *Journal of Nursing Scholarship, 33*(3), 211–216.

Dooks, P. (2001). Diffusion of pain management research into nursing practice. *Cancer Nursing, 24*(2), 99–103.

Ellis, J. (2003). Keeping pediatric patients comfortable. *Nursing, 33*(7), 22.

Griffie, J. (2003). Addressing inadequate pain relief: Effective communication among the health care team is essential. *American Journal of Nursing, 103*(8), 61–63.

Hseish, R., & Lee, W. (2002). One-shot percutaneous electrical nerve stimulation vs. transcutaneous electrical nerve stimulation for low back pain: Comparison of therapeutic effects. *American Journal of Physical Medicine and Rehabilitation, 81*(11), 838–843.

Joint Commission on Accreditation of Healthcare Organizations (2000). *Joint Commission on Accreditation of Healthcare Organizations pain standards for 2001.* Available at *www.jcaho.org.*

Kettelman, K. (1999). Why give more morphine to a dying patient? *Nursing, 29*(11), 54–55.

Krieger, D. (1999). Therapeutic touch in hospice care. *American Journal of Nursing, 99*(4), 46.

LeMone, P., & Burke, K. (2004). *Medical-surgical nursing: Critical thinking in client care* (3rd ed.). Upper Saddle River, NJ: Pearson/Prentice Hall.

Loeb, J. (1999). Pain management in long-term care. *American Journal of Nursing, 99*(2), 48–52.

Love, G. (2000). Electrifying news about iontophoresis. *Nursing, 30*(1), 48–49.

McCaffery, M. (1979). *Nursing management of the patient with pain* (2nd ed.). Philadelphia: J. B. Lippincott.

McCaffery, M. (2003). Switching from IV to PO: Maintaining pain relief in the transition. *American Journal of Nursing, 103*(5), 62–63.

McCaffery, M., & Beebe, A. (1989). *Pain: Clinical manual for nursing practice.* St. Louis: C. V. Mosby.

McCaffery, M., & Ferrell, B. (1999). Opioids and pain management: What do nurses know? *Nursing, 29*(3), 48–52.

McCaffery, M., Ferrell, B., & Pasero, C. (1998). When the physician prescribes a placebo. *American Journal of Nursing, 98*(1), 52–53.

McCaffery, M., & Pasero, C. (1999). *Pain clinical manual* (2nd ed.). St. Louis: C. V. Mosby.

McCaffery, M., & Pasero, C. (2003). Breakthrough pain. *American Journal of Nursing, 103*(4), 83–86.

McHugh, J. M., & McHugh, W. (2000). Pain: Neuroanatomy, chemical mediators, and clinical implications. *AACN Clinical Issues, 11*(2), 168–178.

Melzak, R., & Wall, P. (1968). Gate control theory of pain. In A. Soulairac, J. Cahn & J. Carpentier (Eds). *Pain: Proceedings of the international association on pain.* Baltimore: Williams & Wilkins.

Newshan, G., & Schuller-Civitella, D. (2003). Large clinical study shows value of therapeutic touch program. *Holistic Nursing Practice, 17*(4), 189–192.

Nichols, R. (2003). Pain management in patients with addictive disease: A new position paper provides guidance. *American Journal of Nursing, 103*(3), 87–90.

Nisbet, A. (2003). Alternative approach. Some like it hot! Closing the gate on pain with superficial heat application. *Virginia Nurses Today, 11*(2), 10.

North American Nursing Diagnosis Association. (2003). *NANDA nursing diagnosis: Definitions & classification: 2003–2004.* Philadelphia: Author.

Parke, B. (1998). Realizing the presence of pain in cognitively impaired older adults. *Journal of Gerontological Nursing, 24*(6), 21–28

Pasero, C. (1998a). How aging affects pain management. *American Journal of Nursing, 98*(6), 12–13.

Pasero, C. (1998b). Is laughter the best medicine? *American Journal of Nursing, 98*(12), 12–14.

Pasero, C. (2003a). Pain in the emergency department: Withholding pain medication is not justified. *American Journal of Nursing, 103*(7), 73–74.

Pasero, C. (2003b). Epidural analgesia for postoperative pain: Excellent analgesia and improved patient outcomes after major surgery. *American Journal of Nursing, 103*(10), 62–64.

Pasero, C., Gordon, D., & McCaffery, M. (1999). JCAHO on assessing and managing pain. *American Journal of Nursing, 99*(7), 22.

Pasero, C., & McCaffery, M. (1999). Providing epidural analgesia. *Nursing, 29*(8), 34–39.

Peloso, P. (2000). NSAIDs: A Faustian bargain. *American Journal of Nursing, 100*(6), 34–39.

Pullen, R. (2003), Managing IV patient-controlled analgesia. *Nursing, 33*(7), 24.

Rothrock, J. C. (1999). Laughter: The attitude worth catching. *First Hand, 14*(1), 5–6.

Rush, S. L., & Harr, J. (2001). Evidence-based pediatric nursing: Does it have to hurt? *AACN Clinical Issues, 12*(4), 597–605.

Salmore, R. (2002). Development of a new pain scale: Colorado behavioral numerical pain scale for sedated adult patients undergoing gastrointestinal procedures. *Gastroenterology Nurse 25*(6), 257–262.

Shea, R., Brooks, J., Dayhoff, N., & Keck, J. (2002). Pain intensity and postoperative pulmonary complications among the elderly after abdominal surgery. *Heart & Lung, 31*(6), 440–449.

Sherwood, G., McNeill, J., Starck, P., & Disnard, G. Changing acute pain management outcomes in surgical patients. *AORN, 77*(2), 374–395.

Steefel, L. (2001). Treat pain in any culture. *Nursing Spectrum (Philadelphia), 10*(25), 20–21.

Stoelting, R., & Miller, R. (2000). *Basics of anesthesia* (4th ed.). Philadelphia: Churchill Livingstone.

Tanabe, P., & Buschmann, M. (2000). Emergency nurses' knowledge of pain management principles. *Journal of Emergency Nursing, 26*(4), 299–305.

Wong, D. (2003). Topical local anesthetics. *American Journal of Nursing, 103*(6), 42–44.

World Health Organization (1990). *Cancer pain relief and palliative care: Report of a WHO expert committee.* WHO Tech Rep Series, No. 804. Geneva: WHO.

Nutrition

This chapter will help you develop some of the skills related to nutrition needed to care for the following patients:

Cole Brenau, *age 12, has cystic fibrosis and needs to increase his caloric intake through gastrostomy tube feedings at nighttime.*

Jack Mason, *a 62-year-old man being treated for esophageal cancer, has just received a gastrostomy tube.*

Paula Williams, *age 38, is newly diagnosed with diabetes and is learning to do fingerstick blood glucose monitoring.*

Learning Outcomes

After studying this chapter, the reader should be able to:

1. Insert a nasogastric tube
2. Administer a tube feeding
3. Remove a nasogastric tube
4. Irrigate a nasogastric tube connected to suction
5. Administer medications via a nasogastric tube
6. Care for a gastrostomy tube
7. Monitor blood glucose levels

Key Terms

anorexia: lack or loss of appetite for food

basal metabolism: amount of energy required to carry out involuntary activities of the body at rest

body mass index (BMI): ratio of height to weight that more accurately reflects total body fat stores in the general population (weight in kg/height^2 in meters)

calorie: measure of heat, or energy; kilocalorie, commonly referred to as a calorie, is defined as the amount of heat required to raise 1 kg of water by 1°C

carbohydrate: organic compounds (commonly known as sugars and starches) that are composed of carbon, hydrogen, and oxygen; the most abundant and least expensive source of calories in the diet worldwide

cholesterol: fatlike substance found only in animal tissues that is important for cell membrane structure, a precursor of steroid hormones, and a constituent of bile

enteral nutrition: alternate form of feeding that involves passing a tube into the gastrointestinal tract to allow instillation of the appropriate formula

ketosis: catabolism of fatty acids that occurs when an individual's carbohydrate intake is not adequate; without adequate glucose, the catabolism is incomplete and ketones are formed, resulting in increased ketones

lipid: group name for fatty substances, including fats, oils, waxes, and related compounds

continues

Key Terms (continued)

minerals: inorganic elements found in nature

nasogastric (NG) tube: a tube inserted through the nose and into the stomach

nasointestinal (NI) tube: a tube inserted through the nose and into the upper portion of the small intestine

NPO (nothing by mouth): nothing can be consumed by mouth, including medications, unless ordered otherwise

nutrient: specific biochemical substance used by the body for growth, development, activity, reproduction, lactation, health maintenance, and recovery from illness or injury

nutrition: study of the nutrients and how they are handled by the body, as well as the impact of human behavior and environment on the process of nourishment

obesity: weight greater than 20% above ideal body weight

partial or peripheral parenteral nutrition (PPN): nutritional therapy used for patients who have an inadequate oral intake and require supplementation of nutrients through a peripheral vein

percutaneous endoscopic gastrostomy tube (PEG): a surgically or laparoscopically placed gastrostomy tube

protein: vital component of every living cell; composed of carbon, hydrogen, oxygen, and nitrogen

recommended dietary allowance (RDA): recommendations for average daily amounts of essential nutrients that healthy people should consume over time

residual: as applied to tube feeding, the amount of gastric contents in the stomach after the administration of a tube feeding

total parenteral nutrition (TPN): nutritional therapy that bypasses the gastrointestinal tract; used in patients who cannot take food orally; meets the patient's nutritional needs by way of nutrient-filled solutions administered through a central vein

trans fat: product that results when liquid oils are partially hydrogenated; these oils then become more stable and solid; trans fats raise serum cholesterol levels

triglycerides: predominant form of fat in food and the major storage form of fat in the body; composed of one glyceride molecule and three fatty acids

vitamins: organic substances needed by the body in small amounts to help regulate body processes; are susceptible to oxidation and destruction

Nutrition is a basic human need that changes throughout the life cycle and along the wellness–illness continuum. Food provides nutrition for both the body and the mind. Eating has evolved from being a simple necessity. It may be a source of pleasure, a pastime, a social event, a political statement, a religious symbol, a cultural emblem, or an integral component of medical treatment. As such, food, eating, and nutrition take on different meanings to different people, and changing a person's eating behaviors may be a difficult and slow process.

Because nutrition is vital for life and health, a person's diet should be varied in content to provide all the essential nutrients. Important nutrients, found in food, are needed for the body to function. Poor nutrition can seriously decrease one's level of wellness.

Nutrition is a vital component of nursing. Nurses play a vital role in assessing a patient's nutritional status using many different techniques. Laboratory data also can provide vital clues to nutritional problems.

This chapter discusses the skills needed to care for patients with nutritional needs. Please look over the summary tables and boxes in the beginning of this chapter for a quick review of critical knowledge to assist you in understanding the skills related to nutrition.

TABLE 11-1 Clinical Observations for Nutritional Assessment

Body Area	Signs of Good Nutritional Status	Signs of Poor Nutritional Status
General appearance	Alert, responsive	Listless, apathetic, and cachexic
General vitality	Endurance, energetic, sleeps well, vigorous	Easily fatigued, no energy, falls asleep easily, looks tired, apathetic
Weight	Normal for height, age, body build	Overweight or underweight
Hair	Shiny, lustrous, firm, not easily plucked, healthy scalp	Dull and dry, brittle, loss of color, easily plucked, thin and sparse
Face	Uniform skin color; healthy appearance, not swollen	Dark skin over cheeks and under eyes, flaky skin, facial edema (moon face), pale skin color
Eyes	Bright, clear, moist, no sores at corners of eyelids, membranes moist and healthy pink color, no prominent blood vessels	Pale eye membranes, dry eyes (xerophthalmia); Bitot's spots, increased vascularity, cornea soft (keratomalacia), small yellowish lumps around eyes (xanthelasma), dull or scarred cornea
Lips	Good pink color, smooth, moist, not chapped or swollen	Swollen and puffy (cheilosis), angular lesion at corners of mouth or fissures or scars (stomatitis)
Tongue	Deep red, surface papillae present	Smooth appearance, beefy red or magenta colored, swollen, hypertrophy or atrophy
Teeth	Straight, no crowding, no cavities, no pain, bright, no discoloration, well-shaped jaw	Cavities, mottled appearance (Fluorosis), malpositioned, missing teeth
Gums	Firm, good pink color, no swelling or bleeding	Spongy, bleed easily, marginal redness, recessed, swollen and inflamed
Glands	No enlargement of the thyroid, face not swollen	Enlargement of the thyroid (goiter), enlargement of the parotid (swollen cheeks)
Skin	Smooth, good color, slightly moist, no signs of rashes, swelling, or color irregularities	Rough, dry, flaky, swollen, pale, pigmented, lack of fat under the skin, fat deposits around the joints (xanthomas), bruises, petechiae
Nails	Firm, pink	Spoon shaped (koilonychia), brittle, pale, ridged
Skeleton	Good posture, no malformations	Poor posture, beading of the ribs, bowed legs or knock-knees, prominent scapulas, chest deformity at diaphragm
Muscles	Well developed, firm, good tone, some fat under the skin	Flaccid, poor tone, wasted, underdeveloped, difficulty walking
Extremities	No tenderness	Weak and tender, presence of edema
Abdomen	Flat	Swollen
Nervous system	Normal reflexes, psychological stability	Decrease in or loss of ankle and knee reflexes, psychomotor changes, mental confusion, depression, sensory loss, motor weakness, loss of sense of position, loss of vibration, burning and tingling of the hands and feet (paresthesia)
Cardiovascular system	Normal heart rate and rhythm, no murmurs, normal blood pressure for age	Cardiac enlargement, tachycardia, elevated blood pressure
GI system	No palpable organs or masses (liver edge may be palpable in children)	Hepatosplenomegaly

(Adapted from Dudek, S. G. [2001]. *Nutrition handbook for nursing practice* [4th ed.]. Philadelphia: Lippincott Williams & Wilkins.)

TABLE 11-2 Sources, Functions, and Significance of Carbohydrates, Protein, and Fat

Nutrient	Sources	Functions	Significance
Carbohydrates			
Simple sugars and starch	Fruits Vegetables Grains: rice, pasta, breads, cereals Dried peas and beans Milk (lactose) Sugars: white and brown sugar, honey, molasses, syrup	Provide energy Spare protein so it can be used for other functions Prevent ketosis from inefficient fat metabolism	Provide about 46% of the calories in the typical American diet; many believe carbohydrate intake should be increased to 50%–60% of total calories Low carbohydrate intake can cause ketosis; high simple sugar intake increases the risk for dental caries
Cellulose and other water-insoluble fibers	Whole wheat flour and wheat bran Vegetables: cabbage, peas, green beans, wax beans, broccoli, brussels sprouts, cucumber skins, peppers, carrots Apples	Absorb water to increase fecal bulk Decrease intestinal transit time	Is nondigestible; therefore, it is excreted Helps relieve constipation North Americans are urged to eat more of all types of fiber Excess intake can cause gas, distention, and diarrhea
Water-soluble fibers	Oat bran and oatmeal Dried peas and beans Vegetables Prunes, pears, apples, bananas, oranges	Slow gastric emptying Lower serum cholesterol level Delay glucose absorption	Help improve glucose tolerance in diabetics
Protein	Milk and milk products Meat, poultry, fish Eggs Dried peas and beans Nuts	Tissue growth and repair Component of body framework: bones, muscles, tendons, blood vessels, skin, hair, nails Component of body fluids: hormones, enzymes, plasma proteins, neurotransmitters, mucus Helps regulate fluid balance through oncotic pressure Helps regulate acid–base balance Detoxifies harmful substances Forms antibodies Transports fat and other substances through the blood Provides energy when carbohydrate intake is inadequate	Most North Americans consume twice the RDA (RNI) for protein Experts recommend that we eat less animal protein and more vegetable protein. Protein deficiency is characterized by edema, retarded growth and maturation, muscle wasting, changes in the hair and skin, permanent damage to physical and mental development (in children), diarrhea, malabsorption, numerous secondary nutrient deficiencies, fatty infiltration of the liver, increased risk for infections, and high mortality Except for elderly people, fad dieters, hospitalized patients, and people of low income, protein deficiency is rare in the United States and Canada
Fat	Butter, oils, margarine, lard, salt pork, salad dressings, mayonnaise, bacon Whole milk and whole milk products High-fat meats Nuts	Provides energy Provides structure Insulates the body Cushions internal organs Necessary for the absorption of fat-soluble vitamins	Fat supplies about 37% of total calories in the typical North American diet; experts suggest a reduction to 30% or less of total calories High-fat diets increase the risk for heart disease and obesity and are correlated with an increased risk for colon and breast cancers

(Dudek, S. G. [2001]. *Nutrition handbook for nursing practice* [4th ed.]. Philadelphia: Lippincott Williams & Wilkins.)

BOX 11-1 **Biochemical Data With Nutritional Implications**

- Hemoglobin (normal = 12–18 g/dL)
  decreased → anemia
- Hematocrit (normal = 40–50%)
  decreased → anemia
  increased → dehydration
- Serum albumin (normal = 3.3–5 g/dL)
  decreased → malnutrition (prolonged protein depletion), malabsorption
- Transferrin (normal = 240–480 mg/dL)
  decreased → anemia, protein deficiency
- Total lymphocyte count (normal = greater than 1800)
  decreased → impaired nutritional intake, severe debilitating disease
- Blood urea nitrogen (normal = 17–18 mg/dL)
  increased → starvation, high protein intake, severe dehydration
  decreased → malnutrition, overhydration
- Creatinine (normal = 0.4–1.5 mg/dL)
  increased → dehydration
  decreased → reduction in total muscle mass, severe malnutrition

(Fischbach, F. [2004]. *A manual of laboratory and diagnostic tests* [7th ed.]. Philadelphia: Lippincott Williams & Wilkins.)

BOX 11-2 **Factors That May Affect Nutritional Status**

- Socioeconomic status
- Psychosocial factors
- Medical conditions that involve malabsorption, such as Crohn's disease or cystic fibrosis
- Age
- Medical conditions that may affect desire to eat, such as chemotherapy treatment or pregnancy accompanied by morning sickness
- Culture
- Medications
- Substance abuse
- Religion

SKILL 11-1

Inserting a Nasogastric Tube

The nasogastric (NG) tube is passed through the nose and into the stomach. This type of tube allows the use of the stomach as a natural reservoir for food. NG tubes may also be used to decompress or irrigate the stomach, or to drain fluid or air from the stomach. This application would be used, for example, to allow the intestinal tract to rest and promote healing after bowel surgery. The NG tube can also be used to monitor bleeding in the gastrointestinal (GI) tract or to help treat an intestinal obstruction.

Equipment

- Nasogastric tube of appropriate size (8 to 18 French)
- Stethoscope
- Small basin filled with ice or warm water (optional)
- Water-soluble lubricant
- Normal saline solution (for irrigation only)
- Tongue blade
- Asepto bulb syringe or Toomey syringe (20 to 50 mL)
- Flashlight
- Nonallergenic tape (1″ wide)
- Tissues
- Glass of water with straw
- Topical analgesic (optional)
- Clamp
- Suction apparatus (if ordered)
- Bath towel or disposable pad
- Emesis basin
- Safety pin and rubber band
- Disposable gloves
- Tincture of benzoin
- pH paper

continues

ASSESSMENT

Assess the patency of the patient's nares by asking the patient to occlude one nostril and breathe normally through the other. Select the nostril through which air passes more easily. Also, assess the patient's history for any recent facial trauma or surgeries. Patients with facial fractures or facial surgeries present a higher risk for misplacement into the brain. Many institutions require a physician to place NG tubes in these patients. Auscultate bowel sounds and palpate the abdomen for distention and tenderness. If the abdomen is distended, consider measuring the abdominal girth at the umbilicus to establish a baseline.

NURSING DIAGNOSIS

Determine the related factors for the nursing diagnoses based on the patient's current status. Nursing diagnoses may vary depending on the reason for the NG tube insertion. Possible nursing diagnoses may include:

- Imbalanced Nutrition, Less Than Body Requirements
- Risk for Aspiration
- Impaired Swallowing
- Acute Pain
- Deficient Knowledge

OUTCOME IDENTIFICATION AND PLANNING

The expected outcome to achieve when inserting an NG tube is that the tube is passed into the patient's stomach without any complications. Other outcomes may include the following: the patient demonstrates weight gain, indicating improved nutrition; patient exhibits no signs and symptoms of aspiration; patient rates pain as decreased from prior to insertion; and patient verbalizes an understanding of the reason for NG tube insertion.

IMPLEMENTATION

ACTION	RATIONALE
1. Check physician's order for insertion of NG tube.	This clarifies procedure and type of equipment required.
2. Explain procedure to patient, discussing with patient the need for the NG tube; answer any questions patient may have.	Explanation facilitates patient cooperation.
3. Gather equipment	This provides for organized approach to task.
4. Place a rubber NG tube in a basin with ice for 5 to 15 minutes or place a plastic tube in a basin of warm water, if needed.	Cold stiffens the rubber tube, making it easier to insert. Plastic tube may be placed in warm water to make it more flexible.
5. Perform hand hygiene. Don disposable gloves.	Hand hygiene deters the spread of microorganisms.
6. Assist the patient to high Fowler's position, or elevate the head of the bed 45 degrees, if unable to maintain upright position, and drape chest with bath towel or disposable pad. Have emesis basin and tissues handy.	Upright position is more natural for swallowing and protects against aspiration, if the patient should vomit. Passage of tube may stimulate gagging and tearing of eyes.
7. **Measure the distance to insert tube by placing tip of tube at patient's nostril and extending to tip of ear lobe and then to tip of xiphoid process.** Mark tube with piece of tape.	Measurement ensures that tube will be long enough to enter patient's stomach.
8. Lubricate tip of tube (at least 1″ to 2″) with water-soluble lubricant. Apply topical analgesic to nostril and oropharynx, if ordered, or ask patient to hold ice chips in mouth for several minutes.	Lubrication reduces friction and facilitates passage of the tube into stomach. Water-soluble lubricant will not cause pneumonia if tube accidentally enters the lungs. Topical analgesic or ice acts as a local anesthetic, reducing discomfort. Topical analgesics must be ordered by the physician.

continues

Inserting a Nasogastric Tube (continued)

ACTION

RATIONALE

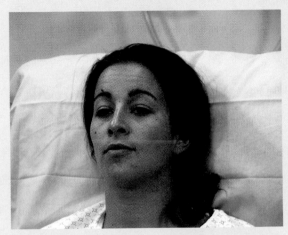

Action 6: Place patient in semi- to high Fowler's position in preparation for tube insertion.

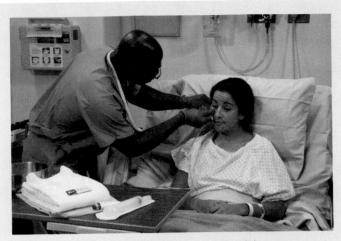

Action 7: Measure NG tube from nostril to tip of ear lobe.

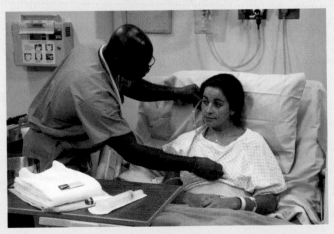

Action 7: Measure NG tube from tip of ear lobe to xiphoid process.

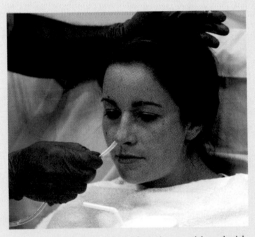

Action 9: Begin insertion with patient positioned with head up.

9. Ask patient to lift head, and insert tube into nostril while directing tube upward and backward. Patient may gag when tube reaches pharynx. Provide tissues for tearing or watering of eyes.

10. **When pharynx is reached, instruct patient to touch chin to chest.** Encourage patient to sip water through a straw or swallow even if no fluids are permitted. Advance tube in downward and backward direction when patient swallows. Stop when patient breathes. **If gagging and coughing persist, check placement of tube with tongue blade and flashlight.** Keep advancing tube until tape marking is reached. **Do not use force. Rotate tube if it meets resistance.**

Following the normal contour of the nasal passage while inserting the tube reduces irritation and the likelihood of mucosal injury. The gag reflex is readily stimulated by the tube. Tears are a natural response as the tube passes into the nasopharynx.

Bringing the head forward helps close the trachea and open the esophagus. Swallowing helps advance the tube, causes the epiglottis to cover the opening of the trachea, and helps to eliminate gagging and coughing. Excessive coughing and gagging may occur if the tube has curled in the back of throat. Forcing the tube may injure mucous membranes.

continues

ACTION	RATIONALE

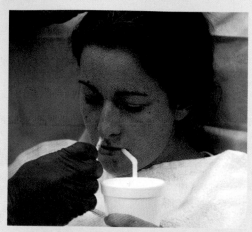

Action 10: Advance tube while patient drops chin to chest and swallows.

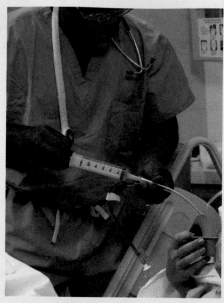

Action 12a: Aspirate to obtain gastric fluid.

11. **Discontinue procedure and remove tube if there are signs of distress, such as gasping, coughing, cyanosis, and inability to speak or hum.**

The tube is in the airway if the patient shows signs of distress and cannot speak or hum.

12. **While keeping one hand on tube, determine that tube is in patient's stomach:**
    a. **Attach syringe to end of tube and aspirate a small amount of stomach contents.**

    b. **Measure the pH of aspirated fluid using pH paper or a meter.**

    c. Visualize aspirated contents, checking for color and consistency.
    d. Obtain radiograph of placement of tube (as ordered by physician).

Keeping one hand on the tube stabilizes it while position is being determined.
a. The tube is in the stomach if its contents can be aspirated; pH of aspirate can then be tested to determine gastric placement.
b. The pH of gastric contents is acidic (4 or less), compared with an average pH of 7.0 or greater for respiratory fluid. Because pH of intestinal fluid also is slightly basic, this method will not effectively differentiate between intestinal fluid and pleural fluid.
c. Gastric fluid can be green with particles, brown if old blood is present, clear or straw-colored; tracheobronchial fluid is usually off-white to tan; pleural fluid can be straw-colored and is usually watery; intestinal fluid is usually light to dark golden-yellow or brownish-green (Metheny & Titler, 2001). A small amount of blood-tinged fluid may be seen immediately after NG insertion.

13. Apply tincture of benzoin to tip of nose and allow to dry. Secure tube with tape to patient's nose. **Be careful not to pull tube too tightly against nose.**
    a. Cut a 4″ piece of tape and split bottom 2″ or use packaged nose tape for NG tubes.
    b. Place unsplit end over bridge of patient's nose.
    c. Wrap split ends under tubing and up and over onto nose.

Tincture of benzoin facilitates attachment of tape. Constant pressure of the tube against the skin and mucous membranes causes tissue injury.

continues

Inserting a Nasogastric Tube (continued)

ACTION

RATIONALE

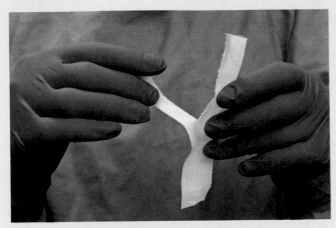

Action 13a: Make a 2″ cut into a 4″ strip of tape.

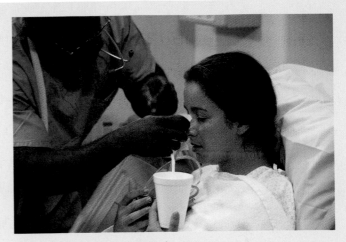

Action 13b: Apply tape to patient's nose.

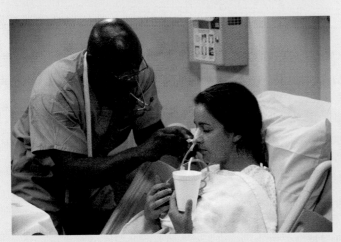

Action 13c: Wrap split ends around NG tube.

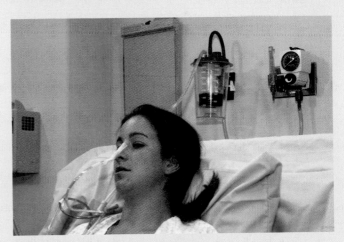

Action 14: Attach NG tube to wall suction.

14. Attach tube to suction or clamp tube and cap it according to the physician's orders.

Suction provides for decompression of stomach and drainage of gastric contents.

15. Secure tube to patient's gown by using rubber band or tape and safety pin. For additional support, tube can be taped onto patient's cheek using a piece of tape. **If double-lumen tube is used, secure vent above stomach level.** Attach at shoulder level.

This prevents tension and tugging on the tube. Securing the double-lumen tube above stomach level prevents seepage of gastric contents and keeps the lumen clear for venting air.

16. Assist with or provide oral hygiene at regular intervals.

Oral hygiene keeps mouth clean and moist and promotes comfort.

17. Remove disposable gloves and perform hand hygiene. Remove all equipment and make patient comfortable.

Hand hygiene deters the spread of microorganisms.

18. Record insertion procedure and type and size of tube, and measure tube from tip of nose to end of tube. Also document a description of gastric contents, including the pH, which naris used, and patient's response.

This facilitates documentation and provides for comprehensive care. Measurement of tube provides a baseline for future comparison.

continues

ACTION   **RATIONALE**

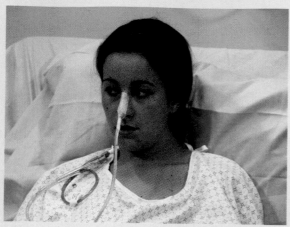

Action 15: Patient with NG tube secured. Note blue vent at patient's shoulder.

> 10/4/06   0945   16 Fr. Salem sump tube inserted via R naris, 20 cm of tube from naris to end of tube; gastric contents aspirated, pH 4, contents light green; patient tolerated without incident; tube attached to low intermittent suction as ordered.—S. Essner, RN

Action 18: Documentation.

EVALUATION

The expected outcome is met when patient exhibits a nasogastric tube placed into the stomach without any complications. In addition, other outcomes are met when patient demonstrates weight gain, indicating improved nutrition; patient remains free of any signs and symptoms of aspiration; patient rates pain as decreased from prior to insertion; and patient verbalizes an understanding of the reason for NG tube insertion.

Unexpected Situations and Associated Interventions

- *As tube is passing through pharynx, patient begins to retch and gag:* This is common during placement of an NG tube. Continue to advance tube. Have the emesis basin nearby in case patient begins to vomit.
- *As tube is passing through pharynx, patient begins to cough, becomes cyanotic, and shows signs of respiratory distress:* **Stop advancing the tube!** The tube is most likely entering the trachea. Pull tube back into nasal area. Allow patient to regain composure. Ask patient to keep chin on chest and swallow as tube is advanced to help prevent the tube from entering the trachea. Begin to advance tube, watching for any signs of respiratory distress.
- *No gastric contents can be aspirated:* If patient is comatose, check oral cavity. If tube is in gastric area, small air boluses may need to be given until gastric contents can be aspirated.

Special Considerations

For insertion of a nasointestinal tube:

- Measure tube from tip of nose to ear lobe and from ear lobe to xiphoid process. Add 8″ to 10″ for intestinal placement. Mark tubing at desired point.
- Place patient on his or her right side. Nasointestinal tube is usually placed in the stomach and allowed to advance through peristalsis through the pyloric sphincter (may take up to 24 hours).
- Administer medications to enhance GI motility, such as metoclopramide (Reglan), if ordered.
- Test pH of aspirate when tube has advanced to marked point to confirm placement in intestine. Confirm position by radiograph. Secure with tape once placement is confirmed.

SKILL 11-2   Administering a Tube Feeding

Depending on the patient's condition and nutritional requirements, a feeding through the NG tube or other GI tube might be ordered. The steps for administering feedings are similar regardless of the tube used.

Feeding can be done on an intermittent or continuous basis. If the order calls for continuous feeding, an external feeding pump is needed to regulate the flow of formula. Intermittent feedings are delivered at regular intervals using gravity for instillation or a feeding pump to administer the formula over a set period of time. Intermittent feedings might also be given as a bolus, using a syringe to instill the formula quickly in one large amount.

Equipment
- Tube feeding at room temperature
- Feeding bag or prefilled tube feeding set
- Stethoscope
- Disposable gloves
- Alcohol preps
- Disposable pad or towel
- Asepto or Toomey syringe
- Enteral feeding pump (if ordered)
- Rubber band
- Clamp (Hoffman or butterfly)
- IV pole
- Water for irrigation

ASSESSMENT

Assess abdomen by auscultating bowel sounds and palpating abdomen. If the abdomen is distended, consider measuring the abdominal girth at the umbilicus.

NURSING DIAGNOSIS

Determine the related factors for the nursing diagnoses based on the patient's current status. The most common nursing diagnosis would be Imbalanced Nutrition, Less Than Body Requirements. Additional nursing diagnoses may include Risk for Aspiration and Deficient Knowledge.

OUTCOME IDENTIFICATION AND PLANNING

The expected outcome to achieve when administering a tube feeding is that the patient will receive the tube feeding without complaints of nausea or episodes of vomiting. Additional expected outcomes may include the following: the patient demonstrates an increase in weight; the patient exhibits no signs and symptoms of aspiration; and the patient verbalizes knowledge related to tube feeding.

IMPLEMENTATION

ACTION	RATIONALE
1. Explain procedure to patient. Use stethoscope to assess bowel sounds.	This facilitates cooperation and provides reassurance for patient. Presence of bowel sounds may indicate functional GI tract.
2. Assemble equipment. Check amount, concentration, type, and frequency of tube feeding on patient's chart. Check expiration date of formula.	This provides for organized approach to task. Checking ensures that correct feeding will be administered. Outdated formula may be contaminated.
3. Perform hand hygiene. Don disposable gloves.	Hand hygiene deters the spread of microorganisms. Gloves protect nurse from exposure to blood or body substances.
4. **Position patient with head of bed elevated at least 30 degrees or as near normal position for eating as possible.**	This position minimizes possibility of aspiration into trachea.

continues

ACTION

RATIONALE

5. Unpin tube from patient's gown. **Check to see that the NG tube is properly located in the stomach,** as described in Skill 11-1, Action 12.

Even when initially positioned correctly, an NG tube left in place can become dislodged between feedings. The instillation of water or nourishment could lead to serious respiratory problems if a gastric tube is in the trachea or a bronchus rather than in the stomach.

6. **Aspirate all gastric contents with a syringe and measure. Return immediately through tube, saving small amount to measure gastric pH.** Flush tube with 30 mL of water for irrigation. Proceed with feeding if amount of residual does not exceed agency policy or physician's guideline. Disconnect syringe from tubing.

This indicates gastric emptying time. **A residual of more than 100 mL from a gastrostomy tube, 200 mL from an NG tube, or more than 10% to 20% above the hourly feeding rate must be reported to the physician.** Fluid should be returned to stomach so as not to cause any fluid or electrolyte losses. If residual is a large amount as indicated by above, confer with physician on whether to discard aspirated contents or to replace them.

7. When using a feeding bag (open system):
   a. Hang bag on IV pole and adjust to about 12″ above the stomach. Clamp tubing.

   a. Proper feeding bag height reduces risk of formula being introduced too quickly

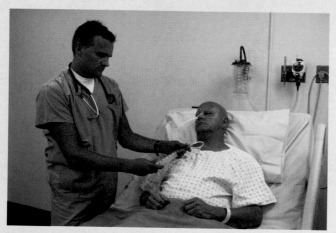

Action 6: Aspirate gastric contents.

b. Cleanse top of feeding container with alcohol before opening it. **Pour formula into feeding bag and allow solution to run through tubing.** Close clamp.
c. Attach feeding setup to feeding tube, open clamp, and regulate drip according to physician's order, or allow feeding to run in over 30 minutes.
d. **Add 30 to 60 mL (1 to 2 oz) of water for irrigation to feeding bag when feeding is almost completed and allow it to run through the tube.**
e. Clamp tubing immediately after water has been instilled. Disconnect from feeding tube. Clamp tube and cover end with sterile gauze secured with a rubber band or apply cap.

b. Cleansing container top with alcohol minimizes risk for contaminants entering feeding bag. Formula displaces air in tubing.
c. Introducing formula at a slow, regular rate allows the stomach to accommodate to the feeding and decreases GI distress.
d. Water rinses the feeding from the tube and helps to keep it patent.
e. Clamping the tube prevents air from entering the stomach. Capping tube deters entry of microorganisms and covering end of tube protects patient and linens from fluid leakage from tube.

continues

Administering a Tube Feeding (continued)

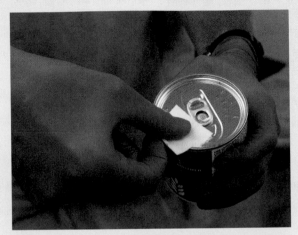

Action 7b: Clean top of feeding container with alcohol before opening it.

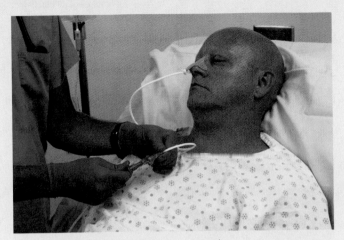

Action 7c: Attach feeding bag tubing to NG tube.

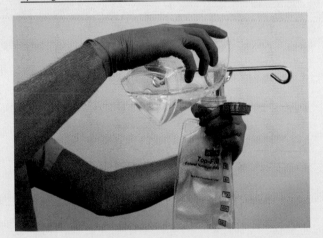

Action 7d: Pour water into feeding bag.

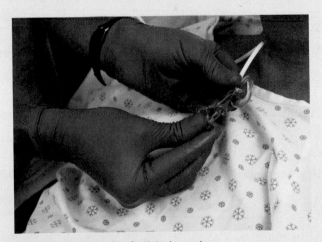

Action 7e: Cap NG tube after it is clamped.

8. When using a large syringe (open system):
    a. Remove plunger from 30- or 60-mL syringe.

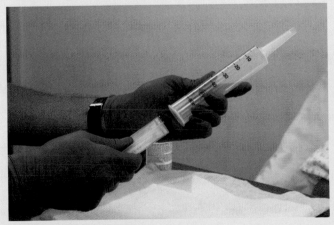

Action 8a: Remove plunger from a 60-cc syringe.

continues

SKILL 11-2   Administering a Tube Feeding (continued)

ACTION

b. Attach syringe to feeding tube, pour premeasured amount of tube feeding into syringe, open clamp, and allow food to enter tube. **Regulate rate, fast or slow, by height of the syringe. Do not push formula with syringe plunger.**

c. **Add 30 to 60 mL (1 to 2 oz) of water for irrigation to syringe when feeding is almost completed, and allow it to run through the tube.**

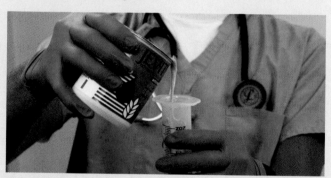

Action 8b: Pour formula into syringe.

d. When syringe has emptied, hold syringe high and disconnect from tube. Clamp tube and cover end with sterile gauze secured with a rubber band, or apply cap.

9. When using prefilled tube feeding set (closed system):
   a. Remove screw on cap and attach administration setup with drip chamber and tubing. Hang set on IV pole and adjust to about 12″ above the stomach. **Clamp tubing and squeeze drip chamber to fill one third to one half of capacity. Release clamp and run formula through tubing.** Close clamp.
   b. Follow actions 7c, 7d, and 7e. Feeding pump may be used with tube feeding setup to regulate drip.

10. When using a feeding pump:
    a. Close flow-regulator clamp on tubing and fill feeding bag with prescribed formula. Amount used depends on agency policy. Place label on container.

    b. Hang feeding container on IV pole. **Allow solution to flow through tubing.**
    c. Connect to feeding pump following manufacturer's directions. Set rate.
    d. **Check residual every 4 to 8 hours.**

RATIONALE

b. Introducing the formula at a slow, regular rate allows the stomach to accommodate to the feeding and decreases GI distress. The higher the syringe is held, the faster the formula flows.

c. Water rinses the feeding from the tube and helps to keep it patent.

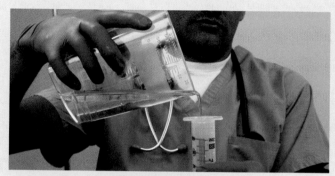

Action 8c: Pour water into almost empty syringe.

d. By holding syringe high, the formula will not backflow out of tube and onto patient. Clamping the tube prevents air from entering the stomach. Capping end of tube deters entry of microorganisms. Covering the end protects patient and linens from fluid leakage from tube.

a. Formula displaces air in tubing.

b. See Rationale 7.

a. Feeding intolerance is less likely to occur with smaller volumes. Hanging smaller amounts of feeding also reduces risk for bacteria growth and contamination of feeding at room temperature (when using open systems).
b. This prevents air from being forced into the stomach or intestines.
c. Feeding pumps vary. A smaller volume of feeding infused continuously may be more easily tolerated by patient.
d. Checking verifies placement of the tube and proper absorption of the feeding and prevents distention which could lead to aspiration.

continues

Administering a Tube Feeding (continued)

ACTION   **RATIONALE**

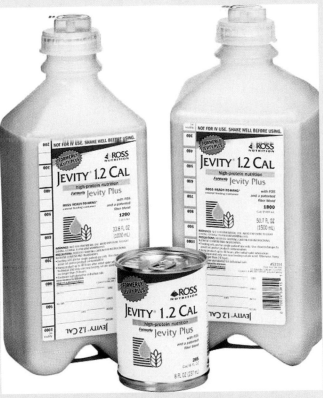

Action 9: Prefilled tube feedings in plastic containers and ready-to-use feeding in a can. (Reprinted with permission from Abbott Laboratories, Ross Products Division.)

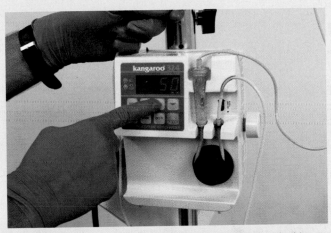

Action 10c: Set up feeding pump with feeding bag and primed tubing.

11. Observe the patient's response during and after tube feeding.

12. **Have patient remain in upright position for at least 30 minutes to 1 hour after feeding.**

13. Wash and clean equipment or replace according to agency policy. Remove gloves and perform hand hygiene.

14. Record type and amount of feeding, residual amount, verification of placement, and patient's response. Monitor blood glucose level, if ordered by physician.

Pain may indicate stomach distention, which may lead to vomiting.

This position minimizes risk for backflow and discourages aspiration, if any reflux or vomiting should occur.

This prevents contamination and deters spread of microorganisms.

This provides accurate documentation of procedure. Many feedings contain high amounts of carbohydrates.

10/29/06 1015   150 mL of (Jevity 1.2 Cal.) administered via bolus feeding. HOB elevated 45°. 30 mL residual aspirated prior to feeding. Aspirate returned to stomach. Tube flushed with 60 mL water with ease. Patient denies any nausea or other stomach upset.—S. Essner, RN

Action 14: Documentation.

continues

SKILL 11-2 Administering a Tube Feeding (continued)

EVALUATION

The expected outcome is achieved when the patient receives the ordered tube feeding without complaints of nausea or episodes of vomiting. The patient demonstrates an increase in weight; the patient remains free of any signs and symptoms of aspiration; and the patient voices knowledge related to tube feeding.

Unexpected Situations and Associated Interventions

- *Tube is found not to be in stomach or intestine:* Tube must be in stomach prior to feeding. If tube is in esophagus, patient is at increased risk for aspiration. See Skill 11-1 for steps to replace tube.
- *When checking for residue, nurse aspirates a large amount:* Before discarding or replacing residue, check with physician. Replacing a large amount may increase patient's risk for vomiting and aspiration, while discarding a large amount may increase patient's risk for metabolic alkalosis. At times the physician will order the nurse to replace half of the residue and recheck in a set amount of time.
- *Patient complains of nausea after tube feeding:* Ensure that head of bed remains elevated and that suction equipment is at bedside. Check medication record to see if any antiemetics have been ordered for patient. Consider notifying the physician for an order for an antiemetic.
- *When attempting to aspirate contents, nurse notes that tube is clogged:* Try using warm water and gentle pressure to remove clog. Carbonated sodas such as Coca Cola and meat tenderizers have not been shown effective in removing clogs in feeding tubes. Tube may have to be replaced. To prevent clogs, ensure that adequate flushing is completed after feedings.

SKILL 11-3 Removing a Nasogastric Tube

When the NG tube is no longer necessary for treatment, the physician will order the tube to be removed. The NG tube is removed as carefully as it was inserted, to provide as much comfort as possible for the patient and to prevent complications. When the tube is removed, the patient must hold his or her breath to prevent aspiration of any secretions or fluid left in the tube as it is removed.

Equipment

- Tissues
- 50-mL syringe (optional)
- Disposable gloves
- Disposable plastic bag
- Bath towel or disposable pad
- Normal saline solution for irrigation (optional)
- Emesis basin

ASSESSMENT

Measure the abdominal girth and auscultate the abdomen for evidence of bowel sounds. Also assess any output from NG tube, noting amount, color, and consistency.

NURSING DIAGNOSIS

Determine the related factors for the nursing diagnoses based on the patient's current status. Possible nursing diagnoses may be Readiness for Enhanced Nutrition and Risk for Aspiration.

OUTCOME IDENTIFICATION AND PLANNING

The expected outcome to achieve when removing a NG tube is that the tube is removed with minimal discomfort to the patient, and the patient maintains an adequate nutritional intake. In addition, the abdomen remains free from distention and tenderness.

continues

Removing a Nasogastric Tube (continued)

IMPLEMENTATION

ACTION	RATIONALE
1. Check physician's order for removal of NG tube.	This ensures correct implementation of physician's order.
2. Explain procedure to patient and assist to semi-Fowler's position.	Explanation facilitates patient cooperation. Sitting position decreases risk of aspiration, if vomiting should occur.
3. Gather equipment.	This provides for organized approach to task.
4. Perform hand hygiene. Don clean disposable gloves.	Hand hygiene deters the spread of microorganisms. Gloves protect nurse's hands from contact with abdominal secretions.
5. Place towel or disposable pad across patient's chest. Give tissues and emesis basin to patient.	This protects patient from contact with gastric secretions. Emesis basin is helpful if patient vomits or gags. Tissues are necessary if patient wants to blow his or her nose when tube is removed.
6. Discontinue suction and separate tube from suction. Unpin tube from patient's gown and carefully remove adhesive tape from patient's nose.	Disconnecting tube from suction and the patient allows for its unrestricted removal.
7. **Attach syringe and flush with 10 mL of water or normal saline solution or clear with 30 to 50 cc of air (optional).**	Air or saline solution clears the tube of feeding or debris.

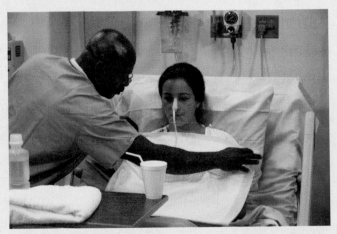

Action 5: Place towel or disposable pad across patient's chest.

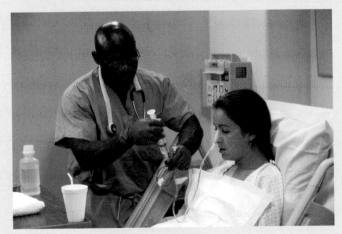

Action 7: Flush NG tube with 10 cc saline.

8. **Instruct patient to take a deep breath and hold it.**	This prevents accidental aspiration of gastric secretions in tube.
9. **Clamp tube with fingers by doubling tube on itself. Quickly and carefully remove tube while patient holds breath.**	Careful removal minimizes trauma and discomfort for patient. Clamping prevents drainage of gastric contents in tube.
10. Dispose of tube per agency policy. Remove gloves and place in bag.	This prevents contamination with microorganisms.
11. Offer mouth care to patient and facial tissue to blow nose.	This provides for comfort.
12. Measure nasogastric drainage in suction device. Remove all equipment and dispose of according to agency policy. Perform hand hygiene.	Measuring nasogastric drainage provides for accurate recording of output. Proper disposal deters spread of microorganisms.

continues

SKILL 11-3   Removing a Nasogastric Tube (continued)

ACTION   **RATIONALE**

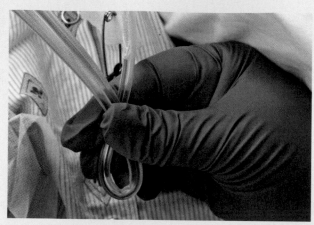

Action 9: Double tube on itself.

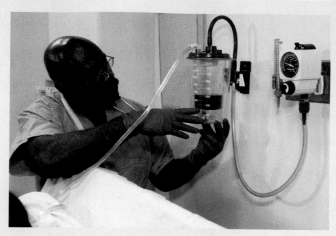

Action 12: Measure nasogastric drainage collection device.

13. Record removal of tube, patient's response, and measurement of drainage. Continue to monitor patient for 2 to 4 hours after tube removal for gastric distention, nausea, or vomiting.

Proper documentation provides for comprehensive care.

> 10/29/06   1320   Nasogastric tube removed
> from L naris without incident. 600 cc of dark
> brown liquid emptied from nasogastric tube.
> Patient's abdomen is 66 cm; abdomen is soft,
> nontender with hypoactive bowel sounds in
> all 4 quadrants.—S. Essner, RN

Action 13: Documentation.

EVALUATION

The expected outcome is met when the patient experiences minimal discomfort and pain on NG tube removal. In addition, the patient's abdomen remains free from distention and tenderness, and the patient verbalizes measures to maintain an adequate nutritional intake.

Unexpected Situations and Associated Interventions

- *Within 2 hours after NG tube removal, patient's abdomen is showing signs of distention:* Notify physician. Physician may order nurse to replace NG tube.
- *Epistaxis occurs with removal of NG tube:* Occlude both nares until bleeding has subsided. Ensure that patient is in upright position. Document epistaxis in patient's medical record.

SKILL 11-4

Irrigating a Nasogastric Tube Connected to Suction

NG tubes can be used to decompress the stomach and to monitor for GI bleeding. The tube is usually attached to suction when used for these reasons. The tube must be kept free from obstruction or clogging and is usually irrigated every 4 to 8 hours.

Equipment
- NG tube connected to continuous or intermittent suction
- Normal saline solution for irrigation
- Disposable gloves
- Stethoscope
- Irrigation set (Asepto or Toomey syringe and container or a 60-mL catheter-tip syringe and cup for irrigating solution)
- Clamp
- Disposable pad or bath towel

ASSESSMENT

Assess suction to ensure that it is running at the prescribed pressure. Measure abdominal girth and auscultate abdomen for evidence of bowel sounds. Also inspect drainage from NG tube, including color, consistency, and amount.

NURSING DIAGNOSIS

Determine the related factors for the nursing diagnoses based on the patient's current status. Possible nursing diagnoses may include Imbalanced Nutrition, Less Than Body Requirements, and Risk for Injury.

OUTCOME IDENTIFICATION AND PLANNING

The expected outcome to achieve when irrigating a patient's NG tube is that the tube will maintain patency with irrigation. In addition, the patient will not experience any trauma or injury.

IMPLEMENTATION

ACTION	RATIONALE
1. Check physician's order for irrigation. Explain procedure to patient.	This clarifies schedule and irrigating solution. An explanation encourages patient cooperation and reduces apprehension.
2. Gather necessary equipment. Check expiration dates on irrigating solution and irrigation set.	This provides for organized approach to task. Agency policy dictates safe interval for reuse of equipment.
3. Perform hand hygiene. Don gloves.	Hand hygiene and gloves deter the spread of microorganisms.
4. Assist patient to semi-Fowler's position, unless this is contraindicated.	This position minimizes risk for aspiration.
5. **Check placement of NG tube** (refer to Skill 11-1, Action 12)	
6. Pour irrigating solution into container. Draw up 30 mL of saline solution (or amount ordered by physician) into syringe.	This delivers measured amount of irrigant through tube. Saline solution compensates for electrolytes lost through nasogastric drainage.
7. Clamp suction tubing near connection site. Disconnect tube from suction apparatus and lay on disposable pad or towel, or hold both tubes upright in nondominant hand.	This protects patient from leakage of nasogastric drainage.
8. Place tip of syringe in tube. **If Salem sump or double-lumen tube is used, make sure that syringe tip is placed in drainage port and not in blue air vent.** Hold syringe upright and gently insert the irrigant (or allow solution to flow in by gravity if agency policy or physician indicates). **Do not force solution into tube.**	Position of syringe prevents entry of air into stomach. Gentle insertion of saline solution (or gravity insertion) is less traumatic to gastric mucosa.

continues

SKILL 11-4   Irrigating a Nasogastric Tube Connected to Suction (continued)

ACTION

RATIONALE

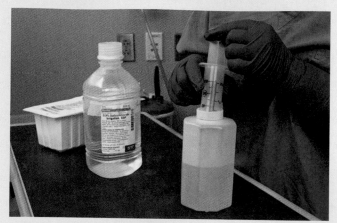

Action 6: Prepare syringe with 30 mL saline for irrigation.

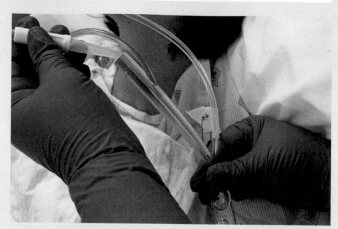

Action 7: Clamp suction tube while disconnecting it from NG tube.

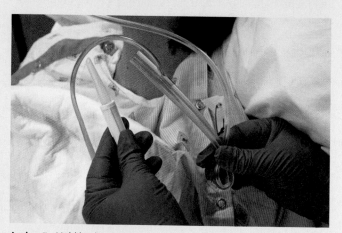

Action 7: Hold both tubes upright to prevent backflow.

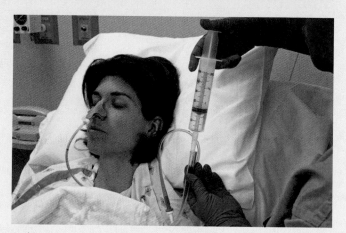

Action 8: Gently instill irrigation.

9. **If unable to irrigate tube, reposition patient and attempt irrigation again. Check with physician if repeated attempts to irrigate tube fail.**

Tube may be positioned against gastric mucosa, making it difficult to irrigate.

10. Withdraw or aspirate fluid into syringe. **If no return, inject 10 to 20 cc of air and aspirate again.**

Injection of air may reposition end of tube.

11. Reconnect tube to suction. Observe movement of solution or drainage.

Observation determines patency of tube and correct operation of suction apparatus.

12. Measure and record amount and description of irrigant and returned solution.

Irrigant placed in tube is considered intake; solution returned is recorded as output.

13. Rinse equipment if it will be reused.

This promotes cleanliness and prepares equipment for next irrigation.

14. Remove gloves. Perform hand hygiene.

Hand hygiene deters the spread of microorganisms.

15. Record irrigation procedure, description of drainage, and patient's response.

This facilitates documentation of procedure and provides for comprehensive care.

continues

Irrigating a Nasogastric Tube Connected to Suction (continued)

ACTION

RATIONALE

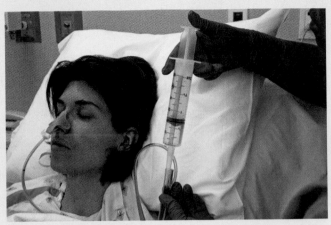

Action 10: Inject 10–20 cc of air into tube.

10/15/06   1100   NG irrigated with 30 mL
of NS. NG reconnected to low intermittent suction. Clear drainage with brown flecks noted
from tube. Patient tolerated irrigation without
incident.—S. Essner, RN

Action 15: Documentation.

EVALUATION

The expected outcome is met when the patient demonstrates a patent and functioning NG tube. In addition, the patient reports no distress with irrigation. The patient remains free of any signs and symptoms of injury or trauma.

Unexpected Situations and Associated Interventions

- *Flush solution is meeting a lot of force when plunger is pushed:* Inject 20 to 30 mL of free air into the abdomen in attempt to reposition the tube and enable the nurse to flush the tube.
- *Tube is connected to suction as ordered, but nothing is draining from tube:* First check the suction canister to ensure that the suction is working appropriately. Disconnect the NG tube from suction and place your thumb over the end of the suction tubing. If there is suction present, the problem lies in the NG tube itself. Next, attempt to flush the tube to ensure patency of the tube.
- *After flushing the tube, the tube is not reconnected to suction as ordered:* Reconnect the tube to suction as soon as error is noticed. Complete any paperwork per institutional policy, such as an incident report.

SKILL 11-5 Administering Medications via a Nasogastric Tube

If a patient cannot take medications orally but has an NG tube in place, the physician may order the medication to be administered via the NG tube. Only medications that can be crushed or mixed with other substances such as food or those in liquid form can be given this way.

Equipment
- 60-mL syringe
- Medications (crushed or in liquid form in oral syringes)
- Water

ASSESSMENT

Research each medication to be given, especially for mode of action, side effects, nursing implications, and whether medication should be given with or without food. Also assess patient's knowledge of medication and the reason for administration. Auscultate the abdomen for evidence of bowel sounds. Percuss and palpate the abdomen for tenderness and distention. Ascertain the time of the patient's last bowel movement and measure abdominal girth.

NURSING DIAGNOSIS

Determine the related factors for the nursing diagnoses based on the patient's current status. Possible nursing diagnoses may include:
- Deficient Knowledge
- Risk for Injury
- Impaired Swallowing

OUTCOME IDENTIFICATION AND PLANNING

The expected outcome to achieve when administering medications via a NG tube is that the patient receives the medication via the tube and experiences the intended effect of the medication. In addition, the patient verbalizes knowledge of the medications given; the patient remains free of any injury; and the NG tube remains patent after the medication administration.

IMPLEMENTATION

ACTION	RATIONALE
1. Check to see if medications to be administered come in a liquid form. **If pills or capsules are to be given, check with pharmacy about crushing or opening capsules.** Ensure that the tube is patent, and irrigate as necessary (see Skill 11-4).	To prevent the tube from becoming clogged, all medications should be given in liquid form whenever possible. Medications in extended-release formulations should not be crushed prior to administration.
2. **Using oral syringes, draw up all medications to be given.** Also draw up a syringe containing 15 to 20 mL of water for each medication to be given.	In many institutions the oral syringes will not fit into the IV tubing. Oral syringes should be used whenever possible to prevent accidental administration of the oral medications into IV tubing.
3. Perform hand hygiene and don gloves. If patient is receiving continuous tube feedings, pause tube feeding pump.	Hand hygiene deters the spread of microorganisms; gloving reduces risky exposure to body fluids. If the pump is not stopped, tube feeding will backflow out of the tube and onto the patient.
4. Fold tube over and clamp with fingers. Disconnect tubing for feeding from NG tube. Insert tip of 60-mL syringe into tube. Release NG tube. Pull plunger back using constant, gentle pressure to check for residue.	Folding the tube over and clamping it prevents any backflow of gastric drainage. Before the medication is administered, assess the stomach for any residual feedings. This indicates gastric emptying time. **A residual of more than 100 mL from a gastrostomy tube, 200 mL from a nasogastric tube, or more than 10% to 20% above the hourly feeding rate must be reported to the physician.**
5. **After noting amount, replace residual back into stomach.**	Fluid should be returned to stomach so as not to cause any fluid or electrolyte losses. If residual is a large amount as indicated by above, confer with physician on whether to discard aspirated contents or replace them.

continues

SKILL
11-5 Administering Medications via a Nasogastric Tube (continued)

ACTION   **RATIONALE**

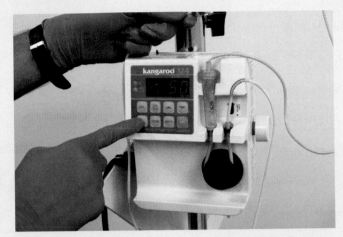

Action 3: Push "pause" button.

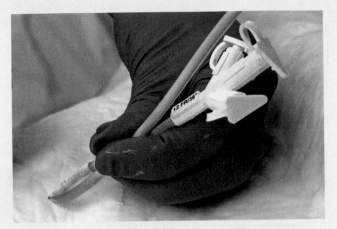

Action 4: Fold tube over on itself to clamp.

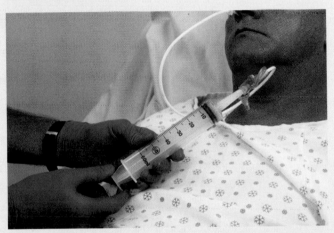

Action 4: Pull back on plunger of 60-mL syringe inserted into NG tube.

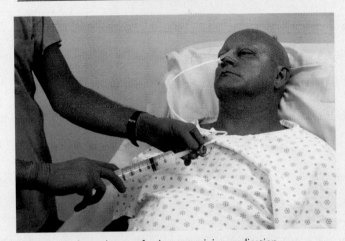

Action 7: Push on plunger of syringe containing medication.

6. Fold NG tube over and clamp with fingers. Remove 60-mL syringe. Apply syringe with first medication to be given.

Folding the tube over and clamping it prevents any backflow of gastric drainage.

7. Release gastric tube and administer the medication. Clamp the gastric tube with fingers and remove syringe. Insert the syringe containing water into the tube and flush the tube with a constant delivery rate.

Folding the tube over and clamping it prevents any backflow of gastric drainage. Flushing between medications prevents any possible interactions between the medications.

8. Fold tubing back over and clamp with fingers. If more medications are to be given, repeat Actions 6 and 7. If no more medications are to be given, reconnect tube feeding. **When last medication is administered, flush tube with 30 mL of water (or according to institution's policy).** Unclamp gastric tube and restart tube feeding.

Flushing between medications prevents any possible interactions between the medications. Adequately flushing tube ensures that tube feeding will not accumulate on inside of tube, causing tube to clog.

9. Remove gloves and perform hand hygiene.

Hand hygiene deters the spread of microorganisms.

10. Record amount of water used to flush tube and document on medication administration record.

This documents procedure and provides for comprehensive care.

continues

SKILL
11-5

SKILL 11-5   Administering Medications via a Nasogastric Tube (continued)

EVALUATION

The expected outcome is met when the patient receives the ordered medications and experiences the intended effects of the medications administered. In addition, the patient demonstrates a patent and functioning NG tube, verbalizes knowledge of the medications given, and exhibits no signs and symptoms of injury.

Unexpected Situations and Associated Interventions

- *Medication enters tube and then tube becomes clogged:* Attach a 10-mL syringe onto end of tube. Pull back and then lightly apply pressure to plunger in a repetitive motion. This may dislodge the medication. If the medication does not move through the tube, notify the physician. The tube may have to be replaced.

SKILL 11-6   Caring for a Gastrostomy Tube

A gastrostomy tube is a tube that is inserted surgically via the abdomen into the stomach. It is used for patients requiring long-term nutritional support. Special care is needed for the insertion site.

Equipment

- Disposable gloves
- Washcloth, towel, and soap
- Cotton-tipped applicator
- Sterile saline solution

ASSESSMENT

Assess gastrostomy tube site, noting any drainage, skin breakdown, or erythema. Check to ensure that the tube is securely stabilized and has not become dislodged. Also, assess the tension of the tube. If there is not enough tension, the tube may leak gastric drainage around exit site. If the tension is too great, the internal anchoring device may erode through the skin.

NURSING DIAGNOSIS

Determine the related factors for the nursing diagnoses based on the patient's current status. Possible nursing diagnoses may include:

- Imbalanced Nutrition, Less Than Body Requirements
- Impaired Skin Integrity
- Risk for Infection
- Deficient Knowledge

OUTCOME IDENTIFICATION AND PLANNING

The expected outcome to achieve when caring for a gastrostomy tube is that the patient ingests an adequate diet and exhibits no signs and symptoms of irritation, excoriation, or infection at the tube insertion site. In addition, the patient will be able to verbalize the care needed for the gastrostomy tube.

IMPLEMENTATION

ACTION	RATIONALE
1. Explain procedure to patient.	Explanation encourages patient cooperation.
2. Perform hand hygiene. Don disposable gloves.	Hand hygiene deters the spread of microorganisms. Gloves protect nurse from exposure to blood or bodily substances.
3. If gastrostomy tube is new and still has sutures holding it in place, dip cotton-tipped applicator into sterile saline solution and gently clean around the insertion site, removing any crust or drainage. If the gastric tube insertion site has healed and the sutures are removed, wet a washcloth	Cleaning new site with sterile saline solution prevents the introduction of microorganisms into the wound. Crust and drainage can harbor bacteria and lead to skin breakdown. Removing soap helps to prevent skin irritation.

continues

SKILL
11-6   Caring for a Gastrostomy Tube (continued)

ACTION   **RATIONALE**

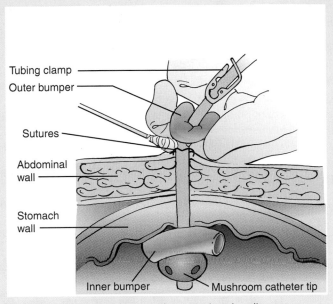

Action 3: Wipe gastric tube site with cotton-tipped applicators.

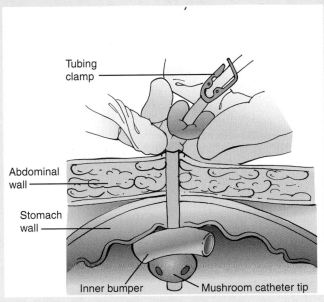

Action 3: Clean site with soap, water, and washcloth.

and apply a small amount of soap onto washcloth. Gently cleanse around the insertion, removing any crust or drainage. **Rinse site, removing all soap.**

4. Pat skin around insertion site dry.

5. If the sutures have been removed, **rotate the guard or external bumper 90 degrees at least once a day.**

6. Remove gloves and perform hand hygiene.

7. Record care given, including appearance of site, any drainage present, and patient's response.

Drying the skin thoroughly prevents skin breakdown.

Rotation of the guard or external bumper prevents skin breakdown and pressure ulcers.

Hand hygiene prevents the spread of microorganisms.

This documents procedure and provides for comprehensive care.

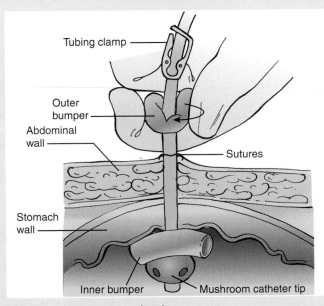

Action 5: Turn or rotate guard 90 degrees.

10/10/06   1145   Gastrostomy tube site cleansed with soap and water. Guard rotated. Skin surrounding site is pink without any signs of skin breakdown. Small amount of clear crust noted on tube. Patient tolerated without incident. Wife at bedside, actively participating in tube care.—S. Essner, RN

Action 7: Documentation.

continues

SKILL 11-6 Caring for a Gastrostomy Tube (continued)

EVALUATION

The expected outcome is met when the patient exhibits a clean, dry, intact gastrostomy tube site without evidence of irritation, excoriation, or infection. Other expected outcomes may include the following: the patient verbalizes no pain when guard is rotated; skin remains pink without any sign of skin breakdown; and the patient participates in care measures.

Unexpected Situations and Associated Interventions

- *Gastrostomy tube is leaking large amount of drainage:* Check tension of tube. If there is a large amount of slack between the internal guard and the external bumper, drainage can leak out of site. Apply gentle pressure to tube while pressing the external bumper closer to the skin. If the tube has an internal balloon holding it in place (similar to a urinary catheter balloon), check to make sure that the balloon is inflated properly.
- *Skin irritation is noted around insertion site:* If the skin is erythematous and appears to be broken down, the culprit could be leakage of gastric fluids from site. Gastric fluids have a low pH and are very acidic. Stop the leakage, as described above, and apply a skin barrier. If the skin has a patchy, red rash, the culprit could be candidiasis (yeast). Notify the physician for an order to apply an antifungal powder. Ensure that the site is kept dry.
- *Site appears erythematous and patient complains of pain at site:* Notify physician; patient could be developing cellulitis at the site.

SKILL 11-7 Monitoring the Blood Glucose Level

Many external feeding formulas contain high amounts of carbohydrates. Patients receiving these types of nutrition or total parenteral nutrition may experience alterations in their ability to regulate blood glucose levels. The monitoring of blood glucose levels is often ordered for these patients. The most common way to determine blood glucose levels is to use a monitoring device with a fingerstick blood sample.

Equipment

- Blood glucose meter
- Sterile lancet
- Cotton balls
- Testing strips
- Disposable gloves
- Alcohol swab or soap and water

ASSESSMENT

Assess the patient's history for indications necessitating the monitoring of blood glucose levels, such as high-carbohydrate feedings, history of diabetes mellitus, or corticosteroid therapy. In addition, assess the patient's knowledge about monitoring blood glucose.

NURSING DIAGNOSIS

Determine the related factors for the nursing diagnoses based on the patient's current status. Possible nursing diagnoses may include:

- Risk for Injury
- Deficient Knowledge
- Anxiety

OUTCOME IDENTIFICATION AND PLANNING

The expected outcome to achieve when monitoring a patient's blood glucose level is that the patient demonstrates a blood glucose level within acceptable parameters. In addition, the patient remains free of injury, demonstrates ability to participate in monitoring, and verbalizes improved comfort with the procedure.

continues

Monitoring the Blood Glucose Level (continued)

IMPLEMENTATION

ACTION

1. Check physician's order for monitoring schedule.
2. Gather equipment.
3. Explain procedure to patient and instruct patient about the need for monitoring blood glucose.

4. Perform hand hygiene. Don disposable gloves.

5. Prepare lancet.
6. Remove test strip from the vial. **Recap container immediately.** Test strips also come individually wrapped. Turn monitor on. **Check that code number on strip matches code number on monitor screen.**

RATIONALE

This confirms times for checking blood glucose.

This provides an organized approach to the task.

Explanations and instructions encourage patient to cooperate.

Hand hygiene deters the spread of microorganisms. Gloves protect nurse from exposure to blood or body fluids.

Aseptic technique maintains sterility.

Immediately recapping protects strips from exposure to humidity, light, and discoloration. Matching code numbers on the strip and glucose monitor ensures that the machine is calibrated correctly.

Action 6: Check test strip from vial.

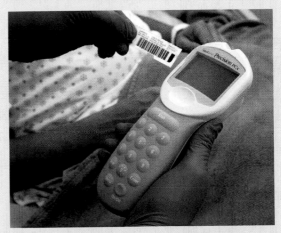

Action 6: Compare code on strip to code on monitor.

7. For adult, massage side of finger toward puncture site.
8. **Have patient wash hands with soap and warm water or cleanse area with alcohol. Dry thoroughly.**

9. Hold lancet perpendicular to skin and prick site with lancet.
10. **Wipe away first drop of blood with cotton ball if recommended by manufacturer of monitor.**

11. Lightly squeeze or milk the puncture site until a hanging drop of blood has formed (check instructions for monitor).
12. **Gently touch drop of blood to pad on test strip without smearing it.**
13. Insert strip into the meter according to directions for that specific device. Some devices require that the drop of blood be applied to a test strip that has already been inserted in the monitor.

Massage encourages blood to flow to the area.

Washing with soap and water or alcohol cleanses the puncture site. Warm water also helps to cause vasodilation.

Holding lancet in proper position facilitates proper skin penetration.

Manufacturers recommend discarding the first drop of blood, which may be contaminated by serum or cleansing product, producing an inaccurate reading.

An appropriate-sized droplet facilitates accurate test results.

Smearing blood on strip may result in inaccurate test results.

Correctly inserted strip allows meter to read blood glucose level accurately.

continues

SKILL 11-7   Monitoring the Blood Glucose Level (continued)

ACTION

RATIONALE

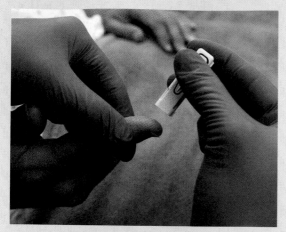

Action 9: Pierce patient's finger with lancet.

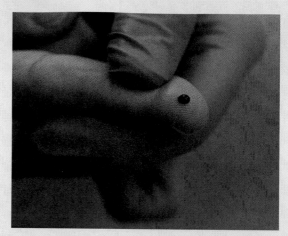

Action 11: Milk patient's finger to get a hanging drop of blood.

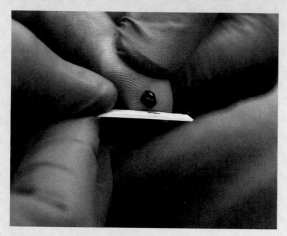

Action 12: Apply drop of blood hanging from patient's finger to test strip.

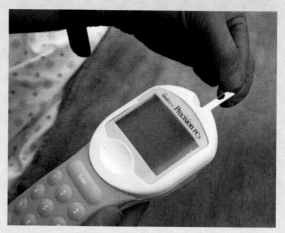

Action 13: Place strip into meter.

14. Press time if directed by manufacturer.	Correct timing produces accurate results.
15. Apply pressure to puncture site with a cotton ball. **Do not use alcohol wipe.**	Pressure causes hemostasis. Alcohol stings and may prolong bleeding.
16. Read blood glucose results and document appropriately at bedside. Inform patient of test result.	Timing depends on type of meter.
17. Turn meter off, dispose of supplies appropriately, and place lancet in sharps container.	Proper disposal prevents exposure to blood and accidental needle sticks.
18. Remove gloves and perform hand hygiene.	Hand hygiene prevents the spread of microorganisms.
19. Record blood glucose result on chart or medication record. Report abnormal results to the physician.	This documents procedure and provides for comprehensive care. Prompt reporting ensures adequate treatment.

continues

Monitoring the Blood Glucose Level (continued)

ACTION	RATIONALE

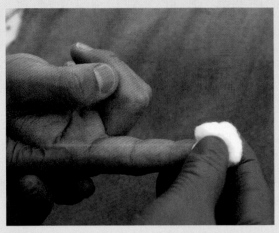

Action 15: Apply pressure to fingerstick area with a cotton ball.

EVALUATION

The expected outcome is met when the patient's blood glucose level is within acceptable limits, the finger is pricked without incident, and an adequate drop of blood is used to monitor the glucose level. In addition, the patient exhibits no signs and symptoms of injury, patient participates in monitoring, and patient verbalizes comfort with the procedure.

Unexpected Situations and Associated Interventions

- *Extremity is pale and cool to the touch:* Begin by warming the extremity. Have adult patients warm their hands by rubbing them together. Warm moist compresses also may be used.
- *Finger is pricked, but even with squeezing of the finger, no drops of blood are being produced:* Feel the pad of the finger, assessing for calluses. Restick patient on a finger that does not have calluses, or a finger with less prominent ones. If the device allows the nurse to adjust the depth of the lancet, adjust for a deeper depth of penetration.

Infant and Child Considerations

- In infants and young children, use the heel to obtain the blood specimen. In an infant, use the outer aspect of the heel.
- If the heel is cool, place a disposable diaper filled with warm water on the foot.

Special Considerations

- In patients with injury or poor circulation to the hands, the ear lobe may be used.
- New devices are being developed to obtain a specimen from the forearm.

■ Developing Critical Thinking Skills

1. Cole Brenau is concerned that his friends may see his gastrostomy tube. He confides to the nurse that he doesn't like the way the tube fits under his clothing. What can be done for him?
2. Jack Mason is concerned about how to clean the gastrostomy tube site and how he can prevent the tube site from getting wet while taking a shower.
3. Paula Williams has begun to do fingerstick blood glucose monitoring and is now complaining of sore fingers.

Bibliography

Barr, S., & Chapman, G. (2002). Perceptions and practices of self-defined current vegetarian, former vegetarian, nonvegetarian women. *Journal of the American Dietetic Association, 102*(3), 354–360.
Bowers, S. (2000). All about tubes: Your guide to enteral feeding devices. *Nursing, 30*(12), 41–47.

Dudek, S. (2001). *Nutrition handbook for nursing practice* (4th ed.). Philadelphia: Lippincott Williams & Wilkins.

Edwards, S., & Metheny, N. (2000). Measurement of gastric residual volume: State of the science. *MedSurg Nursing, 9*(3), 125–128.

Eisenberg, P. (2002). An overview of diarrhea in the patient receiving enteral nutrition. *Gastroenterology Nursing, 25*(3), 95–104.

Fairfield, K., & Fletcher, R. (2002). Vitamins for chronic disease prevention in adults: Scientific review. *JAMA, 287*(23), 3116–3126.

Fellows, L., Miller, E., Frederickson, M., Bly, B., & Felt, P. (2000). Evidence-based practice for enteral feedings: Aspiration prevention strategies, bedside detection, and practice change. *MedSurg Nursing, 9*(1), 27–31.

Flegal, K., Carroll, M., Ogden, C., & Johnson, C. (2002). Prevalence and trends in obesity among U.S. adults, 1999–2000. *JAMA, 288*(14), 1723–1727.

Fischbach, F. (2004). *A manual of laboratory and diagnostic tests* (6th ed.). Philadelphia: Lippincott Williams & Wilkins.

Grant, M., & Martin, S. (2000). Delivery of enteral nutrition. *AACN Clinical Issues, 11*(4), 507–516.

Guigoz, Y., Lauque, S., & Vellas, B. (2002). Identifying the elderly at risk for malnutrition: The mini nutritional assessment. *Clinics in Geriatric Medicine, 18*(4), 735–757.

Heiser, M., & Malaty, H. (2001). Balloon-type versus non-balloon-type replacement percutaneous endoscopic gastrostomy: Which is better? *Gastroenterology Nursing, 24*(2), 58–63.

Kohn-Keeth, C. (2000). How to keep feeding tubes flowing freely. *Nursing, 30*(1), 58–59.

Lord, L. (2001). How to insert a large-bore nasogastric tube. *Nursing, 31*(9), 46–48.

Mackie, S. (2001). PEGS and ethics. *Gastroenterology Nurse, 24*(3), 138–142.

Matlow, A., Wray, R., Goldman, C., Streitenberger, L., Freeman, R., & Kovach, D. (2003). Microbial contamination of enteral feed administration sets in a pediatric institution. *American Journal of Infection Control, 31*(1), 49–53.

McCloskey, J., & Bulechek, J. (1996). *Nursing interventions classification* (NIC) (2nd ed.). St. Louis: C. V. Mosby.

McConnell, E. (2002). Administering medication through a gastrostomy tube. *Nursing, 32*(12), 22.

Metheny, N. (2002). Inadvertent intracranial nasogastric tube placement. *American Journal of Nursing, 102*(8), 25–27.

Metheny, N., & Stewart, B. (2002). Testing feeding tube placement during continuous tube feedings. *Applied Nursing Research, 15*(4), 254–258.

Metheny, N., & Titler, M. (2001). Assessing placement of feeding tubes. *American Journal of Nursing, 101*(5), 36–0045.

Moore, B. (2003). Supersized America: Help your patients regain control of their weight. *Cleveland Clinic Journal of Medicine, 70*(3), 237–240.

O'Brien, B., Davis, S., & Erwin-Toth, P. (1999). G-tube site care: A practical guide. *RN, 62*(2), 52–56.

Schiff, L. (2000). Enhanced enteral feeding formulas. *RN, 63*(9), 77–79.

Stahl, P. (2000). Informing consumers about trans fat labeling. *Journal of the American Dietetic Association, 100*(10), 1132, 1134.

United States Department of Agriculture. (October 1996). The food guide pyramid. Retrieved July 6, 2003, from Access: *http://www.usda.gov/cnpp/pyrabklt.pdf*

Vegetarian Resource Group. How many vegetarians are there? Retrieved July 6, 2003, from: *http://www.vrg.org/journal/vj2000may/2000maypoll.htm*

Urinary Elimination

Focusing on Patient Care

This chapter will help you develop some of the skills needed to care for the following patients:

Ralph Bellows is a 73-year-old man admitted with a stroke. Due to incontinence and skin breakdown, Ralph's physician has ordered the application of a condom catheter.

Grace Halligan, age 24, is pregnant and has been placed on bed rest. She needs to void but cannot get out of bed.

Mike Wimmer, age 36, receives peritoneal dialysis. Mike has noticed that the insertion site around his catheter is becoming tender and reddened.

Learning Outcomes

After studying this chapter, the reader should be able to:

1. Offer and remove a bedpan and urinal
2. Catheterize a female patient's urinary bladder
3. Catheterize a male patient's urinary bladder
4. Irrigate a urinary catheter using a closed system
5. Administer a continuous bladder irrigation
6. Apply a condom catheter
7. Change a stoma appliance on an ileal conduit
8. Collect urine for a urinalysis and urine culture and sensitivity
9. Care for a suprapubic catheter
10. Care for a peritoneal dialysis catheter
11. Care for hemodialysis access

Key Terms

arteriovenous graft: a surgically created passage connecting an artery and a vein, used in hemodialysis

bruit: a sound caused by turbulent blood flow

fenestrated: having a window-like opening

hemodialysis: removal from the body, by means of blood filtration, of toxins and fluid that are normally removed by the kidneys

ileal conduit: a surgical diversion formed by bringing the ureters to the ileum; urine is excreted though a stoma

peritoneal dialysis: removal of toxins and fluid from the body by the principles of diffusion and osmosis; this is accomplished by introducing a solution (dialysate) into the peritoneal cavity

peritonitis: inflammation of the peritoneal membrane

sediment: precipitate found at the bottom of a container of urine

stoma: artificial opening on the body surface

thrill: palpable feeling caused by turbulent blood flow

Elimination from the urinary tract helps to rid the body of waste products and materials that exceed bodily needs. A properly functioning urinary system is essential to physical and emotional well-being and indeed to life itself. Problems associated with urinary elimination, such as urinary incontinence, can be so embarrassing to patients that they may no longer leave their home. Nurses assisting patients with urinary elimination or intervening to resolve health problems related to urination need many specialized skills.

This chapter discusses the skills needed to care for patients with urinary elimination needs. Please look over the summary boxes in the beginning of this chapter for a quick review of critical knowledge to assist you in understanding the skills related to urinary elimination.

BOX 12-1 **Anatomy of the Genitourinary Tract**

- The main components of the urinary tract are the kidneys, ureters, bladder, and urethra.
- The average female urethra is 3.7 to 6.2 cm (1.5″ to 2.5″) long, while the average male urethra is 18 to 20 cm (7″ to 8″) long.

- The male urethra is divided into three segments: cavernous, membranous, and prostatic.
- The average age at which men begin to have prostatic enlargement is 50.

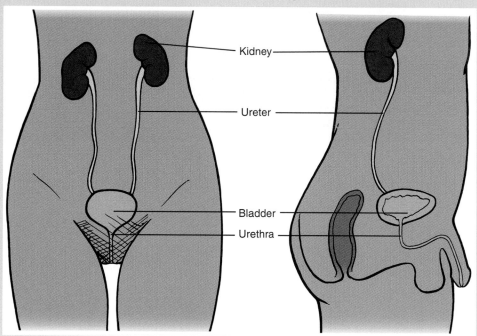

Urinary tract, showing kidneys, ureter, bladder, and urethra.

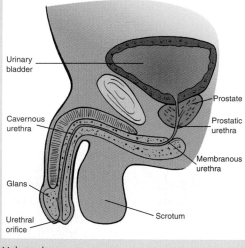

Male urethra.

BOX 12-2 Assessment Techniques for the Urinary System

- Kidneys: Assess by testing for costovertebral tenderness: place one hand over the area where the 12th rib meets the spine, and gently tap with the other hand. If the kidneys are inflamed, the patient will complain of pain. Do not tap hard if you suspect that the area may be tender.
- Bladder: Assess by palpating above the symphysis pubis. Normally the bladder cannot be palpated or percussed if it is empty. If the bladder is distended, it may be palpated or percussed from above the symphysis pubis up to the umbilicus. A full bladder will produce a dull sound upon percussion.
- Urethral orifice: Visually inspect the orifice for any signs of inflammation, discharge, or foul odor. For an uncircumcised patient, retract the foreskin if necessary to visualize the urethral orifice. Place the female patient in the lateral recumbent position for best visualization.

BOX 12-3 Factors Affecting Urinary Elimination

- Fluid intake: The amount of fluid that a person takes in has a direct correlation with the amount of fluid the body puts out.
- Medications: Diuretics and angiotensin-converting enzyme (ACE) inhibitors may lead to an increase in urinary output.
- Caffeine and sodium: Foods and fluids containing caffeine may cause an increase in urinary output, while foods containing high amounts of sodium may cause a decrease in urinary output.
- Urinary diversions: Patients with urinary diversions may have urine that is normally cloudy, with large amounts of sediment.

SKILL 12-1 Offering and Removing a Bedpan or Urinal

Patients who cannot get out of bed because of physical limitations or physician's orders need to use a bedpan or urinal for voiding.

Equipment
- Bedpan or urinal
- Toilet tissue
- Disposable clean gloves
- Cover for bedpan or urinal (disposable waterproof pad or cover)

ASSESSMENT

Determine why the patient needs to use a bedpan or urinal, such as a physician's order for strict bed rest or immobilization. Also assess the patient's degree of limitation and ability to help with activity.

NURSING DIAGNOSIS

Determine the related factors for the nursing diagnoses based on the patient's current status. The two most common nursing diagnoses are Altered Urinary Elimination and Toileting Self-Care Deficit. Other appropriate nursing diagnoses may include:

- Impaired Physical Mobility
- Deficient Knowledge
- Functional Urinary Incontinence

OUTCOME IDENTIFICATION AND PLANNING

The expected outcome to achieve when offering a bedpan or urinal is that the patient is able to void with assistance. Other appropriate outcomes may include the following: the patient maintains continence and demonstrates how to use the bedpan or urinal with assistance.

IMPLEMENTATION

ACTION	RATIONALE
1. Bring bedpan or urinal and other necessary equipment to bedside. Perform hand hygiene. Don disposable gloves.	Having equipment on hand saves time by avoiding unnecessary trips to storage area. Hand hygiene deters the spread of microorganisms. Gloves protect nurse against exposure to blood and body fluids.
2. Warm bedpan, if it is made of metal, by rinsing it with warm water.	A cold bedpan feels uncomfortable and may make it difficult for the patient to void. Plastic bedpans do not require warming.

continues

SKILL 12-1   Offering and Removing a Bedpan or Urinal (continued)

ACTION	RATIONALE
3. If bed is adjustable, place it in high position.	Having the bed in the high position reduces strain on the nurse's back while assisting the patient onto the bedpan.
4. Place bedpan or urinal on chair next to bed or on foot of bed. Fold top linen back just enough to allow placement of bedpan or urinal. If there is no waterproof pad on bedpan and time allows, consider placing a waterproof pad under patient's buttocks before placing bedpan or urinal.	Folding back the linen in this manner minimizes unnecessary exposure while still allowing the nurse to place the bedpan or urinal. The waterproof pad will protect the bed should there be a spill.
5. If patient needs assistance to move onto bedpan, have him or her bend the knees and rest some of his or her weight on the heels. Assist patient by placing one hand under the lower back, and slip bedpan into place with other hand.	The nurse uses less energy when the patient can assist by placing some of his or her weight on the heels.

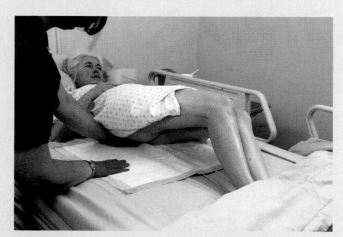

Action 4: Placing waterproof pad under patient's buttocks.

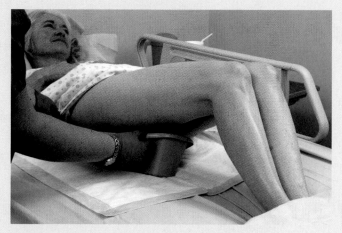

Action 5: Assisting patient to raise self in bed for bedpan.

ACTION	RATIONALE
6. If patient cannot lift, place patient on his or her side with bedpan placed against the buttocks; then roll patient back onto bedpan.	Rolling the patient takes less energy than lifting the patient onto a bedpan.
7. Ensure that bedpan is in proper position and patient's buttocks are resting on rounded shelf of bedpan. For male patients, make sure urinal is properly placed between slightly spread legs with penis positioned in it and urinal resting on bed. If patient has voided more than 500 mL in past, urinal opening should be slightly raised.	Having the bedpan or urinal in the proper position prevents spills onto the bed and prevents injury to the skin from a misplaced bedpan.
8. If permitted, raise head of bed as near to sitting position as tolerated. Cover with bed linens.	This position makes it easier for the patient to void or defecate, avoids strain on the patient's back, and allows gravity to aid in elimination. Covering promotes warmth and privacy.
9. Place call device and toilet tissue within easy reach. Leave patient if it is safe to do so. Use side rails appropriately. Remove gloves and perform hand hygiene.	Falls can be prevented if the patient does not have to reach for items he or she needs. Side rails are an additional safety precaution. Leaving patient alone, if possible, promotes self-esteem and shows respect for privacy.

continues

ACTION

RATIONALE

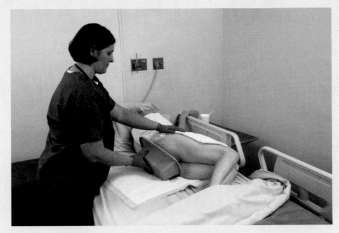

Action 6: Rolling patient on side to place bedpan.

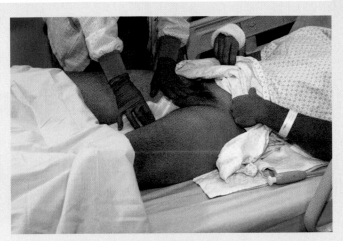

Action 7: Positioning urinal in place for a male patient.

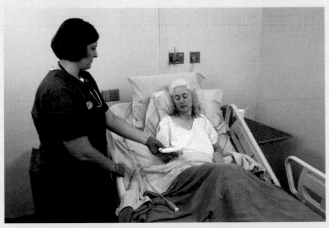

Action 9: Giving patient call light and placing toilet tissue within reach on the bed. Side rails raised.

7/12/06   0730   Patient placed on fracture bedpan with a 2-person assist. Voided large amount dark yellow urine, strong odor noted. Specimen sent for urinalysis as ordered.
—S. Barnes, RN

Action 13: Documentation.

10. Perform hand hygiene and don disposable gloves. Remove bedpan in the same manner in which it was offered, being careful to hold it steady. If patient needs assistance with hygiene, wrap tissue around the hand several times, and **wipe patient clean, using one stroke from the pubic area toward the anal area. Discard tissue, and use more until patient is clean.** Place patient on his or her side and spread buttocks to clean anal area. Cover bedpan.

11. **Do not place toilet tissue in the bedpan if a specimen is required.** Have a receptacle handy for discarding tissue.

12. Offer patient supplies to wash and dry his or her hands, assisting as necessary.

13. Empty and clean bedpan or urinal. Perform hand hygiene. Record according to agency policy. Recording may be done on intake/output record.

Holding the pan steady prevents spills. Cleaning area from front to back minimizes fecal contamination of the vagina and urinary meatus. Cleaning the patient after he or she has used the bedpan prevents offensive odors and irritation to the skin.

Mixing toilet tissue with a specimen makes laboratory examination more difficult and interferes with accurate output measurement.

Washing hands after using the bedpan or urinal helps prevent the spread of microorganisms.

Hand hygiene helps prevent the spread of microorganisms. Documentation is important to maintain communication.

continues

SKILL 12-1 Offering and Removing a Bedpan or Urinal (continued)

EVALUATION

The expected outcome is met when the patient voids using the bedpan or urinal. Other outcomes are met when the patient remains dry, does not experience episodes of incontinence, and demonstrates measures to assist with using the bedpan or urinal.

Special Considerations

- If it is difficult to slide the patient onto the bedpan, apply powder on the resting surfaces of the pan to eliminate friction. However, do not use powder if a specimen is required, because contamination could result.
- A fracture bedpan is usually more comfortable for the patient, but it does not hold as large a volume as the contemporary bedpan.

SKILL 12-2 Catheterizing the Female Urinary Bladder

At times it may be necessary to insert a catheter or tube into the bladder to remove urine. Intermittent catheters, also known as straight catheters, are placed into the bladder for short periods of time (5 to 10 minutes). Those placed into the bladder for extended periods of times are called indwelling catheters or retention or Foley catheters. To keep the catheter in place within the bladder, these catheters have a balloon at the distal end that is inflated after insertion.

Equipment

- Sterile catheter kit that contains:
  - Sterile gloves
  - Sterile drapes (one of which is fenestrated)
  - Sterile catheter
  - Antiseptic solution
  - Lubricant
  - Cotton balls or gauze squares
  - Forceps
  - Prefilled syringe
  - Basin (usually base of kit serves as this)
  - Specimen container
- Flashlight or lamp
- Waterproof disposable pad
- Disposable urine collection bag and drainage tubing (may be connected to sterile indwelling catheter if a closed drainage system is used)
- Velcro leg strap or tape
- Disposable gloves

ASSESSMENT

Assess bladder fullness before performing procedure, either by palpation or with a handheld bladder ultrasound device, and question patient about any allergies, especially to latex and iodine. Ask patient if she has ever been catheterized. If she had an indwelling catheter previously, ask why and for how long it was used. The patient may have urethral strictures that may make insertion more difficult.

NURSING DIAGNOSIS

Determine the related factors for the nursing diagnoses based on the patient's current status. Appropriate nursing diagnoses may include:

- Altered Urinary Elimination
- Urinary Retention
- Total Urinary Incontinence
- Risk for Impaired Skin Integrity

continues

SKILL 12-2   Catheterizing the Female Urinary Bladder (continued)

OUTCOME IDENTIFICATION AND PLANNING

The expected outcome to achieve when inserting a female urinary catheter is that the patient's urinary elimination will be maintained, with a urine output of at least 30 mL/hour, and the patient's bladder will not be distended. Another outcome may be that the patient's skin remains clean, dry and intact, without evidence of irritation or breakdown.

IMPLEMENTATION

ACTION	RATIONALE
1. Assemble equipment. Perform hand hygiene. Explain the skill and its purpose to patient. Discuss any allergies with patient, especially to iodine and latex.	Organization facilitates performance of the task. Hand hygiene deters spread of microorganisms. Explanation encourages patient cooperation and reduces apprehension. Most catheters and gloves in kits are made of latex. Some antiseptic solutions contain iodine.
2. Provide for good light. Artificial light is recommended (use of a flashlight requires an assistant to hold and position it).	Good lighting is necessary to see the meatus clearly.
3. Provide for privacy by closing the curtains or door.	Catheter insertion may be embarrassing for the patient.
4. Assist patient to dorsal recumbent position with knees flexed and feet about 2 feet apart. Drape patient. Or, if preferable, place patient in side-lying position. Slide waterproof drape under patient.	Good visualization of the meatus is important. Embarrassment, chilliness, and tension can interfere with catheter insertion; patient comfort will promote relaxation. The drape will protect bed linens from moisture.
5. **Don gloves. Spread labia well with fingers, and clean area at vaginal orifice with washcloth and warm water, using a different corner of the washcloth with each stroke. Wipe from above orifice downward toward sacrum (front to back).** Rinse and dry. Remove gloves. Perform hand hygiene again.	Gloves reduce the risk of exposure to blood and body fluids. Clean technique decreases the possibility of introducing microorganisms into the bladder.
6. Prepare urine drainage setup if indwelling catheter is to be inserted and if a separate urine collection system is to be used. Secure to bed frame according to manufacturer's directions.	This facilitates connection of the catheter to the drainage system and provides for easy access.
7. **Open sterile catheterization tray on a clean overbed table using sterile technique.**	Placement of equipment near worksite increases efficiency. Sterile technique protects patient and prevents spread of microorganisms.

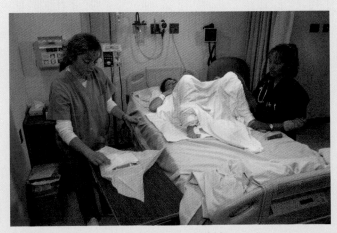

Action 4: Patient in dorsal recumbent position and draped properly.

Action 7: Opening sterile catheter tray at bedside.

continues

ACTION	RATIONALE
8. Put on sterile gloves. Grasp upper corners of drape and unfold drape without touching unsterile areas. Fold back a corner on each side to make a cuff over gloved hands. Ask patient to lift her buttocks and slide sterile drape under her with gloves protected by cuff.	The drape provides a sterile field close to the meatus. Covering the gloved hands will help keep the gloves sterile while placing the drape.
9. A fenestrated sterile drape may be placed over the perineal area, exposing the labia.	The drape expands the sterile field and protects against contamination. Use of a fenestrated drape may limit visualization and is considered optional by some practitioners.
10. Place sterile tray on drape between patient's thighs.	This provides easy access to supplies.
11. Open all supplies:	
a. **If catheter is to be indwelling, test catheter balloon.** Remove protective cap on tip of syringe and attach syringe prefilled with sterile water to injection port. Inject appropriate amount of fluid. If balloon inflates properly, withdraw fluid and leave syringe attached to port.	a. A balloon that does not inflate or that leaks needs to be replaced before insertion.

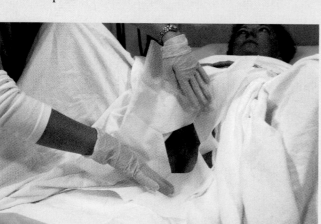

Action 9: Patient with fenestrated drape in place over perineum.

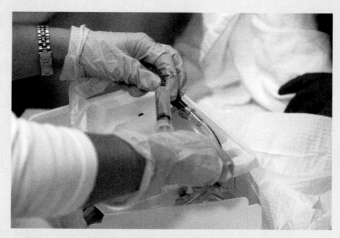

Action 11a: Testing balloon of indwelling catheter with syringe from catheter tray.

b. Fluff cotton balls in tray before pouring antiseptic solution over them. Open specimen container if specimen is to be obtained.	b. It is necessary to open all supplies and prepare for the procedure while both hands are sterile.
c. Lubricate 1″ to 2″ of catheter tip.	c. Lubrication facilitates catheter insertion and reduces tissue trauma.
12. With thumb and one finger of nondominant hand, spread labia and identify meatus. Be prepared to maintain separation of labia with one hand until catheter is inserted and urine is flowing well and continuously.	Smoothing the area immediately surrounding the meatus helps to make it visible. Allowing the labia to drop back into position may contaminate the area around the meatus, as well as the catheter. Your nondominant hand is now contaminated.

continues

Catheterizing the Female Urinary Bladder (continued)

ACTION

RATIONALE

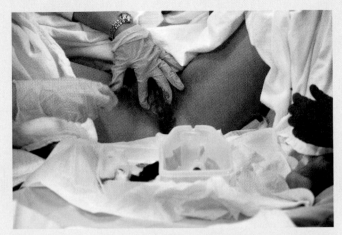

Action 12: Using nondominant hand (gloved) to separate and hold labia open.

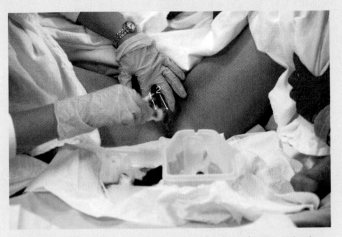

Action 13: Wiping perineum with cotton ball held by forceps. Wipe in one direction from top to bottom.

13. **Using cotton balls held with forceps, move cotton ball from above meatus down toward rectum discarding each cotton ball after one downward stroke. Clean both labial folds and then directly over the meatus, discarding each cotton ball after one downward stroke.**

14. With uncontaminated gloved hand, place drainage end of catheter in receptacle. For insertion of an indwelling catheter that is preattached to sterile tubing and drainage container (closed drainage system), position catheter and setup within easy reach on sterile field. Ensure that clamp on drainage bag is closed.

Moving from an area where there is likely to be less contamination to an area where there is more contamination helps prevent the spread of microorganisms. Cleaning the meatus last helps reduce the possibility of introducing microorganisms into the bladder.

This facilitates drainage of urine and minimizes risk of contaminating sterile equipment.

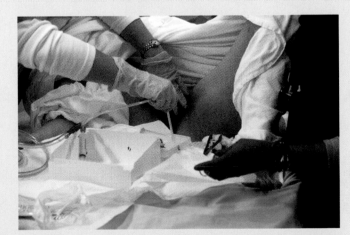

Action 14: Preparing to insert catheter.

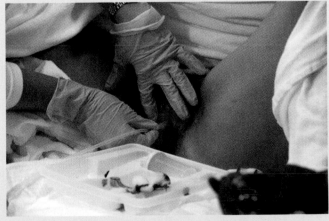

Action 14: Inserting catheter with dominant hand while nondominant hand holds labia apart.

continues

ACTION	RATIONALE
15. **Insert catheter tip into meatus 5 to 7.5 cm (2″ to 3″) or until urine flows. Do not force catheter through urethra into bladder. Ask patient to breathe deeply, and rotate catheter gently if slight resistance is met as catheter reaches external sphincter. For an indwelling catheter, once urine drains, advance catheter another 2.5 to 5.0 cm (1″ to 2″).**	The female urethra is about 3.7 to 6.2 cm (1.5″ to 2.5″) long. Applying force on the catheter is likely to injure mucous membranes. The sphincter relaxes and the catheter can enter the bladder easily when the patient relaxes. Advancing an indwelling catheter an additional 1.3 to 2.5 cm (½″ to 1″) ensures placement in the bladder and facilitates inflation of the balloon without damaging the urethra.
16. Hold catheter securely with nondominant hand while bladder empties. Collect a specimen if required; specimen should be caught in middle of flow. After 50 to 100 mL of urine has drained, place specimen collection device under opening of catheter and allow urine to drain into container. When enough urine has been caught, remove specimen container. Continue drainage according to agency policy.	Withdrawing and reinserting the catheter increases the chances of contaminating it. In general, no more than 750 mL of urine should be removed at one time. Pelvic floor blood vessels may become engorged from the sudden release of pressure, leading to a possible hypotensive episode. This may also cause painful bladder spasms.
17. Remove catheter smoothly and slowly if a straight catheterization was ordered.	This causes less discomfort to the patient.
18. If catheter is to be indwelling:	
a. Inflate balloon according to manufacturer's recommendations. Inject entire volume supplied in prefilled syringe.	a. The balloon anchors the catheter in place in the bladder. Sterile water is used to inflate the balloon as a precaution in case the balloon ruptures.

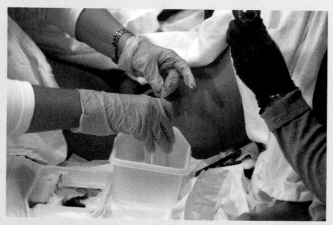

Action 16: Collecting urine in a specimen container.

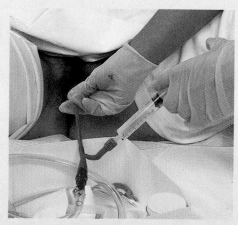

Action 18a: Inflating balloon of indwelling catheter.

b. Tug gently on catheter after balloon is inflated to feel resistance.	b. Improper inflation can cause patient discomfort and malpositioning of catheter.
c. Attach catheter to drainage system if necessary.	c. Closed drainage system minimizes the risk for microorganisms being introduced into the bladder.
d. **Secure to upper thigh with Velcro leg strap or tape. Leave some slack in catheter for leg movement.**	d. Proper attachment prevents trauma to the urethra and meatus from tension on the tubing. Whether to take the drainage tubing over or under the leg depends on gravity flow, patient's mobility, and comfort of the patient.

continues

Catheterizing the Female Urinary Bladder (continued)

ACTION   **RATIONALE**

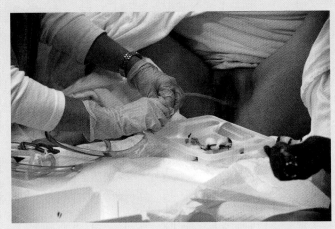

Action 18c: Attaching catheter to drainage bag.

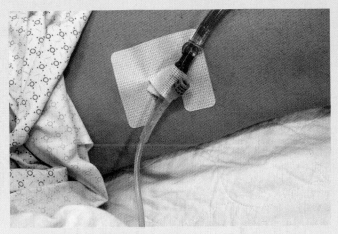

Action 18d: Catheter attached to leg.

e. Check that drainage tubing is not kinked and that movement of side rails does not interfere with catheter or drainage bag.

19. Remove equipment and make patient comfortable in bed. Care for equipment according to agency policy. Send urine specimen to the laboratory promptly or refrigerate it.

20. Perform perineal care as described in Action 5.

21. Remove gloves from inside out. Perform hand hygiene.

22. Record time of catheterization, size of catheter and balloon, amount of urine removed, urine appearance, whether a specimen was sent, and patient's reaction in the medical record; also document urine amount on intake/output flow sheet.

e. This facilitates drainage of urine and prevents the back-flow of urine.

Keeping urine at room temperature may cause micro-organisms, if present, to grow and distort laboratory findings.

Perineal care is done to remove antiseptic solution, which may cause skin irritation.

Contaminated area does not come in contact with hands or wrists. Hand hygiene deters the spread of microorganisms.

A careful record is important for planning the patient's care.

7/14/06 0915   Physician notified of palpable bladder (3 cm below umbilicus) and patient's inability to void. 16 Fr. Foley catheter inserted without difficulty. 10 mL of sterile water injected into balloon port. 700 mL clear yellow urine returned. Patient states, "Oh, I feel much better now." Bladder is no longer palpable. Patient tolerated procedure without incident. —A. Blitz, RN

Action 22: Documentation.

continues

EVALUATION   The expected outcome is met when the catheter, inserted using sterile technique, results in the immediate flow of urine and the bladder is not distended. Other outcomes are met when the patient reports little to no pain on insertion and the perineal area remains clean and dry.

Unexpected Situations and Associated Interventions

- *No urine flow is obtained, and nurse notes that catheter is in vaginal orifice:* Leave catheter in place as a landmark. Obtain fresh sterile gloves and new catheter. Attempt to place new catheter directly above misplaced catheter.
- *Urine flow initially contains a large amount of sediment, and then suddenly stops; bladder remains palpable:* Urinary catheter may be plugged with sediment. After obtaining a physician's order, gently irrigate the catheter.
- *After balloon is inflated, patient voids a large amount around balloon:* Check to make sure that the required amount of solution has been injected into the balloon. Do not overinflate balloon. Leaking around a catheter is a common occurrence when initially inserting catheter owing to large amount of urine pressure. If this continues to happen, a larger catheter may need to be inserted.
- *Patient moves legs during procedure:* If no supplies have been contaminated, ask patient to hold still and continue with procedure. If supplies have been contaminated, stop procedure and start over. If necessary, get an assistant to remind the patient to hold still.
- *Urine flow is initially well established, and urine is clear, but after several hours flow dwindles:* Check tubing for kinking. If patient has changed position, the tubing and drainage bag may need to be moved to facilitate drainage of urine.
- *Patient complains of extreme pain when nurse is inflating balloon:* Stop inflation of balloon. Balloon is most likely still in urethra. Allow solution in balloon to withdraw. Insert catheter an additional 1.3 to 2.5 cm (½" to 1") and slowly attempt to inflate balloon again.

Special Considerations

- If self-catheterization must be performed in the home, clean technique is appropriate. The bladder's natural resistance to the microorganisms normally found in the home makes sterile technique unnecessary. Rubber catheters must be washed thoroughly before boiling for 20 minutes. Dry and store properly for next use.
- If there is not an immediate flow of urine after the catheter has been inserted, several measures may prove helpful:
  - Have the patient take a deep breath, which helps to relax the perineal and abdominal muscles.
  - Rotate the catheter slightly, because a drainage hole may be resting against the bladder wall.
  - Raise the head of the patient's bed to increase pressure in the bladder area.
  - Some catheter kits do not contain the catheter. This allows you to select a catheter and balloon size separately.

SKILL 12-3   Catheterizing the Male Urinary Bladder (Straight and Indwelling)

Catheter insertion for a male patient is performed for the same reasons as for a female. Although the skill is similar, it is important to keep in mind the anatomic differences in the male and female urethra.

Equipment

- Sterile catheter kit that contains:
  Sterile gloves
  Sterile drapes (one of which is fenestrated)
  Sterile catheter
  Antiseptic solution
  Lubricant
  Cotton balls or gauze squares
  Forceps
  Prefilled syringe
  Basin (usually base of kit serves as this)
  Specimen container
- Flashlight or lamp
- Waterproof disposable pad
- Disposable urine collection bag and drainage tubing (may be connected to sterile indwelling catheter if a closed drainage system is used)
- Velcro leg strap or tape

ASSESSMENT

Assess bladder fullness before procedure, either by palpation or with a handheld bladder ultrasound device. Ask patient about any allergies, especially to latex and iodine. Ask patient if he has ever been catheterized. If he had an indwelling catheter previously, ask why and for how long it was used. The patient may have urethral strictures, which may make catheter insertion more difficult. If the patient is 50 or older, ask if he has had any prostate problems. Prostate enlargement typically is noted around the age of 50 years.

NURSING DIAGNOSIS

Determine the related factors for the nursing diagnoses based on the patient's current status. Appropriate nursing diagnoses may include:

- Altered Urinary Elimination
- Urinary Retention
- Total Urinary Incontinence
- Risk for Impaired Skin Integrity

OUTCOME IDENTIFICATION AND PLANNING

The expected outcome to achieve when inserting a male urinary catheter is that the patient's urinary elimination will be maintained, with a urine output of at least 30 mL/hour, and the bladder will not be distended. Another outcome may be that the patient's skin remains clean, dry, and intact, without evidence of irritation or breakdown.

IMPLEMENTATION

ACTION	RATIONALE
1. Follow Actions 1 through 3 for female catheterization in Skill 12-2.	
2. Position patient on his back with thighs slightly apart. Drape patient so that only the area around the penis is exposed.	This prevents unnecessary exposure.
3. Clean the penile area as in Action 5. Follow Actions 5 through 7 for female catheterization in Skill 12-2.	

continues

SKILL 12-3 Catheterizing the Male Urinary Bladder (Straight and Indwelling) (continued)

ACTION	RATIONALE
4. Put on sterile gloves. Open sterile drape and place on patient's thighs. Place fenestrated drape with opening over penis.	This maintains a sterile working area.
5. Place catheter set on or next to patient's legs on sterile drape.	Sterile setup should be arranged so that nurse's back is not turned to it, nor should it be out of the nurse's range of vision.
6. Open all supplies	
a. **If catheter is to be indwelling, test catheter balloon.** Remove protective cap on tip of syringe and attach syringe, prefilled with sterile water, to injection port. Inject appropriate amount of fluid. If balloon inflates properly, withdraw fluid and leave syringe attached to port.	a. A balloon that does not inflate or that leaks must be replaced before insertion.
b. Fluff cotton balls before pouring antiseptic solution over the cotton balls or gauze. Open specimen container if specimen is to be obtained.	b. It is necessary to open all supplies and prepare for the procedure while both hands are sterile.
c. Remove cap from syringe prefilled with lubricant.	
7. Lift penis with nondominant hand, which is then considered contaminated. **Retract foreskin in uncircumcised patient. Clean area at meatus with cotton ball held with forceps. Use circular motion, moving from meatus toward base of penis for three cleansings.**	The hand touching the penis becomes contaminated. Cleansing the area around the meatus and under the foreskin in the uncircumcised patient helps prevent infection. Moving from the meatus toward the base of the penis prevents bringing microorganisms to the meatus.

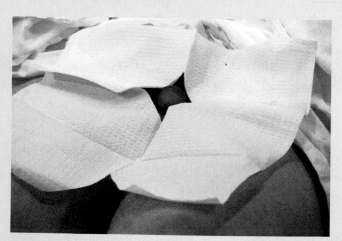

Action 4: Patient lying supine with fenestrated drape over penis.

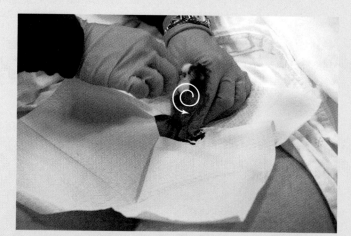

Action 7: Lifting penis with gloved nondominant hand and cleaning meatus with cotton ball held with forceps in gloved dominant hand.

8. Hold penis with slight upward tension and perpendicular to patient's body. Gently insert tip of syringe with lubricant into urethra and instill the 10 mL of lubricant. If kit does not have a prefilled syringe, lubricate catheter tip.	The lubricant causes the urethra to distend slightly and facilitates passage of the catheter without traumatizing the lining of the urethra.

continues

Catheterizing the Male Urinary Bladder (Straight and Indwelling) (continued)

ACTION	RATIONALE

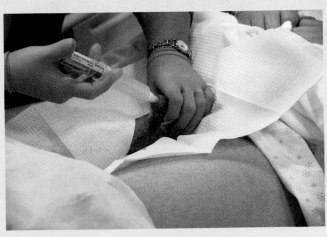

Action 8: Inserting syringe with lubricant into urethra.

9. With dominant hand, place drainage end of catheter in receptacle. For insertion of an indwelling catheter that is preattached to sterile tubing and a drainage container (closed drainage system), position catheter and setup with easy reach on sterile field. Ensure that clamp on drainage bag is closed.

This facilitates drainage of urine and minimizes risk of contamination of sterile equipment.

10. Ask patient to bear down as if voiding. Insert tip into meatus. Advance catheter 15 to 20 cm (6" to 8") or until urine flows. **Do not use force to introduce catheter. If catheter resists entry, ask patient to breathe deeply and rotate catheter slightly. For an indwelling catheter, once urine drains, advance catheter to bifurcation of catheter. Once balloon is inflated, catheter may be gently pulled back into place. Replace foreskin over catheter.** Lower penis.

Bearing down eases the passage of the catheter through the urethra. The male urethra is about 20 cm long. Having the patient take deep breaths or twisting the catheter slightly may ease the catheter past resistance at the sphincters. Advancing an indwelling catheter to the bifurcation ensures its placement in the bladder and facilitates inflation of the balloon without damaging the urethra.

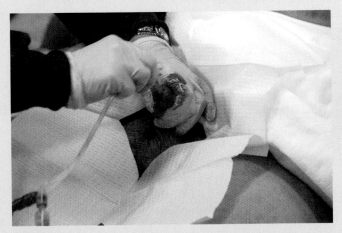

Action 10: Inserting catheter with gloved dominant hand.

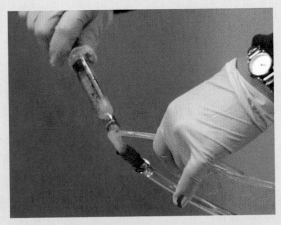

Action 10: Inflating balloon.

continues

Catheterizing the Male Urinary Bladder (Straight and Indwelling) (continued)

ACTION	RATIONALE
11. Follow Actions 16 to 20 for female catheterization in Skill 12-2, except that the catheter may be secured to the upper thigh or lower abdomen with the penis directed toward patient's chest. Leave enough slack in catheter to prevent tension.	This is done to prevent irritation at the angle of the penis and scrotum. Slack left in the catheter allows for penile erection, which can occur naturally during sleep.
12. Remove gloves from inside out. Perform hand hygiene.	Contaminated area does not come in contact with hands or wrists. Hand hygiene deters the spread of microorganisms.
13. Record time of catheterization, catheter and balloon size, amount of urine removed, urine appearance, whether a specimen was sent, and patient's reaction to the procedure in the medical record. Also document urine amount on the intake/output flow sheet.	A careful record is important for planning the patient's care.

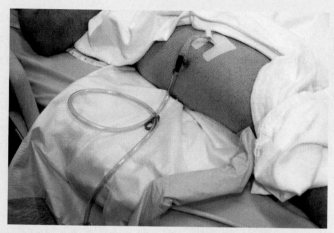

Action 11: Catheter in place and taped to patient's upper thigh.

7/14/06   0915   Physician notified of palpable bladder (3 cm below umbilicus) and patient's inability to void. 16 Fr. Foley catheter inserted without difficulty. 10 mL of sterile water injected into balloon port. 700 mL clear yellow urine returned. Patient states, "Oh, I feel much better now." Bladder is no longer palpable. Patient tolerated procedure without incident. —A. Blitz, RN

Action 13: Documentation.

EVALUATION

The expected outcome is met when the catheter, inserted using sterile technique, results in the immediate flow of urine and the patient's bladder is not distended. Other outcomes are met when the patient reports little to no pain on insertion and the perineal area remains clean and dry.

Unexpected Situations and Associated Interventions

- *Patient complains of intense pain when nurse begins to inflate balloon:* Stop inflation. Be sure to insert catheter all the way in to the bifurcation. The balloon is probably still in the urethra. Damage to the urethra can result if balloon is inflated in urethra.
- *Nurse cannot insert catheter past 3" to 4"; rotating the catheter and having patient breathe deeply are of no help:* If still unable to place catheter, notify physician. Repeated catheter placement attempts can traumatize the urethra. Physician may order and insert a Credé catheter.
- *Patient is obese and has retracted penis:* Have assistant available to hold patient's penis up and back. The catheter still needs to be inserted to the bifurcation; the length of the urethra has not changed.

continues

SKILL 12-3   Catheterizing the Male Urinary Bladder (Straight and Indwelling) (continued)

- *Urine flow initially contains a large amount of sediment and then suddenly stops; bladder remains palpable:* Catheter may be plugged with sediment. After obtaining a physician's order, gently irrigate the catheter.
- *After balloon is inflated, patient voids a large amount around balloon:* Make sure that the required amount of solution has been injected into the balloon. Do not overinflate balloon. Leaking around the catheter is a common occurrence when initially inserting catheter due to large amount of urine pressure. If this continues to happen, a larger catheter may need to be inserted.
- *Patient moves legs during procedure:* If no supplies have been contaminated, ask patient to hold still, and continue with procedure. If supplies have been contaminated, stop procedure and start over. The nurse may want to get an assistant to remind the patient to hold still.
- *Urine flow is initially well established, and urine is clear, but after several hours urine flow dwindles:* Check tubing for kinking. If patient has changed position, the tubing and drainage bag may need to be moved to facilitate drainage of urine.

Special Considerations

- If resistance is met while inserting catheter and rotating does not help, do not use force. Enlargement of the prostate gland is commonly seen in men over age 50. A special crook-tipped catheter called a Credé catheter may be required to maneuver past the prostate gland.

SKILL 12-4   Irrigating the Catheter Using the Closed System

Indwelling catheters at times require irrigation, or flushing, with solution to restore or maintain the patency of the drainage system. Sediment or debris as well as blood clots might block the catheter, preventing the flow of urine out of the catheter. Irrigations might also be used to instill medications that will act directly on the bladder wall. Irrigating a catheter through a closed system is preferred to opening the catheter because opening the catheter could lead to contamination and infection.

Equipment

- Sterile basin or container
- Sterile irrigating solution (at room temperature or warmed to body temperature)
- 30- to 60-mL syringe with 18- or 19-gauge blunt-ended needle
- Gauze squares or cotton balls with disinfectant or alcohol swabs
- Bath blanket
- Disposable gloves
- Waterproof drape

ASSESSMENT

Check to ensure that a physician's order has been written, including the type of solution to use for the irrigation. Before performing the procedure, assess bladder fullness either by palpation or with a handheld bladder ultrasound device.

NURSING DIAGNOSIS

Determine the related factors for the nursing diagnoses based on the patient's current status. An appropriate nursing diagnosis is Altered Urinary Elimination. Other nursing diagnoses, such as Risk for Infection, may also require this procedure.

OUTCOME IDENTIFICATION AND PLANNING

The expected outcome to achieve when performing a closed catheter irrigation is that the patient exhibits the free flow of urine through the catheter. Other outcomes may include the following: the patient's bladder is not distended and the patient remains free of any signs and symptoms of infection.

continues

SKILL 12-4

Irrigating the Catheter Using the Closed System (continued)

IMPLEMENTATION

ACTION	RATIONALE
1. Assemble equipment. Perform hand hygiene. Explain procedure and its purpose to patient.	Organization facilitates performance of task. Hand hygiene deters the spread of microorganisms. Explanation encourages patient cooperation and reduces apprehension.
2. Provide privacy by closing the curtains or door and draping patient with bath blanket.	The procedure may be embarrassing for the patient.
3. Assist patient to comfortable position and expose aspiration port on catheter setup. Place waterproof drape under catheter and aspiration port.	This provides visualization. Drape protects patient and bed from leakage.
4. Open sterile supplies. Pour sterile solution into sterile basin. Aspirate irrigant (30 to 60 mL) into sterile syringe and attach capped, sterile, blunt-ended needle. Don gloves.	This prevents the spread of microorganisms and contact with blood or body fluids.

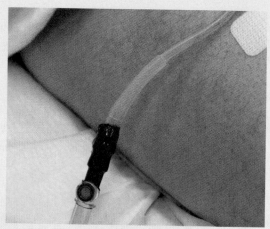

Action 3: Aspiration port on catheter.

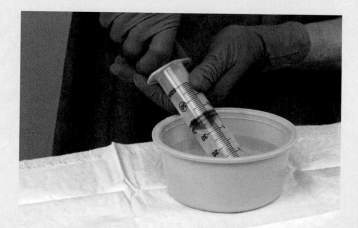

Action 4: Drawing up irrigant from sterile basin into a 30- to 60-mL syringe.

5. **Wipe aspiration port with alcohol swabs or gauze square with antiseptic solution.**	This prevents the spread of microorganisms.
6. Clamp or fold catheter tubing distal to aspiration port.	This directs the irrigating solution into the bladder.

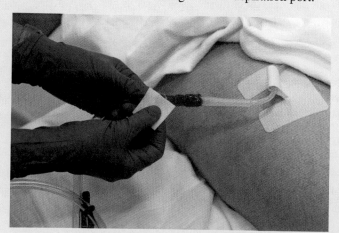

Action 5: Wiping port on catheter.

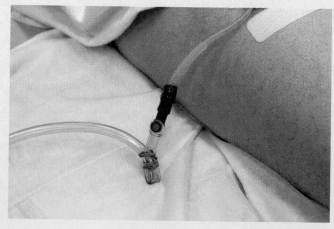

Action 6: Urinary catheter with drainage tubing clamped or folded below port.

continues

Irrigating the Catheter Using the Closed System (continued)

ACTION	RATIONALE
7. Remove cap and insert needle into port. Gently instill solution into catheter.	Gentle irrigation prevents damage to bladder lining.
8. Remove needle from port. Unclamp or unfold tubing and allow irrigant and urine to drain. Repeat procedure as necessary.	Gravity aids drainage of urine and irrigant from the bladder.

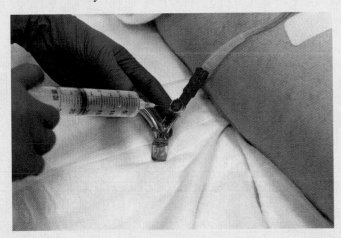

Action 7: Inserting syringe into port.

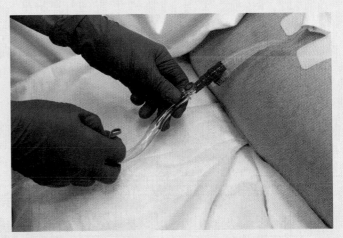

Action 8: Fluid draining through tubing into drainage bag.

9. Remove equipment and discard uncapped needle and syringe in appropriate receptacle. Remove gloves and perform hand hygiene. Make patient comfortable.	This provides accurate documentation of the procedure.
10. Assess patient's response to procedure and quality and amount of drainage with irrigation. Document on patient's chart.	This provides accurate documentation of the procedure.

7/22/06 1630   Urinary catheter irrigated with 500 mL of normal saline. All of irrigation returned plus 200 mL of cloudy urine. Patient tolerated procedure without incident. Order received to notify physician if urine output <30 mL per hour.—A. Blitz, RN

Action 10: Documentation.

11. Record amount of irrigant used on intake/output record. Subtract this from urine output when totaled.	Subtracting irrigant total from drainage in urine collection bag provides accurate recording of urine output.

EVALUATION   The expected outcome is met when urine flows freely through the catheter after the irrigation solution is introduced without resistance or pain. The irrigant plus urine is returned into the drainage bag. Other outcomes may include the following: the bladder is not distended and the patient remains free of any signs and symptoms of infection.

**UNEXPECTED
SITUATIONS
AND ASSOCIATED
INTERVENTIONS**

- *Irrigation solution will not enter the catheter:* Do not force the solution into the catheter. Notify physician. Prepare to change catheter.
- *Tubing was not clamped before introducing irrigation solution:* Repeat irrigation. If the tubing is not clamped, the irrigation solution will drain into the urinary drainage bag and not enter the catheter.

Giving a Continuous Bladder Irrigation

Indwelling catheters sometimes require continuous irrigations to prevent blood clots and other debris from blocking the catheter. Irrigation also may be used to administer medications. Often the patient will have a triple-lumen or three-way catheter in place to maintain a closed system.

Equipment

- Sterile irrigating solution (at room temperature or warmed to body temperature), usually 200-mL bags
- Sterile tubing with drip chamber and clamp for connection to irrigating solution
- IV pole
- IV pump (if bladder is being irrigated with a solution containing medication)
- Three-way indwelling catheter in place in patient's bladder
- Indwelling catheter drainage setup (tubing and collection bag)
- Bath blanket
- Disposable gloves

ASSESSMENT

Verify physician's order for continuous bladder irrigation. Also assess the catheter to ensure that it has an irrigation port (if the patient has an indwelling catheter already in place). Review the patient's medical record for and ask the patient about any allergies to medications.

NURSING DIAGNOSIS

Determine the related factors for the nursing diagnoses based on the patient's current status. Appropriate nursing diagnoses may include Altered Urinary Elimination and Risk for Infection.

OUTCOME IDENTIFICATION AND PLANNING

The expected outcome to achieve when giving a continuous bladder irrigation is that the patient exhibits free-flowing urine through the catheter. Initially clots or debris may be noted. These should decrease over time, with the patient ultimately exhibiting urine that is free of clots or debris. Other outcomes would include the following: the continuous bladder irrigation begins without incident; drainage is greater than the hourly amount of irrigation solution being placed in bladder; and the patient exhibits no signs and symptoms of infection.

IMPLEMENTATION

ACTION	IMPLEMENTATION
1. Explain procedure and its purpose to patient.	Explanation encourages patient cooperation and reduces apprehension.
2. Assemble equipment and double-check physician's order.	Organization facilitates performance of tasks. Double-checking the order ensures that the correct procedure is to be performed.
3. Perform hand hygiene.	Hand hygiene deters the spread of microorganisms.
4. Provide privacy by closing curtains or door and draping patient with bath blanket.	Procedure may be embarrassing for patient.
5. Prepare sterile irrigation bag for use as directed by manufacturer. Secure clamp and attach sterile tubing with drip chamber to container. Hang bag on IV pole 2.5 to 3 feet above level of patient's bladder. Release clamp and remove protective cover on end of tubing without contaminating it. Allow solution to flush tubing and remove air. Reclamp.	Irrigation solution continuously bathes the lining of the bladder and keeps the catheter patent. Flushing the tubing before irrigation clears air from the tubing that might cause bladder distention.
6. **Don gloves. Using sterile technique, attach irrigation tubing to irrigation port of three-way indwelling catheter.** If a closed system is used, tubing may already be connected to irrigation port on catheter.	Sterile technique prevents the spread of microorganisms into the bladder.

continues

SKILL 12-5   **Giving a Continuous Bladder Irrigation** (continued)

ACTION

RATIONALE

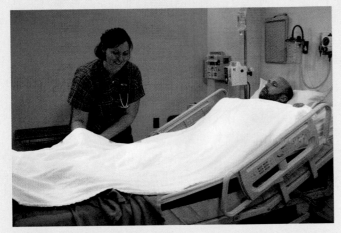

Action 4: Ensuring patient's privacy.

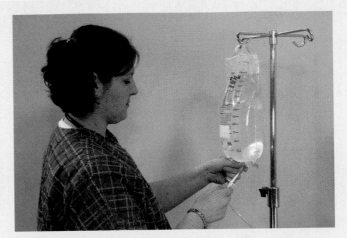

Action 5: Spiking bag with tubing for irrigation.

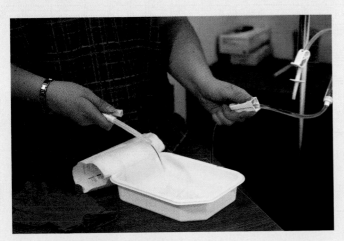

Action 5: Regulating flow clamp to prime tubing.

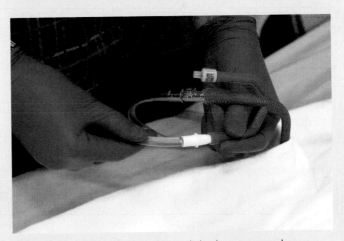

Action 6: Attaching irrigation tubing to irrigation port on catheter.

7. Release clamp on irrigation tubing and regulate flow according to physician's order. At times, the physician may order the bladder irrigation to be done with a medicated solution. In these cases, use an IV pump to regulate the flow.

8. As irrigation is completed, clamp tubing. **Do not allow drip chamber to empty. Disconnect empty bag and attach full irrigation bag.** Continue as ordered by physician.

9. Assess patient's response to procedure and quality and amount of drainage. Document on patient's chart.

10. Record amount of irrigant used on intake/output record. Don gloves and empty drainage collection bag as each new container is hung and recorded.

11. Remove gloves and perform hand hygiene.

This allows for continual gentle irrigation without causing discomfort to the patient. An IV pump regulates the flow of the medication.

This eliminates the need to separate tubing from the catheter and clear air from the tubing. Opening the drainage system provides access for microorganisms.

This provides accurate documentation of the procedure.

This ensures accurate recording of urine output. Gloves protect against exposure to blood, body fluids, and microorganisms.

Hand hygiene deters the spread of microorganisms.

continues

ACTION   **RATIONALE**

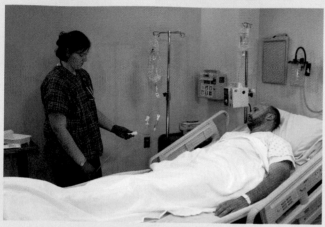

Action 7: Regulating irrigation flow rate using flow clamp.

7/14/06   1330   *Foley catheter replaced
with 3-way Foley catheter. Continuous bladder irrigation with normal saline at 100
mL/hour begun. Patient tolerated procedure
without incident. Drainage from bladder
slightly cloudy. —A. Blitz, RN*

Action 9: Documentation.

EVALUATION

The expected outcome is met when urine flows freely through the catheter. Effectiveness of therapy is determined by the urine characteristics. Upon completion of the therapy with a continuous bladder irrigation, the patient should exhibit urine that is clear, without evidence of clots or debris. Other outcomes would include the following: the continuous bladder irrigation begins without incident; drainage is greater than the hourly amount of irrigation solution being placed in bladder; and the patient exhibits no signs and symptoms of infection.

Unexpected Situations and Associated Interventions

- *Continuous bladder irrigation begins and hourly drainage is less than amount of irrigation being given:* Palpate for bladder distention. If patient is lying supine, rolling the patient onto a side may help increase the amount of drainage. Check to make sure that the tubing is not kinked.
- *Bladder irrigation is not flowing at ordered rate, even with clamp wide open:* Raise the bag 3″ to 6″ and then check flow of irrigation solution. Frequently check flow rate of irrigation solution.

Special Considerations

- At times, the physician may want the bladder irrigated with a solution containing a medication. Ensure that you follow the Five Rights for medication administration with every change of the irrigation fluid bag.

SKILL 12-6   Applying a Condom Catheter

A condom catheter is an alternative to an indwelling catheter in male patients who cannot control urination voluntarily. The condom catheter is applied externally to the penis. The risk for urinary tract infection with a condom catheter is lower than the risk associated with an indwelling urinary catheter.

Equipment

- Condom sheath in appropriate size
- Bath blanket
- Reusable leg bag with tubing or urinary drainage setup
- Elastic strip or Velcro (optional)
- Basin of warm water and soap
- Disposable gloves
- Washcloth and towel

ASSESSMENT

Assess patient's knowledge of need for catheter. Ask patient about any allergies, especially to latex or tape. Assess the size of the patient's penis to ensure that the appropriate-sized condom is used. Inspect the skin in the groin and scrotal area, noting any areas of redness, irritation, or breakdown. If any areas are observed, notify the physician.

NURSING DIAGNOSIS

Determine the related factors for the nursing diagnoses based on the patient's current status. Possible nursing diagnoses may include:

- Altered Urinary Elimination
- Risk for Impaired Skin Integrity
- Total Incontinence
- Functional Urinary Incontinence

OUTCOME IDENTIFICATION AND PLANNING

The expected outcome to achieve when applying a condom catheter is that the patient's urinary elimination will be maintained, with a urine output of at least 30 mL/hour, and the bladder is not distended. Other outcomes may include the following: the patient's skin remains clean, dry, and intact, without evidence of irritation or breakdown.

IMPLEMENTATION

ACTION	RATIONALE
1. Explain procedure to patient. Obtain a latex-free condom if patient is allergic to latex.	This provides reassurance and promotes patient cooperation. If patient is allergic to latex, a latex-free condom catheter must be used. Some condom catheters have adhesive on the inside. If the patient has a tape allergy, the patient may have an allergy to this adhesive.
2. Prepare urinary drainage setup or reusable leg bag for attachment to condom sheath.	This provides for an organized approach to the task.
3. Perform hand hygiene.	Hand hygiene deters the spread of microorganisms.
4. Assist patient to supine position. Close curtain or door. Use bath blanket and sheet to expose only the patient's genital area.	This provides privacy.
5. Don disposable gloves. Trim any long pubic hair that is in contact with penis.	Trimming pubic hair prevents pulling of hair by adhesive without the risk of infection associated with shaving.
6. Wash genital area with soap and water, rinse, and dry thoroughly. **If patient is uncircumcised, retract foreskin and clean glans of penis. Replace foreskin.**	Washing removes urine, secretions, and microorganisms. The penis must be clean and dry to minimize skin irritation. If the foreskin is left retracted, it may cause venous congestion in the glans of the penis, leading to edema.

continues

ACTION   **RATIONALE**

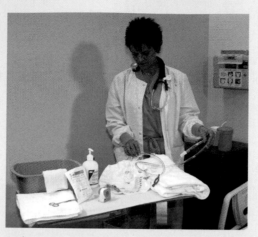

Action 2: Preparing urinary drainage setup.

7. Roll condom sheath outward onto itself. Grasp penis firmly with nondominant hand. Apply condom sheath by rolling it onto penis with dominant hand. **Leave 2.5 to 5 cm (1″ to 2″) of space between tip of penis and end of condom sheath.**

Rolling the condom sheath outward allows for easier application. The space prevents irritation to tip of penis and allows free drainage of urine.

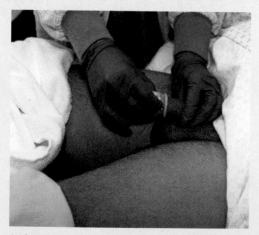

Action 7: Grasping penis firmly and unrolling condom sheath onto penis.

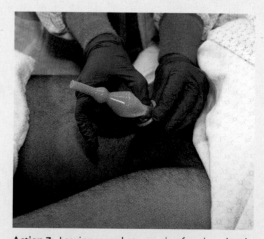

Action 7: Leaving space between tip of penis and end of condom sheath.

8. Apply elastic or Velcro strap snugly but not too tightly. Do not allow elastic or Velcro to come in contact with skin.

The elastic or Velcro strap should secure the condom sheath but not interfere with blood circulation to the penis.

9. Connect condom sheath to drainage setup. Avoid kinking or twisting drainage tubing.

The collection device keeps the patient dry. Kinked tubing encourages backflow of urine.

10. Remove equipment. Place patient in a comfortable, safe position. Perform hand hygiene.

This provides a safe, comfortable setting for the patient. Hand hygiene deters the spread of microorganisms.

continues

Applying a Condom Catheter (continued)

ACTION

RATIONALE

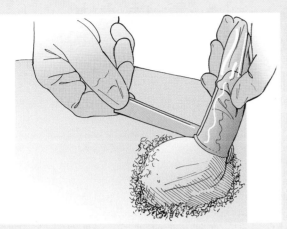

Action 8: If applicable, apply Velcro strap (or elastic strap) snugly.

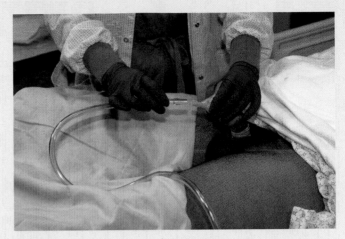

Action 9: Attaching condom to drainage setup.

11. Assess patient's response and record observations on patient's chart.

This provides accurate documentation and observation of urine output.

> 7/12/06 1910   Order received for placement of condom catheter. Medium-sized condom cath placed. 200 mL of clear urine returned. Patient's sacral area remains erythematous. Patient tolerated procedure without incident. —A. Blitz, RN

Action 11: Documentation.

EVALUATION

The expected outcome is met when the condom catheter is applied without incident, urine is observed in the drainage bag, and the patient's skin remains clean and dry.

Unexpected situations and Associated Interventions

- *Condom catheter leaks with every voiding:* Check size of condom catheter. If it is too big or too little, it may leak. Check space between tip of penis and end of condom sheath. If this space is too small, the urine has no place to go and will leak out.
- *Condom catheter will not stay on patient:* Ensure that condom catheter is correct size and that penis is thoroughly dried before applying condom catheter. Remind patient that condom catheter is in place, so that patient does not tug at tubing. Make sure elastic or Velcro strap is in place. If the patient has a retracted penis, a condom catheter may not be the best choice; there are pouches made for patients with a retracted penis.
- *When assessing patient's penis, nurse finds a break in skin integrity:* Do not reapply condom catheter. Allow skin to be open to air as much as possible. If institution has a wound, ostomy, and continence nurse, a consult would be in order.

Changing a Stoma Appliance on an Ileal Conduit

A patient with an ileal conduit requires an appliance to collect the urine that drains from the stoma continuously. Proper application minimizes the risk for skin breakdown around the stoma.

Equipment

- Basin with warm water, soap, towel
- Sterile 2 × 2 gauze squares
- Washcloth or cotton balls
- Skin protectant or barrier
- Ostomy bag cut to the correct stoma size (with adhesive-backed faceplate if available)
- Graduated container
- Ostomy belt (optional)
- Adhesive cement (optional for reusable pouches)
- Disposable gloves

ASSESSMENT

Assess current ileal conduit appliance, looking at product style, condition of appliance, and stoma (if bag is clear). Inspect the skin surrounding the ileal conduit. Determine the patient's knowledge of care of the ileal conduit.

NURSING DIAGNOSIS

Determine the related factors for the nursing diagnoses based on the patient's current status. Possible nursing diagnoses may include:

- Altered Urinary Elimination
- Risk for Impaired Skin Integrity
- Deficient Knowledge
- Disturbed Body Image

OUTCOME IDENTIFICATION AND PLANNING

The expected outcome to achieve when changing a patient's urinary stoma appliance is that the stoma appliance is applied correctly to the skin to allow urine to drain freely. Other outcomes may include the following: the patient will exhibit a healthy pink stoma with intact skin surrounding the stoma; the patient will demonstrate knowledge of how to apply the pouch; and the patient verbalizes positive self-image.

IMPLEMENTATION

ACTION	RATIONALE
1. Explain procedure and encourage patient to observe or participate if possible. Have patient perform hand hygiene. Provide privacy.	Explaining the procedure and having the patient observe or assist encourages self-acceptance.
2. Assemble equipment.	Organization facilitates performance of task.
3. Perform hand hygiene and don disposable gloves.	Hand hygiene deters the spread of microorganisms. Gloves protect nurse from blood, body fluid, and microorganisms.
4. Have patient sit or stand if able to assist with skill or assume supine position in bed.	These positions result in fewer abdominal folds and facilitate removal and application of the device.
5. Empty pouch being worn into graduated container (before removing if it is reusable and not attached to straight drainage).	Emptying the pouch before handling it reduces the likelihood of spilling the excretions. The physician may have ordered recording of intake and output.
6. Gently remove pouch faceplate from skin by pushing skin from appliance rather than pulling appliance from skin.	The seal between the surface of the faceplate and the skin must be broken before the faceplate can be removed. Harsh handling of the appliance can damage the skin and impair the development of a secure seal in the future.

continues

Changing a Stoma Appliance on an Ileal Conduit (continued)

ACTION	RATIONALE

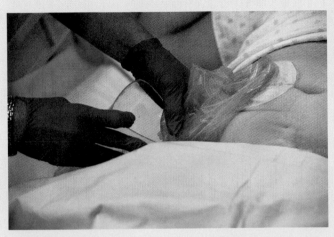

Action 5: Emptying pouch into graduated container.

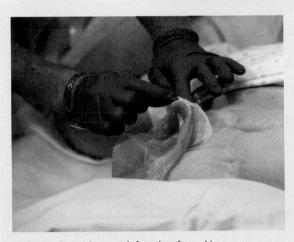

Action 6: Removing pouch faceplate from skin.

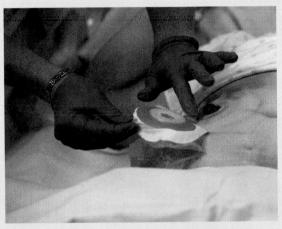

Action 6: Pushing skin from appliance rather than pulling appliance from skin.

7. Discard pouch appropriately if disposable, or wash reusable pouch in lukewarm soap and water and allow to air dry.

Thorough cleaning and airing of the appliance reduce odor and deterioration of appliance. For esthetic and infection control purposes, used appliances should be discarded appropriately.

8. **Clean skin around stoma with soap and water or a commercial cleaner using a washcloth or cotton balls. Remove all old adhesive from skin; an adhesive remover may be used.**

Cleaning the skin removes excretions and old adhesive and skin protectant. Excretions or a buildup of other substances can irritate and damage the skin.

9. Gently pat area dry. Make sure skin around stoma is thoroughly dry. Assess stoma and condition of surrounding skin.

Careful drying prevents trauma to skin and stoma. An intact, properly applied urinary collection device protects skin integrity. Any change in color and size of the stoma may indicate circulatory problems.

10. Place a gauze square or two over stoma opening.

Continuous drainage must be absorbed to keep skin dry during appliance change.

continues

SKILL
12-7   **Changing a Stoma Appliance on an Ileal Conduit** (continued)

ACTION   **RATIONALE**

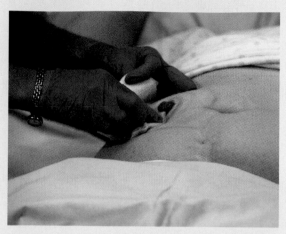

Action 8: Cleaning stoma area with soap and water and washcloth.

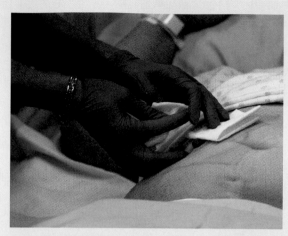

Action 10: Placing one or two gauze squares over opening.

11. Apply skin protectant to a 5-cm (2″) radius around the stoma, and allow it to dry completely, which takes about 30 seconds.

12. If necessary, enlarge size of faceplate opening to fit stoma.

The skin needs protection from the excoriating effect of the excretion and appliance adhesive. Allowing the protectant to dry completely enhances its effectiveness.

The appliance should fit snugly around the stoma, with only ⅟₁₆″ to ⅛″ of skin visible around the opening. A faceplate opening that is too small can cause trauma to the stoma. If the opening is too large, exposed skin will be irritated by urine.

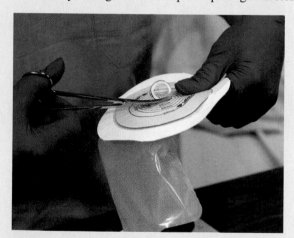

Action 12: If necessary, cut faceplate of stoma bag to enlarge it.

13. Remove gauze squares from stoma before applying pouch. Apply adhesive to faceplate or remove protective covering from disposable faceplate, carefully position appliance, and press it in place, moving from the center outward.

14. Secure optional belt to appliance and around patient.

15. Remove or discard equipment and assess patient's response to procedure. Remove gloves and perform hand hygiene.

The appliance is effective only if it is properly positioned and securely adhered. Commercial deodorants may be used if odor is a problem.

An elasticized belt helps support the appliance for some people.

The patient's response may indicate acceptance of the ostomy as well as the need for health teaching. Hand hygiene deters the spread of microorganisms.

continues

ACTION   **RATIONALE**

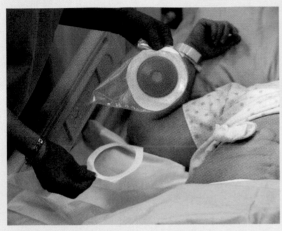

Action 13: Removing protective covering from faceplate.

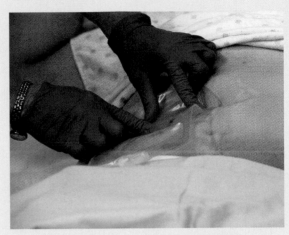

Action 13: Applying faceplate over stoma and press it in place, moving from center outward.

16. Record appearance of stoma and surrounding skin as well as patient's reaction to procedure.

A careful record is important for planning the patient's care.

> 7/23/06 1245   Ileal conduit appliance changed. Mr. Jones present. Mrs. Jones asking questions about care for ileal conduit, states, "I don't know if I'll ever be able to care for this thing at home." Tearful at times. Patient encouraged to express feelings. Patient agreed to talk with wound, ostomy, and continence nurse about concerns. Mr. Jones very supportive, also asking appropriate questions. Patient states would like to watch change one more time before she attempts to do it. Stoma is pink, peristomal skin intact, drainage cloudy with small amount of mucus.—A. Blitz, RN

Action 16: Documentation.

EVALUATION

The expected outcome is met when the ileal conduit appliance is changed without trauma to stoma or peristomal skin, or leaking; urine is draining freely into the appliance; the skin surrounding the stoma is clean, dry, and intact; and the patient shows an interest in learning to perform the pouch change and verbalizes positive self-image.

Unexpected Situations and Associated Interventions

- *Nurse removes appliance and finds area of skin excoriated:* If institution has a wound, ostomy, and incontinence nurse, a consult may be needed. Cleanse the skin thoroughly and pat dry. Apply products made for excoriated skin before placing appliance over stoma. Frequently check faceplate to ensure that a seal has formed and that there is no leakage. Document the excoriation in the patient's chart.
- *Faceplate is leaking after applying new appliance:* Remove appliance, clean the skin, and start over.
- *Nurse is ready to place faceplate and notices that opening is cut too large:* Discard appliance and begin over. A faceplate that is cut too big may lead to excoriation of the skin.

SKILL 12-8   Collecting a Urine Specimen for Culture

Collecting a urine specimen for culture is an assessment measure to determine the characteristics of a patient's urine. A specimen collected for culture is collected midstream to provide a specimen that most closely reflects the characteristics of the urine being produced by the body.

Equipment

- Moist towelette or alcohol wipe (for specimen collection from an indwelling catheter)
- Disposable gloves
- Sterile specimen container
- Adhesive collection bag (infants)
- Syringe with blunt-tipped needle (for specimen collection from a catheter)

ASSESSMENT

After verifying the physician's order for specimen collection, ask patient about any medications that he or she is taking, because medications may affect the results of the test. Assess for any signs and symptoms of a urinary tract infection, such as burning, pain (dysuria), or frequency. Ask the patient to describe the urine odor, clarity, and color. During the physical examination, palpate the bladder and costovertebral angle for tenderness.

NURSING DIAGNOSIS

Determine the related factors for the nursing diagnoses based on the patient's current status. Possible nursing diagnoses may include:

- Altered Urinary Elimination
- Anxiety
- Deficient Knowledge

OUTCOME IDENTIFICATION AND PLANNING

The expected outcome to be met when collecting a urine specimen for culture is that an adequate amount of urine is obtained from the patient without contamination. Other outcomes include the following: the patient exhibits minimal anxiety during specimen collection and demonstrates ability to collect a clean urine specimen.

IMPLEMENTATION

ACTION	RATIONALE

For the Adult Patient Who Is Capable of Self-Care:

1. Explain procedure to patient, including performing of hand hygiene before and after specimen collection. Instruct patient to wipe perineal area from front to back or meatus of penis with moist towelette. Instruct male patient who is not circumcised to retract foreskin and clean glans of penis.

Cleaning the perineal area or penis reduces the risk for contamination of the specimen, which should be as clean as possible.

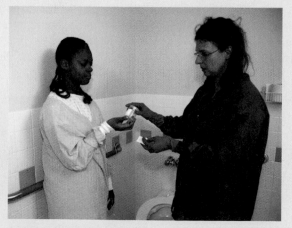

Action 1: Instructing patient about use of specimen cup and cleansing towelettes.

continues

SKILL 12-8 Collecting a Urine Specimen for Culture (continued)

ACTION	RATIONALE
2. **Have patient void about 25 mL into toilet, stop stream, collect specimen (10 to 20 mL is more than enough), and then finish voiding. Tell patient not to touch the inside of the container or the lid.**	Collecting a midstream specimen ensures that fresh urine is analyzed. Some urine may have collected in the urethra from the last void. By voiding a little before collecting the specimen, the specimen will contain only fresh urine.
3. Have patient place lid on container. Don gloves and label container with patient's name, date, time, and person collecting specimen.	Placing lid on container helps to keep specimen clean and prevents spills. Gloves reduce the risk of exposure to body fluids. Labeling the container provides valuable information to the laboratory and ensures accurate reporting of results.
4. Place container in biohazard bag. Remove gloves and perform hand hygiene.	Transporting specimen in biohazard bag prevents exposure of other healthcare workers to pathogens. Hand hygiene deters the spread of microorganisms.

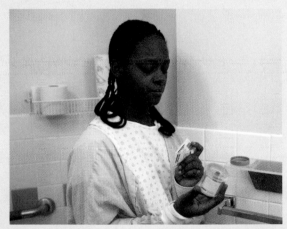

Action 2: Instruct patient not to touch inside of container or lid.

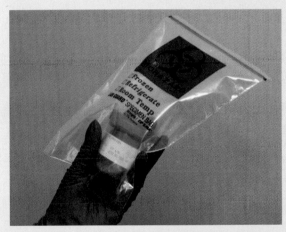

Action 4: Placing labeled urine specimen in biohazard transport bag.

5. Transport specimen to laboratory as soon as possible. If unable to take specimen to laboratory immediately, refrigerate it.	If not refrigerated immediately, urine may act as a culture medium, allowing bacteria to multiply and skewing the results of testing. Refrigeration prevents the bacteria from multiplying.
6. Document specimen sent, odor, amount (if known), color, and clarity of urine.	A careful record is important for planning the patient's care.

7/10/06 2200   Patient instructed to collect midstream urine sample. 70 mL of cloudy, odorless, yellow urine sent to laboratory.
—A. Blitz, RN

Action 6: Documentation.

For Very Young Children and Infants:

7. Explain steps to a young child, if old enough, and to the parents. Talk to child at child's level, stressing that no pain will be involved.	Explanation at the child's level helps to promote cooperation. Knowing that the procedure is not painful helps to relieve anxiety and fear.
8. Perform hand hygiene and don disposable gloves.	Hand hygiene deters the spread of microorganisms. Gloves protect nurse from contact with microorganisms.

continues

SKILL 12-8   Collecting a Urine Specimen for Culture (continued)

ACTION	RATIONALE
9. If the child is old enough, follow the steps as for an adult. For an infant, remove the diaper. Perform thorough perineal care: for girls, spread labia and cleanse area; for boys, retract foreskin if intact and cleanse glans of penis. Pat skin dry.	The specimen needs to be as clean as possible. Skin needs to be dry for adhesive bag to stick.
10. Remove paper backing from adhesive faceplate. Apply faceplate over labia or over penis. Gently push faceplate so that seal forms on skin. **Take care to not contaminate inside of bag when applying, because it is considered sterile.**	Since child cannot void on command and specimen needs to be as aseptic as possible, using a urine collection bag is a less traumatic way to obtain a sterile urine specimen. At times the physician may order insertion of an intermittent (straight) catheter to obtain a specimen.

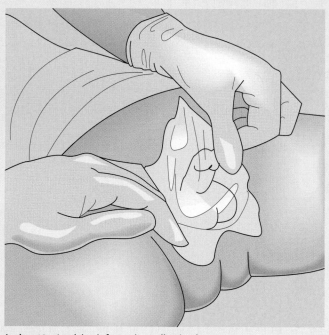

Action 10: Applying infant urine collection bag.

11. Apply clean diaper over bag. Remove gloves and perform hand hygiene. **Check bag frequently to see whether child has voided.**	Applying a diaper over the bag prevents child from removing bag. Frequent checking is necessary to ensure as fresh a specimen as possible. Since the urine is not a midstream catch and the bag comes in contact with the child's skin, a small amount of contaminants may be present. To prevent these contaminants from skewing the laboratory test, the specimen must be refrigerated or sent to the laboratory as soon as possible. Some specimen bags have a divider to prevent urine from flowing back over the child's skin.
12. As soon as enough urine is in collection bag, perform hand hygiene and don gloves. Gently remove bag by pushing skin away from bag. Using sterile scissors, cut corner of bag and pour urine into sterile container.	Pushing skin away from bag reduces skin trauma. Sterile scissors must be used to prevent the contact with any other pathogens. Do not pour urine out of application hole because this area has been grossly contaminated with epithelial cells.

continues

SKILL 12-8 Collecting a Urine Specimen for Culture (continued)

ACTION	RATIONALE
13. Perform perineal care and reapply diaper.	Cleansing the area will remove any adhesive remaining from collection bag.
14. Follow Actions 3 through 6 in the adult section of the procedure.	

For the Patient with an Indwelling Urinary Catheter:

ACTION	RATIONALE
15. Explain procedure to patient. Organize equipment at bedside.	This provides reassurance and promotes patient cooperation. Organization improves efficiency.
16. Perform hand hygiene and don disposable gloves.	Hand hygiene deters the spread of microorganisms. Gloves protect nurse from any microorganisms in urine.
17. Clamp or kink off drainage tubing near urinary catheter distal to the port. Remove lid from specimen container, keeping the inside of the container and lid free from contamination.	The drainage tubing can be clamped with the plastic clamp provided on tubing. This ensures the collection of an adequate amount of fresh urine. The container needs to remain sterile so as not to contaminate the urine.
18. **Cleanse aspiration port with alcohol wipe and allow port to air dry.**	Cleaning with alcohol deters entry of microorganisms when the needle punctures the port.
19. Insert the blunt-tipped needle into the port. Slowly aspirate enough urine for specimen (usually 5 mL is adequate). Remove blunt-tipped needle from port.	Using a blunt-tipped needle prevents a needlestick. Collecting urine from the port ensures that the specimen will contain fresh urine.

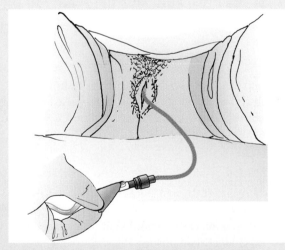

Action 18: Cleaning port on catheter with alcohol wipe.

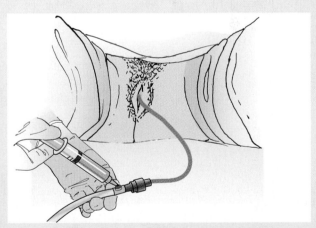

Action 19: Inserting blunt-tipped needle attached to 5-cc syringe into port on catheter.

ACTION	RATIONALE
20. Slowly inject urine into specimen container. Replace lid on container. Dispose of needle and syringe appropriately.	If the urine is injected quickly into the container, it may splash out of the container or into the nurse's eyes.
21. Perform Actions 3 through 6 in the adult section of this procedure.	

continues

Collecting a Urine Specimen for Culture (continued)

EVALUATION

The expected outcome is met when a clean urine specimen is collected and sent to the laboratory. Other outcomes may include the following: the patient demonstrated the proper technique for specimen collection and stated that anxiety is lessened.

Unexpected Situations and Associated Interventions

- *Patient cannot provide a large enough urine sample:* Offer patient fluids to drink, although drinking too much fluid may dilute the urine, invalidating the test. Patient may return later in day to supply sample. Offer patient assistance with the next void.
- *When checking urine collection bag on an infant, nurse notes that bag has fallen off and the child has voided into the diaper:* Remove the bag, perform perineal care, and apply a new collection bag.
- *The patient missed voiding into the specimen container but did void into the specimen hat:* Do not use this urine as a sample for a culture; it could be heavily contaminated with bacteria and give a misleading result. Attempt to collect urine with next void. Offer patient assistance when trying to collect sample.

Special Considerations

- For many urine tests, such as a urinalysis, drug testing, or diabetes testing, the specimen does not need to be sterile and does not need to be collected as a midstream specimen. However, in the case of urinalysis, if the specimen shows nitrates and white blood cells, a culture of a urine specimen may be ordered.
- Since the first voiding of the day contains the highest bacterial counts, collect this sample whenever possible.

Caring for a Suprapubic Catheter

A suprapubic catheter is inserted surgically into the bladder and is used to divert urine from the urethra when injury, stricture, prostatic obstruction, or surgery has compromised the flow of urine through the urethra. A suprapubic catheter places the patient at a lesser risk for injury than does use of a long-term indwelling urinary catheter.

Equipment

- Washcloth
- Gentle soap
- Disposable gloves
- Tape
- Drainage sponge (if necessary)

ASSESSMENT

Assess the current suprapubic catheter and bag, looking at the condition of the catheter and the drainage bag connected to catheter and the product style. Inspect the site around the suprapubic catheter, looking for drainage, erythema, or excoriation. Assess patient's knowledge of caring for a suprapubic catheter.

NURSING DIAGNOSIS

Determine the related factors for the nursing diagnoses based on the patient's current status. Possible nursing diagnoses may include:

- Altered Urinary Elimination
- Risk for Impaired Skin Integrity
- Deficient Knowledge

OUTCOME IDENTIFICATION AND PLANNING

The expected outcomes to be achieved when caring for a suprapubic catheter are that the patient eliminates adequate amounts of urine and the skin around the catheter remains free of redness, irritation, and excoriation. In addition, the patient demonstrates the ability to provide care to the suprapubic catheter site and to state observations about the site.

continues

SKILL 12-9

Caring for a Suprapubic Catheter (continued)

IMPLEMENTATION

ACTION	RATIONALE

1. Explain procedure and encourage patient to observe or participate if possible. Provide privacy.

Explanation helps to reduce anxiety. Observing or assisting with procedure encourages self-acceptance.

2. Assemble equipment.

Organization facilitates performance of task.

3. Perform hand hygiene and don disposable gloves.

Hand hygiene deters the spread of microorganisms. Gloves protect nurse from blood, body fluid, and microorganisms.

4. Wet washcloth and soap with warm water. Gently cleanse around suprapubic exit site. Remove any encrustations. If this is a new suprapubic catheter, use cotton-tipped applicators and sterile saline for cleaning until incision has healed.

Using a gentle soap helps to protect the skin. The exit site is the most common area of skin irritation with a suprapubic catheter. If encrustations are left on the skin, they provide a medium for bacteria and an area of skin irritation.

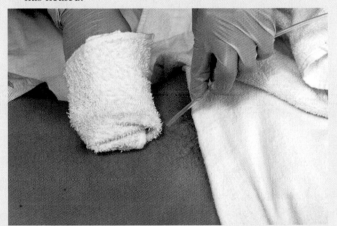

Action 4: Cleaning area around catheter site with soap and water.

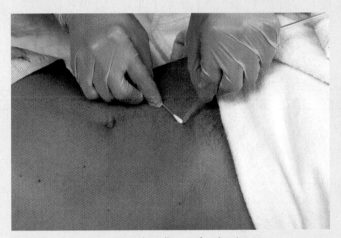

Action 4: Using cotton-tipped applicators for cleaning.

5. Rinse area of all soap. Pat dry.

If left on the skin, soap can cause irritation. The skin needs to be kept dry to prevent any irritation.

6. If exit site has been draining, place small drain sponge around catheter to absorb any drainage. Be prepared to change this sponge throughout the day, depending on the amount of drainage. Do not cut a 4×4 to make a drain sponge.

A small amount of drainage from the exit site is normal. The sponge needs to be changed when it becomes saturated to prevent skin irritation and breakdown. The fibers from the cut 4×4 may enter the exit site and cause irritation or infection.

7. Form a loop in tubing and place tape on abdomen.

The tape absorbs any tugging, instead of the skin or bladder.

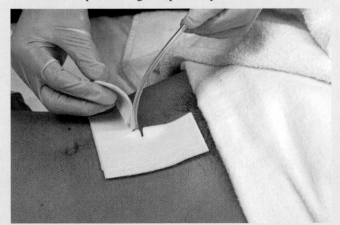

Action 6: Applying small drain sponge around catheter.

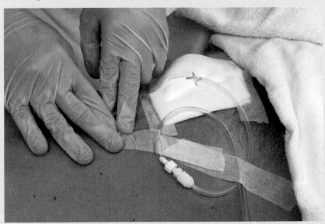

Action 7: Forming a loop in tubing and taping to abdomen.

continues

ACTION	RATIONALE
8. Remove or discard equipment and assess patient's response to procedure. Remove gloves and perform hand hygiene.	The patient's response may indicate acceptance of the catheter or the need for health teaching. Hand hygiene deters the spread of microorganisms.
9. Record appearance of catheter exit site and surrounding skin, urine amount and characteristics, as well as patient's reaction to procedure.	A careful record is important for planning the patient's care.

7/12/06   1845   *Suprapubic catheter care performed. Patient assisted in care. Skin is slightly erythematous on R side where catheter was taped. Catheter taped to L side. Small amount of yellow, clear drainage noted on drain sponge. Patient would like to try to go without drain sponge at this time. Instructions given to call nurse if amount of drainage increases. Moderate amount of clear yellow urine continues to drain from catheter into collection bag. —A. Blitz, RN*

Action 9: Documentation.

EVALUATION

The expected outcome is met when the site remains clean and dry without redness, irritation, or excoriation as the suprapubic catheter drains urine. Other outcomes may include the following: the patient demonstrates ability to participate in suprapubic site care and can verbalize important observations related to the site.

Unexpected Situations and Associated Interventions

- *When cleaning site, catheter becomes dislodged and pulls out:* Notify physician. If this is a well-healed site, a new catheter can be easily placed. If this is a new suprapubic, the physician may want to assess for any trauma to the bladder wall.
- *Exit site is extremely excoriated:* Consult wound, ostomy, and incontinence nurse for evaluation. A skin protectant or barrier may need to be applied, as well as more frequent cleansing of the area and changing of the drain sponge (if applied).

Special Considerations

- If suprapubic is not draining into bag but instead has a valve at the end of the catheter, open the valve at least every 6 hours (or more frequently depending on institutional policy) to drain.

Caring for a Peritoneal Dialysis Catheter

Peritoneal dialysis is a method of removing fluid and wastes from the body of a patient with kidney failure. A catheter inserted into the peritoneal space allows a special fluid (dialysate) to be infused and then drained from the body. The site of insertion is a potential site for infection, so meticulous care is needed.

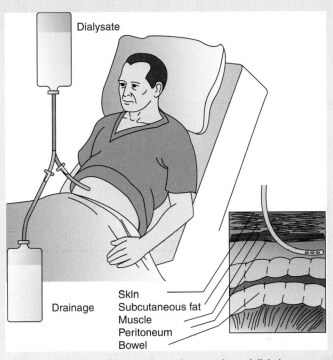

Dialysate

Drainage

Skin
Subcutaneous fat
Muscle
Peritoneum
Bowel

In peritoneal dialysis and in acute intermittent peritoneal dialysis, dialysate is infused into the peritoneal cavity by gravity, after which the clamp on the infusion line is closed. After a dwell time (when the dialysate is in the peritoneal cavity), the drainage tube is unclamped and the fluid drains from the peritoneal cavity, again by gravity. A new container of dialysate is infused as soon as drainage is complete. The duration of the dwell time depends on the type of peritoneal dialysis.

Equipment

- Face masks (two)
- Sterile gloves
- Nonsterile gloves
- Hydrogen peroxide
- Sterile 4×4 gauze (three)
- Sterile basin
- Povidone–iodine swabs
- Sterile drain sponge

ASSESSMENT

Inspect peritoneal dialysis catheter exit site for any erythema, drainage, tenderness, swelling, skin irritation or breakdown, or leakage. Assess abdomen for any tenderness by palpating (checking for signs of peritonitis). Assess patient's knowledge about measures to care for exit site.

NURSING DIAGNOSIS

Determine the related factors for the nursing diagnoses based on the patient's current status. Possible nursing diagnoses may include:

- Risk for Impaired Skin Integrity
- Altered Urinary Elimination
- Deficient Knowledge
- Excess Fluid Volume
- Deficient Fluid Volume

continues

SKILL 12-10   Caring for a Peritoneal Dialysis Catheter (continued)

OUTCOME IDENTIFICATION AND PLANNING

The expected outcomes to achieve when performing care for a peritoneal dialysis catheter are as follows: the peritoneal dialysis catheter dressing change is completed using aseptic technique without trauma to the site or patient; the site is clean, dry, and intact without evidence of inflammation or infection; and the patient exhibits fluid balance and participates in care as appropriate.

IMPLEMENTATION

ACTION	RATIONALE
1. Explain procedure to patient. Close curtain or door.	Explanation provides reassurance and promotes patient cooperation. Closing curtain or door provides privacy.
2. Gather equipment. Perform hand hygiene and don nonsterile gloves.	This provides for an organized approach to the task. Hand hygiene deters the spread of microorganisms. Gloves protect nurse from microorganisms.
3. Assist patient to supine position. Expose abdomen.	The supine position is usually the best way to gain access to the peritoneal dialysis catheter.
4. Don face mask; have patient put on face mask.	The face masks deter the spread of microorganisms.
5. Gently remove old dressing, noting odor, amount and color of drainage, leakage, and condition of skin around catheter.	Drainage, leakage, and skin condition can indicate problems with the catheter, such as infection.
6. Remove nonsterile gloves. Set up sterile field. Open packages. Place two sterile 4×4s in basin with hydrogen peroxide. Leave one sterile 4×4 opened on sterile field. Don sterile gloves.	Until catheter site has healed, site should be dressed using aseptic technique.
7. Gently palpate area surrounding exit site with gauze soaked in hydrogen peroxide.	By gently palpating, the nurse may discover any abdominal tenderness or more drainage, which may indicate an infection.
8. Pick up catheter with nondominant hand. **With the hydrogen peroxide-soaked gauze, cleanse around the skin around the exit site using a circular motion, starting at the exit site and then slowly going outward 3″ to 4″.**	The hydrogen peroxide can help to cleanse the skin and remove any drainage or crust from the wound.
9. Continue to hold catheter with nondominant hand. After skin has dried, apply povidone–iodine to catheter, **beginning at exit site, going around catheter, and then moving up to end of catheter.**	Povidone–iodine offers long-acting protection from microorganisms.
10. Place drain sponge around exit site. Then place a 4×4 over exit site. Secure edges of gauze pad with tape. Some institutions recommend placing a transparent dressing over the gauze pads instead of tape.	The drain sponge and 4×4 are used to absorb any drainage from the exit site.
11. Remove sterile gloves and perform hand hygiene.	This deters the spread of microorganisms.
12. Document dressing change, including condition of skin surrounding exit site, drainage, or odor, as well as patient's reaction to procedure.	A careful record is important for planning the patient's care.

7/22/06   1530   Peritoneal dialysis catheter dressing changed; skin surrounding catheter slightly erythematous but remains intact. Small amount of clear drainage without odor noted on drain sponge. Pt asking appropriate questions regarding dressing change.
—A. Blitz, RN

Action 12: Documentation.

continues

SKILL 12-10   **Caring for a Peritoneal Dialysis Catheter** (continued)

EVALUATION	The expected outcome is met when the peritoneal dialysis catheter dressing change is completed using aseptic technique without trauma to the site or patient; the site is clean, dry, and intact, without evidence of redness, irritation, or excoriation; the patient's fluid balance is maintained; and the patient verbalizes appropriate measures to care for the site.

Unexpected Situations and Associated Interventions	• *Patient complains of pain when nurse palpates abdomen, purulent or cloudy drainage is present, or foul odor is noted when old dressing is removed:* Notify physician immediately. Any of these signs could indicate a site infection or peritonitis. • *Nurse notes that old dressing is saturated with clear fluid:* Replace dressing to prevent skin breakdown. Notify physician. A frequent complication is leaking from exit site. Frequently check dressing, especially after patient has had solution placed in the abdominal cavity.
Special Considerations	• Once site is healed, some physicians do not require patients to wear a dressing unless the site is leaking. The patient may shower with the catheter but needs to cleanse the area around the exit site after showering.

SKILL 12-11   **Caring for a Hemodialysis Access (Arteriovenous Fistula or Graft)**

Hemodialysis, a method of removing fluid and wastes from the body, requires the creation of a fistula or graft. The fistula or graft requires care by specialized personnel. Accessing a hemodialysis arteriovenous graft or fistula should be done only by specially trained healthcare team members. The following information should be taught to the patient to ensure that he or she cares for the site at home.

Equipment	• Stethoscope
ASSESSMENT	Ask the patient how much he or she knows about caring for the site. Ask the patient to describe important observations to be made.
NURSING DIAGNOSIS	Determine the related factors for the nursing diagnoses based on the patient's current status. The primary nursing diagnosis is Deficient Knowledge. Another nursing diagnosis may be Risk for Injury.
OUTCOME IDENTIFICATION AND PLANNING	The expected outcomes to achieve when caring for a hemodialysis catheter are that the patient verbalizes appropriate care measures and observations to be made and the graft or fistula remains patent.

IMPLEMENTATION

ACTION	RATIONALE
1. Inspect area over access site for any redness, warmth, tenderness, or blemishes. **Palpate over access site, feeling for a thrill or vibration. Auscultate over access site with bell of stethoscope, listening for a bruit or vibration.**	Inspection, palpation, and auscultation aid in determining the patency of the hemodialysis access.

continues

ACTION	RATIONALE

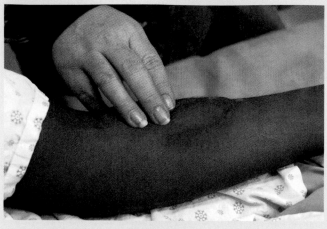

Action 1: Palpate access site for thrill.

ACTION	RATIONALE
2. Ensure that a sign is placed over head of bed informing the healthcare team which arm is affected. Do not perform a venipuncture or start an IV on the access arm.	The affected arm should not be used for any other procedures such as obtaining blood pressure, which could lead to clotting of the graft or fistula. Venipuncture or IV access could lead to an infection of the affected arm and could cause the loss of the graft or fistula.
3. Instruct patient not to sleep with access arm under head or body.	This could lead to clotting of the fistula or graft.
4. Instruct patient not to lift heavy objects with or put pressure on the access arm. The patient should not carry heavy bags (including purses) on the shoulder of the access arm.	This could lead to clotting of the fistula or graft.
5. Document assessment findings and any patient education performed.	A careful record is important for planning the patient's care.

EVALUATION   The expected outcome is met when the access site has an audible bruit and a palpable thrill; the site is without erythema, warmth, skin blemishes, or pain; and the patient verbalizes appropriate information about caring for the access site and observations to report.

Unexpected Situations and Associated Interventions

- *Thrill is not palpable or bruit is not audible:* Notify the physician at once. The thrill and bruit are caused by arterial blood flowing into the vein. If these signs are not present, the access may be clotting off.
- *Site is warm to touch, erythematous, or painful or has a skin blemish:* Notify the physician. These signs can indicate a site infection.

■ Developing Critical Thinking Skills

1. When checking Ralph Bellow's condom catheter, the nurse notices that although the catheter is still in place, Mr. Bellow's bed is soaked with urine and there is very little urine in the catheter tubing. What should the nurse do?
2. Grace Halligan is asking to go to the bathroom; she says, "I don't think I can go on a bedpan." The nurse rechecks the physician's orders and notices that Grace is on strict bed rest. How can the nurse help alleviate Grace's concerns about using a bedpan?
3. Mike Wimmer notices that his peritoneal dialysis catheter insertion site is reddened and tender. He phones the nurse to ask what should be done. What should the nurse tell Mike?

Bibliography

American Nephrology Nurses' Association, East Holly Avenue/Box 56, Pitman, NJ, 08071-0056; (856) 256-2320; *http://www.anna.org*

Blazys, D. (1999). Clinical nurses' forum: Urinary catheterization. *Journal of Emergency Nursing, 25*(4), 300–301.

Burns, C., Brady, M., Dunn, A., et al. (2000). *Pediatric primary care: a handbook for nurse practitioners* (2nd ed.). Philadelphia: W. B. Saunders.

Casteel, L., Clodfelter, J., Russell, C., et al. (1998). Maintaining healthy peritoneal dialysis catheter access. *Dialysis & Transplantation, 27*(1), 22–24.

Hanchett, M. (2002). Techniques for stabilizing urinary catheters: Tape may be the oldest method, but it's not the only one. *American Journal of Nursing, 102*(3), 44–48.

McConnell, E. (2001). Applying a condom catheter. *Nursing, 31*(1), 70.

McConnell, E. (2002). Protecting a hemodialysis fistula. *Nursing, 32*(11), 18.

National Kidney and Urologic Diseases Information Clearinghouse, 3 Information Way, Bethesda, MD, 2092-3580; (301) 907-8906; *http://kidney.niddk.nigh.gov*

Phipps, W., Sands, J., & Marek, J. (2003). *Medical-surgical nursing: concepts & clinical practice* (7th ed.). St. Louis: C. V. Mosby.

Sienty, M., & Dawson, N. (1999). Preventing urosepsis from indwelling urinary catheters. *American Journal of Nursing, 99*(1), 24C–24H.

Slugg, A. (2000). A scanner can help restore continence in LTC patients. *RN, 63*(2), 16.

Smeltzer, S., & Bare, B. (2004). *Brunner & Suddarth's textbook of medical surgical nursing* (10th ed.). Philadelphia: Lippincott Williams & Wilkins.

Smith, D. (1999). Gauging bladder volume. *Nursing, 29*(12), 52–53.

Bowel Elimination

Focusing on Patient Care

This chapter will help you develop some of the skills related to bowel elimination necessary to care for the following patients:

Hugh Levens is a 64-year-old man who has been placed on a bowel program after a fall left him paralyzed from the waist down.

Isaac Greenberg, age 4, has been diagnosed with a viral gastroenteritis. The physician has ordered that all of his stools be tested for occult blood.

Maria Blakely, age 26, has recently received an ileostomy. She is having problems with her appliances and is concerned about excoriation.

Learning Outcomes

After studying this chapter, the reader should be able to:

1. Test stool for occult blood
2. Insert a rectal tube
3. Administer a cleansing enema
4. Administer a retention enema
5. Administer a return-flow enema
6. Remove stool digitally
7. Apply a fecal incontinence pouch
8. Change and empty an ostomy bag
9. Irrigate a colostomy
10. Collect a stool specimen

Key Terms

colostomy: artificial opening that permits feces from the colon to exit through the stoma

constipation: passage of dry, hard stools

defecation: emptying of the large intestine; also called a bowel movement

diarrhea: passage of excessively liquid, nonformed stool

enema: introduction of a solution into the large intestine

fecal impaction: prolonged retention or an accumulation of fecal material that forms a hardened mass in the rectum

flatus: intestinal gas

hemorrhoids: abnormally distended veins in the anal area

ileostomy: artificial opening created to allow liquid fecal content from the ileum to be eliminated through the stoma

occult blood: blood that is hidden in the stool

ostomy: general term that refers to an artificial opening; usually used to refer to an opening created for the excretion of body wastes

stoma: opening created by bringing the intestinal mucosa out to the abdominal wall and suturing it to the skin

continues

Key Terms (continued)

suppository: a conical or oval solid substance shaped for easy insertion into a body cavity and designed to melt at body temperature

vagal stimulus or response: stimulation of the vagus nerve that causes an increase in parasympathetic stimulation, triggering a decrease in heart rate

Valsalva maneuver: voluntary contraction of the abdominal wall muscles, fixing of the diaphragm, and closing of the glottis that increases intra-abdominal pressure and aids in expelling feces

Elimination of the waste products of digestion is a natural process critical for human functioning. Patients differ widely in their expectations about bowel elimination, their usual pattern of defecation, and the ease with which they speak about bowel elimination or bowel problems. Although most people have experienced minor acute bouts of diarrhea or constipation, some patients experience severe or chronic bowel elimination problems affecting their fluid and electrolyte balance, hydration, nutritional status, skin integrity, comfort, and self-concept. Because many patients experience illnesses that affect bowel elimination or are undergoing diagnostic testing and pharmacologic or surgical treatments that affect bowel functioning, nurses play an integral role in the prevention, careful assessment, management, and correction of potential complications arising from altered bowel elimination.

This chapter will cover skills to assist the nurse in promoting and assisting with bowel elimination. Please look over the summary boxes at the beginning of this chapter for a quick review of critical knowledge to assist you in understanding the skills related to bowel elimination.

BOX 13-1 Anatomy of the Gastrointestinal Tract

- The GI tract begins with the mouth and continues to the esophagus, the stomach, the small intestine, and the large intestine. It ends at the anus.
- From the mouth to the anus, the GI tract is approximately 9 m (30 feet) long.
- The small intestine consists of the duodenum, jejunum, and ileum.

- The large intestine consists of the cecum, colon (ascending, transverse, descending, and sigmoid), and rectum.
- Accessory organs of the GI tract include the teeth, salivary glands, gallbladder, liver, and pancreas.

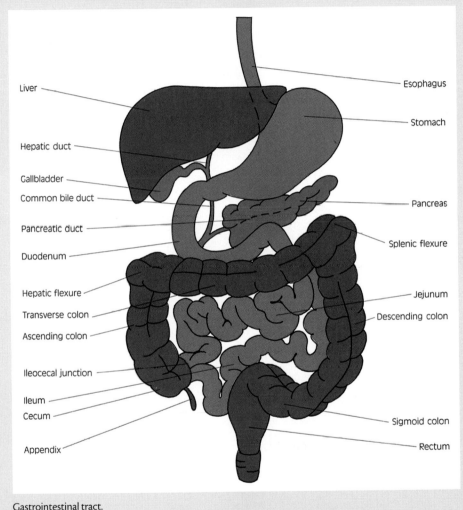

Gastrointestinal tract.

BOX 13-2 Assessment Techniques for the Abdomen

- Place patient in a supine position with knees slightly flexed.
- When assessing an infant or toddler, you may want to place the child on the parent's lap to prevent the child from becoming upset and crying.
- Perform the abdominal assessment in the following sequence: inspection, auscultation, percussion, palpation.
  - Inspection: Observe contour of abdomen; note any changes in skin or evidence of scars; inspect for any masses, bulges, or areas of distention.
  - Auscultation: Listen, using an orderly clockwise approach, in all abdominal quadrants with the diaphragm of the stethoscope; listen for bowel sounds (high-pitched, gurgling, and soft); note the frequency of bowel sounds (should be 5 to 34 sounds per minute).
  - Percussion: Percuss, using an orderly clockwise approach in all abdominal quadrants; expect to hear tympany over most regions.
  - Palpation: Lightly palpate over abdominal quadrants, first checking for any areas of pain or discomfort. Proceed to deep palpation, noting any muscular resistance, tenderness, enlargement of organs, or masses.

BOX 13-3 Factors That Affect Bowel Elimination

- Mobility: Movement and exercise help to move stool through the bowel.
- Diet: Foods high in fiber help keep stool moving through the intestines. High fluid intake keeps stools from becoming dry and hard. Fluid also helps fiber to keep stool soft and bulky.
- Medications: Antibiotics and laxatives may cause stool to become loose and more frequent. Diuretics may lead to dry, hard, and less frequent stools.
- Intestinal diversions: Ileostomies normally have liquid, foul-smelling stool. Sigmoid colostomies normally have pasty, formed stool.

SKILL 13-1   Testing Stool for Occult Blood

Occult blood in the stool refers to blood that is hidden in the specimen or that cannot be seen on gross examination. Certain conditions, such as ulcer disease, inflammatory bowel disorders, and colon cancer, place the patient at risk for intestinal bleeding. Testing for occult blood uses a simple reagent substance to detect the presence of the enzyme peroxidase in the hemoglobin molecule.

Equipment

- Disposable gloves
- Washcloth, soap, and towel
- Wooden applicator
- Hemoccult testing card and developer
- Water-soluble lubricant (for digital rectal examination)

ASSESSMENT

Assess patient for any blood in perineal area, including hemorrhoids, menstruation, urinary tract infection, or vaginal or rectal tears. Blood may be from a source other than the gastrointestinal tract. Investigate the patient's diet: a diet high in rare meat, liver, melon, broccoli, cauliflower, radishes, or turnips may produce false-positive results on Hemoccult testing, and a diet high in vitamin C can cause false-negative results.

NURSING DIAGNOSIS

Determine the related factors for the nursing diagnoses based on the patient's current status. Several nursing diagnoses may be appropriate, including:

- Deficient Knowledge
- Constipation
- Diarrhea
- Bowel Incontinence
- Anxiety
- Pain

OUTCOME IDENTIFICATION AND PLANNING

The expected outcome to achieve when testing a patient's stool for occult blood is that a stool sample will be obtained and the patient will demonstrate ability to test stool (if indicated), with the stool testing negative for occult blood. Other outcomes may include the following: the patient verbalizes a decrease in anxiety related to the testing and the patient tolerates testing without a large amount of discomfort or embarrassment.

IMPLEMENTATION

ACTION	RATIONALE
1. Discuss with patient the need for a stool sample. Explain to patient the process by which the stool will be collected, either from a bowel movement or from a digital rectal examination. If specimen is from a bowel movement, instruct patient not to urinate or discard toilet paper with the stool, which may contaminate the specimen. Gather necessary equipment. If stool sample	Discussion and explanation help to allay some of the patient's anxiety and prepare the patient for what to expect. Organization facilitates performance of tasks.

continues

Testing Stool for Occult Blood (continued)

ACTION

is to be obtained from digital rectal examination, proceed to Action 2. If stool sample is to be collected from a bowel movement, proceed to Action 9.

2. If digital rectal examination is to be performed, perform hand hygiene and put on nonsterile gloves.

3. If patient is able to stand, instruct patient to bend over examination table or bed placed at a comfortable height. If patient is bedridden, place in Sims or side-lying position.

4. **Generously lubricate 1" to 1.5" of finger with water-soluble lubricant to be inserted into anus to collect stool sample.**

5. Ask patient to take a large, deep breath through the nose and exhale through the mouth.

6. After separating buttocks with nondominant hand, gently insert lubricated finger of dominant hand 1" to 2" into rectum while lightly palpating for any stool.

7. Remove finger. Apply stool to one window of Hemoccult testing card.

8. **Apply stool to second window of Hemoccult testing card from different place on glove than first sample.** Skip to Actions 12 through 16.

9. If patient is to defecate for the stool sample, assist patient to bathroom or bedside commode or place on bedpan. **Instruct patient not to void or discard toilet paper into stool collection container.**

10. Perform hand hygiene and put on disposable gloves.

11. **With wooden applicator, apply a small amount of stool onto one window of Hemoccult testing card. With opposite end of wooden applicator, obtain another sample of stool from another area and apply a small amount of stool onto second window of Hemoccult card.**

RATIONALE

Hand hygiene deters the spread of microorganisms. Gloves protect nurse from microorganisms in the feces.

By positioning the patient in a comfortable position, it may be easier for the patient to relax while the sample is being obtained.

Lubrication facilitates passage of the finger through the anal sphincter and prevents injury to the mucosa.

The patient will concentrate on following directions, and this may help patient to relax anal sphincter.

Insertion into the rectum provides a sample for testing.

Stool must be applied to the card so that it can be tested.

Two separate areas of the same stool sample are tested in case there is trace blood from a hemorrhoid or fissure.

Contaminants such as toilet paper or urine may void testing.

Hand hygiene deters the spread of microorganisms. Gloves protect nurse from microorganisms in feces.

Two separate areas of the same stool sample are tested in case there is trace blood from a hemorrhoid or fissure. By using opposite ends of the wooden applicator, cross-contamination is avoided.

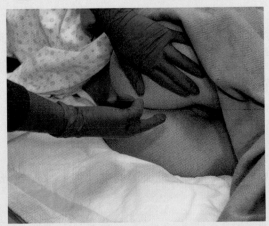

Action 6: Separating buttocks with nondominant hand and getting ready to insert lubricated finger into rectum.

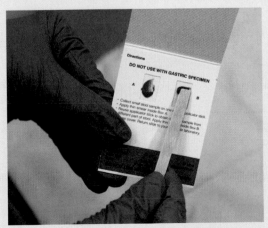

Action 11: Using wooden applicator to transfer stool specimen to window of testing card.

continues

SKILL 13-1 Testing Stool for Occult Blood (continued)

ACTION	RATIONALE
12. Close flap over stool samples.	Closing the flap prevents contamination of the samples.
13. Open flap on opposite side of card and **place two drops of developer over each window and wait the time stated in the manufacturer's instructions.**	The developer will react with any blood in the stool. Following the manufacturer's instructions promotes accuracy of results.
14. Observe card for any blue areas.	Any blue coloring on the card indicates a test positive for blood.
15. Discard Hemoccult testing slide. Remove disposable gloves from inside out and discard. Perform hand hygiene.	Proper removal of gloves and hand hygiene reduce the risk of transmission of microorganisms.

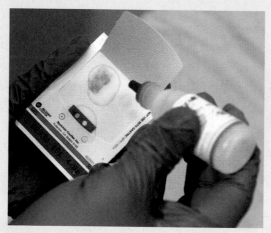

Action 13: Applying developer to card windows.

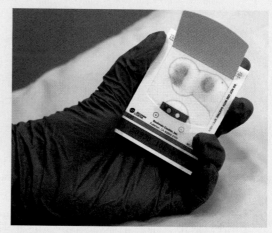

Action 14: Observing windows on card for blue areas.

16. Document testing results.	Documentation provides a means of communicating the results.

07/12/06   1040   Stool tested for occult blood.
Result (+). Physician notified.—K. Sanders, RN.

Action 16: Documentation.

EVALUATION

The expected outcome is met when the stool tests negative for occult blood and the patient tolerates testing without a large amount of discomfort or embarrassment. If the patient is to obtain the stool sample on his or her own, another outcome is met when the patient is able to collect the stool and place it correctly on the card.

Unexpected Situations and Associated Interventions

- *Stool is positive for occult blood:* If stool is positive for occult blood, the results should be documented and the primary care provider notified.
- *One window tests positive, while the second window tests negative:* This could indicate that the blood is from a source other than the gastrointestinal tract. These results should be documented and the primary care provider notified.

Inserting a Rectal Tube

Gases can build up in the stomach or intestine, causing flatulence. Moving about in bed or ambulating can help to promote peristalsis and the escape of gas. However, when these measures are ineffective, the physician may order a rectal tube to be inserted. The tube helps to stimulate peristalsis and provides a passageway for gas to escape.

Equipment

- Disposable gloves
- Washcloth, soap, and towel
- Rectal tube (size 22 to 34 French for adults, 12 to 18 French for children)
- Water-soluble lubricant
- Disposable waterproof pad
- Tape
- Urinal (optional)

ASSESSMENT

Assess the rectal area for any fissures, hemorrhoids, sores, or rectal tears. If any of these are noted, added care should be taken while inserting tube. Assess the results of the patient's laboratory work, specifically the platelet count and white blood cell (WBC) count. A normal platelet count is 150,000 to 400,000/mm^3. A platelet count of less than 20,000 may seriously compromise the patient's ability to clot blood. A rectal catheter may irritate the gastrointestinal mucosa, causing bleeding or bowel perforation. A low WBC count places the patient at risk for infection, such as rectal abscess. Therefore, any unnecessary procedures that would place the patient at risk for bleeding or infection should not be performed. Measure the patient's abdominal girth with a tape measure at the umbilicus before inserting the tube. This measurement provides a baseline upon which to evaluate the effectiveness of the tube insertion. Measure again after the rectal tube has been removed, noting any decrease in abdominal girth.

Percuss and palpate the abdomen. Normal abdominal percussion will elicit tympany (a resonant sound). With excessive flatus, hyperresonance typically is noted. A dull sound may be elicited due to fluid or a mass. The abdomen should be soft and nontender. With increased flatulence or diarrhea, the abdomen may be firm, distended, or painful to deep and light palpation. Have the patient rate his or her level of pain before the rectal tube is inserted, and then compare this rating after the rectal tube is removed.

Assess pulse before and during rectal tube insertion. The rectal tube may stimulate a vagal response, which increases parasympathetic stimulation, causing a decrease in heart rate.

NURSING DIAGNOSIS

Determine the related factors for the nursing diagnoses based on the patient's current status. A common nursing diagnosis is Acute Pain. Another nursing diagnosis may be Risk for Injury.

OUTCOME IDENTIFICATION AND PLANNING

The expected outcome to achieve when inserting a rectal tube is that the patient will verbalize a decrease in the level of pain experienced due to passage of flatus. Flatus will be expelled from rectum and the patient's abdominal girth will decrease. The patient remains free of any signs and symptoms of injury to the intestinal mucosa and rectum.

IMPLEMENTATION

ACTION	RATIONALE
1. Explain to patient technique for insertion of rectal tube and rationale for insertion. Gather equipment.	Explanation helps to decrease anxiety and promote cooperation. Organization facilitates performance of tasks.
2. Perform hand hygiene and put on nonsterile gloves.	Hand hygiene deters the spread of microorganisms. Gloves protect nurse from microorganisms in feces.
3. Place patient in side-lying position. Drape patient properly to provide privacy and warmth.	The patient's comfort and warmth will help him or her relax.
4. **Lubricate approximately 4″ (10 cm) of the rectal tube with water-soluble lubricant (see following page).**	Lubrication reduces irritation to mucous membranes on insertion.

continues

SKILL 13-2 Inserting a Rectal Tube (continued)

ACTION

RATIONALE

5. Separate buttocks so that anus is visible. Have patient take a slow, deep breath, inhaling through nose and exhaling through mouth. **Gently insert the rectal tube beyond the anal canal into the rectum approximately 4″ (10 cm) for an adult.** Use a shorter distance for a child, depending on the patient's size.

To remove flatus and to help stimulate peristalsis, the tube must be inserted into the rectum. The patient will concentrate on following directions, and this may help the patient to relax the anal sphincter.

6. Secure waterproof pad to end of rectal tube, or place end of rectal tube into urinal.

This will prevent any stool from leaking onto patient or bedding.

7. **Leave rectal tube in place for no longer than 20 minutes.** Tube may be taped in place.

The tube will no longer act as a stimulant for peristalsis and may cause intestinal mucosal trauma if left in place longer.

8. **Monitor patient for any change in heart rate while tube is in place.**

The rectal tube may stimulate a vagal response, which increases parasympathetic stimulation, causing a decrease in heart rate. If a decrease in heart rate is noted, the rectal tube may need to be removed.

9. If patient is able, have him or her assume the prone or knee-chest position.

Gas is lighter than fluids and solids and thus will rise.

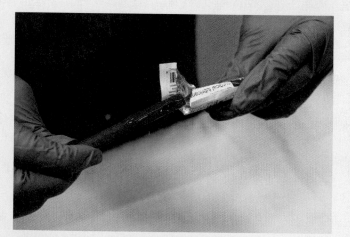

Action 4: Lubricating rectal tube.

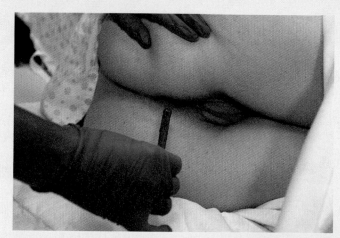

Action 5: Separating the patient's buttocks, getting ready to insert rectal tube.

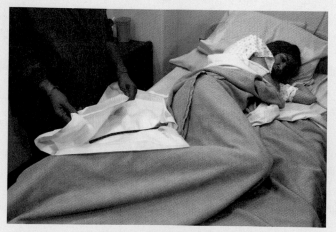

Action 6: Securing waterproof pad to end of rectal tube already inserted.

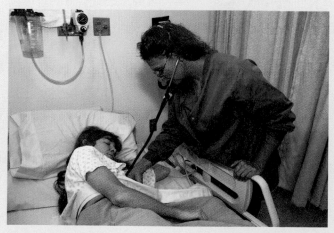

Action 8: Assessing patient's apical heart rate with stethoscope.

continues

Inserting a Rectal Tube (continued)

ACTION

RATIONALE

10. Replace nonsterile gloves if they have been removed.

Gloves protect nurse from microorganisms in feces.

11. Have patient take a slow, deep breath, inhaling through nose and exhaling through mouth, while removing rectal tube.

The patient will concentrate on following directions, and this may help patient to relax anal sphincter.

12. Wrap contaminated end of rectal tube in paper towel and discard.

Wrapping the end contains any feces that may be on the tip.

13. Clean perineal area.

Cleaning promotes comfort and helps to maintain skin integrity.

14. Remove disposable gloves from inside out and discard. Perform hand hygiene.

Proper glove removal keeps contaminated portion contained within the glove; hand hygiene deters the spread of micro-organisms.

15. Reassess abdomen (girth measurement, percussion, palpation).

If any flatus or stool was removed, changes from baseline may be noted.

16. Document size of rectal tube used; length of time tube was left in place; color, amount, and consistency of any stool removed; any changes noted in abdominal girth, abdominal assessment, or complaints of pain; patient's positions during procedure; and patient's reaction to procedure.

Documentation promotes continuity of care and communication.

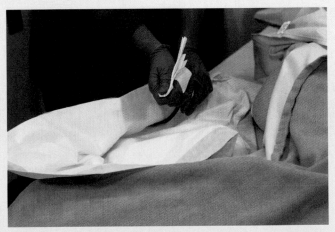

Action 12: Nurse wrapping contaminated rectal tube in paper towel to discard.

07/10/06 1145   Patient placed into side-lying Sims position. Rectal tube 22 Fr. inserted and left in place for 15 minutes. Small amount of brown, soft stool removed. Patient's abdominal girth 42 cm prior to rectal tube; abdominal girth 40.5 cm after removal of tube. Abdomen remains slightly distended but is softer to palpation. Denies any pain. Patient tolerated procedure without incident.
—K. Sanders, RN

Action 16: Documentation.

EVALUATION

The expected outcome is met when flatus is expelled from rectum, patient demonstrates a decrease in abdominal girth measurement, and patient states that pain is significantly decreased. Patient exhibits no signs and symptoms of injury to the intestinal mucosa and rectum.

Unexpected Situations and Associated Interventions

- *Abdominal girth has not changed and patient is still uncomfortable:* The rectal tube may be used intermittently every 2 to 3 hours, as ordered. Through repeated use, peristalsis may increase; however, irritation to gastrointestinal mucosa also increases with repeated use. Use caution to prevent irritation when using tube repeatedly.

SKILL 13-3   Administering a Cleansing Enema

Cleansing enemas are given to remove feces from the colon. They are classified as large-volume and small-volume cleansing enemas. Large-volume enemas are also known as hypotonic or isotonic, depending on the solution used. Small-volume enemas are also known as hypertonic enemas. This skill addresses administering a large-volume enema.

Equipment

- Solution as ordered by the physician at a temperature of 105° to 110°F (40° to 43°C) for adults in the appropriate amount (amount will vary depending on type of solution, patient's age, and patient's ability to retain the solution. Average cleansing enema for an adult may range from 750 to 1,000 mL.)
- Disposable enema set
- Water-soluble lubricant
- IV pole
- Necessary additives as ordered (eg, soap, salt)
- Waterproof pad
- Bath thermometer (if available)
- Bath blanket
- Bedpan and toilet tissue
- Disposable gloves
- Paper towel
- Washcloth, soap, and towel

ASSESSMENT

Assess the patient's abdomen, including auscultating for bowel sounds, percussing, and palpating. Since the goal of a cleansing enema is to increase peristalsis, which should increase bowel sounds, the nurse will assess the abdomen before and after the enema. Inspect the rectal area for any fissures, hemorrhoids, sores, or rectal tears. If any of these are noted, added care should be taken while administering enema. Check the results of the patient's laboratory work, specifically the platelet count and white blood cell (WBC) count. A normal platelet count ranges from 150,000 to 400,000/mm^3. A platelet count of less than 20,000 may seriously compromise the patient's ability to clot blood. Therefore, any unnecessary procedures that would place patient at risk for bleeding or infection should not be performed. A low WBC count places the patient at risk for infection.

NURSING DIAGNOSIS

Determine the related factors for the nursing diagnoses based on the patient's current status. Appropriate nursing diagnoses may include:

- Acute Pain
- Constipation
- Risk for Constipation
- Risk for Injury

OUTCOME IDENTIFICATION AND PLANNING

The expected outcome to be met when administering a cleansing enema is that the patient expels feces and reports a decrease in pain and discomfort. In addition, the patient remains free of any evidence of trauma to the rectal mucosa.

IMPLEMENTATION

ACTION	RATIONALE
1. Verify physician's orders, gather necessary equipment, and explain procedure to patient, including where he or she will defecate. Have a bedpan, commode, or nearby bathroom ready for use.	Verifying the physician's order is crucial to ensuring that the proper enema is administered to the right patient. Organization facilitates performance of tasks. Explanation helps to minimize anxiety. The patient is better able to relax and cooperate if he or she is familiar with the procedure and knows everything is in readiness when the urge to defecate is felt. Defecation usually occurs within 5 to 15 minutes.

continues

Administering a Cleansing Enema (continued)

ACTION	RATIONALE

2. Warm solution in amount ordered, and check temperature with a bath thermometer if available. (If bath thermometer is not available, warm to room temperature or slightly higher, and test on inner wrist.) If tap water is used, adjust temperature as it flows from faucet.

Warming the solution prevents chilling the patient, adding to the discomfort of the procedure.

3. Perform hand hygiene.

Hand hygiene deters the spread of microorganisms.

4. Add enema solution to container. Release clamp and allow fluid to progress through tube before reclamping.

This causes any air to be expelled from the tubing. Although allowing air to enter the intestine is not harmful, it may further distend the intestine.

5. Position waterproof pad under patient.

The waterproof pad protects bed linen.

6. Provide for privacy. Position and drape the patient on the left side (Sims position) with anus exposed on the back, as dictated by patient comfort and condition.

The patient's comfort and warmth help him or her relax. The exact position of the patient has not been found to alter the results of an enema significantly.

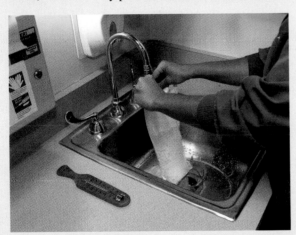

Action 2: Preparing enema bag.

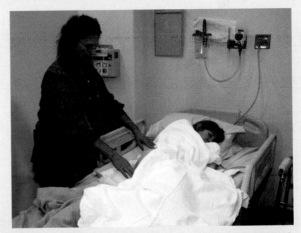

Action 6: Assisting patient to side-lying position (Sims position).

7. Put on nonsterile gloves.

Gloves protect nurse from microorganisms in feces.

8. **Elevate solution so that it is no higher than 45 cm (18″) above level of anus.** Plan to give the solution slowly over a period of 5 to 10 minutes. The container may be hung on an IV pole or held in the nurse's hands at the proper height. (See photo, next page).

Gravity forces the solution to enter the intestine. The amount of pressure determines the rate of flow and pressure exerted on the intestinal wall. Giving the solution too quickly causes rapid distention and pressure, poor defecation, or damage to the mucous membrane.

9. **Generously lubricate end of rectal tube for 5 to 7 cm (2″ to 3″).** A disposable enema set may have a prelubricated rectal tube.

Lubrication facilitates passage of the rectal tube through the anal sphincter and prevents injury to the mucosa.

10. Lift buttock to expose anus. **Slowly and gently insert the enema tube 7 to 10 cm (3″ to 4″). Direct it at an angle pointing toward the spine, not bladder (see photo, next page).** Ask patient to take several deep breaths.

Good visualization of the anus helps prevent injury to tissues. The anal canal is about 2.5 to 5 cm (1″ to 2″) long. The tube should be inserted past the external and internal sphincters, but further insertion may damage intestinal mucous membrane. The suggested angle follows the normal intestinal contour and thus will help to prevent perforation of the bowel. Slow insertion of the tube minimizes spasms of the intestinal wall and sphincters. Deep breathing helps relax the anal sphincters.

continues

SKILL 13-3   Administering a Cleansing Enema (continued)

ACTION   **RATIONALE**

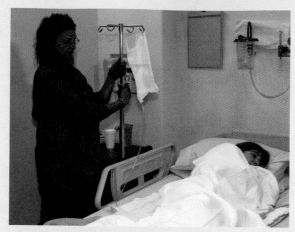

Action 8: Placing enema solution container approximately 18" above patient (on IV pole).

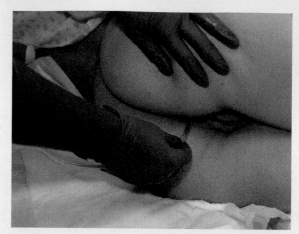

Action 10: Inserting enema tip into anus, directing tip toward umbilicus.

11. If resistance is met while inserting tube, permit a small amount of solution to enter, withdraw tube slightly, and then continue to insert it. **Do not force entry of the tube.** Ask patient to take several deep breaths.

Resistance may be due to spasms of the intestine or failure of the internal sphincter to open. The solution may help to reduce spasms and relax the sphincter, thus making continued insertion of the tube safe. Forcing a tube may injure the intestinal mucosa wall. Taking deep breaths helps relax the anal sphincter.

12. **Introduce solution slowly over a period of 5 to 10 minutes.** Hold tubing all the time that solution is being instilled.

Introducing the solution slowly helps prevent rapid distention of the intestine and a desire to defecate.

13. Clamp tubing or lower container if patient has desire to defecate or cramping occurs. Patient also may be instructed to take small, fast breaths or to pant.

These techniques help relax muscles and prevent premature expulsion of the solution.

14. After solution has been given, clamp tubing and remove tube. Have paper towel ready to receive tube as it is withdrawn. **Have patient retain solution until urge to defecate becomes strong,** usually in about 5 to 15 minutes.

This amount of time usually allows muscle contractions to become sufficient to produce good results.

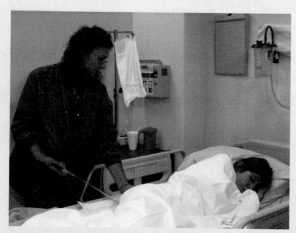

Action 12: Regulating flow rate of solution.

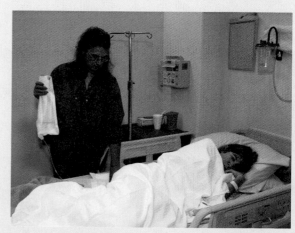

Action 13: Holding bag lower to slow flow of enema solution.

continues

Administering a Cleansing Enema (continued)

ACTION	RATIONALE
15. Remove nonsterile gloves from inside out and discard.	This protects nurse from contact with any microorganisms.
16. When patient has a strong urge to defecate, place him or her in a sitting position on a bedpan or assist to commode or bathroom. Stay with patient or have call light readily accessible.	The sitting position is most natural and facilitates defecation. Fall prevention is a high priority due to the urgency of reaching the commode.
17. Record character of stool and patient's reaction to enema. Remind patient not to flush commode before nurse inspects results of enema.	The nurse needs to observe and record the results. Additional enemas may be necessary if physician has ordered enemas "until clear."
18. Assist patient if necessary with cleaning of anal area. Offer washcloths, soap, and water for handwashing.	Cleaning the anal area and proper hygiene deter the spread of microorganisms.
19. Leave the patient clean and comfortable. Care for equipment properly.	Bacteria that grow in the intestine can be spread to others if equipment is not properly cleaned.
20. Perform hand hygiene.	Hand hygiene deters the spread of microorganisms.
21. Document the following: amount and type of enema solution used; amount, consistency, and color of stool; pain assessment rating; assessment of perineal area for any irritation, tears, or bleeding; and patient's reaction to procedure.	Proper documentation facilitates continuity of care and ensures communication.

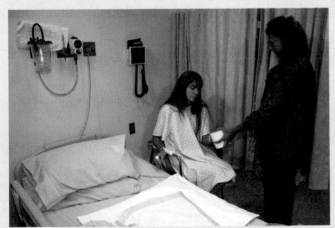

Action 16: Offering toilet tissue to patient on bedside commode.

7/22/06   1310   800 mL warm tap water enema given via rectum. Large amount of soft, brown stool returned. No irritation, tears, or bleeding noted in perineal area. Patient complained of "stomach cramping" relieved when enema was released. Rates pain as 0 after evacuation of enema.—K. Sanders, RN

Action 21: Documentation.

EVALUATION

The expected outcome is met when peristalsis is increased so that the patient expels feces and reports a decrease in pain and discomfort. In addition, the patient exhibits no evidence of trauma to the rectal mucosa.

Unexpected Situations and Associated Interventions

- *Solution does not flow into rectum:* Reposition rectal tube. If solution will still not flow, remove tube and check for any fecal contents.
- *Patient cannot retain enema solution for adequate amount of time:* Patient may need to be placed on bedpan in the supine position while receiving enema. The head of the bed may be elevated 30 degrees for the patient's comfort.
- *Patient cannot tolerate large amount of enema solution:* Amount and length of administration may have to be modified if patient begins to complain of pain.
- *Patient complains of severe cramping with introduction of enema solution:* Lower solution container and check temperature and flow rate. If the solution is too cold or flow rate too fast, severe cramping may occur.

continues

SKILL 13-3 Administering a Cleansing Enema (continued)

Infant and Child Considerations	• When administering an enema to a child, ensure that the volume of solution is appropriate and the solution is at a temperature of 100°F (37.7°C).
Older Adult Considerations	• Older adult patients who cannot retain the enema solution should receive the enema while on the bedpan in the supine position. For comfort, the head of the bed can be elevated 30 degrees if necessary and pillows used appropriately.
Special Considerations	• If enema has been ordered to be given "until clear," check with the physician before administering more than three enemas. Severe fluid and electrolyte imbalances may occur if the patient receives more than three cleansing enemas. Results are considered clear whenever there are no more pieces of stool in enema return. The solution may be colored but still considered a clear return.

SKILL 13-4 Administering a Retention Enema

Retention enemas are ordered for various reasons. *Oil retention* enemas help to lubricate the stool and intestinal mucosa, making defecation easier. *Carminative* enemas help to expel flatus from the rectum and relieve distention secondary to flatus. *Medicated* enemas are used to administer a medication rectally. *Antihelmintic* enemas are administered to destroy intestinal parasites. *Nutritive* enemas are administered to replenish fluids and nutrition rectally.

Equipment

- Enema solution (varies depending on reason for enema), often prepackaged commercially prepared solutions
- Nonsterile gloves
- Waterproof pad
- Bath blanket
- Washcloth, soap, and towel
- Bedpan or commode
- Toilet tissue
- Water-soluble lubricant (if needed)

ASSESSMENT

Assess abdomen, including auscultating for bowel sounds, percussing, and palpating. Inspect rectal area for any fissures, hemorrhoids, sores, or rectal tears. If any of these are noted, added care should be taken while administering enema. Check the results of the patient's laboratory tests, specifically the platelet count and white blood cell (WBC) count. A normal platelet count is 150,000 to 400,000/mm³. A platelet count of less than 20,000 may seriously compromise the patient's ability to clot blood. A low WBC count increases the patient's risk for infection. Therefore, any unnecessary procedures that would place the patient at risk for bleeding or infection should not be performed.

NURSING DIAGNOSIS

Determine the related factors for the nursing diagnoses based on the patient's current status. Appropriate nursing diagnoses may include Constipation and Risk for Injury. Depending on the reason for the retention enema, other nursing diagnoses may include:

- Acute Pain
- Risk for Infection
- Imbalanced Nutrition, Less Than Body Requirements

OUTCOME IDENTIFICATION AND PLANNING

The expected outcome to be met is that the patient expels feces and experiences no evidence of trauma to the rectal mucosa. Other outcomes may include: patient verbalizes a decrease in pain after enema; patient demonstrates signs and symptoms indicative of a resolving infection; and patient exhibits signs and symptoms of adequate nutrition.

continues

Administering a Retention Enema (continued)

IMPLEMENTATION

ACTION	RATIONALE
1. Verify physician's orders, explain to patient procedure and rationale for enema, including where he or she will defecate, and have a bedpan, commode, or nearby bathroom ready for use. Gather equipment. Allow solution to warm to room temperature.	A retention enema is considered a medication and requires an order. Explanation decreases patient anxiety and facilitates cooperation. The patient will be better able to relax and cooperate if he or she is familiar with the procedure and knows everything is in readiness when the urge to defecate is felt. Organization facilitates performance of tasks. A cold solution can cause intestinal cramping.
2. Perform hand hygiene.	Hand hygiene deters the spread of microorganisms.
3. Position waterproof pad under patient.	The pad protects bed linen.
4. Provide privacy. Position and drape patient on left side (Sims position) with anus exposed on the back, as dictated by patient comfort and condition.	The patient's comfort and warmth help him or her relax. The exact position of the patient has not been found to alter results of an enema significantly.
5. Put on nonsterile gloves.	This protects nurse from microorganisms in feces.
6. Remove cap of prepackaged enema solution and ensure that rectal tube is prelubricated. If not, apply a generous amount of lubricant to the tube.	Lubrication is necessary to minimize trauma on insertion.
7. Lift buttock to expose anus. **Slowly and gently insert rectal tube 7 to 10 cm (3″ to 4″). Direct it at an angle pointing toward the spine. Ask patient to take several deep breaths.**	Good visualization of the anus helps prevent injury to tissues. The anal canal is about 2.5 to 5 cm (1″ to 2″) long. The tube should be inserted past the external and internal sphincters, but further insertion may damage intestinal mucous membrane. The suggested angle follows the normal intestinal contour and thus will help to prevent perforation of the bowel. Slow insertion of the tube minimizes spasms of the intestinal wall and sphincters. Deep breathing helps relax the anal sphincters.
8. If resistance is met while inserting tube, permit a small amount of solution to enter, withdraw tube slightly, and then continue to insert it. **Do not force entry of tube.**	Resistance may be due to spasms of the intestine or failure of the internal sphincter to open. The solution may help to reduce spasms and relax the sphincter, thus making continued insertion of the tube safe. Forcing a tube may injure the intestinal mucosa wall.
9. Slowly squeeze enema container, emptying entire contents.	Compressing the container slowly allows the solution to enter the rectum and prevent rapid distention of the intestine and a desire to defecate.

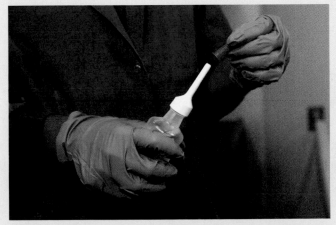

Action 6: Removing cap from prepackaged enema solution container.

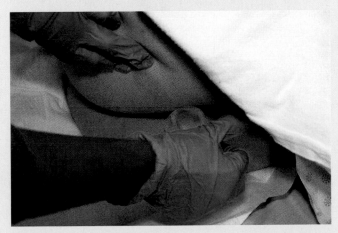

Action 9: Slowly squeezing container.

continues

ACTION	RATIONALE
10. **Remove container while keeping it compressed.**	If container is released, a vacuum will form, allowing some of the enema solution to re-enter the container.
11. **Instruct patient to retain enema solution for at least 30 minutes or as indicated.**	Solution needs to dwell for at least 30 minutes to provide quality results.
12. Remove nonsterile gloves from inside out and discard.	This protects nurse from contact with any microorganisms.
13. When patient has a strong urge to defecate, place him or her in a sitting position on bedpan or assist to commode or bathroom. Stay with patient or have call light readily accessible.	The sitting position is most natural and facilitates defecation. Fall prevention is a high priority due to the urgency of reaching the commode.
14. Remind patient not to flush commode before nurse inspects results of enema. Record character of stool and patient's reaction to enema.	The nurse needs to observe and record the results.
15. Assist patient if necessary with cleaning of anal area (putting on gloves if necessary). Offer washcloths, soap, and water for handwashing.	Proper cleansing deters spread of microorganisms and promotes hygiene.
16. Leave patient clean and comfortable. Care for equipment properly.	Bacteria that grow in the intestine can be spread to others if equipment is not properly cleaned.
17. Perform hand hygiene.	Hand hygiene deters the spread of microorganisms.
18. Document the following: amount and type of enema solution used; amount, consistency, and color of stool; pain assessment rating; assessment of perineal area for any irritation, tears, or bleeding; and patient's reaction to procedure.	Documentation promotes continuity of care and ensures communication.

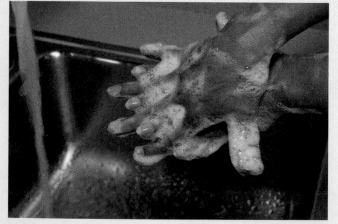

Action 17: Perform hand hygiene.

6/26/06   100 mL of mineral oil administered as enema via rectum. Small amount of firm, black stool returned. Small (approx. 1 cm) tear noted at 2 o'clock position on anus. No erythema or bleeding noted. Physician notified of tear and stool color. Patient tolerated without incident. Reports pain at 2 on a 0 to 10 rating scale after enema evacuated.
—K. Sanders, RN

Action 18: Documentation.

EVALUATION

The expected outcome is met when the patient expels feces without evidence of trauma to the rectal mucosa. Depending on the reason for the retention enema, other outcomes met may include: patient verbalizes a decrease in pain after enema; patient demonstrates signs and symptoms indicative of a resolving infection; and patient exhibits signs and symptoms of adequate nutrition.

Unexpected Situations and Associated Interventions

- *Solution does not flow into rectum:* Reposition rectal tube; if solution still will not flow, remove and check for any fecal contents.
- *Patient cannot retain enema solution for adequate amount of time:* Patient may need to be placed on bedpan in supine position while receiving enema. The head of the bed may be elevated 30 degrees for the patient's comfort.

SKILL 13-5   Administering a Return-Flow Enema (Harris Flush)

A return-flow enema, also called a Harris flush, is prescribed to aid in expelling flatus. With this type of enema, a small amount of solution is instilled and then allowed to return to the solution container. This sequence is repeated several times. The back-and-forth action of the solution stimulates peristalsis, thereby aiding in expelling flatus.

Equipment

- Disposable enema set
- Water-soluble lubricant
- Waterproof pad
- Bath thermometer (if available)
- Bath blanket
- Bedpan or commode
- Toilet tissue
- Disposable gloves
- Paper towel
- Washcloth, soap, and towel
- Solution (as ordered by physician), usually 100 to 200 mL at a temperature of 105° to 110°F (40° to 43°C) for an adult

ASSESSMENT

Percuss and palpate abdomen, noting any areas of distention or tenderness. Normally, abdominal percussion will elicit tympany (a resonant sound); when excessive flatus is present, hyperresonance will be noted. The abdomen should be soft and nontender on palpation. With increased flatulence or diarrhea, the abdomen may be firm, distended, or painful to deep and light palpation. Measure the abdominal girth with tape measure at umbilicus. Then measure again after the enema, noting any decrease in the abdominal girth. Inspect the rectal area for any fissures, hemorrhoids, sores, or rectal tears. If any of these are noted, added care should be taken while inserting rectal tube. Check the results of the patient's laboratory tests, specifically the platelet count and white blood cell (WBC) count. A normal platelet count is 150,000 to 400,000/mm^3. A platelet count of less than 20,000 may seriously compromise the patient's ability to clot blood. A low WBC count increases the patient's risk for infection. Therefore, any unnecessary procedures that would place the patient at risk for bleeding or infection should not be performed.

NURSING DIAGNOSIS

Determine the related factors for the nursing diagnoses based on the patient's current status. A common nursing diagnosis would be Acute Pain. Another nursing diagnosis may be Risk for Injury.

OUTCOME IDENTIFICATION AND PLANNING

The expected outcome to achieve when administering a return-flow enema is that the patient will verbalize a decrease in the level of pain experienced due to passage of flatus. Flatus will be expelled from the rectum and the abdominal girth will decrease. The patient remains free of any signs and symptoms of injury to the intestinal mucosa and rectum.

IMPLEMENTATION

ACTION	RATIONALE
1. Verify physician's orders. Explain need for enema to patient, including where he or she will defecate. Have a bedpan, commode, or nearby bathroom ready for use. Gather necessary equipment.	Verification of the order ensures the patient's safety. Explanation aids in minimizing patient anxiety and encourages cooperation and relaxation because the patient is familiar with what is to occur and knows that everything is in readiness when the urge to defecate is felt. Organization facilitates performance of tasks.
2. Warm solution in amount ordered, and check temperature with a bath thermometer if available. (If bath thermometer is not available, warm to room temperature or slightly higher, and test on inner wrist.) If tap water is used, adjust temperature as it flows from faucet.	Warming the solution prevents chilling and minimizes patient discomfort.

continues

ACTION	RATIONALE
3. Perform hand hygiene.	Hand hygiene deters the spread of microorganisms.
4. Add enema solution to container. Release clamp and allow fluid to progress through tube before reclamping.	This causes any air to be expelled from the tubing. Although allowing air to enter the intestine is not harmful, it may further distend the intestine.
5. Position waterproof pad under patient.	The waterproof pad protects bed linen.
6. Provide privacy. Position and drape patient on left side (Sims position) with anus exposed on the back, as dictated by patient comfort and condition.	The patient's comfort and warmth help him or her relax. The exact position of the patient has not been found to alter the results of an enema significantly.
7. Put on nonsterile gloves.	This protects nurse from microorganisms in feces.
8. Generously lubricate end of rectal tube for 5 to 7 cm (2″ to 3″) with water-soluble lubricant.	This facilitates passage of the rectal tube through the anal sphincter and prevents injury to the mucosa.
9. Lift buttock to expose anus. Slowly and gently insert enema tube 7 to 10 cm (3″ to 4″). Direct it at an angle pointing toward the spine. Ask patient to take several deep breaths.	Good visualization of the anus helps prevent injury to tissues. The anal canal is about 2.5 to 5 cm (1″ to 2″) long. The tube should be inserted past the external and internal sphincters, but further insertion may damage intestinal mucous membrane. The suggested angle follows the normal intestinal contour and thus will help to prevent perforation of the bowel. Slow insertion of the tube minimizes spasms of the intestinal wall and sphincters. Deep breathing helps relax the anal sphincters.
10. **Elevate solution so that it flows freely into rectum and sigmoid colon.**	Gravity forces the solution to enter the intestine.
11. If resistance is met while inserting tube, permit a small amount of solution to enter, withdraw tube slightly, and then continue to insert it. Do not force entry of tube.	Resistance may be due to spasms of the intestine or failure of the internal sphincter to open. The solution may help to reduce spasms and relax the sphincter, thus making continued insertion of the tube safe. Forcing a tube may injure the intestinal mucosa wall. Taking deep breaths helps relax the anal sphincter.

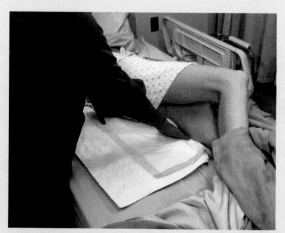

Action 5: Positioning waterproof pad under patient.

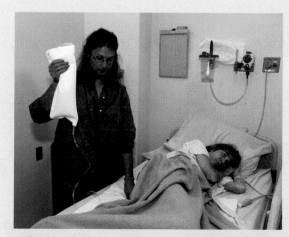

Action 10: Elevating solution container to allow free flow of solution.

continues

Administering a Return-Flow Enema (Harris Flush) (continued)

ACTION	RATIONALE
12. **After all solution has been given, lower container and allow solution to flow back into container. Repeat this process of allowing solution to flow into rectum, then back into container, five or six times.**	This process stimulates peristalsis and aids in the expelling of flatus.
13. If solution becomes thick with feces, replace with fresh solution.	Solution will clog rectal tube if it becomes too thick.
14. Clamp enema set and remove. Wrap in paper towel.	Clamping set before removal prevents the solution from flowing out of the tubing. Wrapping the tubing in a paper towel prevents solution from dripping on bed or floor.

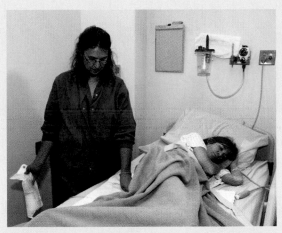

Action 12: Lowering solution to allow solution to flow back into container.

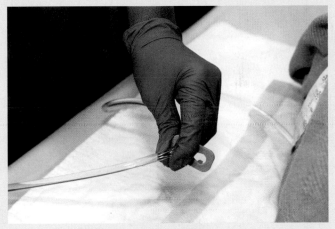

Action 14: Clamping tubing before tubing is removed.

15. Allow contaminated solution to flow into toilet, and dispose of enema set; if patient feels urge to defecate, assist patient onto bedpan or to the commode.	Due to increased peristalsis, patient may need to defecate.
16. Assist patient if necessary with cleaning of anal area. Offer washcloth, soap, and water for handwashing.	Cleaning deters the spread of microorganisms and promotes hygiene.
17. Remove nonsterile gloves from inside out and discard.	This protects nurse from contact with any microorganisms.
18. Perform hand hygiene.	Hand hygiene deters the spread of microorganisms.
19. Document the following: amount and type of enema solution used; amount, consistency, and color of stool; pain assessment rating; assessment of perineal area for any irritation, tears, or bleeding; changes in abdominal girth or abdominal percussion; and patient's reaction to procedure.	Documentation promotes continuity of care and ensures communication.

6/13/06   1515   750 mL of tap water administered as enema via rectum. Solution allowed to flow back five times prior to release. Large amount of soft, brown stool returned. Perineal area without any irritation, erythema, or bleeding. Abdominal girth remains 46 cm. Patient complained of "stomach cramping" while solution flowing into rectum. Stated, "My stomach feels better now that I've had a bowel movement." Rates pain as 2 on a scale of 0 to 10.—K. Sanders, RN

Action 19: Documentation.

continues

SKILL 13-5   Administering a Return-Flow Enema (Harris Flush) (continued)

EVALUATION

The expected outcome is met when peristalsis increases so that patient expels flatus, patient demonstrates a decreased abdominal girth, and patient states that pain is significantly decreased. Patient also exhibits no signs and symptoms of injury to the intestinal mucosa and rectum.

Unexpected Situations and Associated Interventions

- *Solution does not flow into rectum:* Reposition enema tube; if solution will still not flow, remove tube and check for any fecal contents.
- *Patient complains of severe cramping with introduction of enema solution:* Lower the solution container and check temperature and flow rate. If the solution is too cold or flow rate too fast, severe cramping may occur.

SKILL 13-6   Digital Removal of Stool

When a patient develops a fecal impaction (prolonged retention or an accumulation of fecal material that forms a hardened mass in the rectum), the stool must sometimes be broken up manually. Digital removal of stool is typically ordered when attempts to pass the stool voluntarily or enemas have been ineffective in moving the stool. Patient discomfort and irritation of the rectal mucosa may occur.

Equipment

- Disposable gloves
- Water-soluble lubricant
- Waterproof pad
- Bedpan
- Toilet paper, washcloth, and towel
- Sitz bath (optional)

ASSESSMENT

Verify the time of the patient's last bowel movement by asking the patient and checking the patient's medical record. Assess the abdomen, including auscultating for bowel sounds, percussing, and palpating. Inspect the rectal area for any fissures, hemorrhoids, sores, or rectal tears. If any of these are noted, added care should be taken while removing stool. Check the results of the patient's laboratory tests, specifically the platelet count and white blood cell (WBC) count. A normal platelet count is 150,000 to 400,000/mm^3. A platelet count of less than 20,000 may seriously compromise the patient's ability to clot blood. A low WBC count increases the patient's risk for infection. Therefore, any unnecessary procedures that would place the patient at risk for bleeding or infection should not be performed.

NURSING DIAGNOSIS

Determine the related factors for the nursing diagnoses based on the patient's current status. An appropriate nursing diagnosis may be Constipation. Other nursing diagnoses may include Acute Pain and Risk for Injury.

OUTCOME IDENTIFICATION AND PLANNING

The expected outcome to achieve when digitally removing stool is that the patient will expel feces with assistance and complaints of pain will be decreased. In addition, the patient will remain free of any signs and symptoms of trauma.

continues

Digital Removal of Stool (continued)

IMPLEMENTATION

ACTION	RATIONALE
1. Verify physician's order. Explain procedure to patient, discussing signs and symptoms of a slow heart rate. Instruct patient to alert you if any of these symptoms are felt during the procedure.	Digital removal of stool is considered an invasive procedure and requires a physician's order. Explanation helps to minimize anxiety and foster cooperation. Rectal stimulation may cause a vagal response.
2. Gather necessary equipment.	Organization facilitates performance of task.
3. Perform hand hygiene.	Hand hygiene deters the spread of microorganisms.
4. Place patient in a side-lying position, draping with bath blanket so only buttocks are exposed.	This position provides for best visualization of anus. Providing privacy and warmth will help patient to relax.
5. Place waterproof pad under buttocks.	The waterproof pad protects linens from becoming soiled.
6. Put on nonsterile gloves.	This protects nurse from microorganisms in feces. The GI tract is not a sterile environment.
7. **Generously lubricate forefinger with water-soluble lubricant and insert finger gently into anal canal pointing toward the spine.**	Lubrication reduces irritation of the rectum. The presence of the finger added to the mass tends to cause discomfort for the patient if the work is not done slowly and gently.
8. **Work the finger around and into the hardened mass to break it up and then remove pieces of it.** Instruct patient to bear down, if possible, while extracting feces to ease in removal. Place extracted stool in bedpan.	Fecal mass may be large and may need to be removed in smaller pieces.

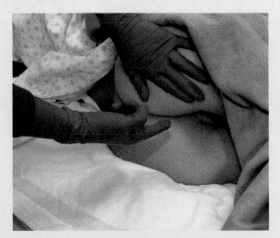

Action 7: Inserting lubricated forefinger of dominant hand into anal canal.

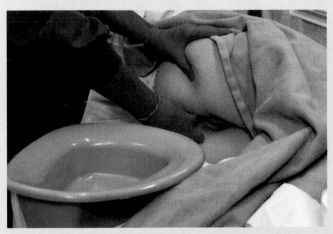

Action 8: Inserting gloved finger and gently moving to break up stool.

9. **Remove impaction at intervals if it is severe. Instruct patient to alert you if he or she begins to feel light-headed or nauseated. If patient reports either symptom, stop removal and assess patient.**	This helps to prevent discomfort, irritation, and vagal nerve stimulation.

continues

ACTION

RATIONALE

10. Assist patient if necessary with cleaning of anal area. Offer washcloths, soap, and water for handwashing. If patient is able, offer sitz bath.

Cleaning deters the transmission of microorganisms and promotes hygiene. Sitz bath may relieve the irritated perianal area.

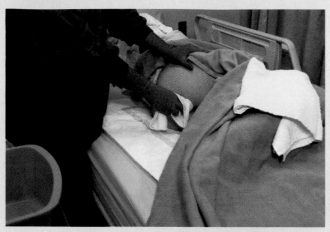

Action 10: Helping to clean anal area with washcloth and soap.

11. Remove nonsterile gloves from inside out and discard.

This protects nurse from contact with any microorganisms.

12. Perform hand hygiene.

Hand hygiene deters the spread of microorganisms.

13. Document the following: color, consistency, and amount of stool removed; condition of perianal area after procedure; pain assessment rating; patient's reaction to procedure.

Documentation promotes continuity of care and ensures communication.

6/29/06   Large amount of hard, brown stool removed with digital exam. Perineal area remains free from tears, erythema, or bleeding. Patient denied any lightheadedness or nausea during procedure. Rates pain at 1 on a scale of 0 to 10.—K. Sanders, RN

Action 13: Documentation.

EVALUATION

The expected outcome is met when the fecal impaction is removed without stimulation of the vagus nerve. The patient voices a decrease in pain and discomfort and exhibits no evidence of trauma to the rectal mucosa.

Unexpected Situations and Associated Interventions

- *Patient complains of being dizzy, lightheaded, or nauseated or begins to vomit:* Stop digital stimulation immediately. Vagal nerve might have been stimulated. Assess heart rate and blood pressure. Notify physician.
- *Patient experiences a large amount of pain during procedure:* Stop procedure and notify physician.

Applying a Fecal Incontinence Pouch

A fecal incontinence pouch is used to protect the perianal skin from excoriation due to repeated exposure to liquid stool. Although best used before excoriation occurs, a skin barrier can be applied if excoriation already is present.

Equipment
- Fecal incontinence pouch
- Disposable gloves
- Washcloth and towel
- Urinary drainage (Foley) bag
- Scissors (optional)
- Bath blanket

ASSESSMENT

Assess the amount and consistency of stool being passed. Also assess the frequency. Inspect the perianal area for any excoriation or hemorrhoids.

NURSING DIAGNOSIS

The primary nursing diagnosis for the patient would be Bowel Incontinence. Other possible nursing diagnoses may include:

- Risk for Impaired Skin Integrity
- Impaired Skin Integrity
- Risk for Infection

OUTCOME IDENTIFICATION AND PLANNING

The expected outcome to achieve when applying a fecal incontinence pouch is that the patient expels feces into the pouch and maintains intact perianal skin. Other outcomes may include the following: patient demonstrates a decrease in the amount and severity of excoriation and remains free of any signs and symptoms of infection.

IMPLEMENTATION

ACTION	RATIONALE
1. Gather necessary equipment. Discuss reason for fecal incontinence bag with patient.	Organization facilitates performance of task. Discussion promotes cooperation and helps to minimize anxiety.
2. Perform hand hygiene.	Hand hygiene deters the spread of microorganisms.
3. Place patient in side-lying position, draping with bath blanket so only buttocks are exposed.	This position provides for best visualization of anus. Providing privacy and warmth will help patient to relax.
4. Put on nonsterile gloves. Cleanse perianal area. Pat dry thoroughly.	Gloves protect nurse from microorganisms in feces. The GI tract is not a sterile environment. Skin must be dry for pouch to adhere securely.
5. Trim perianal hair if needed.	It may be uncomfortable if the perianal hair is pulled by adhesive from the fecal pouch. Trimming with scissors minimizes the risk for infection compared with shaving.
6. Remove paper backing from adhesive of pouch. (See next page for Action 6–8 photos.)	Removing the paper backing is necessary so that the pouch can adhere to the skin.
7. With nondominant hand, separate buttocks. **Apply fecal pouch to anal area with dominant hand, ensuring that opening of bag is over anus.**	Opening should be over anus so that stool empties into bag and does not stay on patient's skin, which could lead to skin breakdown.
8. Release buttocks. Attach connector of fecal incontinence pouch to urinary drainage bag. **Hang urinary drainage bag below patient.**	Bag must be dependent for stool to drain into bag.
9. Remove nonsterile gloves from inside out and discard.	This protects nurse from contact with any microorganisms.
10. Perform hand hygiene.	Hand hygiene deters the spread of microorganisms.
11. Document the following: date and time fecal pouch was applied; appearance of perianal area; color of stool; intake and output (amount of stool out); patient's reaction to procedure.	Documentation promotes continuity of care and ensures communication.

continues

Applying a Fecal Incontinence Pouch (continued)

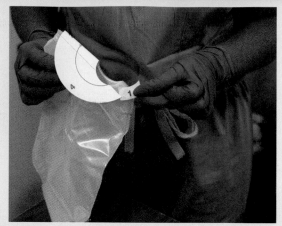

Action 6: Removing paper backing from adhesive of rectal pouch.

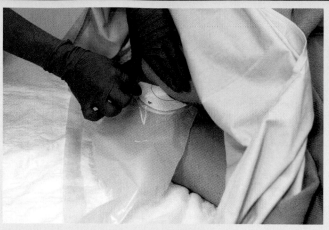

Action 7: Applying pouch over anal opening.

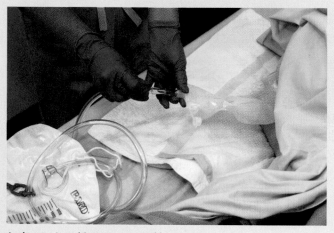

Action 8: Attaching connector of fecal pouch to tubing of drainage bag.

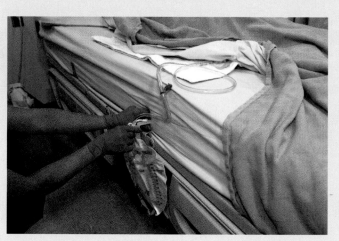

Action 8: Checking that drainage bag is below the level of the patient.

8/13/06. 1210   Perineal area slightly erythematous. Fecal incontinence bag applied
due to incontinence of large amounts of liquid stool and possible skin breakdown. Approximately 90 cc of liquid brown stool noted
in drainage bag.—K. Sanders, RN.

Action 11: Documentation.

continues

EVALUATION

The expected outcome is met when the fecal pouch contains feces that have drained, and perineal skin breakdown is prevented. If the patient had perianal skin breakdown before the pouch was applied, the expected outcome is met when the patient demonstrates a decrease in the amount and severity of excoriation and remains free of any signs and symptoms of infection.

Unexpected Situations and Associated Interventions

- *Perianal area becomes excoriated:* Skin barrier may be applied before fecal pouch to protect skin.
- *Stool does not drain from pouch into urinary drainage bag:* Stool may be too thick. If stool no longer drains from pouch into drainage bag, remove pouch to prevent perianal skin breakdown.
- *Stool is leaking from around sides of fecal pouch:* Remove pouch and clean the area well before applying a new pouch.

Special Considerations

- Remove fecal pouch at least every 72 hours to check for signs of skin breakdown.

SKILL
13-8   Changing and Emptying an Ostomy Appliance or Pouch

Patients with certain chronic illnesses or those who have undergone certain surgical procedures require bowel diversion techniques to enable them to have an appropriate elimination pattern. Such a diversion is commonly known as an ostomy (a surgical opening made through the abdominal wall that connects part of the intestinal tract to the abdominal opening, allowing fecal elimination). Ileostomies drain liquid stool; colostomies typically drain formed stool. Ostomy appliances or pouches are applied to the opening to collect stool. Ostomy appliances or pouches should be emptied promptly, usually when they are one-third to one-half full. If they are allowed to fill up, they may leak or become detached from the skin. Ostomy appliances are available in a one-piece or two-piece system and are usually changed every 3 to 7 days, although this could be done more often.

Equipment

- Clean ostomy appliance or pouch
- Gauze pad
- Closure clamp (called a tail)
- Plastic bag
- Disposable gloves
- Stoma measuring guide
- Water or special solution to clean pouch
- Toilet or bedpan
- Scissors
- Toilet tissue
- Protective skin barrier (optional)
- Adhesive solvent (optional)
- Cleansing products (warm water, mild soap [optional], towel, and washcloth)
- Disposable pad (optional)
- Deodorant for pouch (optional)

continues

Changing and Emptying an Ostomy Appliance or Pouch (continued)

ASSESSMENT

Assess peristomal skin for any breakdown, irritation, or signs and symptoms of infection such as from *Candida albicans* (yeast). Assess stoma for color and size. The stoma should appear pink and moist. In addition, assess the amount, color, consistency, and odor of stool from ostomy. If patient previously had an ostomy, ask patient what type of appliances or pouches he or she uses.

**NURSING
DIAGNOSIS**

Determine the related factors for the nursing diagnoses based on the patient's current status. Appropriate nursing diagnoses may include:

- Risk for Impaired Skin Integrity
- Deficient Knowledge
- Disturbed Body Image
- Ineffective Coping
- Constipation
- Diarrhea

**OUTCOME
IDENTIFICATION
AND PLANNING**

The expected outcome to be met when changing and emptying an ostomy appliance or pouch is that the patient exhibits no signs and symptoms of peristomal skin breakdown. Other outcomes may include the following: patient demonstrates ability to participate in ostomy appliance care; patient demonstrates positive coping skills; patient expels stool that is appropriate in consistency and amount for the ostomy location.

IMPLEMENTATION

ACTION	RATIONALE
1. Gather necessary equipment.	Organization facilitates performance of tasks.
2. Perform hand hygiene and apply nonsterile gloves.	Hand hygiene deters the spread of microorganisms. Gloves protect nurse from microorganisms in feces.
3. Explain procedure to patient.	The patient is better able to cooperate and learn the technique when he or she is aware of the procedure.
4. Provide privacy. Assist patient to a comfortable sitting or lying position in bed or a standing or sitting position in the bathroom. To empty a pouch, proceed to Action 11. To change a pouch, continue with Action 5.	Either position should allow the patient to view the procedure in preparation for learning to perform it independently. Lying flat or sitting upright facilitates smooth application of the appliance.
5. Empty the partially filled appliance or pouch into a bedpan if it is drainable.	Emptying the contents before removal prevents accidental spillage of fecal material. Appliances or pouches that are too full can detach or leak.
6. **Slowly remove appliance, beginning at the top, while keeping abdominal skin taut.** If any resistance is felt, use warmth or adhesive solvent to facilitate removal. Discard disposable appliance or pouch in plastic bag.	Careful removal protects the underlying skin from damage and minimizes discomfort for the patient. Solvent is rarely necessary to ease removal.
7. Use toilet tissue to remove any excess stool from stoma. Cover stoma with gauze pad. Gently wash and pat dry peristomal skin. Mild soap may be used to cleanse peristomal skin, but be sure to rinse all soap before reapplying pouch. **Do not apply lotion to peristomal area.**	Soap may not be recommended because it may be irritating to the peristomal skin; check your institution's policy. Toilet tissue, used gently, will not damage the stoma. The gauze absorbs any drainage from the stoma while the skin is being prepared. Lotion will prevent a tight adhesive seal.
8. Assess appearance of peristomal skin and stoma. **A moist, reddish-pink stoma is considered normal.**	Any change in normal appearance may indicate either anemia (pale stoma) or altered circulation (bluish-purple color), and the physician should be notified.

continues

Changing and Emptying an Ostomy Appliance or Pouch (continued)

ACTION	RATIONALE

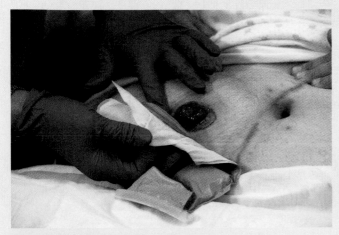

Action 6: Removing appliance.

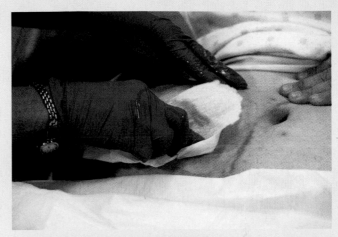

Action 7: Using toilet tissue to wipe around stoma.

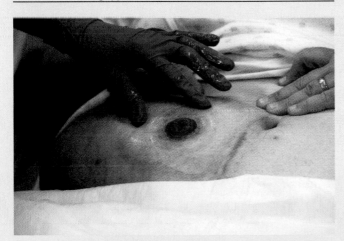

Action 8: Assessing stoma and peristomal skin.

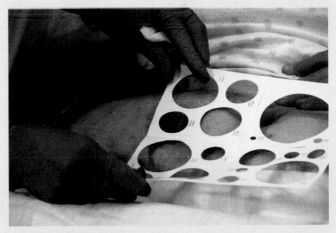

Action 9a: Using template to measure size of stoma.

9. Apply one-piece or two-piece system:
   a. Select size for stoma opening by using the measurement guide (template).
   b. Trace same size circle on the back and center the skin barrier. (See next page for photos illustrating Actions 9b–9f.)
   c. **Use scissors to cut an opening 1/4″ to 1/8″ larger than stoma.**
   d. Remove backing of protective skin barrier. Apply additional skin protection as necessary.
   e. Remove gauze pad covering stoma.
   f. **Ease barrier and appliance or pouch onto abdomen and over stoma,** and gently press onto skin while smoothing out creases or wrinkles. Hold in place for 3 minutes.

Placing the system as a unit over the stoma makes application easier. The opening is cut slightly larger to prevent irritation to the stoma as peristalsis occurs, but not large enough for skin to become excoriated. Smooth application of the appliance or pouch prevents escape of odor and feces. The warmth from the nurse's hands facilitates a tight seal.

continues

ACTION

RATIONALE

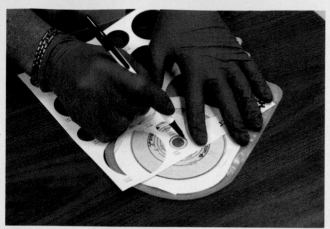

Action 9b: Tracing the same sized circle on the back and center of skin barrier.

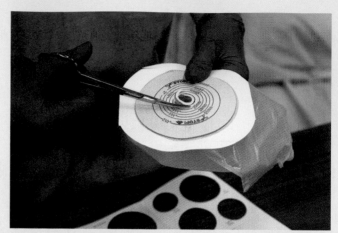

Action 9c: Cutting opening on skin barrier about 1/8″ to 1/4″ larger than circle traced.

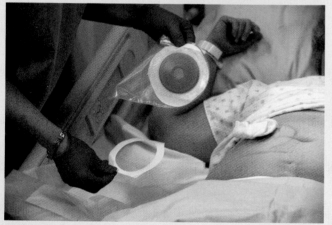

Action 9d: Removing backing of skin barrier.

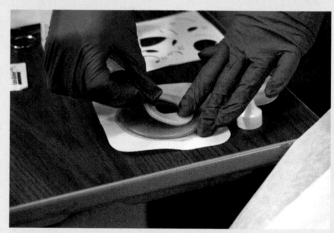

Action 9d: Attaching additional skin protection.

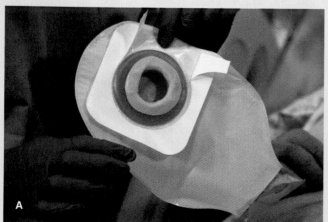

A

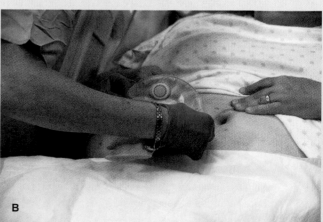

B

Action 9f: Applying skin barrier and appliance together (**A**) onto abdomen over stoma (**B**).

continues

ACTION	RATIONALE
10. Close bottom of appliance or pouch by folding the end upward and using clamp or clip that comes with product. Continue with Action 15.	A tightly sealed appliance will not leak and cause embarrassment and discomfort for the patient.

To Empty the Appliance or Pouch

ACTION	RATIONALE
11. Plan to drain appliance or pouch when it is one-third to one-half full. Remove clamp and fold end of pouch upward like a cuff.	Allowing the appliance or pouch to fill more than one-half full increases its weight and makes it more likely to separate or loosen from the skin. Creating a cuff before emptying prevents additional soilage and odor.

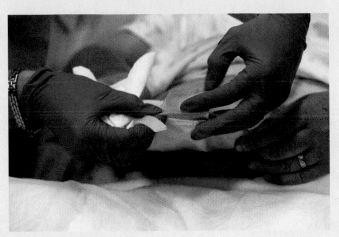

Action 10: Closing bottom of pouch.

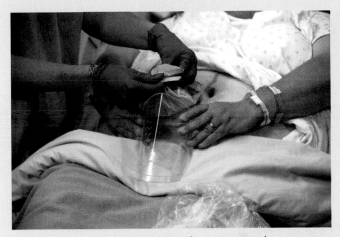

Action 11: Removing clamp, getting ready to empty pouch.

ACTION	RATIONALE
12. Empty contents into bedpan, toilet, or measuring device. Rinse appliance or pouch with tepid water or water mixed with a drop of mouthwash administered with a squeeze bottle. (Actions 12, 13, and 17 are illustrated on following page.)	Rinsing the inside provides a cleaner appearance and minimizes odor.
13. Wipe the lower 2″ of the appliance or pouch with toilet tissue.	Drying the lower section removes any additional fecal material, thus decreasing odor problems.
14. Uncuff edge of appliance or pouch and apply clip or clamp.	The edge of the appliance or pouch should remain clean. The clamp secures closure.
15. Dispose of used equipment according to agency policy. Remove nonsterile gloves from inside out and discard.	This protects nurse from contact with any microorganisms.
16. Perform hand hygiene.	Hand hygiene deters the spread of microorganisms.
17. Document appearance of stoma, condition of peristomal skin, characteristics of drainage (amount, color, consistency, unusual odor), and patient's reaction to procedure.	Documentation promotes continuity of care and ensures communication.

continues

Changing and Emptying an Ostomy Appliance or Pouch (continued)

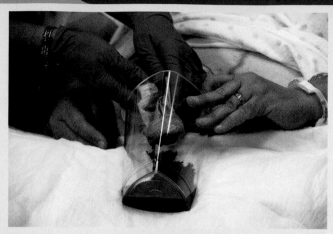

Action 12: Emptying pouch into a measuring device.

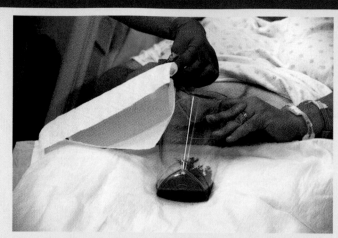

Action 13: Wiping lower 2″ of pouch with toilet tissue.

> 7/22/06 1630   Colostomy bag changed
> due to leakage. Stoma is pink, moist, and flat
> against abdomen. No erythema or excoriation
> of surrounding skin. Moderate amount of
> pasty, brown stool noted in bag. Patient ask-
> ing appropriate questions during bag appli-
> cation. States, "I'm ready to try the next one."
> —K. Sanders, RN.

Action 17: Documentation.

EVALUATION

The expected outcomes are met when the patient tolerates the procedure without pain and the peristomal skin remains intact without excoriation. Odor is contained within the closed system. The patient participates in ostomy appliance care, demonstrates positive coping skills, and expels stool that is appropriate in consistency and amount for the location of the ostomy.

Unexpected Situations and Associated Interventions

- *Peristomal skin is excoriated or irritated:* Make sure that appliance is not cut too large. Skin that is exposed inside of the ostomy appliance will become excoriated. Apply additional skin protection under ostomy appliance until skin is healed.
- *Patient continues to notice odor:* Check system for any leaks or poor adhesion. Clean outside of bag thoroughly when emptying. Odor control products are sold wherever ostomy supplies are located.
- *Bag continues to come loose or fall off:* Cleanse skin thoroughly with soap that does not contain a moisturizer. A skin prep may need to be applied to promote better adhesion.
- *Stoma is protruding into bag:* This is called a prolapse. Have patient rest for 30 minutes. If stoma is not back to normal size within that time, notify physician. If stoma stays prolapsed, it may twist, resulting in impaired circulation to the stoma.

Irrigating a Colostomy

Irrigations may be used to help promote regular evacuation of feces from some colostomies. These colostomies typically are located in the right lower portion of the colon.

Equipment
- Disposable irrigation system and irrigation sleeve
- Waterproof pad
- Bedpan or toilet
- Water-soluble lubricant
- IV pole
- Disposable gloves
- Lukewarm solution at a temperature of 105° to 110°F (40° to 43°C) (as ordered by physician; normally tap water)
- Washcloth, soap, and towels
- Paper towel
- New appliance if needed

ASSESSMENT

Ask patient if he or she has been experiencing any abdominal discomfort. Ask patient about date of last irrigation and whether there have been any changes in stool pattern or consistency. If patient irrigates his or her ostomy at home, ask if he or she has any special routines during irrigation, such as reading the newspaper or listening to music. Also determine how much solution patient typically uses for irrigation. The normal amount of irrigation fluid varies but is usually around 750 to 1,000 mL for an adult. If this is a first irrigation, the normal irrigation volume is around 250 to 500 mL.

Assess ostomy, ensuring that the diversion is a colostomy. Ileostomies are never irrigated because the fecal content is liquid and cannot be controlled. Note placement of ostomy on abdomen, color and size of ostomy, color and condition of stoma, and amount and consistency of stool.

NURSING DIAGNOSIS

Determine the related factors for the nursing diagnoses based on the patient's current status. Possible nursing diagnoses may include:
- Deficient Knowledge
- Anxiety
- Constipation
- Ineffective Coping
- Disturbed Body Image

OUTCOME IDENTIFICATION AND PLANNING

The expected outcome to be met when irrigating a colostomy is that the patient demonstrates ability to participate in care. The patient voices increased confidence with ostomy care; soft formed stool is expelled; and the patient demonstrates positive coping mechanisms.

IMPLEMENTATION

ACTION	RATIONALE
1. Assemble necessary equipment (see next page for illustration). Warm solution in amount ordered. If tap water is used, adjust temperature as it flows from faucet.	Organization facilitates task performance. If the solution is too cool, patient may experience cramps or nausea.
2. Explain procedure to patient and plan where he or she will receive irrigation. Assist patient onto bedside commode or into nearby bathroom.	Unlike a cleansing enema, the patient cannot hold the irrigation solution. A large immediate return of irrigation solution and stool usually occurs.
3. Perform hand hygiene.	Hand hygiene deters the spread of microorganisms.
4. Add irrigation solution to container. Release clamp and allow fluid to progress through tube before reclamping.	This causes any air to be expelled from the tubing. Although allowing air to enter the intestine is not harmful, it may distend the intestine, causing gas pains.

continues

ACTION

RATIONALE

5. Hang container so that bottom of bag will be at patient's shoulder level when seated.

Gravity forces the solution to enter the intestine. The amount of pressure determines the rate of flow and pressure exerted on the intestinal wall.

6. Put on disposable gloves.

This protects nurse from microorganisms in feces.

7. Remove appliance and attach irrigation sleeve. **Place drainage end into toilet bowl or bedpan.**

The irrigation sleeve directs all irrigation fluid and stool into the toilet or bedpan for easy disposal.

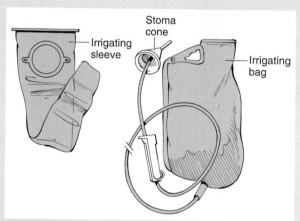

Action 1: Irrigating sleeve and bag.

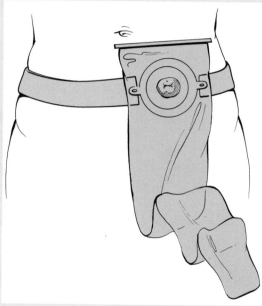

Action 7: Positioning of irrigation sleeve on abdomen.

8. Lubricate end of cone with water-soluble lubricant.

This facilitates passage of the cone into the stoma opening.

9. Insert the cone into the stoma. **Introduce solution slowly over a period of 5 minutes.** Hold tubing (or if patient is able, allow patient to hold tubing) all the time that solution is being instilled. Control rate of flow by closing or opening the clamp.

If the irrigation solution is administered too quickly, the patient may experience nausea and cramps due to rapid distention and increased pressure in the intestine.

10. **Hold cone in place for an additional 10 seconds after fluid is infused.**

This will allow a small amount of dwell time for the irrigation solution.

11. Remove cone. Patient should remain seated on toilet or bedside commode.

An immediate return of solution and stool will usually occur, followed by a return in spurts for up to 45 more minutes.

12. After majority of solution has returned, allow patient to clip (close) bottom of irrigating sleeve and continue with daily activities.

An immediate return of solution and stool will usually occur, followed by a return in spurts for up to 45 more minutes.

13. After solution has stopped flowing from stoma, remove irrigating sleeve and cleanse skin around stoma opening with mild soap and water. Gently pat peristomal skin dry.

Peristomal skin must be clean and free of any liquid or stool prior to application of new appliance.

continues

ACTION   **RATIONALE**

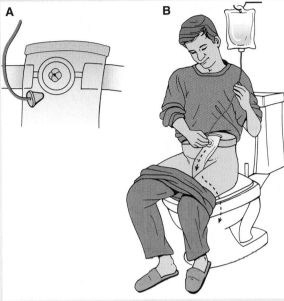

Action 9: Colostomy irrigation. **(A)** Inserting irrigation cone.
(B) Instilling irrigating fluid with sleeve in place.

14. Attach new appliance to stoma (see Skill 13-8) if
    needed.

15. Document the procedure, including the amount of irri-
    gating solution used; color, amount, and consistency of
    stool returned; condition of stoma; degree of patient
    participation; and patient's reaction to irrigation.

Patient is now done with colostomy irrigation and ready to
continue daily activities.

Documentation promotes continuity of care and enhances
communication.

> 8/1/06   0945   1,000 mL of warmed tap
> water used to irrigate colostomy. Large
> amount of pasty, dark brown stool returned.
> Patient performed procedure with small
> amount of assistance from nurse. Stoma is
> pink and moist with no signs of bleeding.
> Patient tolerated procedure without incident.
> New ostomy bag applied.—K. Sanders, RN

Action 15: Documentation.

EVALUATION   The expected outcome is achieved when the irrigation solution flows easily into the stoma
opening and irrigation solution and feces empty from ostomy into irrigating sleeve. The
patient participates in irrigation with increasing confidence and demonstrates positive coping
mechanisms.

**Unexpected Situations
and Associated
Interventions**

• *Irrigation solution is not flowing or is flowing at a slow rate:* Check clamp on tubing to
make sure that tubing is open. Gently manipulate cone in stoma; if stool or tissue is
blocking opening of cone, this may block flow of fluid. Remove cone from stoma, clean
the area, and gently reinsert.

SKILL
13-10   Collecting a Stool Specimen

A stool specimen may be ordered as a means of evaluating the feces, for example for ova, parasites, or other pathogens that may be causing diarrhea.

Equipment
- Tongue blade (two)
- Clean specimen container (or container with preservatives for ova and parasites)
- Biohazard bag

ASSESSMENT

Assess the patient's understanding of the need for the test and the requirements of the test. Ask the patient when his or her last bowel movement was, and check the patient's medical record for this information.

NURSING DIAGNOSIS

Determine the related factors for the nursing diagnoses based on the patient's current status. An appropriate nursing diagnosis may be Deficient Knowledge. Other nursing diagnoses may include Diarrhea and Anxiety.

OUTCOME IDENTIFICATION AND PLANNING

The expected outcome to achieve when collecting a stool specimen is that an uncontaminated specimen is obtained and sent to the laboratory promptly. Additional outcomes that may be appropriate include the following: the patient demonstrates ability to collect stool specimen and verbalizes a decrease in anxiety related to stool collection.

IMPLEMENTATION

ACTION	RATIONALE
1. Gather necessary equipment. Place disposable collection container (hat) in toilet or bedside commode to catch stool without urine. Instruct patient not to discard toilet paper with stool. Tell patient to call you as soon as bowel movement is completed.	Organization facilitates performance of task. Placing a container in the toilet or bedside commode aids in obtaining a clean stool specimen uncontaminated by urine. Explanation helps to alleviate anxiety and facilitate cooperation.
2. Perform hand hygiene and put on gloves.	Hand hygiene deters the spread of microorganisms. Gloves protect nurse from microorganisms in feces.
If Random Stool Collection is Needed:	
3. After patient has passed a stool, use a clean tongue blade to obtain specimen, and place it in a dry, clean, urine-free container.	Due to the nature of the testing, no preservatives are needed for the stool. The container does not have to be sterile, since stool is not sterile. To ensure accurate results, the stool should be free of urine or menstrual blood.
4. Collect as much of the stool as possible to send to the laboratory. If patient is wearing a diaper, the stool may be collected from diaper.	Different tests and laboratories require different amounts of stool. Collecting as much as possible helps to ensure that the laboratory has an adequate amount of specimen for testing.
5. Place lid on container, label with patient's data, and place container in small biohazard bag.	All specimens sent to the laboratory should include the following information: patient's name and ID number, test ordered, date and time collected, and initials of person collecting specimen. Packaging the specimen in a biohazard bag prevents the person transporting the container from coming in contact with any pathogens that may be present in stool.
6. Remove gloves from inside out.	This protects nurse from contact with any microorganisms.
7. Perform hand hygiene.	Hand hygiene deters the spread of microorganisms.
8. **Transport specimen to laboratory while stool is still warm. If immediate transport is impossible, check with laboratory personnel or policy manual as to whether refrigeration is contraindicated.**	Most tests have better results with fresh stool. Different tests may require different preparation if the test is not immediately completed. Some tests will be compromised if the stool is refrigerated.

continues

Collecting a Stool Specimen (continued)

ACTION	RATIONALE

If Stool Is Collected for Ova and Parasites:

9. Follow above steps. Do not refrigerate specimen. Some institutions require ova and parasite specimens to be placed in container filled with preservatives; check institutional policy.

Refrigeration will affect parasites. Ova and parasites are best detected in warm stool.

10. Document amount, color, and consistency of stool sent.

Documentation promotes continuity of care and communication, alerting healthcare team members that ordered test has been sent.

7/12/06   2045   *Large amount of pasty, green stool sent to laboratory for ova and parasite testing.*—K. Sanders, RN

Action 10: Documentation.

EVALUATION

The expected outcome is met when the patient passes a stool that is not contaminated by urine or menstrual blood and is placed in a clean container. The specimen is transported appropriately to the laboratory. The patient participates in stool collection and verbalizes feelings of diminished anxiety related to the procedure.

Unexpected Situations and Associated Interventions

- *Patient is menstruating or has discarded toilet paper into commode with stool:* Call laboratory to discuss possible effects on test results. Not all tests will be affected by contaminants. The laboratory may accept the specimen even with the contaminant. Make notation on order card that goes to laboratory with specimen.
- *Specimen is inadvertently left on counter instead of being sent to laboratory:* Call laboratory to discuss possible effects on test results. Not all tests will be affected by leaving the specimen on the counter for a period of time. The laboratory may accept the specimen even though it has been sitting out. Make sure that the time on the card is the actual time the specimen was obtained.

■ Developing Critical Thinking Skills

1. While you are digitally removing feces from Hugh Levens, he suddenly complains of feeling light-headed. You note that he is now diaphoretic. What should you do?
2. Isaac Greenberg is having such uncontrollable watery diarrhea that he is wearing a diaper. When you try to obtain a stool sample to test for occult blood, no stool is present due to the absorbency of the diaper. How could you obtain a sample with the next stool?
3. Maria Blakely has noted that an area of peristomal skin is becoming erythematous and excoriated. She asks you whether she should cut her ostomy bag bigger so that the adhesive does not irritate this skin. How should you reply?

Bibliography

Ahmed, D., Karch, A., & Karch, F. (2000). Hidden factors in occult blood testing. *American Journal of Nursing, 100*(12), 25.

Ball, E. (2000). Part two: A teaching guide for continent ileostomy. *RN, 63*(12), 35–40.

Black, P. (2000). Practical stoma care. *Nursing Standard, 14*(41), 47–55.

Bryant, D., & Fleischer, I. (2000). Changing an ostomy appliance. *Nursing, 30*(11), 51–55.

Erwin-Toth, P. (2001). Caring for a stoma is more than skin deep. *Nursing, 31*(5), 36–40.

Interpreting abnormal abdominal sounds. (2000). *Nursing, 30*(6), 28.

McConnell, E. (2000). Myths & facts about rectal catheters. *Nursing, 30*(1), 73.

McConnell, E. (2002). Clinical do's & don'ts: Changing an ostomy appliance. *Nursing, 32*(3), 17.

Secord, C., Jackman, M., & Wright, L. (2001). Adjusting to life with an ostomy. *Canadian Nurse, 97*(1), 29–32.

Smeltzer, S., & Bare, B. (2004). *Brunner & Suddarth's textbook of medical-surgical nursing* (10th ed.). Philadelphia: Lippincott Williams & Wilkins.

Thompson, J. (2000). Part one: A practical ostomy guide. *RN, 63*(11), 61–68.

Weeks, S., Hubbartt, S., & Michaels, T. (2000). Keys to bowel success. *Rehabilitation Nursing, 25*(2), 66–69.

Oxygenation

Focusing on Patient Care

This chapter will help you develop some of the skills related to oxygenation necessary to care for the following patients:

Scott Mingus, age 12, who has a mediastinal chest tube after thoracic surgery

Saranam Srivastava, age 35, who has chest tube after a motor vehicle accident

Paula Cunningham, age 72, who is intubated and needs to be suctioned through her endotracheal tube

Learning Outcomes

After studying this chapter the reader should be able to:

1. Use a pulse oximeter.
2. Teach a patient to use an incentive spirometer.
3. Teach a patient to use a metered-dose inhaler.
4. Administer medication via a small-volume nebulizer.
5. Collect a sputum specimen.
6. Obtain arterial blood gases.
7. Provide chest tube care.
8. Assist with chest tube removal.
9. Administer oxygen by nasal cannula.
10. Administer oxygen by mask.
11. Use an oxygen hood.
12. Use an oxygen tent.
13. Insert an oropharyngeal airway.
14. Suction the nasopharynx and oropharynx.
15. Insert a nasal airway.
16. Suction a tracheostomy.
17. Provide tracheostomy care.
18. Retape an endotracheal tube.
19. Suction an endotracheal tube using an open and closed system.
20. Collect a sputum specimen via suctioning an endotracheal tube.
21. Use a bag and mask to deliver oxygen.

Key Terms

adventitious breath sounds: abnormal breath sound heard over the lungs

alveoli: small air sacs at the end of the terminal bronchioles that are the site of gas exchange

atelectasis: incomplete expansion or collapse of a part of the lungs

bronchial breath sounds: breath sounds heard over the trachea; high in pitch and intensity, with expiration being longer than inspiration

bronchodilator: medication that relaxes contractions of smooth muscles of the bronchioles

bronchovesicular breath sounds: normal breath sounds heard over the upper anterior chest and intercostal area

cilia: microscopic hairlike projections that propel mucus toward the upper airway so that it can be expectorated

crackles: fine crackling sounds made as air moves through wet secretions in the lungs

dyspnea: difficult or labored breathing

endotracheal tube: polyvinylchloride airway that is inserted through the nose or mouth into the trachea using a laryngoscope

expiration: act of breathing out

extubation: removal of a tube (in this case an endotracheal tube)

fraction of inspired oxygen (FIO$_2$): concentration of oxygen delivered

hemothorax: blood in the pleural space around the heart

hyperventilation: condition in which there is more than the normal amount of air entering and leaving the lungs

hypoxia: inadequate amount of oxygen available to the cells

hypoventilation: decreased rate or depth of air movement into the lungs

inspiration: act of breathing in

metered-dose inhaler (MDI): device that delivers a controlled dose of medication with each compression of the canister

nasal cannula: disposable plastic device with two protruding prongs for insertion into the nostrils; used to administer oxygen

nebulizer: method of delivering medication by dispersing fine particles of medication into the deeper passages of the respiratory tract

pulse oximetry: noninvasive technique that measures the oxygen saturation (SpO$_2$) of arterial blood

pleurae: membranes that cover the lungs

pleural effusion: fluid in the pleural space

pneumothorax: air in the pleural space

spirometer: instrument used to measure lung capacity and volume; one type is used to encourage deep breathing (incentive spirometry)

subcutaneous emphysema: small pockets of air trapped in the subcutaneous tissue; usually found around chest tube insertion sites

surfactant: lipoprotein produced by the alveolar epithelium, reduces surface tension, allowing alveolar sacs to open easily

thoracentesis: aspiration of fluid or air from the pleural space

tracheostomy: curved tube inserted into an artificial opening made into the trachea; comes in varied angles and multiple sizes

ventilation: exchange of gases

vesicular breath sounds: normal sound of respiration heard on auscultation over peripheral lung areas

wheezes: continuous high-pitched squeaks or musical sounds made as air moves through a narrowed or partially obstructed airway

Most people take respiratory function for granted, but it is necessary for life. Living cells require oxygen. The air passages must remain patent (open) for oxygen to enter the system. Any condition that interferes with normal functioning must be minimized or eliminated to prevent pulmonary distress, which could lead to death.

Normal functioning depends on essentially three factors:
- The integrity of the airway system to transport air to and from the lungs
- A properly functioning alveolar system in the lungs to oxygenate venous blood and to remove carbon dioxide from the blood
- A properly functioning cardiovascular and hematologic system to carry nutrients and wastes to and from body cells

This chapter will cover the skills necessary for the nurse to promote oxygenation. Please look over the summary figures, tables, and boxes in the beginning of this chapter for a quick review of critical knowledge to assist you in understanding the skills related to oxygenation.

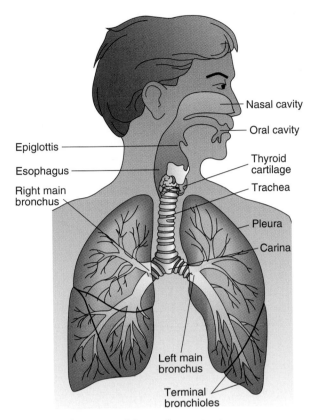

FIGURE 14-1 The organs of the respiratory tract.

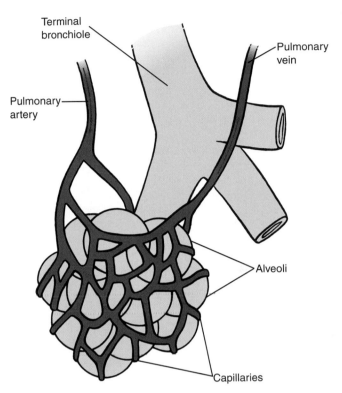

FIGURE 14-2 Alveoli and the intrapulmonary system where gas exchange occurs. The terminal bronchioles lead into the alveoli. Air in the alveoli and blood in the capillaries are separated by only a very thin partition, which is readily crossed by diffusing gases. The pulmonary artery carries unoxygenated blood to the capillaries, and the pulmonary veins return oxygenated blood to the left side of the heart.

TABLE 14-1 Respiratory Variations in the Life Cycle

	Infant (Birth–1 year)	Early Childhood (1–5 years)	Late Childhood (6–12 years)	Aged Adult (65+ years)
Respiratory rate	30–60 breaths/min	20–40 breaths/min	15–25 breaths/min	16–20 breaths/min
Respiratory pattern	Abdominal breathing, irregular in rate and depth	Abdominal breathing, irregular	Thoracic breathing, regular	Thoracic, regular
Chest wall	Thin, little muscle, ribs and sternum easily seen	Same as infant's but with more subcutaneous fat	Further subcutaneous fat deposited, structures less prominent	Thin, structures prominent
Breath sounds	Loud, harsh crackles at end of deep inspiration	Loud, harsh expiration longer than inspiration	Clear inspiration is longer than expiration	Clear
Shape of thorax	Round	Elliptical	Elliptical	Barrel shaped or elliptical

TABLE 14-2 Oxygen Delivery Systems

Method	Amount Delivered FiO2 (Fraction Inspired Oxygen)	Priority Nursing Interventions
Nasal cannula	*Low Flow* 1 L/min = 24% 2 L/min = 28% 3 L/min = 32% 4 L/min = 36% 5 L/min = 40% 6 L/min = 44%	Check frequently that both prongs are in patient's nares. Never deliver more than 2–3 L/min to patient with chronic lung disease.
Simple mask	*Low Flow* 6–10 L/min = 35%–60% (5 L/min is minimum setting)	Monitor patient frequently to check placement of the mask. Support patient if claustrophobia is a concern. Secure physician's order to replace mask with nasal cannula during meal time.
Partial rebreather mask	*Low Flow* 6–15 L/min = 70%–90%	Set flow rate so that mask remains two thirds full during inspiration. Keep reservoir bag free of twists or kinks.
Nonrebreather mask	*Low Flow* 6–15 L/min = 60%–100%	Maintain flow rate so reservoir bag collapses only slightly during inspiration. Check that valves and rubber flaps are functioning properly (open during expiration and closed during inhalation). Monitor SaO2 with pulse oximeter.
Venturi mask	*High Flow* 4–10 L/min = 24%–55%	Requires careful monitoring to verify FiO2 at flow rate ordered. Check that air intake valves are not blocked.

BOX 14-1 Arterial Blood Gas Results

pH Acidotic <7.35–7.45>
Alkalotic
CO_2 Alkalotic <35–45 mm Hg>
Acidotic

HCO_3 Acidotic <22–26 mEq/L>
Alkalotic

BOX 14-2 Interpreting ABGs

1. Is pH acidic or alkalotic?
   <7.35 acidic
   >7.40 alkalotic
2. Is CO_2 higher or lower than normal? (respiratory component)
   <35 lower (alkalotic)
   >45 higher (acidic)
3. Is HCO_3 higher or lower than normal? (metabolic component)
   <22 lower (acidic)
   >26 higher (alkalotic)
4. Look at the results from Step 2 and 3. The cause for the change in pH will match up with the pH. If the pH is acidic and the CO_2 is higher (acidic) with a higher HCO_3 (alkalotic), then the cause for the change in the pH is the CO_2 or respiratory acidosis. If the pH is alkalotic and the CO_2 is normal with a higher HCO_3 (alkalotic), then the cause for the change in the pH is the HCO_3 or metabolic alkalosis.
5. Check for compensation.

   If the pH is out of the 7.35 to 7.45 range, and either the CO_2 or the HCO_3 is outside normal limits with the other component (CO_2 or HCO_3) within normal limits, the patient is not compensating. The body has not reached the point where it is attempting to put the pH back into the normal range.

7.32 pH (acidic), 48 CO_2 (acidic), 24 HCO_3 (normal) = respiratory acidosis without compensation
7.49 pH (alkalotic), 38 CO_2 (normal), 30 HCO_3 (alkalotic) = metabolic alkalosis without compensation

If the pH is out of the 7.35 to 7.45 range, with the CO_2 and the HCO_3 outside normal limits, the patient is attempting to compensate. The body has reached the point where it is attempting to put the pH back into the normal range, but since the pH is not back within its normal range, this is referred to as partial compensation.

7.30 pH (acidic), 32 CO_2 (alkalotic), 18 HCO_3 (acidic) = metabolic acidosis with partial compensation
7.48 pH (alkalotic), 30 CO_2 (alkalotic), 18 HCO_3 (acidic) = respiratory alkalosis with partial compensation

If the pH is within normal limits (7.35 to 7.45) and both the CO_2 and the HCO_3 are outside their normal ranges, the patient is in total compensation. In the case you would use 7.40 as the cutoff point (<7.40 acidic, >7.40 alkalotic).

7.37 pH (acidic), 48 CO_2 (acidic), 28 HCO_3 (alkalotic) = respiratory acidosis with total compensation
7.42 pH (alkalotic), 48 CO_2 (acidic), 29 HCO_3 (alkalotic) = metabolic alkalosis with total compensation

SKILL 14-1 — Using a Pulse Oximeter

The pulse oximeter is a noninvasive way of monitoring the oxygen saturation of arterial blood.

Equipment

- Pulse oximeter with probe
- Nail polish remover (if necessary)

ASSESSMENT

Assess the patient's skin temperature and color, including the color of the nail beds. Temperature is a good indicator of blood flow. Warm skin indicates adequate circulation. In a well-oxygenated patient, the skin and nail beds are usually pink. Skin that is bluish or dusky indicates hypoxia. Also check capillary refill: prolonged capillary refill indicates a reduction in blood flow. Auscultate the lungs. Patients with clear lung sounds are expected to have a higher saturation than patients with coarse or wheezing lung sounds.

NURSING DIAGNOSIS

Determine the related factors for the nursing diagnosis based on the patient's current status. Appropriate nursing diagnoses may include:

- Ineffective Tissue Perfusion
- Impaired Gas Exchange
- Ineffective Airway Clearance
- Activity Intolerance

Other nursing diagnoses also may require the use of this skill, such as Decreased Cardiac Output, Excess Fluid Volume, Anxiety, and Risk for Aspiration.

OUTCOME IDENTIFICATION AND PLANNING

The expected outcome to achieve when caring for a patient with a pulse oximeter is that the patient will exhibit arterial blood oxygen saturation within acceptable parameters, or greater than 95%.

IMPLEMENTATION

ACTION	RATIONALE
1. Explain procedure to patient.	Explanation relieves anxiety and facilitates cooperation.
2. Perform hand hygiene.	Hand hygiene deters the spread of microorganisms.
3. Select an adequate site for application of the sensor.	
a. Use the patient's index, middle, or ring finger.	a. Inadequate circulation can interfere with the oxygen saturation (SpO_2) reading.

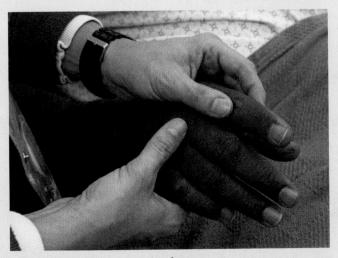

Action 3a: Selecting an appropriate finger.

continues

SKILL 14-1   Using a Pulse Oximeter (continued)

ACTION

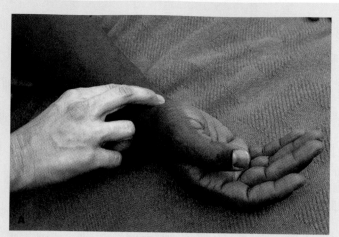

Action 3b: Assessing pulse.

RATIONALE

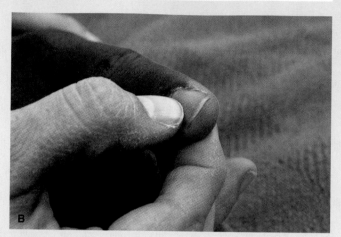

Action 3b: Assessing capillary refill.

b. Check the proximal pulse and capillary refill at the pulse closest to the site.

c. If circulation at site is inadequate, consider using the earlobe or bridge of nose.

d. Use a toe only if lower extremity circulation is not compromised.

4. Use proper equipment:

a. If one finger is too large for the probe, use a smaller one. A pediatric probe may be used for a small adult.

b. Use probes appropriate for patient's age and size.

c. Check if patient is allergic to adhesive. A nonadhesive finger clip or reflectance sensor is available.

5. Prepare the monitoring site:

a. Cleanse the selected area and allow it to dry.

b. Remove nail polish and artificial nails after checking manufacturer's instructions.

6. **Apply probe securely to skin. Make sure that the light-emitting sensor and the light-receiving sensor are aligned opposite each other (not necessary to check if placed on forehead or bridge of nose).**

7. Connect the sensor probe to the pulse oximeter and check operation of the equipment (audible beep, fluctuation of bar of light or waveform on face of oximeter).

8. Set alarms on pulse oximeter. Check manufacturer's alarm limits for high and low pulse rate settings.

b. Brisk capillary refill and a strong pulse indicate that circulation to the site is adequate.

c. These alternate sites are highly vascular alternatives.

d. Peripheral vascular disease is common in lower extremities.

a. Inaccurate readings can result if probe or sensor is not attached correctly.

b. Probes come in adult, pediatric, and infant sizes.

c. A reaction may occur if patient is allergic to adhesive substance.

Skin oils, dirt, or grime on the site, polish, and artificial nails can interfere with the passage of light waves.

Secure attachment and proper alignment promote satisfactory operation of the equipment and accurate recording of the SpO_2.

Audible beep represents the arterial pulse, and fluctuating waveform indicates the strength of the pulse. A weak signal will produce an inaccurate recording of the SpO_2. Tone of beep reflects SpO_2 reading. If SpO_2 drops, tone becomes lower in pitch.

Alarm provides additional safeguard and signals when high or low limits have been surpassed.

continues

ACTION   RATIONALE

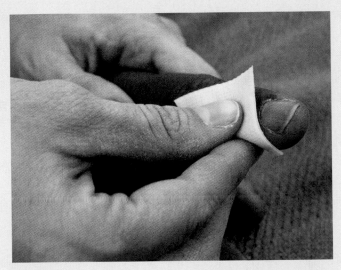

Action 5: Cleaning the area.

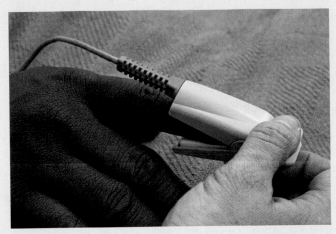

Action 6: Attaching probe to patient's finger.

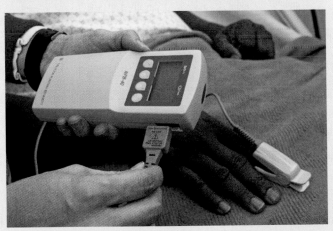

Action 7: Connecting sensor probe to unit.

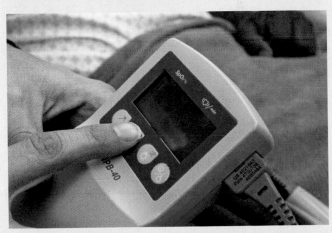

Action 8: Checking alarms.

9. **Check oxygen saturation at regular intervals as ordered by physician and signaled by alarms. Monitor hemoglobin level.**

Monitoring SpO_2 provides ongoing assessment of patient's condition. A low hemoglobin level may be satisfactorily saturated yet inadequate to meet a patient's oxygen needs.

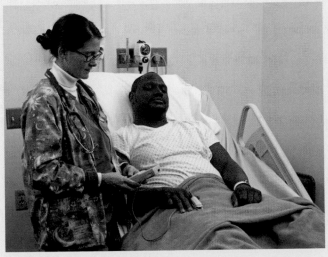

Action 9: Reading pulse oximeter.

continues

ACTION

RATIONALE

10. Remove sensor on a regular basis and check for skin irritation or signs of pressure (every 2 hours for spring tension sensor or every 4 hours for adhesive finger or toe sensor).

Prolonged pressure may lead to tissue necrosis. Adhesive sensor may cause skin irritation.

11. Evaluate any malfunctions or problems with equipment.

   a. For absent or weak signal, check vital signs and patient condition. If satisfactory, check connections and circulation to site.

   a. Hypotension makes an accurate recording difficult. Equipment (restraint, blood pressure cuff) may compromise circulation to site and cause venous blood to pulsate, giving an inaccurate reading. If extremity is cold, cover with a warm blanket.

   b. For inaccurate reading, check prescribed medications and history of circulatory disorders. Try device on a healthy person to see if problem is equipment-related or patient-related.

   b. Drugs that cause vasoconstriction interfere with accurate recording of oxygen saturation.

   c. If bright light (sunlight or fluorescent light) is suspected of causing equipment malfunction, cover probe with a dry washcloth.

   c. Bright light can interfere with operation of light sensors and cause unreliable report.

12. Document and report SpO_2 appropriately.

Documentation ensures continuity of care and ongoing assessment record.

> 9/03/06   Pulse oximeter placed on right hand; reading 98% on 2 L via nasal cannula.
> —C. Bausler, RN

Action 12: Documentation.

EVALUATION

The expected outcome is met when the patient exhibits an oxygen saturation level of 95% or greater and heart rate that correlates with the pulse.

Special Considerations

• Portable units are available for use in the home or an outpatient setting.

Infant and Child Considerations

• For infants, the oximeter probe may be placed on the foot.

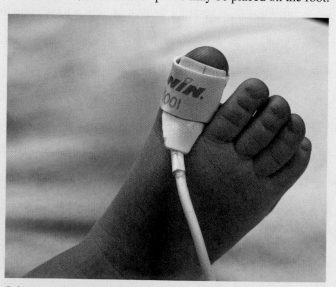

Oximetry probe on infant's foot.

SKILL
14-2

Teaching Patient to Use an Incentive Spirometer

Incentive spirometry keeps the alveoli from collapsing so that gas exchange can occur and secretions can be cleared and expectorated. This intervention offers immediate positive reinforcement to the patient for his or her breathing efforts.

Equipment
- Incentive spirometer

ASSESSMENT
Assess the patient for pain and prepare to administer pain medication if deep breathing may cause pain. Assess lung sounds to establish a baseline and determine the effectiveness of incentive spirometry. Incentive spirometry encourages patients to take deep breaths; lung sounds may be diminished before using the incentive spirometer. Assess oxygen saturation, which may increase due to alveoli inflation.

NURSING DIAGNOSIS
Determine the related factors for the nursing diagnosis based on the patient's current status. Appropriate nursing diagnoses may include:

- Ineffective Breathing Pattern
- Impaired Gas Exchange
- Acute Pain
- Activity Intolerance
- Risk for Injury
- Risk for Infection
- Deficient Knowledge

Other nursing diagnoses may require the use of this skill.

OUTCOME IDENTIFICATION AND PLANNING
The expected outcome to achieve when instructing a patient in using the incentive spirometer is that the patient will demonstrate increased lung expansion with clear breath sounds. Other outcomes that may be appropriate include the following: patient demonstrates increased oxygen saturation level, patient reports adequate control of pain during use, and patient demonstrates steps for use of spirometer.

IMPLEMENTATION

ACTION	RATIONALE
1. Perform hand hygiene.	Hand hygiene deters the spread of microorganisms.
2. Assist patient to an upright or semi-Fowler's position if possible. Remove dentures if they fit poorly. Administer pain medication if needed. **If patient has recently undergone abdominal surgery, place a pillow over the abdomen for splinting.**	Upright position facilitates lung expansion. Dentures may inhibit patient from taking deep breaths if patient is concerned that dentures may fall out. Pain may decrease patient's ability to take deep breaths. Deep breaths may cause patient to cough.
3. Demonstrate how to steady the device with one hand and hold mouthpiece with other hand. If patient cannot use hands, nurse may assist patient with the incentive spirometer.	This allows the patient to remain upright, visualize the volume of each breath, and stabilize the device.
4. Instruct patient to exhale normally and then place lips securely around the mouthpiece.	Patient should fully empty lungs so that maximum volume may be inhaled.
5. **Instruct patient to inhale slowly and as deeply as possible through the mouthpiece without using nose (if desired, a nose clip may be used).**	Inhaling through the nose would provide an inaccurate measurement of inhalation volume.
6. **Tell patient to hold breath and count to three.** Check position of gauge to determine progress and level attained. If patient begins to cough, use pillow to help splint patient's abdomen.	Holding breath for 3 seconds helps the alveoli to re-expand. Volume on incentive spirometry should increase with practice.

continues

SKILL 14-2 Teaching Patient to Use an Incentive Spirometer (continued)

ACTION   **RATIONALE**

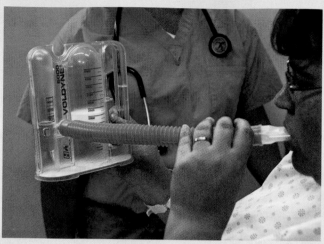

Action 5: Patient using incentive spirometer.

ACTION	RATIONALE
7. Instruct patient to remove lips from mouthpiece and exhale normally. **If patient becomes light-headed during the process, tell him or her to stop and take a few normal breaths before resuming incentive spirometry.**	Deep breaths may change the CO_2 level, leading to light-headedness.
8. Encourage patient to do incentive spirometry 5 to 10 times every 1 to 2 hours if possible.	This helps to re-inflate the alveoli and prevent atelectasis due to hypoventilation.
9. Document that incentive spirometry was done, number of repetitions, and average volume. If patient coughs, document whether cough is productive or nonproductive. If cough is productive, document consistency, amount, and color of sputum.	This provides accurate documentation and provides for comprehensive care.

> 9/8/06   Incentive spirometry performed × 10, volume 1,500 mL obtained; patient with nonproductive cough during incentive spirometry.—C. Bausler, RN

Action 9: Documentation.

EVALUATION

The expected outcome is met when the patient demonstrates the steps for use correctly and exhibits improved lung sounds that are clear and equal in all lobes. In addition, the patient demonstrates an increase in oxygen saturation levels and verbalizes the importance of and need for incentive spirometry.

Unexpected Situations and Associated Interventions

- *Patient tells you he or she has done incentive spirometry before you entered the room:* If you don't believe that the patient is doing incentive spirometry, auscultate lung sounds. The patient will need to take 6 to 10 deep breaths during the auscultation.
- *Volume inhaled is decreasing:* Assess patient's pain and anxiety level. Patient may have pain and not be inhaling fully, or patient may have experienced pain previously during incentive spirometry and have an increased anxiety level. If ordered, medicate patient when pain is present. Discuss fears with patient and encourage him or her to inhale fully or to increase the volume by 100 each time incentive spirometry is performed.
- *Patient attempts to blow into incentive spirometer:* Compare the incentive spirometer to a straw. Remind patient to inhale before beginning each time.

Instructing Patient to Use a Metered-Dose Inhaler (MDI)

Many medications to help with respiratory problems may be delivered via the respiratory system. A metered-dose inhaler (MDI) allows the medication to be absorbed rapidly through the lung tissue, reducing systemic side effects.

Equipment

- Medication
- Spacing mechanism or holding chamber (optional)

ASSESSMENT

Assess patient's lung sounds. Frequently patients will have wheezes or coarse lung sounds before medication administration. If ordered, assess oxygen saturation level before medication administration. The oxygenation level will usually increase after the medication is administered. Assess patient's ability to manage an MDI; young and older patients may have dexterity problems.

NURSING DIAGNOSIS

Determine related factors for the nursing diagnosis based on the patient's current status. Appropriate nursing diagnoses may include:

- Ineffective Airway Clearance
- Ineffective Breathing Pattern
- Impaired Gas Exchange
- Deficient Knowledge
- Risk for Activity Intolerance

OUTCOME IDENTIFICATION AND PLANNING

The expected outcome to achieve when using an MDI is that the patient receives the medication. Other outcomes that may be appropriate include the following: patient demonstrates improved lung expansion and breath sounds; respiratory status is within acceptable parameters; and patient demonstrates correct use of MDI.

IMPLEMENTATION

ACTION	RATIONALE
1. Explain procedure to patient.	Explanation relieves anxiety and facilitates cooperation.
2. Perform hand hygiene.	Hand hygiene deters the spread of microorganisms.

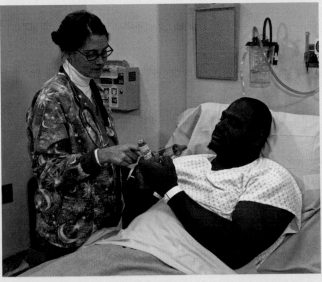

Action 1: Talking with patient about MDI.

continues

SKILL 14-3   Instructing Patient to Use a Metered-Dose Inhaler (MDI) (continued)

ACTION	RATIONALE
3. **Remove the mouthpiece cover and shake inhaler well.**	The medication and propellant may separate when the canister is not in use. Shaking well ensures that the patient is receiving the correct dosage of medication.

Spacer Technique

4. Attach the mouthpiece of the inhaler to the spacer.	Use of a spacer is preferred because it can deliver higher amounts of the medication.
5. Instruct patient to take a deep breath and exhale. Have patient place the spacer's mouthpiece into mouth, grasping securely with teeth and lips. Have patient inhale slowly and deeply through the mouth. **Depress the canister (actuator) about one fourth or one third of the way through the inspiration.**	The patient should exhale as much as possible so that he or she can take a larger amount of air in. The spacer will hold the medication in suspension for a short period so that the patient can receive more of the prescribed medication than if it had been projected into the air.

Non-Spacer Technique

6. Have patient hold the inhaler 1″ to 2″ in front of open mouth, or have patient place mouthpiece into mouth, grasping it securely with teeth and lips (closed mouth). Instruct patient to take a deep breath and exhale. Have the patient inhale slowly and deeply through the mouth. Press down on the medication canister while continuing to inhale a full breath.	The open-mouth technique helps to prevent some of the medication from being lost in the oral cavity. The closed-mouth technique should not be used with oral steroids due to the risk of thrush infections.

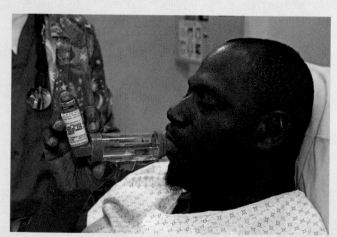

Action 5: Using an MDI with a spacer.

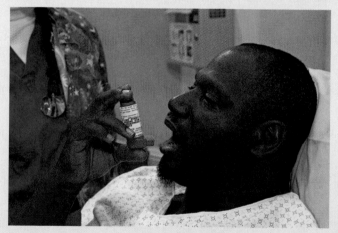

Action 6: Preparing to use an MDI without spacer.

7. **Instruct patient to hold the breath for 5 to 10 seconds, or as long as possible, and then to exhale slowly through pursed lips.**	This allows a longer absorption time for the medication.
8. **Wait 1 to 5 minutes before administering the next puff.**	This ensures that both puffs are absorbed as much as possible.
9. After the prescribed amount of puffs has been administered, have patient remove spacer (if used) and replace the cap on the mouthpiece.	By replacing the cap, the patient is preventing any dust or dirt from entering the inhaler and being propelled into the bronchioles.
10. **Reassess lung sounds, oxygenation saturation if ordered, and respirations.**	Lung sounds and oxygenation saturation may improve after MDI use. Respirations may decrease after MDI use.

continues

Instructing Patient to Use a Metered-Dose Inhaler (MDI) (continued)

ACTION	RATIONALE
11. Perform hand hygiene.	Hand hygiene deters the spread of microorganisms.
12. Document respiratory rate, oxygen saturation, and lung sounds.	Documentation ensures continuity of care and ongoing assessment record.

9/29/06   Wheezes noted in all lobes of lungs before albuterol MDI, O_2 saturation 92%, respiratory rate 24 breaths per minute. After albuterol treatment, lung sounds are clear and equal in all lobes, O_2 saturation 97%, respiratory rate 18 breaths per minute.
—C. Bausler, RN

Action 12: Documentation.

EVALUATION

The expected outcome is met when the patient demonstrates improved lung sounds and ease of breathing. In addition, patient demonstrates correct use of MDI and verbalizes correct information about medication therapy associated with MDI use.

Unexpected Situations and Associated Interventions

- *Patient uses MDI, but symptoms are not relieved:* Check to make sure that the inhaler still contains medication. The patient may have received only propellant, without medication.
- *Patient is unable to use MDI:* Many companies have adaptive devices that allow patients to use MDIs.
- *Patient reports that relief of symptoms has decreased, even with increased number of puffs:* Have patient demonstrate technique that he or she is using. Many patients develop poor habits over time. Poor administration technique can lead to a decrease in effectiveness and a need for an increased dosage of medication.

Special Considerations

- Spacers and inhalers should be cleaned at least weekly with warm water or soaked in a vinegar solution (1 pint of water to 2 oz vinegar) for 20 minutes. Rinse with clean water and allow to air-dry.
- If the medication being administered is a steroid, the patient should rinse the mouth with water after administration to prevent a thrush infection.
- Patients should know how to tell when medication levels are getting low. The most reliable method is to look on the canister and see how many puffs the canister contains. Divide this number by the number of puffs used daily to ascertain how many days the MDI will last. For instance, if the MDI contains 200 puffs and the patient takes 6 puffs per day, the MDI should last for 33 days. The flotation method is also used, but it is not reliable. The patient places the medication canister into a bowl of water. If the canister is full, it will sink to the bottom; if it is empty, it will float horizontally on the top of the water; if it is half-full, it will float vertically. To protect the ozone layer, all MDIs are changing the type of propellant used. The flotation method may not work with the new inhalers.

Infant and Child Considerations

- Young children usually require a spacer to use an MDI.
- Many medications can also be administered as a nebulizer (see Skill 14-4).

SKILL 14-4   Administering Medication Via a Small-Volume Nebulizer

Many medications to help with respiratory problems may be delivered via the respiratory system using a small-volume nebulizer. As with MDIs, medications are absorbed rapidly through the lung tissue, reducing the risk for systemic effects.

Equipment

- Medication
- Nebulizing tubing and chamber
- Air compressor or oxygen hookup
- Sterile saline (if not premeasured)

ASSESSMENT

Assess patient's lung sounds as a baseline to determine effectiveness of therapy. Often patients have wheezes or coarse lung sounds before medication administration. If ordered, assess patient's oxygenation saturation level before medication administration. The oxygenation level will usually increase after the medication has been administered.

NURSING DIAGNOSIS

Determine related factors for the nursing diagnosis based on the patient's current status. Appropriate nursing diagnoses may include:

- Deficient Knowledge
- Ineffective Airway Clearance
- Risk for Activity Intolerance
- Ineffective Breathing Pattern
- Impaired Gas Exchange

OUTCOME IDENTIFICATION AND PLANNING

The expected outcome to achieve when administering medication via a small-volume nebulizer is that the patient receives the medication. Other outcomes that may be appropriate include the following: patient exhibits improved lung sounds and respiratory effort; patient demonstrates steps for use of nebulizer and understanding of the need for the medication regimen.

IMPLEMENTATION

ACTION	RATIONALE
1. Explain procedure to patient.	Explanation relieves anxiety and facilitates cooperation.
2. Perform hand hygiene.	Hand hygiene deters the spread of microorganisms.
3. Gather equipment. Check physician's order for medication.	The physician's order is the legal record of medication orders for each agency.
4. Remove the nebulizer cup from the device and open it. Place premeasured unit-dose medication in the bottom section of the cup or use a dropper to place concentrated dose of medication in cup and add prescribed fluid to dilute it.	To get enough volume to make a fine mist, normal saline must be added to the concentrated medication.
5. Screw the top portion of the nebulizer cup back in place and attach the cup to the nebulizer. Attach one end of tubing to the stem on the bottom of the nebulizer cuff and the other end to the air compressor or oxygen source.	Air or oxygen must be forced through the nebulizer to form a fine mist.

continues

Administrating Medication Via a Small-Volume Nebulizer (continued)

ACTION	RATIONALE

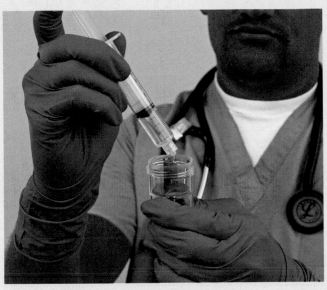

Action 4: Putting medication into nebulizer chamber.

6. Turn on the air compressor or oxygen. Check that a fine medication mist is produced by opening the valve. Have patient place mouthpiece into mouth and grasp securely with teeth and lips.

If there is no fine mist, make sure that medication has been added to the cup and that the tubing is connected to the air compressor or oxygen outlet. Adjust flow meter if necessary.

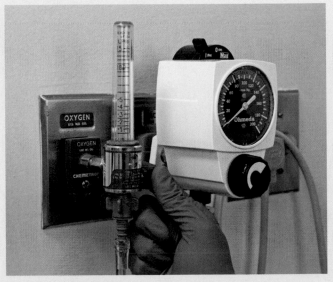

Action 6: Adjust flow rate.

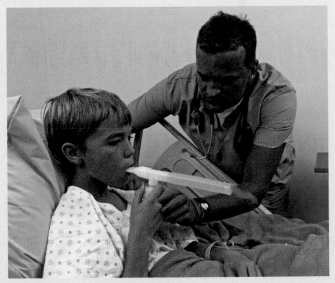

Action 6: Using nebulizer for treatment.

continues

ACTION	RATIONALE
7. **Instruct patient to inhale slowly through the mouth (a nose clip may be necessary if patient is also breathing through nose). Hold each breath for 5 to 10 seconds, or as long as possible, before exhaling.**	While the patient inhales and holds the breath, the medication comes in contact with the respiratory tissue and is absorbed. The longer the breath is held, the more medication can be absorbed.
8. **Continue this inhalation technique until all medication in the nebulizer cup has been aerosolized (usually about 15 minutes). Once the fine mist decreases in amount, gently flick the sides of the nebulizer cup.**	Once the fine mist stops, the medication is no longer being aerosolized. By gently flicking the cup sides, any medication that is stuck to the sides is knocked into the bottom of the cup, where it can become aerosolized.
9. If desired, have the patient gargle with tap water after using nebulizer. Rinse the equipment in warm water and allow to air-dry on a clean towel.	The buildup of medication can affect how the medication is delivered as well as attract bacteria.
10. **Reassess lung sounds, oxygenation saturation if ordered, and respirations.**	Lung sounds and oxygenation saturation may improve after nebulizer use. Respirations may decrease after nebulizer use.
11. Clean equipment in warm water. Perform hand hygiene.	Hand hygiene deters the spread of microorganisms.
12. Document respiratory rate, oxygen saturation, and lung sounds.	Documentation ensures continuity of care and ongoing assessment record.

> 9/29/06   0900   Lung sounds before al-
> buterol nebulizer were wheezes all lobes, O_2 sat-
> uration 92%, respiratory rate 24 breaths per
> minute. After albuterol treatment, lung
> sounds are clear and equal in all lobes, O_2 sat-
> uration 97%, respiratory rate 18 breaths per
> minute.—C. Bausler, RN

Action 5: Documentation.

EVALUATION

The expected outcome is met when the patient receives the medication and exhibits improved lungs sounds and respiratory effort. In addition, the patient demonstrates correct steps for use and verbalizes an understanding of the need for the medication.

Unexpected Situations and Associated Interventions

- *Patient reports that nebulizer doesn't smell or taste the way it usually does:* Double-check to make sure that medication was added to nebulizer cup.

Infant and Child Considerations

- A small child may use a mask instead of a mouthpiece.

SKILL
14-5

Collecting a Sputum Specimen

A sputum specimen may be ordered if a bacterial, viral, or fungal infection of the pulmonary system is suspected.

Equipment
- Sterile sputum specimen container
- Disposable gloves
- Goggles or safety glasses

ASSESSMENT
Assess patient's lung sounds. Patients with a productive cough may have coarse, wheezing, or diminished lung sounds. Monitor oxygen saturation levels, because patients with excessive pulmonary secretions may have decreased oxygen saturation. Assess patient's level of pain. Consider administering pain medication before obtaining the sample, since patient will have to cough.

NURSING DIAGNOSIS
Determine the related factors for the nursing diagnosis based on the patient's current status. Appropriate nursing diagnoses may include:
- Risk for Infection
- Acute Pain
- Ineffective Airway Clearance

OUTCOME IDENTIFICATION AND PLANNING
The expected outcome to achieve when collecting a sputum specimen is that the patient produces an adequate sample from the lungs. Other outcomes that may be appropriate include the following: airway patency is maintained; oxygen saturation increases; patient demonstrates understanding about the need for specimen collection; and patient demonstrates improved respiratory status.

IMPLEMENTATION

ACTION	RATIONALE
1. Explain procedure to patient. If patient may have pain with coughing, administer pain medication if ordered. If patient can perform task without assistance after instruction, leave container at bedside with instructions to call nurse as soon as specimen is produced.	This provides reassurance and promotes cooperation.
2. Assemble equipment.	This provides for organized approach.
3. Perform hand hygiene.	Hand hygiene deters the spread of microorganisms.
4. Don disposable gloves and goggles.	The gloves and goggles prevent the spread of pathogens to the nurse.
5. Adjust bed to comfortable working position. Lower side rail closer to you. Place patient in semi-Fowler's position. **Have patient rinse mouth with water before beginning procedure.**	The semi-Fowler's position will help the patient to cough and expectorate the sputum specimen. Water will rinse the oral cavity of any food particles.
6. **Instruct patient to inhale deeply and cough.** If patient has had abdominal surgery, assist patient to splint abdomen.	The specimen will need to come from the lungs; saliva is not acceptable. Splinting helps to reduce the pain in the abdominal incision.
7. If patient produces sputum, open the lid to the container and have patient expectorate specimen into container.	The specimen needs to come from the lungs; saliva is not acceptable.
8. If patient believes he or she can produce more specimen, have patient repeat the procedure.	This gives the laboratory more specimen to work with.

continues

ACTION	**RATIONALE**
9. Close lid to container. Offer oral hygiene to patient.	Oral hygiene helps to remove pathogens from the oral cavity.
10. Remove gloves. Perform hand hygiene.	Hand hygiene deters the spread of microorganisms.
11. Label container with patient's name, time specimen was collected, any antibiotics administered within the past 24 hours, route of collection, and any other information required by agency policy.	This helps the laboratory to log the specimen correctly.
12. Record the time the specimen was collected and sent and the nature and amount of secretions. Note the character of patient's respirations before and after sputum collection. Note on the laboratory request form any antibiotics administered in the past 24 hours.	This provides accurate documentation and provides for comprehensive care.

> 9/13/06   1015   *Sputum specimen ob-*
> *tained; patient has moderate amount of*
> *thick, yellow sputum; specimen sent to lab for*
> *culture and sensitivity.*—C. Bausler, RN

Action 12: Documentation.

EVALUATION

The expected outcome is met when the patient expectorates sputum and it is collected in a sterile container and sent to the laboratory as soon as possible. In addition, the patient maintains a patent airway and demonstrates understanding about the rationale for the specimen collection.

Unexpected Situations and Associated Interventions

- *Patient produced a specimen but did not tell you, so you don't know how long the specimen has been sitting at the bedside:* Phone laboratory and ask if a new specimen should be obtained. Most specimens should be sent to the laboratory as soon as possible to ensure that pathogens have not been affected.
- *Patient spits saliva into container, without specimen from lungs:* Instruct patient that specimen needs to come from the lungs. Discard contaminated container and place new container at the bedside.

Special Considerations

- If nasopharyngeal suctioning is required to obtain a specimen, see Skill 14-14, with the following additions. Connect the specimen container to the tubing during Action 7e. Do not flush catheter with normal saline unless <1 mL is in the container.

Drawing Arterial Blood Gases

Arterial blood gases (ABGs) are obtained to determine the adequacy of oxygenation and ventilation and to assess acid–base status. The most common site for sampling arterial blood is the radial artery; other arteries may be used, but most institutions require a physician's order to obtain the sample from another artery.

ABG analysis evaluates ventilation by measuring blood pH and the partial pressures of arterial oxygen (PaO_2) and partial pressure of arterial carbon dioxide ($PaCO_2$). Blood pH measurement reveals the blood's acid–base balance. PaO_2 indicates the amount of oxygen that the lungs deliver to the blood, and $PaCO_2$ indicates the lungs' capacity to eliminate carbon dioxide. ABG samples can also be analyzed for oxygen content and saturation and for bicarbonate values. A respiratory technician or specially trained nurse can collect most ABG samples, but a physician usually performs collection from the femoral artery. An Allen's test should always be performed before sticking the radial artery to determine whether the ulnar artery delivers sufficient blood to the hand and fingers in case there is damage to the radial artery during the blood draw.

Equipment

- ABG kit, *or* heparinized 10-mL syringe with 22G 1″ needle attached
  If syringe is not heparinized:
  - 10-mL glass syringe
  - 20G 1 ¼″ needle
  - 22G 1″ needle
  - 1-mL ampule of aqueous heparin (1:1,000)
  - Cap for hub of syringe (or rubber stopper for needle)
  - 2″ × 2″ gauze pad
  - Band-Aid
  - Alcohol or povidone–iodine wipes
  - Label
- Cup or bag of ice
- Gloves
- Laboratory request form
- Rolled towel

ASSESSMENT

Review the patient's medical record and plan of care for information about the need for an ABG. Assess the patient's cardiac status, including heart rate, blood pressure, and auscultation of heart sounds. Also assess the patient's respiratory status, including respiratory rate, excursion, lung sounds, and use of oxygen, including the amount being used, if ordered. Determine the adequacy of peripheral blood flow to the extremity to be used by performing the Allen's test. If Allen's test reveals no or little collateral circulation to the hand, do not perform an arterial stick to that artery. Assess the patient's radial pulse. If you are unable to palpate the radial pulse, consider using the other wrist.

Assess the patient's understanding about the need for specimen collection. Ask the patient if he or she has ever felt faint, sweaty, or nauseated when having blood drawn.

NURSING DIAGNOSIS

Determine the related factors for the nursing diagnoses based on the patient's current status. Appropriate nursing diagnoses may include:

- Acute Pain
- Risk for Injury
- Impaired Gas Exchange
- Decreased Cardiac Output
- Ineffective Airway Clearance
- Anxiety
- Fear

Many other nursing diagnoses may require the use of this skill.

continues

OUTCOME IDENTIFICATION AND PLANNING

The expected outcome to achieve when obtaining an ABG specimen is the blood is obtained from the artery without damage to the artery. Other outcomes that may be appropriate include: the patient will experience minimal pain and anxiety during the procedure and the patient demonstrates understanding of the need for the ABG specimen.

IMPLEMENTATION

ACTION	RATIONALE
1. Check the patient's identification and confirm the patient's identity. Tell the patient you need to collect an arterial blood sample, and explain the procedure. Tell the patient that the needlestick will cause some discomfort but that he or she must remain still during the procedure. Check the chart to make sure the patient hasn't been suctioned within the past 15 minutes.	Explanation facilitates cooperation and provides reassurance for patient. Suctioning may change the oxygen saturation and is a temporary change not to be confused with baseline for the patient.
2. Gather equipment and provide privacy. Label the syringe clearly with the patient's name and room number, the physician's name, the date and time of collection, and initials of the person performing the ABG. If not already done, heparinize the syringe and needle:	This provides for an organized approach to the task. Heparinizing the syringe and needle prevents the sample from clotting.
a. Attach the 20G needle to the syringe; open the ampule of heparin and withdraw all the heparin into the syringe.	
b. Hold the syringe upright and pull the plunger back slowly to about the 7-mL mark. Rotate the barrel while pulling the plunger back to allow the heparin to coat the inside surface of the syringe. Then slowly force the heparin toward the hub of the syringe and expel all but about 0.1 mL of the heparin.	
c. To heparinize the needle, first replace the 20G needle with the 22G needle. Then hold the syringe upright, tilt it slightly, and eject the remaining heparin.	
3. Perform hand hygiene.	Hand hygiene deters the spread of microorganisms.
4. If the patient is on bed rest, ask him or her to lie in a supine position, with the head slightly elevated and the arms at the sides. Ask the ambulatory patient to sit in a chair and support the arm securely on an armrest or a table. Place a waterproof pad under the site and a rolled towel under the wrist.	Positioning the patient comfortably helps minimize anxiety. Using a rolled towel under the wrist provide for easy access to the insertion site.
5. **Perform Allen's test prior to obtaining a specimen from the radial artery:**	Allen's testing assesses patency of the ulnar and radial arteries.
a. Have the patient clench the wrist to minimize blood flow into the hand.	
b. Using your index and middle fingers, press on the radial and ulnar arteries. Hold this position for a few seconds.	

continues

Drawing Arterial Blood Gases (continued)

ACTION	RATIONALE
c. Without removing your fingers from the arteries, ask the patient to unclench the fist and hold the hand in a relaxed position. The palm will be blanched because pressure from your fingers has impaired the normal blood flow.	
d. Release pressure on the ulnar artery. If the hand becomes flushed, which indicates that blood is filling the vessels, it is safe to proceed with the radial artery puncture. If the hand doesn't flush, perform the test on the other arm.	
6. Perform hand hygiene again and put on gloves.	Hand hygiene and gloving deter the spread of micro-organisms.
7. Locate the radial artery and lightly palpate it for a strong pulse.	If you push too hard during palpation, the radial artery will be obliterated and hard to palpate.
8. Clean the site with an alcohol or povidone–iodine pad (if the patient is not allergic). **Don't wipe off the povidone–iodine with alcohol, because alcohol cancels the effect of povidone–iodine.** Wipe in a circular motion, spiraling outward from the center of the site. If using alcohol, apply it with friction for 30 seconds or until the final pad comes away clean. Allow the skin to dry.	Site cleansing prevents potentially infectious skin flora from being introduced into the vessel during the procedure.
9. Stabilize the hand with the wrist extended over the rolled towel. Palpate the artery with the index and middle fingers of one hand while holding the syringe over the puncture site with the other hand. **Do not directly touch the area to be stuck.**	Stabilizing the hand and palpating the artery with one hand while holding the syringe in the other provides better access to the artery. Palpating the area to be stuck would contaminate the clean area.
10. Hold the needle bevel up at a 45-degree angle at the site of maximal pulse impulse and the shaft parallel to the path of the artery. (When puncturing the brachial artery, hold the needle at a 60-degree angle.)	The proper angle of insertion ensures correct access to the artery. The artery is shallow and does not require a deeper angle to penetrate.
11. Puncture the skin and arterial wall in one motion. Watch for blood backflow in the syringe. The pulsating blood will flow into the syringe. Do not pull back on the plunger. Fill the syringe to the 5-mL mark.	The blood should enter the syringe automatically due to arterial pressure.
12. After collecting the sample, withdraw the syringe while your nondominant hand is beginning to place pressure proximal to the insertion site with the 2″ × 2″ gauze. Press a gauze pad firmly over the puncture site until the bleeding stops—at least 5 minutes. **If the patient is receiving anticoagulant therapy or has a blood dyscrasia, apply pressure for 10 to 15 minutes; if necessary, ask a coworker to hold the gauze pad in place while you prepare the sample for transport to the laboratory, but do not ask the patient to hold the pad.**	If insufficient pressure is applied, a large, painful hematoma may form, hindering future arterial puncture at the site.

continues

ACTION	RATIONALE
13. When the bleeding stops, apply a small adhesive bandage or small pressure dressing (fold a 2″ × 2″ gauze into fourths and firmly apply tape, stretching the skin tight).	Applying a dressing also prevents arterial hemorrhage and extravasation into the surrounding tissue, which can cause a hematoma.
14. Once the sample is obtained, check the syringe for air bubbles. If any appear, remove them by holding the syringe upright and slowly ejecting some of the blood onto a 2″ × 2″ gauze pad.	Air bubbles can affect the laboratory values.
15. Remove the needle and place the closed cap on the syringe or insert the needle attached to syringe into a rubber stopper. Gently rotate the syringe to ensure that heparin is well distributed. Insert the syringe into a cup or bag of ice.	This prevents the sample from leaking and keeps air out of the syringe, because blood will continue to absorb oxygen and will give a false reading if allowed to have contact with air. Heparin prevents blood from clotting. Ice prevents the blood from degrading.
16. Attach a properly completed laboratory request form and send the sample to the laboratory immediately.	Blood must be evaluated immediately for accurate results.
17. Remove gloves and perform hand hygiene.	Hand hygiene deters the spread of microorganisms.
18. Continue to monitor the patient's vital signs, and monitor the extremity for signs and symptoms of circulatory impairment such as swelling, discoloration, pain, numbness, or tingling. Watch for bleeding at the puncture site.	Frequent monitoring allows for early detection and prompt intervention should problems arise.
19. Document results of Allen's test, time the sample was drawn, patient's temperature, arterial puncture site, amount of time pressure was applied to the site to control bleeding, type and amount of oxygen therapy, if any, the patient was receiving, pulse oximetry, respiratory rate, and respiratory effort.	Documentation ensures continuity of care and provides an ongoing assessment record.

9/22/06 1245   Allen's test positive. Arterial blood gas obtained using R radial artery. Pressure applied to site for 5 minutes. Patient receiving 3 L/NC oxygen, pulse ox 94%, respirations even/unlabored, respiratory rate 18 breaths per minute, patient denies dyspnea.—C. Bausler, RN

Action 12: Documentation.

EVALUATION   The expected outcome is met when an arterial blood specimen is obtained and the patient reports minimal pain during the procedure. In addition, the site remains free of injury, without evidence of hematoma formation, and the patient verbalizes the rationale for the specimen collection.

continues

SKILL
14-6   **Drawing Arterial Blood Gases** (continued)

Unexpected Situations and Associated Interventions

- *While you are attempting to puncture the artery, the patient complains of severe pain:* Using too much force may cause the needle to touch bone, causing the patient pain. Too much force may also result in advancing the needle through the opposite wall of the artery. If this happens, slowly pull the needle back a short distance and check to see if blood returns. If blood still fails to enter the syringe, withdraw the needle completely and restart procedure.
- *You cannot obtain a specimen after two attempts from the same site:* Stop. Do not make more than two attempts from the same site. Probing the artery may injure it and the radial nerve.
- *Blood won't flow into the syringe:* Typically, this occurs as a result of arterial spasm. Replace the needle with a smaller one and try the puncture again. A smaller-bore needle is less likely to cause arterial spasm.
- *After inserting the needle, you note that the syringe is filling sluggishly with dark purple blood:* If the patient is in critical condition, this may be arterial blood. But if the patient is awake and alert with a pulse oximeter reading of 99%, you have most likely obtained a venous sample. Discard the sample and redraw.
- *The patient is on warfarin (Coumadin) therapy:* Expect to hold pressure on the puncture site for at least 10 minutes. If pressure is not held long enough, a hematoma may form, place pressure on the artery, and decrease the flow of blood.
- *The patient cannot keep the wrist extended or lying flat:* Obtain a small armboard, as used for IV securement, and a roll of gauze. Place the roll of gauze under the patient's wrist. Tape the fingers and forearm to the armboard. This will keep the wrist in an extended position during the blood draw.
- *Blood was drawn without incident, but now, 2 hours later, the patient is complaining of tingling in the fingers and the hand is cool and pale:* Notify the physician. An arterial thrombosis may have formed. If not treated, the thrombosis can lead to necrosis of tissue on the extremity.
- *Puncture site continues to ooze:* If the site is not actively bleeding, consider placing a small pressure bandage on the insertion site. This will prevent the artery from continuing to ooze. Continually check the site for bleeding and assess the extremity to ensure that blood flow is adequate.
- *The Allen's test is negative:* Try the other extremity. If the other extremity has a positive result (collateral circulation), use that extremity. If the Allen's test is negative in both extremities, notify the physician.

Special Considerations

- If the patient is receiving oxygen, make sure that this therapy has been underway for at least 15 minutes before collecting an arterial blood sample. Also be sure to indicate on the laboratory request slip the amount and type of oxygen therapy the patient is receiving. Also note the patient's current temperature, most recent hemoglobin level, and current respiratory rate. If the patient is receiving mechanical ventilation, note the fraction of inspired oxygen and tidal volume.
- If the patient isn't receiving oxygen, indicate that he or she is breathing room air.
- If the patient has just received a nebulizer treatment, wait about 20 minutes before collecting the sample.
- If necessary, anticipate using 1% lidocaine solution to anesthetize the puncture site (requires a physician's order). Consider such use of lidocaine carefully because it can delay the procedure. The patient may be allergic to the drug, or the resulting vasoconstriction may prevent successful puncture.
- Arterial blood and other blood samples may be obtained from an arterial line (see Chapter 16).

Chest tubes may be inserted to drain fluid (pleural effusion), blood (hemothorax), or air (pneumothorax) from the pleural space. The chest tube may be connected to suction or a seal to prevent air from re-entering the pleural space.

Equipment

- Bottle of sterile normal saline or water
- Two pairs of padded Kelly clamps
- Pair of nonsterile scissors
- Disposable gloves
- Foam tape or bands

ASSESSMENT

Assess the patient's respiratory status, including respiratory rate and oxygen saturation. If chest tube is not functioning appropriately, the patient may become tachypneic and hypoxic. Assess the patient's lung sounds. The lung sounds over the chest tube site may be diminished due to the presence of fluid, blood, or air. Also assess the patient for pain. Many patients report pain at the chest tube insertion site and request medication for the pain. Assess the patient's knowledge of the chest tube to ensure that he or she understands the rationale for the chest tube.

NURSING DIAGNOSIS

Determine the related factors for the nursing diagnosis based on the patient's current status. An appropriate nursing diagnosis is Risk for Impaired Gas Exchange. Other appropriate nursing diagnoses may include:

- Risk for Activity Intolerance
- Deficient Knowledge
- Acute Pain

OUTCOME IDENTIFICATION AND PLANNING

The expected outcome to achieve when caring for a chest tube is the patient will not experience any respiratory distress. Other outcomes that may be appropriate include the following: patient understands need for the chest tube; patient will have adequate pain control at chest tube insertion site; lung sounds will be clear and equal bilaterally; and patient will be able to increase activity tolerance gradually.

IMPLEMENTATION

ACTION	RATIONALE
1. Explain procedure to patient.	Explanation relieves anxiety and facilitates cooperation.
2. Perform hand hygiene and don gloves.	Hand hygiene and gloving deter the spread of microorganisms.
3. Move gown to expose chest tube insertion site. **Observe the dressing around the chest tube insertion site and ensure that it is occlusive.** All connections should be securely taped. Gently palpate around the insertion site, feeling for any subcutaneous emphysema (this will feel crunchy under your fingers).	If the dressing is not occlusive, air can leak into the space, causing displacement of the lung tissue. Subcutaneous emphysema will be absorbed by the body after the chest tube is removed. At times, subcutaneous emphysema can cause discomfort to the patient.

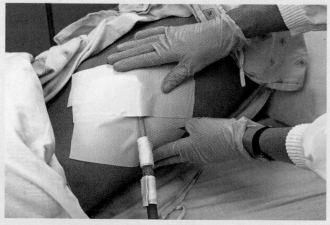

Action 3: Identifying chest tube insertion site.

continues

SKILL 14-7 Providing Care of a Chest Tube (continued)

ACTION	RATIONALE
4. Check drainage tubing to ensure that there are no dependent loops or kinks. The drainage collection device must be positioned below the tube insertion site.	Dependent loops or kinks in the tubing can prevent the tube from draining appropriately. The drainage collection device must be positioned below the tube insertion site so that drainage can move out of the tubing and into the collection device.
5. **Ensure that a bottle of sterile water or normal saline is at the bedside at all times.**	Chest tubes should never be clamped except to change the drainage system. If the chest tube becomes accidentally disconnected from the drainage system, place the end of the chest tube into the sterile solution. This prevents more air from entering the pleural space through the chest tube but allows for any air that does enter the pleural space, through respirations, to escape once pressure builds up.
6. If the chest tube is ordered to be to suction, assess the amount of suction set on the chest tube against the amount of suction ordered. **Look for any bubbling or tidaling in the suction chamber.** The chest tube may be connected to a Heimlich valve, which is a one-way valve to let air out but not in.	If suction is set too low, the amount needs to be increased to ensure that enough negative pressure is placed in the pleural space to drain the pleural space sufficiently. If suction is set too high, the amount needs to be decreased to prevent any damage to the fragile lung tissue. Gentle bubbling in the suction chamber indicates that suction is being applied to assist drainage. Continuous bubbling may indicate a leak in the system. Tidaling is normal. Tidaling is the constant rise and fall of the pressure produced when the patient's own respirations cause a change of pressure in the thoracic cavity.
7. Measure drainage output at the end of each shift by marking the level on the container or placing a small piece of tape at the drainage level to indicate date and time. The amount should be a running total, because the drainage system is never emptied. If the drainage system fills, it will be removed and a new one placed.	The drainage system would lose its negative pressure if it were opened; therefore, companies have made the drainage system large enough to hold several days worth of drainage to prevent the need to interrupt the suction.

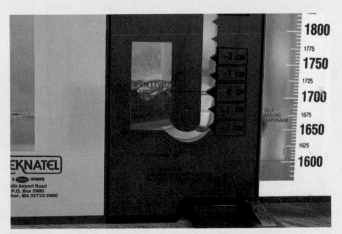

Action 6: Bubbling (tidaling) in the suction chamber

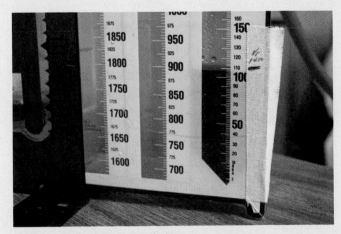

Action 7: Drainage marked on device.

continues

ACTION	RATIONALE

To Change the Drainage System

8. Obtain two pairs of padded Kelly clamps, new drainage system, and bottle of sterile water. Follow manufacturer's directions to add water to suction system if called for.

This provides for an organized approach.

9. **Apply Kelly clamps 1.5" to 2.5" from insertion site and 1" apart, going opposite directions.**

This prevents air from entering the pleural space through the chest tube.

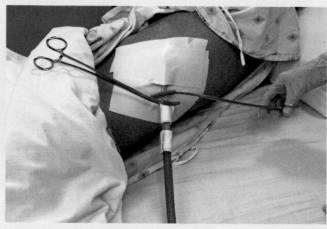

Action 9: Using padded clamps on chest tube.

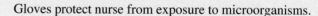

10. Prepare new drainage system. Don disposable gloves.

Gloves protect nurse from exposure to microorganisms.

11. Remove the suction from the drainage system. Unroll the band or use scissors to cut away any foam tape on connection of chest tube and drainage system. Using a slight twisting motion, remove the drainage system. **Do not pull on the chest tube.**

Removing suction permits application to new system. In many institutions, bands or foam tape are placed where the chest tube meets the drainage system to ensure that the chest tube and the drainage system remain connected. Due to the negative pressure, a slight twisting motion may be needed to separate the tubes. The chest tube is sutured in place, so make sure you don't tug on the chest tube and dislodge it.

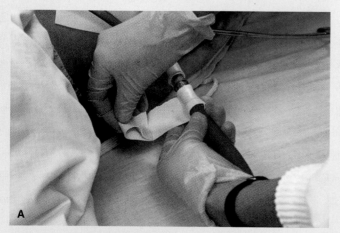

A

Action 11: Unrolling the foam tape.

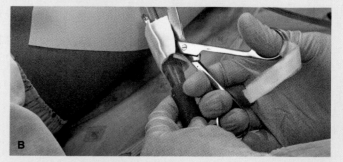

B

Action 11: Cutting the foam tape.

continues

Providing Care of a Chest Tube (continued)

ACTION	RATIONALE

12. **Keeping the end of the chest tube sterile, insert the end of the new drainage system into the chest tube.** Reconnect suction if ordered. Apply plastic bands or foam tape to chest tube/drainage system connection site. Remove Kelly clamps.

Chest tube is sterile. Tube must be reconnected to suction to form a negative pressure and allow for re-expansion of lung or drainage of fluid. Bands or foam tape help prevent the separation of the chest tube from the drainage system. If Kelly clamps remain in place, another pneumothorax may form.

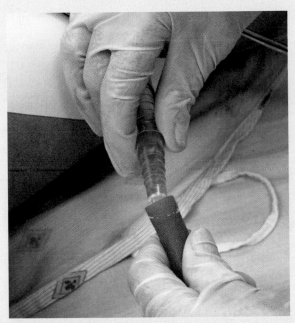

Action 12: Attaching new drainage tube.

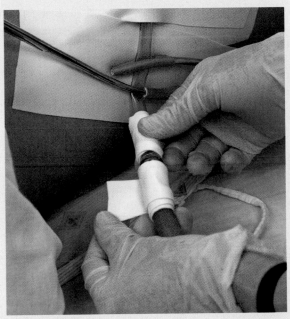

Action 12: Applying foam tape.

13. Assess drainage system for continuous bubbling, tidaling, and amount of suction applied.

Continuous bubbling may indicate a leak in the system. Tidaling is a normal function of the chest tube. The suction needs to be checked to make sure there has not been a change with the new drainage system.

14. Remove gloves. Perform hand hygiene.

This deters the spread of microorganisms.

15. Document the site of the chest tube, amount and type of drainage, amount of suction applied, and any bubbling, tidaling, or subcutaneous emphysema noted. Document the type of dressing in place and the patient's pain level as well as any measures performed to relieve the patient's pain.

Documentation ensures continuity of care and ongoing assessment record.

> 9/10/06 1805   Chest tube R lower portion of rib cage, axillary line; draining moderate amount of serosanguineous fluid; suction at 20 cm H$_2$0 noted; gentle bubbling and tidaling noted in suction chamber; small amount of subcutaneous emphysema noted around insertion site, patient denies any pain; occlusive dressing remains intact.—C. Bausler, RN

Action 15: Documentation.

continues

EVALUATION

The expected outcome is met when the patient remains free of signs and symptoms of respiratory distress and exhibits clear and equal lung sounds. In addition, the patient verbalizes adequate pain relief, gradually increases activity tolerance, and demonstrates understanding of the need for the chest tube.

Unexpected Situations and Associated Interventions

- *The chest tube becomes separated from the drainage device:* Don gloves. Open the sterile normal saline or water and attempt to insert the chest tube into the bottle while not contaminating the chest tube. Assess the patient for any signs of respiratory distress. Notify physician. Do not leave the patient. Anticipate the need for a new drainage system and a chest x-ray.

- *The chest tube becomes dislodged:* Don gloves. Apply an occlusive dressing. There is a controversy in the literature over whether the occlusive dressing should be a sterile Vaseline-impregnated gauze covered with an occlusive tape or a sterile 4″ × 4″ folded and covered with an occlusive tape. (An example of an occlusive tape would be foam tape or the clear dressing used to cover IV insertion sites.) Assess the patient for any signs of respiratory distress. Notify physician. Anticipate the need for a chest x-ray. The physician will determine whether the chest tube needs to be replaced.

- *While assessing the chest tube, you notice that the suction chamber is not tidaling:* Check for kinked tubing or a clot in the tubing. Note the amount of suction that the chest tube is set on. If there is a clot in the tubing, some institutions allow you to "milk" the tubing. To milk the tubing, grasp the tubing and squeeze quickly, then let go. "Stripping" the tubing is not recommended. Stripping the tubing entails grasping the tubing firmly and sliding the hand down the tubing toward the drainage device. This increases the negative pressure in the pleural space and causes damage to the fragile lung tissue. If the suction is not set appropriately, adjust until the ordered amount is achieved.

- *While assessing the chest tube, you notice that the suction chamber is continuously bubbling:* Check for any leaks in the system, starting at the dressing and working toward the drainage device. Once the dressing has been inspected, clamp the tube with a Kelly clamp. If the drainage device is still continuously bubbling, clamp the drainage tubing with a Kelly clamp (this can help to determine if the air leak is in the chest tube itself or in the drainage tubing).

- *Drainage exceeds 100 mL/hr or becomes bright red:* Notify physician immediately. This can indicate fresh bleeding.

- *Chest tube drainage suddenly decreases and the suction chamber is not tidaling:* Notify physician immediately. This could signal that the tube is blocked.

SKILL 14-8   Assisting With Removal of a Chest Tube

The physician will determine when the chest tube is ready for removal by evaluating the chest x-ray and assessing the patient and the amount of drainage.

Equipment
- Disposable gloves
- Suture removal kit (tweezers and scissors)
- Sterile Vaseline-impregnated gauze or pair of 4×4s
- Occlusive tape such as foam tape

ASSESSMENT

Assess the patient's respiratory status, including respiratory rate and oxygen saturation level. This provides a baseline for comparison after the tube is removed. If the patient begins to have respiratory distress, he or she will usually become tachypneic and hypoxic. Assess the patient's lung sounds. The lung sounds over the chest tube site may be diminished due to the tube. Assess the patient for pain. Many patients report pain at the chest tube insertion site and request medication for the pain. If the patient has not recently received pain medication, it may be given before the chest tube removal to decrease the pain felt with the procedure. Assess the patient's knowledge of the chest tube to ensure that he or she understands the rationale for the tube.

NURSING DIAGNOSIS

Determine the related factors for the nursing diagnosis based on the patient's current status. Appropriate nursing diagnoses may include:
- Deficient Knowledge
- Acute Pain
- Impaired Skin Integrity

OUTCOME IDENTIFICATION AND PLANNING

The expected outcome to achieve when caring for a patient after removal of a chest tube is that the patient will remain free of respiratory distress. Other outcomes that my be appropriate include the following: the insertion site will remain clean and dry without evidence of infection; patient will state adequate pain control during the chest tube removal; lung sounds will be clear and equal bilaterally; and patient will be able to increase activity tolerance gradually.

IMPLEMENTATION

ACTION	RATIONALE
1. Explain procedure to patient.	Explanation relieves anxiety and facilitates patient cooperation.
2. Perform hand hygiene.	Hand hygiene deters the spread of microorganisms.
3. Administer pain medication.	Most patients report discomfort during chest tube removal. **Premedicate patient 10 to 15 minutes before chest tube removal.**
4. Don gloves.	Gloves help to protect nurse from pathogens.
5. Provide reassurance to patient while physician removes dressing.	The removal of the dressing can increase the patient's anxiety level. Offering reassurance may make the patient feel more secure.
6. **After physician has removed chest tube and secured occlusive dressing, assess patient's lung sounds, respiratory rate, oxygen saturation, and pain level.**	In most institutions, physicians remove chest tubes, but some institutions train nurses to remove chest tubes. Once the tube is removed, the patient's respiratory status will need to be assessed to ensure that no distress is noted.
7. Anticipate the physician ordering a chest x-ray.	The physician may want a chest x-ray taken to evaluate the status of the lungs after chest tube removal.

continues

ACTION	RATIONALE
8. Dispose of equipment appropriately. Remove and dispose of gloves. Perform hand hygiene.	Hand hygiene deters the spread of microorganisms.
9. Document the patient's respiratory rate, oxygen saturation, lung sounds, total chest tube output, and status of dressing.	Documentation ensures continuity of care and ongoing assessment record.

9/16/06   1950   Procedure explained to patient. Morphine sulfate 2 mg IV given. Physician at bedside, R midaxillary lower lobe chest tube removed. Lung sounds clear, slightly diminished over R lower lobe. Respirations 16 breaths per minute; oxygen saturation at 97%. 322 mL of serosanguineous drainage noted in drainage device; Vaseline gauze applied over insertion site covered by foam tape. Patient denies pain or respiratory distress.—C. Bausler, RN

Action 9: Documentation.

EVALUATION

The expected outcome is met when the patient exhibits no signs and symptoms of respiratory distress after the chest tube is removed. In addition, the patient verbalizes adequate pain control; lung sounds are clear and equal; and the patient's activity level gradually increases.

Unexpected Situations and Associated Interventions

- *Patient experiences respiratory distress after chest tube removal:* Auscultate lung sounds. Diminished or absent lung sounds could be a sign that the lung has not fully reinflated or that the fluid has returned. Notify physician immediately. Anticipate an order for a chest x-ray with possible reinsertion of a chest tube.
- *Chest tube dressing becomes loosened:* The chest tube dressing should be changed at least every 24 hours or per agency policy so that the nurse can assess the site for erythema and drainage. Replace the occlusive dressing using a sterile technique. The dressing should remain occlusive for at least 3 days.

Administering Oxygen by Nasal Cannula

Oxygen can be delivered to the patient through a variety of devices. Each has a specific function and oxygen concentration. The device selected is based on the patient's condition and oxygen needs. A nasal cannula is used to deliver from 25 mL per minute to 6 L per minute of oxygen.

Equipment

- Flow meter connected to oxygen supply
- Humidifier with sterile distilled water (optional low-flow system)
- Nasal cannula and tubing
- Gauze to pad tubing over ears (optional)

ASSESSMENT

Assess patient's oxygen saturation level before starting oxygen therapy to provide a baseline to evaluate the effectiveness of oxygen therapy. Assess patient's respiratory status, including respiratory rate, effort, and lung sounds. Note any signs of respiratory distress, such as tachypnea, nasal flaring, use of accessory muscles, or dyspnea.

NURSING DIAGNOSIS

Determine the related factors for the nursing diagnosis based on the patient's current status. Appropriate nursing diagnoses may include:

- Impaired Gas Exchange
- Ineffective Breathing Pattern
- Ineffective Airway Clearance

Other nursing diagnoses that may be appropriate include:

- Risk for Activity Intolerance
- Decreased Cardiac Output
- Excess Fluid Volume

OUTCOME IDENTIFICATION AND PLANNING

The expected outcome to achieve when administering oxygen via a nasal cannula is that the patient will exhibit an oxygen saturation level within acceptable parameters. Other outcomes that may be appropriate include the following: patient will not experience dyspnea; patient will demonstrate effortless respirations in the normal range for age group, without evidence of nasal flaring or use of accessory muscles.

IMPLEMENTATION

ACTION	RATIONALE
1. Explain procedure to patient and review safety precautions necessary when oxygen is in use. Place "no smoking" signs in appropriate areas.	Oxygen supports combustion.
2. Perform hand hygiene.	Hand hygiene deters the spread of microorganisms.
3. **Connect nasal cannula to oxygen setup with humidification, if one is in use.** Adjust flow rate as ordered by physician. Check that oxygen is flowing out of prongs.	Oxygen forced through a water reservoir is humidified before it is delivered to the patient, thus preventing dehydration of the mucous membranes. Low-flow oxygen does not require humidification.
4. Place prongs in patient's nostrils. Adjust according to type of equipment: a. Over and behind each ear with adjuster comfortably under chin or b. Around the patient's head	Correct placement of the prongs and fastener facilitates oxygen administration and patient comfort.

continues

SKILL 14-9   **Administering Oxygen by Nasal Cannula** (continued)

ACTION	RATIONALE
5. Place gauze pads at ear beneath the tubing as necessary. Adjust cannula as necessary.	Pads reduce irritation and pressure and protect the skin.

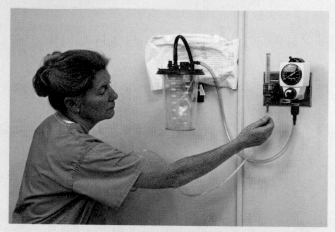

Action 3: Connecting cannula to oxygen source.

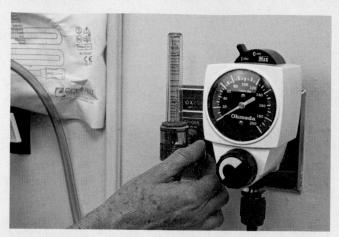

Action 3: Adjusting flow rate.

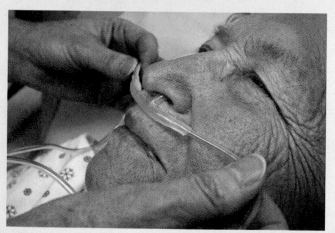

Action 4: Applying cannula to nares.

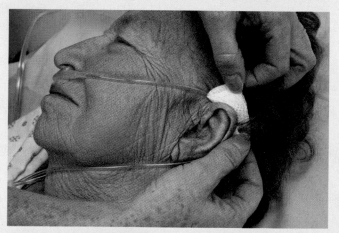

Action 5: Placing gauze pad at ears.

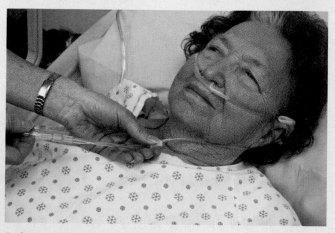

Action 5: Adjusting cannula if needed.

continues

Administering Oxygen by Nasal Cannula (continued)

ACTION	RATIONALE
6. **Encourage patient to breathe through the nose, with mouth closed.**	Nose breathing provides for optimal delivery of oxygen to patient.
7. Perform hand hygiene.	Hand hygiene deters the spread of microorganisms.
8. Assess and chart patient's response to therapy.	Patient's respirations, color, breathing pattern, and chest movements indicate effectiveness of oxygen therapy.
9. Remove and clean the cannula and assess nares at least every 8 hours, or according to agency recommendations. Check nares for evidence of irritation or bleeding.	The continued presence of the cannula causes irritation and dryness of the mucous membranes. Water-soluble lubricant counteracts the drying effects of oxygen.
10. Document the amount of oxygen applied, the patient's respiratory rate, oxygen saturation, and lung sounds.	Documentation ensures continuity of care and ongoing assessment record.

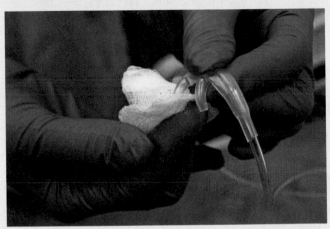

Action 9: Cleaning cannula when indicated.

9/17/06 1300   Oxygen via nasal cannula
applied at 2 L/min. Humidification in place.
Pulse oximeter before placing oxygen 92%;
after oxygen at 2 L/min 98%. Respirations
even and unlabored. Chest rises symmetrically. No nasal flaring or retractions noted.
Lung sounds clear and equal all lobes.
—C. Bausler, RN

Action 10: Documentation.

EVALUATION

The expected outcome is met when the patient demonstrates an oxygen saturation level within acceptable parameters. In addition, the patient remains free of dyspnea, nasal flaring, or accessory muscle use and demonstrates respiratory rate and depth within normal ranges.

Unexpected Situations and Associated Interventions

- *Patient was fine on oxygen delivered by nasal cannula but now is cyanotic, and the pulse oximeter reading is <93%:* Check to see that the oxygen tubing is still connected to the flow meter and the flow meter is still on the previous setting. Someone may have stepped on the tubing, pulling it from the flow meter, or the oxygen may have accidentally been turned off. Assess lung sounds to note any changes.
- *Areas over ear or back of head are reddened:* Ensure that areas are adequately padded and that tubing is not pulled too tight. If available, a skin care team may be able to offer some suggestions.
- *When dozing, patient begins to breathe through the mouth:* Temporarily place the nasal cannula near the mouth. If this does not raise the pulse oximeter reading, you may need to obtain an order to switch the patient to a mask while sleeping.

Home Care Considerations

- Oxygen administration may need to be continued in the home setting. Portable oxygen concentrators are used most frequently. Caregivers require instruction concerning safety precautions with oxygen use and need to understand the rationale for the specific liter flow of oxygen.

SKILL 14-10   Administering Oxygen by Mask

When a patient requires a higher concentration of oxygen than a nasal cannula can deliver (6 L or 44% oxygen concentration), an oxygen mask is used. There are several different types of masks.

Equipment

- Flow meter connected to oxygen supply
- Humidifier with sterile distilled water
- Face mask specified by physician
- Gauze to pad elastic band (optional)

ASSESSMENT

Assess patient's oxygen saturation level before starting oxygen therapy to provide a baseline for determining the effectiveness of therapy. Assess patient's respiratory status, including respiratory rate and depth and lung sounds. Note any signs of respiratory distress, such as tachypnea, nasal flaring, use of accessory muscles, or dyspnea.

NURSING DIAGNOSIS

Determine the related factors for the nursing diagnosis based on the patient's current status. Appropriate nursing diagnoses may include:

- Impaired Gas Exchange
- Ineffective Breathing Pattern
- Ineffective Airway Clearance

Many other nursing diagnoses may be appropriate, possibly including:

- Risk for Activity Intolerance
- Decreased Cardiac Output
- Excess Fluid Volume

OUTCOME IDENTIFICATION AND PLANNING

The expected outcome to achieve when administering oxygen via face mask is that patient exhibits an oxygen saturation level within acceptable parameters. Other outcomes that may be appropriate include the following: patient will remain free of signs and symptoms of respiratory distress, and respiratory status, including respiratory rate and depth, will be in the normal range for the patient's age.

IMPLEMENTATION

ACTION	RATIONALE
1. Explain procedure to patient and review safety precautions necessary when oxygen is in use. Place "no smoking" signs in appropriate areas.	Oxygen supports combustion. Explanation alleviates anxiety.
2. Perform hand hygiene.	Hand hygiene deters the spread of microorganisms.
3. Attach face mask to oxygen setup with humidification. Start the flow of oxygen at the specified rate. For a mask with a reservoir, allow oxygen to fill the bag before placing the mask over patient's nose and mouth.	Oxygen forced through a water reservoir is humidified before it is delivered to the patient, thus preventing dehydration of the mucous membranes. A reservoir bag must be inflated with oxygen because the bag is the source of oxygen supply for the patient.
4. Position face mask over patient's nose and mouth. Adjust it with the elastic strap so that the mask fits snugly but comfortably on the face. Adjust the flow rate.	A loose or poorly fitting mask will result in oxygen loss and decreased therapeutic value. Masks may cause a feeling of suffocation, and the patient needs frequent attention and reassurance.
5. Use gauze pads to reduce irritation to ears and scalp.	Pads reduce irritation and pressure and protect the skin.
6. Perform hand hygiene.	Hand hygiene deters the spread of microorganisms.

continues

Administering Oxygen by Mask (continued)

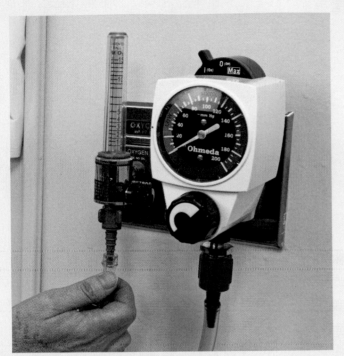

Action 3: Connecting face mask to oxygen source.

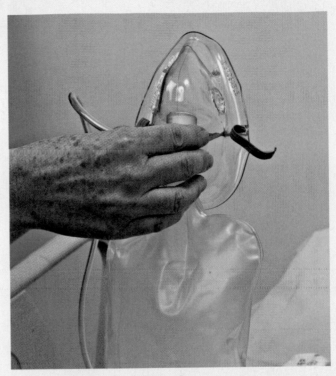

Action 3: Allowing oxygen to fill the bag.

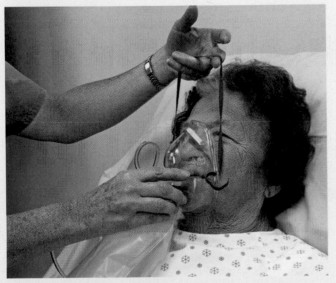

Action 4: Applying face mask over nose and mouth.

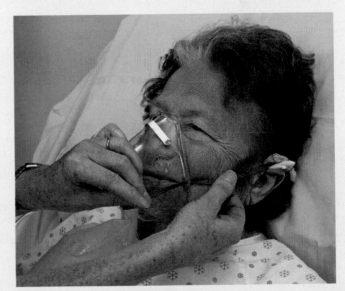

Action 4: Adjusting elastic straps.

continues

SKILL
14-10   Administering Oxygen by Mask (continued)

ACTION   **RATIONALE**

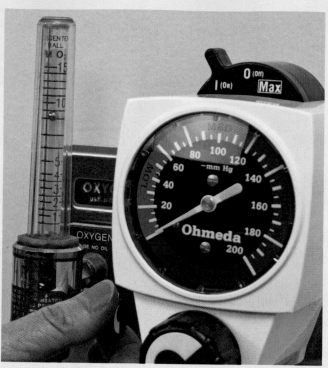

Action 4: Adjusting flow rate.

7. **Remove the mask and dry the skin every 2 to 3 hours if the oxygen is running continuously. Do not use powder around the mask.**

The tight-fitting mask and moisture from condensation can irritate the skin on the face. There is a danger of inhaling powder if it is placed on the mask.

8. Assess and chart patient's response to therapy.

Patient's respiratory rate and pattern, color, and so forth indicate effectiveness of oxygen therapy.

9. Document type of mask used, amount of oxygen used, oxygen saturation level, lung sounds, and rate/pattern of respirations.

> 9/22/06   Oxygen via nonrebreather face mask applied at 12 L/minute. Patient's skin is pink after O₂ applied. Pulse oximeter before oxygen placement 88%; after oxygen started, oxygen saturation increased to 98%. Respirations even and unlabored. Chest rises symmetrically. Respiratory rate 18 breaths per minute. Patient denies dyspnea.—C. Bausler, RN

Action 9: Documentation.

EVALUATION

The expected outcome is met when the patient exhibits an oxygen saturation level within acceptable parameters. In addition, the patient demonstrates an absence of respiratory distress and accessory muscle use and exhibits respiratory rate and depth within normal parameters.

continues

Unexpected Situations and Associated Interventions

- *Patient was previously fine but now is cyanotic, and the pulse oximeter reading is <93%:* Check to see that the oxygen tubing is still connected to the flow meter and the flow meter is still on the previous setting. Someone may have stepped on the tubing, pulling it from the flow meter, or the oxygen may have accidentally been turned off. Assess lung sounds for any changes.

- *Areas over ear or back of head are reddened:* Ensure that areas are adequately padded and that tubing is not pulled too tight. If available, a skin care team may be able to offer some suggestions.

Special Considerations

- Different types of face masks are available for use. Refer to Table 14-2 for more information.

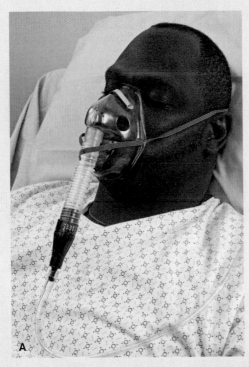

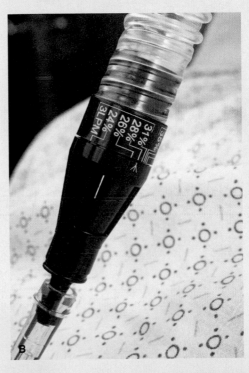

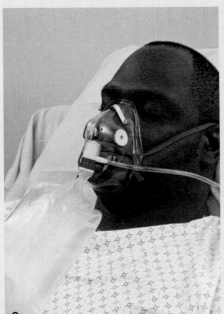

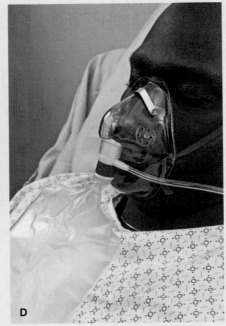

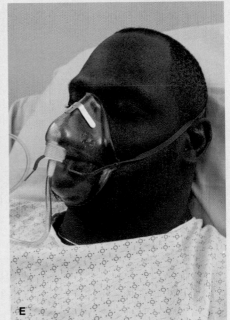

Types of oxygen masks. (**A**) Venturi mask. (**B**) Dial on Venturi mask. (**C**) Nonrebreather mask. (**D**) Partial rebreather mask (**E**) Simple face mask.

continues

SKILL 14-10   Administering Oxygen by Mask (continued)

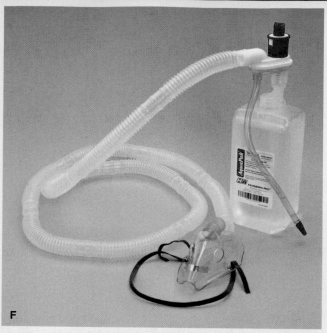

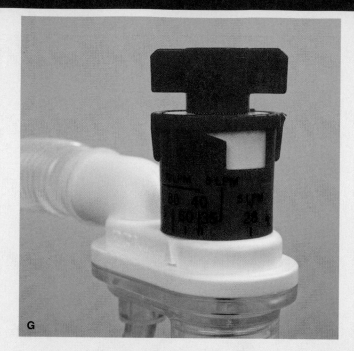

(F) High-flow oxygen face mask and bottle. **(G)** High-flow oxygen meter.

SKILL 14-11   Using an Oxygen Hood

Oxygen hoods are generally used to deliver oxygen to infants at rates approaching 100% (Wong et al., 2001). The oxygen hood is placed over the infant's head and shoulders. The hoods are made of hard plastic or vinyl with a metal frame.

Equipment

- Oxygen source
- Oxygen hood
- Oxygen analyzer
- Humidification device

ASSESSMENT

Assess the patient's lung sounds. Secretions may cause the patient's oxygen demand to increase. Assess the oxygen saturation level. The physician will usually order a baseline for the pulse oximeter (ie, deliver oxygen to keep pulse ox >95%). Assess skin color. A pale or cyanotic patient may not be receiving enough oxygen. Assess patient for any signs of respiratory distress such as nasal flaring, grunting, or retractions; oxygen-depleted patients often exhibit these signs.

NURSING DIAGNOSIS

Determine the related factors for the nursing diagnosis based on the patient's current status. Appropriate nursing diagnoses may include:

- Impaired Gas Exchange
- Ineffective Breathing Pattern
- Ineffective Airway Clearance

continues

Using an Oxygen Hood (continued)

Many other nursing diagnoses may be appropriate, possibly including:

- Risk for Activity Intolerance
- Decreased Cardiac Output
- Excess Fluid Volume
- Risk for Impaired Skin Integrity

OUTCOME IDENTIFICATION AND PLANNING

The expected outcome to achieve when administering oxygen via hood is that the patient exhibits an oxygen saturation level within acceptable parameters. Other outcomes that may be appropriate include the following: patient will remain free of signs and symptoms of respiratory distress; respiratory status, including respiratory rate and depth, will be in the normal range for the patient's age; and patient's skin will be pink, dry, and without evidence of breakdown.

IMPLEMENTATION

ACTION	RATIONALE
1. Explain procedure to patient and review safety precautions necessary when oxygen is in use. Place "no smoking" signs in appropriate areas.	Oxygen supports combustion.
2. Perform hand hygiene.	Hand hygiene deters the spread of microorganisms.
3. Place hood on crib. Connect humidifier to oxygen source in the wall. Insert oxygen tubing from humidifier into hole in the back of the oxygen hood. Adjust flow rate as ordered by physician. Check that oxygen is flowing into hood.	Oxygen forced through a water reservoir is humidified before it is delivered to the patient, thus preventing dehydration of the mucous membranes.
4. Turn analyzer on. **Place oxygen analyzer probe in hood.**	The analyzer will give an accurate reading of the concentration of oxygen in the hood or bed.
5. Adjust oxygen flow as necessary. Once oxygen levels reach the prescribed amount, place hood over patient's head.	Patient will receive oxygen once placed under the hood.

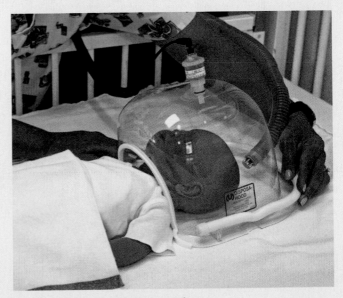

Action 5: Increasing oxygen based on sensor readings.

Action 5: Placing oxygen hood over infant.

continues

SKILL
14-11   Using an Oxygen Hood (continued)

ACTION	RATIONALE
6. If using the soft vinyl hood, roll small blankets or towels and place around edges where hood meets crib if needed to keep oxygen concentration at desired level. **Do not block hole in top of hood if present. If using a vinyl hoods, the hole covering may need to be removed.**	The blankets help keep the edges of the hood sealed and prevent oxygen from escaping. This hole allows for the escape of carbon dioxide; blocking it may cause a buildup of carbon dioxide in the hood.
7. Instruct family members not to raise edges of the hood.	Every time the hood is raised, oxygen is released.
8. Frequently check bedding and patient's head for moisture.	The humidification delivered in an oxygen hood makes cloth moist, which would be uncomfortable for the patient.
9. Perform hand hygiene.	Hand hygiene deters the spread of microorganisms.
10. Document amount of oxygen applied, respiratory rate, oxygen saturation level, and lung sounds.	Documentation ensures continuity of care and ongoing assessment record.

9/17/06   Patient placed under oxygen hood at 35%. Pulse oximeter reading before placing under hood at 92%; increased to 99% after hood placement. Respirations even, unlabored, and symmetrical. No nasal flaring or retractions noted. Lung sounds clear and equal all lobes.—C. Bausler, RN

Action 10: Documentation.

EVALUATION

The expected outcome is met when the patient exhibits an oxygen saturation level within acceptable parameters. In addition, the patient remains free of dyspnea, nasal flaring, grunting, or use of accessory muscles when breathing, and respirations remain in normal range for age.

Unexpected Situations and Associated Interventions

- *It is difficult to maintain oxygen at desired level:* Ensure that edges of hood are in contact with crib pad. If necessary, roll small blankets or towels and put around edges to prevent escape of oxygen. If you need to reach the baby's head for medication administration, feedings, and so forth, group procedures together so that the hood remains in place for longer consecutive periods of time. Consider recalibrating the analyzer according to the manufacturer's directions.

Special Considerations

- The nurse and family can offer visual stimulation to the infant. Brightly colored toys or pictures of family members may be placed on or around the hood, as long as they do not block the exhalation hole.

Using an Oxygen Tent

Oxygen tents are often used in children who will not leave a face mask or nasal cannula in place. The oxygen tent gives the patient freedom to move in the bed or crib while humidified oxygen is being delivered. However, it is difficult to keep the tent closed, since the child may want contact with his or her parents; it is difficult to maintain a consistent level of oxygen; and it is difficult to deliver oxygen at a higher rate than 30% to 50%. Frequent assessment of the child's pajamas and bedding is necessary because the humidification quickly creates moisture, leading to damp clothing and linens.

Equipment

- Oxygen source
- Oxygen tent
- Humidifier compatible with tent
- Oxygen analyzer

ASSESSMENT

Assess the patient's lung sounds. Secretions may cause the patient's oxygen demand to increase. Assess the oxygen saturation level. The physician will usually order a baseline for the pulse oximeter (ie, deliver oxygen to keep pulse ox >95%). Assess skin color. A pale or cyanotic patient may not be receiving enough oxygen. Assess patient for any signs of respiratory distress such as nasal flaring, grunting, or retractions; oxygen-depleted patients often exhibit these signs.

**NURSING
DIAGNOSIS**

Determine the related factors for the nursing diagnosis based on the patient's current status. Appropriate nursing diagnoses may include:

- Impaired Gas Exchange
- Ineffective Breathing Pattern
- Ineffective Airway Clearance

Many other nursing diagnoses may be appropriate, possibly including:
- Risk for Activity Intolerance
- Decreased Cardiac Output
- Excess Fluid Volume
- Risk for Impaired Skin Integrity

**OUTCOME
IDENTIFICATION
AND PLANNING**

The expected outcome to achieve when administering oxygen via hood is that the patient exhibits an oxygen saturation level within acceptable parameters. Other outcomes that may be appropriate include the following: patient will remain free of signs and symptoms of respiratory distress; respiratory status, including respiratory rate and depth, will be in the normal range for the patient's age; and patient's skin will be pink, dry, and without evidence of breakdown.

IMPLEMENTATION

ACTION	RATIONALE
1. Explain procedure to patient and review safety precautions necessary when oxygen is in use. Place "no smoking" signs in appropriate areas.	Oxygen supports combustion.
2. Perform hand hygiene.	Hand hygiene deters the spread of microorganisms.
3. Place tent over crib or bed. Connect the humidifier to the oxygen source in the wall. Insert oxygen tubing connected to the humidifier inside tent, out of patient's reach. Adjust flow rate as ordered by physician. Check that oxygen is flowing into tent.	Oxygen forced through a water reservoir is humidified before it is delivered to the patient, thus preventing dehydration of the mucous membranes.

continues

SKILL 14-12   **Using an Oxygen Tent** (continued)

ACTION	RATIONALE

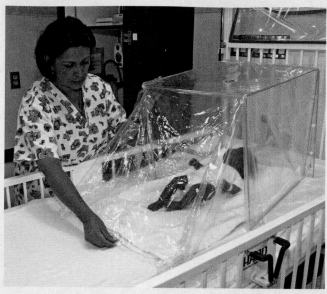

Action 3: Placing tent in or over crib.

4. Turn analyzer on. Place oxygen analyzer probe in tent, out of patient's reach.

5. Adjust oxygen as necessary. Once oxygen levels reach the prescribed amount, place patient in the bed.

6. Tuck tent edges under blanket rolls.

The analyzer will give an accurate reading of the concentration of oxygen in the crib or bed.

Patient will receive oxygen once placed in the tent.

The blanket helps keep the edges of the tent flap from coming up and letting oxygen out.

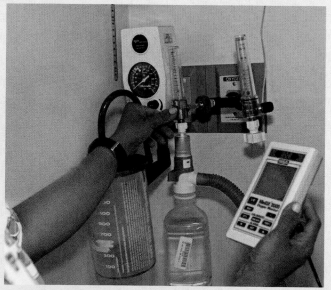

Action 5: Adjusting oxygen flow.

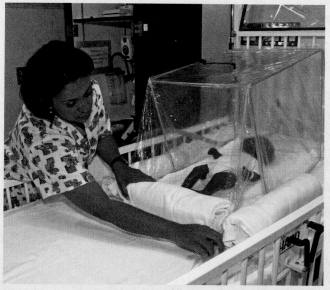

Action 6: Tucking edges under blanket rolls.

continues

Using an Oxygen Tent (continued)

ACTION	RATIONALE
7. **Encourage patient and family members to keep tent flap closed.**	Every time the tent flap is opened, oxygen is released.
8. Frequently check bedding and patient's pajamas for moisture.	The large amount of humidification delivered in an oxygen tent quickly makes cloth moist, which would be uncomfortable for the patient.
9. Perform hand hygiene.	Hand hygiene deters the spread of microorganisms.
10. Document amount of oxygen applied, respiratory rate, oxygen saturation, and lung sounds.	Documentation ensures continuity of care and ongoing assessment record.

9/17/06   Patient placed in oxygen tent at 45%. Pulse oximeter reading before placing in tent 92%; increased to 98% after placing in tent. Respirations even, unlabored, and symmetrical. No nasal flaring or retractions noted. Lung sounds clear and equal all lobes.
—C. Bausler, RN

Action 10: Documentation.

EVALUATION

The expected outcome is met when the patient exhibits an oxygen saturation level within acceptable parameters. In addition, the patient remains free of dyspnea, nasal flaring, grunting, or use of accessory muscles when breathing; and respirations remain in normal range for age.

Unexpected Situations and Associated Interventions

- *Child refuses to stay in tent:* Parent may play games in tent with child if this will help child to stay in tent. Alternative methods of oxygen delivery may need to be considered if child still refuses to stay in tent.
- *It is difficult to maintain an oxygen level above 40% in the tent:* Ensure that flap is closed and edges of tent are tucked under blanket. Check oxygen delivery unit to ensure that the rate has not been changed. Encourage patient to leave flaps closed. If still a problem, analyzer may need to be replaced or recalibrated.

SKILL
14-13   **Inserting an Oropharyngeal Airway**

The oropharyngeal airway can help protect the airway of an unconscious patient by preventing the tongue from falling back against the posterior pharynx and blocking it. The nurse can insert this device at the bedside with little to no trauma to the unconscious patient.

Equipment

- Oropharyngeal airway
- Disposable gloves
- Airway
- Goggles or face shield (optional)
- Flashlight (optional)

ASSESSMENT

Assess patient's level of consciousness and ability to protect the airway. Assess amount and consistency of oral secretions. Auscultate lung sounds. If the tongue is occluding the airway, lung sounds may be diminished.

NURSING DIAGNOSIS

Determine related factors for the nursing diagnosis based on the patient's current status. Appropriate nursing diagnoses may include:

- Risk for Aspiration
- Ineffective Airway Clearance
- Risk for Injury

Many other nursing diagnoses may require the use of this skill.

OUTCOME IDENTIFICATION AND PLANNING

The expected outcome to achieve when inserting an oral airway is that the patient will sustain a patent airway. Other outcomes that may be appropriate include the following: the patient remains free of aspiration and injury.

IMPLEMENTATION

ACTION	RATIONALE
1. Gather equipment. Explain procedure to patient and family.	Explanation alleviates fears. Even though patient appears unconscious, the nurse should explain what is happening.
2. Perform hand hygiene.	Hand hygiene deters the spread of microorganisms.
3. Measure the oropharyngeal airway for correct size.	The oropharyngeal airway is measured by holding the airway on the side of the patient's face. The airway should reach from the opening of the mouth to the back angle of the jaw (ear).

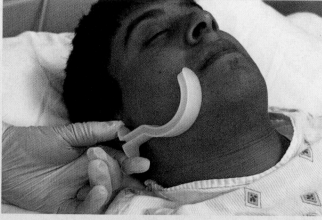

Action 3: Measuring for oropharyngeal airway.

continues

ACTION	RATIONALE
4. Don disposable gloves.	Gloves protect against pathogens.
5. **Check mouth for any loose teeth, candy, or dentures.**	During insertion, the airway may push any foreign objects in the mouth to the back of the throat.
6. Position patient on his or her back with neck hyper-extended (unless this is contraindicated).	This position facilitates airway insertion.
7. Open patient's mouth by using your thumb and index finger to gently pry teeth apart. **Insert the airway with the curved tip pointing up toward the roof of the mouth.**	This is done to advance the tip of the airway past the tongue, toward the back of the throat.
8. Slide the airway across the tongue to the back of the mouth. Rotate the airway 180 degrees as it passes the uvula (a flashlight can be used to confirm the position of the airway with the curve fitting over the tongue).	This is done to shift the tongue anteriorly, thereby allowing the patient to breathe through and around the airway.
9. Ensure accurate placement and adequate ventilation by auscultating breath sounds.	If the airway is placed correctly, lung sounds should be audible and equal in all lobes.

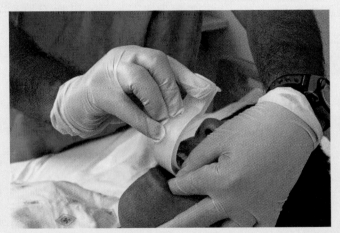

Action 7: Slide the airway in.

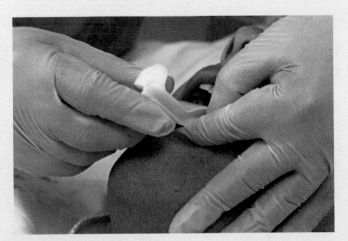

Action 8: Flip the airway.

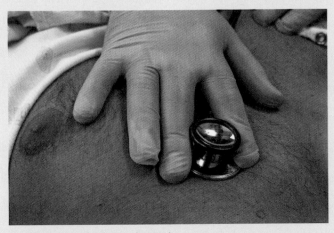

Action 9: Auscultating breath sounds.

continues

ACTION	RATIONALE
10. Position patient on his or her side when airway is in place.	This position also helps keep the tongue out of the posterior pharynx area, as well as helping to prevent aspiration if the unconscious patient should vomit.
11. Remove the airway for a brief period every 4 hours. Provide mouth care and rinse airway before reinserting it.	This helps to prevent pressure ulcers in the mouth and to keep the airway open.
12. Remove gloves and perform hand hygiene.	Hand hygiene deters the spread of microorganisms.
13. Document the placement of the airway as well as lung sounds and pulse oximetry level.	Documentation ensures continuity of care and ongoing assessment record.

9/22/06   1210   Size 4 oropharyngeal airway inserted. Patient placed on left side. Lung
sounds clear and equal all lobes. Pulse oximeter 98% on room air.—C. Bausler, RN

Action 13: Documentation.

EVALUATION

The expected outcome is met when the patient exhibits a patent airway with oxygen saturation levels >95%. In addition, the patient remains free of trauma and aspiration.

Unexpected Situations and Associated Interventions

- *The patient awakens:* Remove the oral airway once the patient is awake because it may be uncomfortable. Awake patients can usually protect their airway.
- *The tongue is sliding back into the posterior pharynx, causing respiratory difficulties:* Don disposable gloves and remove the airway. Make sure the airway is the appropriate size for the patient.
- *Patient vomits as oropharyngeal airway is inserted:* Quickly position patient onto his or her side to prevent aspiration. Remove oral airway. Suction mouth if needed.

Special Considerations

- Wearing gloves, remove the airway briefly every 4 hours to provide mouth care. Also assess the mouth and tongue for tissue irritation and ulceration.
- When reinserting the oropharyngeal airway, attempt to insert it on the other side of the mouth. This helps to prevent the tongue and mouth from irritation.
- Suction secretions, as needed, by manipulating around and through the oropharyngeal airway.

Suctioning the Nasopharyngeal and Oropharyngeal Airways

Some patients need help removing secretions from their airways. A suction device is needed for this action.

Equipment

- Portable or wall suction unit with tubing
- Sterile suction catheter with Y-port in appropriate size (for adults, 12F to 16F)
- Sterile water or saline
- Sterile disposable container
- Sterile gloves
- Towel or waterproof pad
- Goggles or eye shield if splashing is likely.

ASSESSMENT

Assess lung sounds. Patients who need to be suctioned usually have coarse lung sounds. Assess oxygenation saturation level. Oxygen saturation usually decreases when a patient needs to be suctioned. Assess respiratory status, including respiratory rate and depth. Patients may become tachypneic when they need to be suctioned. Assess patient for signs of respiratory distress, such as nasal flaring, retractions, or grunting.

NURSING DIAGNOSIS

Determine the related factors for the nursing diagnosis based on the patient's current status. An appropriate nursing diagnosis is Ineffective Airway Clearance. Many other nursing diagnoses may require the use of this skill.

OUTCOME IDENTIFICATION AND PLANNING

The expected outcome to achieve when suctioning the nasopharyngeal or oropharyngeal area is that the patient will exhibit a clear, patent airway. Other outcomes that may be appropriate include the following: patient will exhibit an oxygen saturation level within acceptable parameters; patient will demonstrate a respiratory rate and depth within age-acceptable range; and patient will remain free of any signs of respiratory distress, including retractions, nasal flaring, or grunting.

IMPLEMENTATION

ACTION	RATIONALE
1. Determine the need for suctioning. **For postoperative patient, administer pain medication before suctioning.**	To minimize trauma to airway mucosa, suctioning should be done only when secretions have accumulated or adventitious breath sounds are audible. Suctioning stimulates coughing, which is painful for patients with surgical incisions.

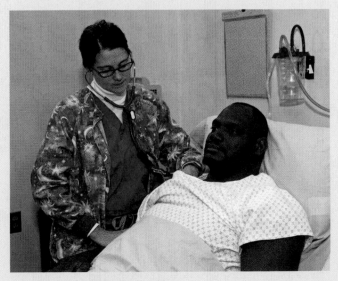

Action 1: Assess need for suctioning.

continues

ACTION	RATIONALE
2. Explain procedure to patient.	This provides reassurance and promotes cooperation.
3. Assemble equipment.	This provides for organized approach.
4. Perform hand hygiene.	Hand hygiene deters the spread of microorganisms.
5. Adjust bed to comfortable working position. Lower side rail closer to you. If patient is conscious, place him or her in a semi-Fowler's position. **If patient is unconscious, place him or her in the lateral position, facing you.**	A sitting position helps the patient to cough and makes breathing easier. Gravity also facilitates catheter insertion. The lateral position prevents the airway from becoming obstructed and promotes drainage of secretions.
6. Place towel or waterproof pad across patient's chest.	This protects bed linens.
7. **Turn suction to appropriate pressure:**	Negative pressure must be at a safe level, or pneumothorax may occur.
a. For a wall unit for an adult: 100 to 120 mm Hg	
b. For a portable wall unit for an adult: 10 to 15 cm Hg	

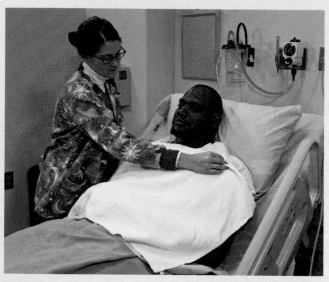

Action 5: Preparing the patient for suctioning.

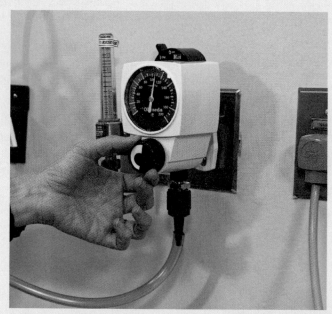

Action 7a: Adjusting wall suction.

8. **Open sterile suction package. Set up sterile container, touching only the outside surface, and pour sterile saline into it.**	Sterile normal saline or water is used to lubricate the outside of the catheter, thus minimizing irritation of mucosa during introduction.
9. Don sterile gloves. **The dominant hand that will handle the catheter must remain sterile, while the nondominant hand is considered clean rather than sterile.**	Handling the sterile catheter using a sterile glove helps prevent introducing organisms into the respiratory tract; the clean glove protects the nurse from microorganisms.
10. With sterile gloved hand, pick up sterile catheter and connect to suction tubing that is held with unsterile hand.	Sterility can be maintained.
11. Moisten the catheter by dipping it into the container of sterile saline. Occlude Y-tube to check suction.	Lubricating the inside of the catheter with saline helps move secretions in the catheter.
12. Estimate the distance from the ear lobe to the nostril and place thumb and forefinger of gloved hand at that point on the catheter.	Proper measurement ensures that catheter remains in pharynx rather than trachea.

continues

SKILL 14-14 Suctioning the Nasopharyngeal and Oropharyngeal Airways (continued)

ACTION

RATIONALE

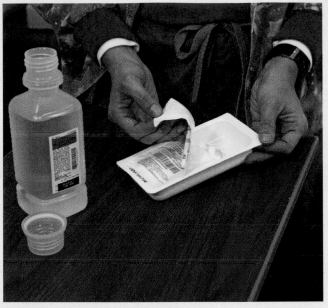

Action 8: Setting up sterile suctioning field.

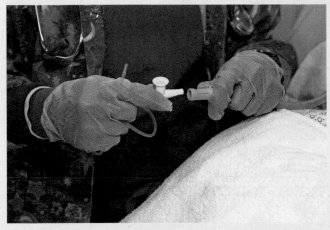

Action 10: Connecting catheter to tubing.

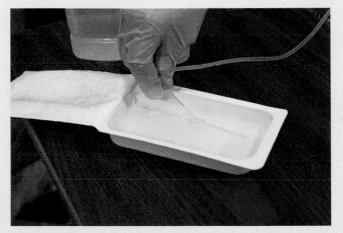

Action 11: Dipping catheter into sterile saline.

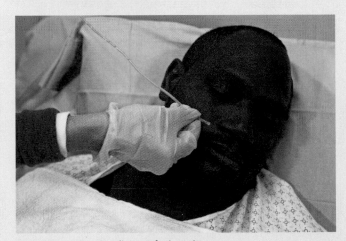

Action 12: Estimating distance for insertion.

13. **Gently insert catheter with suction off by leaving vent on Y-connector open.** Slip catheter gently along floor of an unobstructed nostril toward trachea to suction nasopharynx. Or, insert catheter along the side of the mouth toward trachea to suction oropharynx. Never apply suction as the catheter is introduced.

14. Apply suction by intermittently occluding the suctioning port with your thumb, and gently rotate the catheter as it is being withdrawn. **Do not suction for more than 10 to 15 seconds at a time.**

Using suction while inserting the catheter can cause trauma to the mucosa and removes oxygen from the respiratory tract. Coughing is induced when the trachea is touched. This helps the patient raise secretions.

Turning the catheter as it is withdrawn helps clean all surfaces of the respiratory passageways. Suctioning for longer than 10 to 15 seconds robs the respiratory tract of oxygen, which may result in hypoxia.

continues

ACTION

RATIONALE

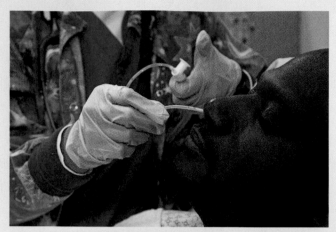

Action 13: Inserting catheter into nares.

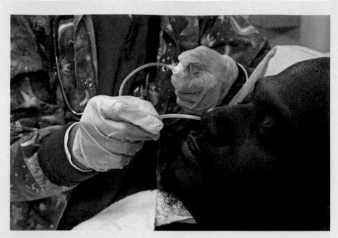

Action 14: Suctioning nasopharynx.

15. Flush catheter with saline and repeat suctioning as needed and according to patient's tolerance.

Flushing clears catheter and lubricates it for next insertion.

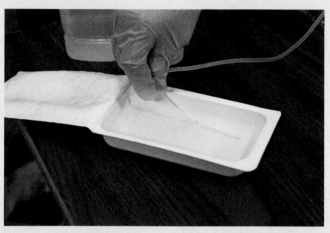

Action 15: Rinsing catheter.

16. **Allow at least a 20- to 30-second interval if additional suctioning is needed. Alternate the nares if repeated suctioning is required. Do not force catheter through the nares. Encourage patient to cough and deep breathe between suctionings.** Suction the oropharynx.

Normal breathing between suctioning helps compensate for any hypoxia induced by the suctioning.

17. When suctioning is completed, remove gloves inside out and dispose of gloves, catheter, and container with solution in proper receptacle. Perform hand hygiene.

Hand hygiene prevents transmission of microorganisms.

continues

ACTION	RATIONALE

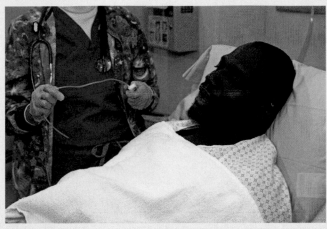

Action 16: Assessing while patient is coughing and deep breathing.

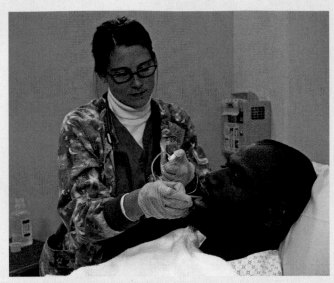

Action 16: Suctioning oropharynx.

18. Use auscultation to listen to chest and breathing sounds to assess effectiveness of suctioning.

Listening to chest and breathing sounds helps determine whether the respiratory passageways are clear of secretions.

19. Record the time of suctioning and the nature and amount of secretions. Also note the character of the patient's respirations before and after the suctioning.

Keeping records of nursing measures used helps assess, evaluate, and coordinate care.

20. Offer oral hygiene after suctioning.

Respiratory secretions that are allowed to accumulate in the mouth are irritating to mucous membranes and unpleasant for the patient.

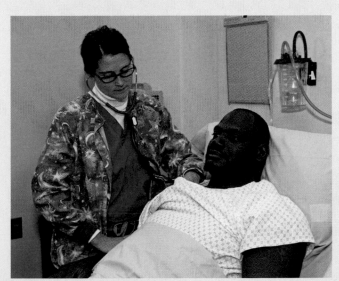

Action 18: Auscultating lung sounds.

9/17/06 1440   Lung sounds coarse in lower lobes, wheezes noted in upper lobes bilaterally. Respirations 24 breaths per minute. Intercostal retractions noted. Nasopharyngeal suction completed with 12F catheter. Large amount of thick, yellow secretions obtained. After suctioning lung sounds clear in all lobes, respirations 18 breaths per minute, no intercostal retractions noted.—C. Bausler, RN

Action 19: Documentation.

continues

SKILL 14-14   Suctioning the Nasopharyngeal and Oropharyngeal Airways (continued)

EVALUATION

The expected outcome is met when the patient exhibits a clear and patent airway. In addition, the oxygen saturation level is within acceptable parameters and the patient has no signs and symptoms of respiratory distress, such as nasal flaring, grunting, or retractions.

Unexpected Situations and Associated Interventions

- *The catheter or sterile glove touches an unsterile surface:* Stop the procedure. If the gloved hand is still sterile, ask for someone to open another catheter, or remove the gloves and start the procedure over.
- *Patient begins to cough and appears cyanotic:* This is normal. Do not suction for longer than 10 to 15 seconds and replace oxygen source. Leave adequate time between suctionings so that patient can compensate for any hypoxia induced by suctioning.
- *Patient vomits during suctioning:* If the patient needs to be suctioned again, change catheters. The catheter may be contaminated by vomit, and you do not want to pass it into the lungs. Turn patient to the side and elevate the head of the bed.
- *Secretions appear to be stomach contents:* Ask the patient to extend the neck slightly. This helps to prevent the tube from passing into the esophagus.
- *Epistaxis is noted with continued suctioning:* Notify physician and anticipate the need for a nasal trumpet (see Skill 14-15). The nasal trumpet will protect the nasal mucosa from further trauma related to suctioning.

Infant and Child Considerations

- For infants, use a 6F to 8F catheter; for children, use an 8F to 10F catheter.
- Set wall unit suction at 50 to 95 mm Hg for an infant and 95 to 110 mm Hg for a child. Set portable suction at 2 to 5 mm Hg for an infant and 5 to 10 mm Hg for a child.

SKILL 14-15   Inserting a Nasal Airway

Nasal airways are frequently referred to as nasal trumpets. These airways may be indicated if the teeth are clenched, the tongue is enlarged, or the patient needs frequent nasopharyngeal suctioning. The nasal airway is a route from the nares to the pharynx.

Equipment

- Nasal airway (average adult size is 28F)
- Disposable gloves
- Water-soluble lubricant
- Mask (if necessary)
- Goggles (if necessary)

ASSESSMENT

Assess patient's lung sounds. If lung sounds are diminished, patient may need nasal airway to keep airway patent. If lung sounds are coarse or wheezing is noted, patient may need the nasal airway to help with suctioning. Assess patient's respiratory rate and effort. If patient is not getting enough air or if patient needs to be suctioned, the respiratory rate will generally increase and the patient may have retractions, nasal flaring, and grunting. Assess the oxygen saturation level. If the patient is not getting enough air or if the patient needs to be suctioned, the oxygen saturation level will generally decrease.

continues

SKILL 14-15 | Inserting a Nasal Airway (continued)

NURSING DIAGNOSIS

Determine related factors for the nursing diagnosis based on the patient's current status. Appropriate nursing diagnoses may include:

- Risk for Aspiration
- Ineffective Airway Clearance
- Risk for Activity Intolerance
- Risk for Impaired Skin Integrity
- Risk for Infection
- Risk for Injury

OUTCOME IDENTIFICATION AND PLANNING

The expected outcome to achieve when inserting a nasal airway is that the patient will sustain and maintain a patent airway. Other outcomes that may be appropriate include the following: the patient demonstrates a respiratory rate and depth within normal limits and equal, clear lung sounds bilaterally.

IMPLEMENTATION

ACTION	RATIONALE
1. Gather equipment. Explain procedure to patient.	Explanation alleviates fears.
2. Perform hand hygiene.	Hand hygiene deters the spread of microorganisms.
3. **Measure the nasopharyngeal airway for correct size.**	The nasopharyngeal airway size is measured by holding the airway on the side of the patient's face. The airway should reach from the tragus of the ear to the nostril plus 1″.
4. Don disposable gloves. If patient is coughing or has copious secretions, a mask and goggles may also be worn.	Gloves and safety equipment protect against pathogens.
5. Adjust bed to a comfortable working level. Lower side rail closer to you. If patient is awake and alert, position patient supine in semi-Fowler's position. If patient is not conscious or alert, position patient in a side-lying position.	By raising the head of the bed or placing patient in the side-lying position, the nurse is helping to protect the airway if the patient should vomit during the placement of the nasopharyngeal airway.
6. Lubricate the nasopharyngeal airway generously with the water-soluble lubricant, covering the airway from the tip to the guard rim.	The water-soluble lubricant helps to protect the mucosa as the airway is glided in place.

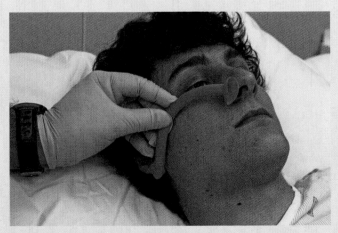

Action 3: Measuring the nasopharyngeal airway.

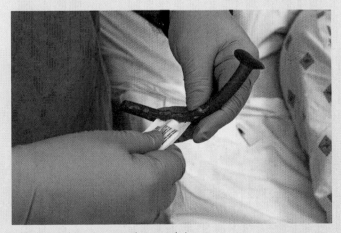

Action 6: Lubricating nasopharyngeal airway.

continues

ACTION	RATIONALE
7. Gently insert the airway into the nares until the rim is touching the nares. If resistance is met, stop and try other nares.	The airway should not be forced into the nares. The skin should not be blanched or appear stretched due to the nasopharyngeal airway.

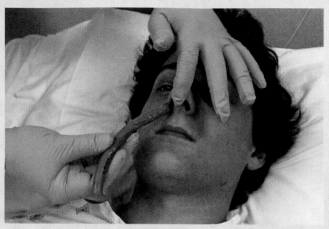

Action 7: Inserting nasopharyngeal airway.

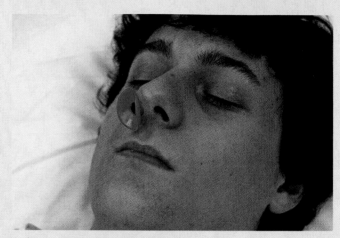

Action 7: Nasopharyngeal airway inserted.

8. **Remove the airway and place in other naris at least every 24 hours.**	The nasopharyngeal airway may lead to skin breakdown if left in place for too long.
9. If patient needs to be suctioned, follow steps in Skill 14-14. Ensure that the suction catheter is lubricated with water before suctioning to prevent any trauma to mucosa. Document the placement of the nasopharyngeal airway, including size of airway, nares placed in, and respiratory status before and after placement.	

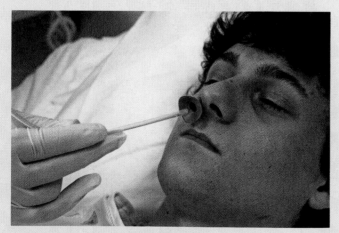

Action 9: Inserting suction catheter into nasopharyngeal airway.

9/12/06   0430   24F nasal trumpet placed in right nares due to nasal mucosa trauma from frequent suctioning. Patient suctioned for copious amount of thin, white secretions after nasopharyngeal airway placement. Lung sounds prior to suctioning course throughout; after suctioning lung sounds clear all lobes. Respirations even/unlabored.—C. Bausler, RN

Action 9: Documentation.

continues

SKILL 14-15   Inserting a Nasal Airway (continued)

EVALUATION

The expected outcome is met when the patient maintains a clear, patent airway with minimal to no secretions. In addition, the patient exhibits an oxygen saturation level >95% and respiratory rate remains in the normal range. The patient experiences no trauma when suctioned.

Unexpected Situations and Associated Interventions

- *Patient becomes tachypneic and anxious when nasal trumpet is placed:* Discuss with patient feelings regarding the nasal trumpet. Some patients feel claustrophobic when the nasal trumpet is in place. Patient may need to be sedated, if ordered, or reassurance may be needed until patient becomes accustomed to the airway. If patient does not relax, the physician may need to be notified and the airway discontinued.
- *When removing the nasopharyngeal airway, you note skin breakdown on the nares:* The size of the nasopharyngeal airway may need to be assessed. The airway may be too big, causing pressure on the skin surrounding the nares. Replace the airway in the opposite nares with a smaller-sized airway.

SKILL 14-16   Suctioning the Tracheostomy

Some patients need help removing secretions from their airways. For patients who have a tracheostomy, secretions commonly build up, necessitating suctioning.

Equipment

- Portable or wall suction unit with tubing
- Sterile suction catheter with Y-port in appropriate size (12F to 16F for an adult)
- Sterile water or saline
- Sterile disposable container
- Sterile and disposable gloves
- Towel or waterproof pad
- Goggles (or safety glasses) and mask
- Gown (optional)
- Resuscitation bag connected to 100% oxygen

ASSESSMENT

Auscultate lung sounds. Patients who need to be suctioned usually have coarse lung sounds. Assess oxygenation saturation level, which usually decreases when a patient needs to be suctioned. Assess respirations. Patients may become tachypneic when they need to be suctioned. Assess patient for signs of respiratory distress, such as nasal flaring, retractions, or grunting.

NURSING DIAGNOSIS

Determine the related factors for the nursing diagnosis based on the patient's current status. Appropriate nursing diagnoses may include:

- Ineffective Airway Clearance
- Risk for Aspiration
- Impaired Gas Exchange
- Ineffective Breathing Pattern

OUTCOME IDENTIFICATION AND PLANNING

The expected outcome to achieve when suctioning the tracheostomy is that the patient will demonstrate a clear, patent airway. Other outcomes that may be appropriate include the following: oxygenation saturation level will increase; respiratory status will remain within acceptable parameters; and patient will remain free of any signs of respiratory distress, such as retractions, nasal flaring, or grunting.

continues

IMPLEMENTATION

ACTION	RATIONALE

1. Explain procedure to patient. Reassure patient you will interrupt procedure if he or she indicates respiratory difficulty. **For postoperative patient, administer pain medication before suctioning.**

Explanation facilitates cooperation and provides reassurance for patient. Any procedure that compromises respiration is frightening for the patient. Suctioning stimulates coughing, which is painful for patients with surgical incisions.

2. Gather equipment and provide privacy for patient.

This provides for an organized approach.

3. Perform hand hygiene.

Hand hygiene deters spread of microorganisms.

4. Assist patient to semi-Fowler's or Fowler's position if conscious. If patient is unconscious, place him or her in the lateral position facing you.

Sitting position helps patient to cough and breathe more easily. This position also uses gravity to aid in catheter insertion. Lateral position prevents the airway from becoming obstructed and promotes drainage of secretions.

5. **Turn suction to appropriate pressure:** in adults, 100 to 120 mm Hg for a wall unit and 10 to 15 cm Hg for a portable unit.

Negative pressure must be at safe level, or damage to tracheal mucosa may occur.

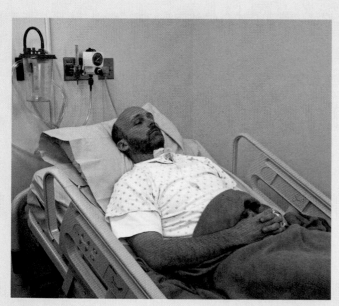

Action 4: Patient in semi-Fowler's position.

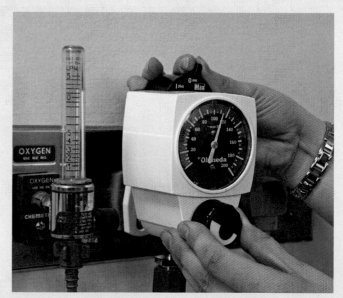

Action 5: Turning suction device to the appropriate pressure.

6. Place clean towel, if being used, or waterproof pad across patient's chest. Don goggles, mask, and gown, if necessary.

Towel protects patient and bed linens. Wearing protective equipment protects nurse against contamination of mucous membranes.

7. Open sterile kit or set up equipment and prepare to suction:

   a. Place sterile drape, if available, across patient's chest.

   b. Open sterile container and place on bedside table or overbed table without contaminating inner surface. Pour sterile saline into it.

   c. **Hyperoxygenate patient using manual resuscitation bag or sigh mechanism on mechanical ventilator.**

   a. Drape protects patient and bed linens.

   b. This maintains sterile setup.

   c. This prevents hypoxemia, which can occur during suctioning.

continues

Suctioning the Tracheostomy (continued)

ACTION	RATIONALE

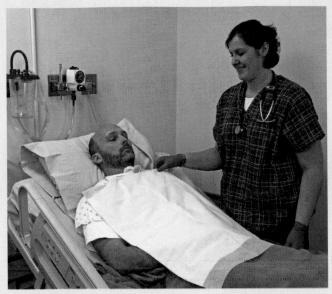

Action 6: Placing waterproof pad across patient's chest.

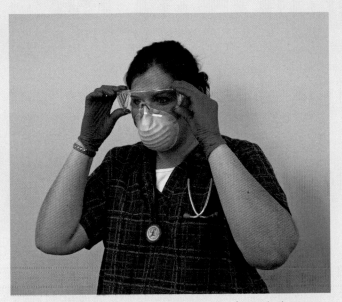

Action 6: Donning gloves and mask in preparation for suctioning.

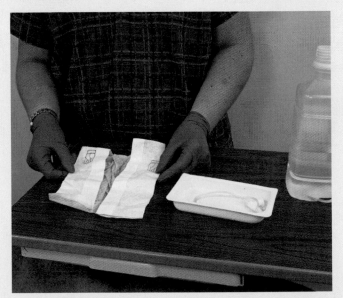

Action 7b: Setting up sterile tray.

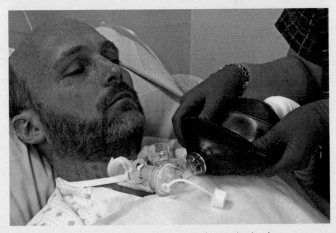

Action 7c: Hyperoxygenating using a manual resuscitation bag.

d. **Don sterile gloves, or one sterile glove on dominant hand and clean glove on nondominant hand.**

e. Connect sterile suction catheter to suction tubing that is held with unsterile gloved hand.

d. Gloves maintain sterility of procedure and protect the nurse from microorganisms.

e. Sterile technique helps prevent introduction of organisms into the respiratory tract.

continues

ACTION	RATIONALE

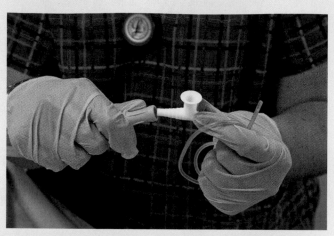

Action 7e: Connecting suction catheter to the suction tubing.

8. Holding catheter with sterile dominant hand, moisten by dipping it into the container of sterile saline or water, unless it is one of the newer silicone catheters that do not require lubrication. Check suction on catheter by occluding the Y-port.

Lubricating the inside of catheter with saline helps move secretions in the catheter. Silicone catheters do not require lubrication.

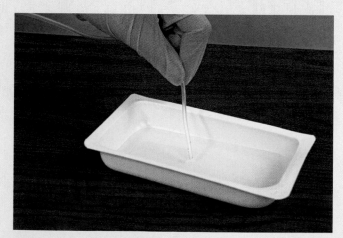

Action 8: Moistening catheter in saline solution.

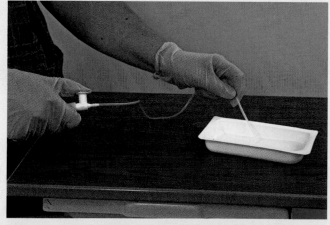

Action 8: Occluding Y-port to check for proper suction.

9. Remove oxygen delivery setup with unsterile gloved hand if it is still in place.

10. Using sterile gloved hand, gently and quickly insert catheter into trachea. **Advance about 10 to 12.5 cm (4″ to 5″), or until patient coughs. Do not occlude Y-port when inserting catheter.**

This exposes tracheostomy tube without contaminating sterile gloved hand.

Suctioning when inserting catheter can cause trauma to mucosa and removes oxygen from the respiratory tract.

continues

Suctioning the Tracheostomy (continued)

ACTION

11. **Apply intermittent suction by occluding Y-port with thumb of unsterile gloved hand. Gently rotate catheter with thumb and index finger of sterile gloved hand as catheter is being withdrawn. Do not allow suctioning to continue for more than 10 seconds. Hyperventilate three to five times between suctionings, or encourage patient to cough and deep breathe between suctionings.**

12. Flush the catheter with saline and repeat suctioning as needed and according to patient's tolerance. **Allow patient to rest at least 1 minute between suctionings, and replace oxygen delivery setup if necessary. Limit number of suctionings to three.**

RATIONALE

Turning the catheter while withdrawing it helps clean surfaces of respiratory tract and prevents injury to tracheal mucosa. Suctioning for longer than 10 seconds may result in hypoxia. Hyperventilation reoxygenates the lungs.

Flushing cleans and clears catheter and lubricates it for next insertion. Allowing a time interval between suctionings and replacing oxygen delivery setup helps compensate for hypoxia induced by the suctioning. Irritation from multiple suctionings results in an increased amount of secretions.

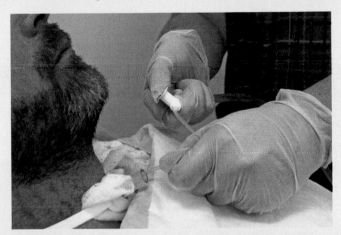

Action 11: Applying intermittent suction while withdrawing catheter.

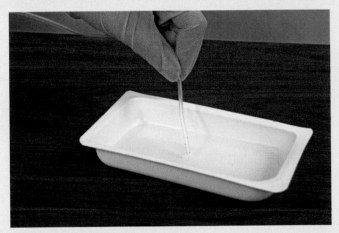

Action 12: Flushing catheter.

13. When procedure is completed, turn off suction and disconnect catheter from suction tubing. Remove gloves inside out and dispose of gloves, catheter, and container with solution in proper receptacle. Perform hand hygiene.

This prevents transmission of microorganisms.

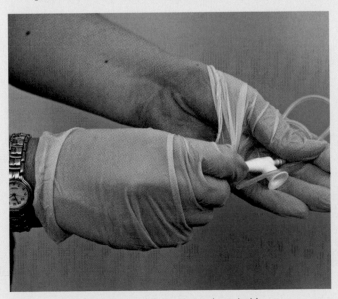

Action 13: Removing gloves while keeping catheter inside.

continues

Suctioning the Tracheostomy (continued)

ACTION	RATIONALE
14. Adjust patient's position. Reapply oxygen supply if indicated. Auscultate chest to evaluate breath sounds.	Auscultation helps determine whether respiratory passage-ways have been cleared of secretions.
15. Record the time of suctioning and the nature and amount of secretions. Also note the character of patient's respirations before and after suctioning.	This provides accurate documentation and provides for comprehensive care.
16. Offer oral hygiene.	Respiratory secretions that accumulate are irritating to mucous membranes and unpleasant for the patient.

9/1/06 1515   Lung sounds coarse lower lobes, wheezes upper lobes bilaterally. Respirations 24 breaths per minute. Intercostal retractions noted. Nasopharyngeal suction completed with 12F catheter. Large amount of thick, yellow secretions obtained. Specimen for culture collected and sent. After suctioning lung sounds clear all lobes, oxygen saturation at 97%, respirations 18 breaths per minute, no intercostal retractions noted.—C. Bausler, RN

Action 15: Documentation.

EVALUATION

The expected outcome is met when the patient exhibits a patent, clear tracheostomy without evidence of trauma or respiratory distress such as nasal flaring, grunting, or retractions. In addition, the patient's oxygen saturation level remains within acceptable parameters.

Unexpected Situations and Associated Interventions

- *Secretions are blood-tinged when suctioning:* Notify physician. Some physicians will order the catheter not to be passed past the tip of the tracheostomy to prevent damage to the trachea mucosa.
- *Patient coughs hard enough to dislodge tracheostomy:* Spare tracheostomy and obturator should be kept at bedside. Insert obturator into tracheostomy and reinsert tracheostomy into stoma. Remove obturator. Secure ties and auscultate lung sounds. Palpate for any subcutaneous emphysema.
- *Lung sounds do not improve greatly and oxygen saturation remains low after three suctionings:* Allow patient time to recover from previous suctioning. If needed, hyper-oxygenate again. Resuction patient and assess whether the oxygen saturation increases, lung sounds improve, and secretion amount decreases.

Infant and Child Considerations

- For infants, use a 6F to 8F suction catheter; for children, use an 8F to 10F catheter.
- For infants, set wall unit suction at 50 mm Hg; for children, set wall unit at 95 to 110 mm Hg.
- For infants, set portable suction at 2 to 5 cm Hg; for children, set portable unit at 5 to 10 cm Hg.

SKILL 14-17 Providing Tracheostomy Care

A tracheostomy tube is inserted for a variety of reasons: to replace an endotracheal tube, to provide a method to mechanically ventilate the patient, to bypass an upper airway obstruction, or to remove tracheobronchial secretions. Because the respiratory tract is sterile and the tracheostomy provides a direct opening, meticulous care is necessary.

Equipment

- Disposable gloves
- Sterile gloves
- Goggles or face shield (optional)
- Sterile tracheostomy cleaning kit (if available)
  or
  - Sterile basins (two)
  - Sterile brush/pipe cleaners
  - Sterile cotton-tipped applicators
- Sterile cleaning solutions:
  - Hydrogen peroxide
  - Normal saline solution
- Replacement inner cannula (if available)
- Sterile suction catheter and glove set
- Commercially prepared tracheostomy dressing or sterile non-cotton-filled 4″ × 4″ gauze pad, additional sterile gauze pad
- Tracheostomy ties (twill tape or Velcro)
- Scissors
- Plastic disposal bag

ASSESSMENT

Assess insertion site for any redness or purulent drainage; if present, these may signify an infection. Assess patient for pain. If tracheostomy is fresh, pain medication may be needed before performing tracheostomy care. Assess lung sounds and oxygen saturation levels. Lung sounds should be equal in all lobes with an oxygen saturation level >93%. If tracheostomy is dislodged, lung sounds and oxygen saturation level will diminish. Inspect the area on the posterior portion of the neck for any skin breakdown that may result from irritation or pressure from tracheostomy ties.

NURSING DIAGNOSIS

Determine the related factors for the nursing diagnosis based on the patient's current status. Appropriate nursing diagnoses may include:

- Impaired Skin Integrity
- Risk for Infection
- Ineffective Airway Clearance
- Risk for Aspiration

OUTCOME IDENTIFICATION AND PLANNING

The expected outcome to achieve when performing tracheostomy care is that the patient will exhibit a tracheostomy site free from drainage and skin breakdown. Other outcomes that may be appropriate include the following: oxygen saturation levels will be within acceptable parameters and patient will have no evidence of respiratory distress.

continues

IMPLEMENTATION

ACTION	RATIONALE

1. Explain procedure to patient.

   Explanation facilitates cooperation and provides reassurance for patient.

2. If tracheostomy tube has just been suctioned, remove soiled dressing from around tube and discard with gloves when they are removed.

   Suctioning prevents secretions from accumulating in inner cannula and occluding airway.

3. Perform hand hygiene and open necessary supplies.

   Hand hygiene deters spread of microorganisms.

Cleaning a Nondisposable Inner Cannula

4. Prepare supplies before cleaning inner cannula

   a. Open tracheostomy care kit and separate basins, touching only the edges. If kit is not available, open two sterile basins.

      a. Basins are sterile receptacles for cleaning solutions.

   b. Fill one basin 0.5″ (1.25 cm) deep with hydrogen peroxide.

      b. Hydrogen peroxide helps remove dry, encrusted secretions.

   c. Fill other basin 0.5″ (1.25 cm) deep with saline.

      c. Saline rinses and removes hydrogen peroxide and lubricates the outer surface of the inner cannula for easier reinsertion.

   d. Open sterile brush or pipe cleaners if they are not already available in a cleaning kit. Open additional sterile gauze pad.

      d. Sterile brush or pipe cleaner provides friction to clean inner surface of cannula.

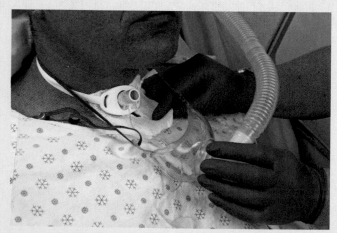

Action 2: Removing soiled dressing.

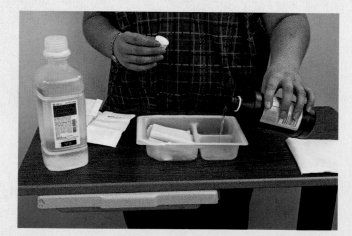

Action 4: Preparing sterile field.

5. Don disposable gloves.

   Gloves protect against exposure to blood and body substances.

6. Remove the oxygen source if one is present. Rotate the lock on the inner cannula in a counterclockwise motion to release it.

   Releasing the lock permits removal of the inner cannula.

7. Gently remove the inner cannula and carefully drop it in the basin with hydrogen peroxide. Remove gloves and discard.

   Soaking in hydrogen peroxide loosens dry, hardened secretions.

continues

SKILL 14-17 Providing Tracheostomy Care (continued)

ACTION

RATIONALE

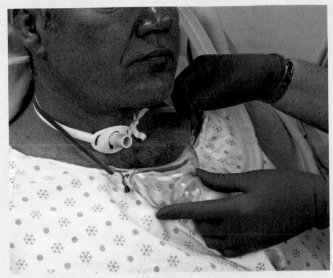

Action 6: Removing oxygen source if one is present.

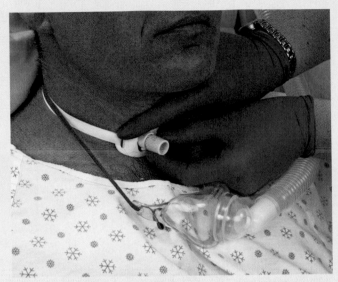

Action 6: Rotating inner cannula while stabilizing outer cannula.

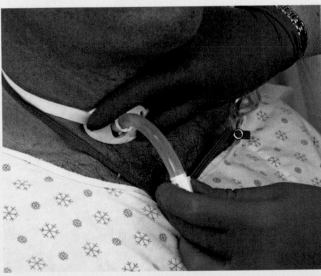

Action 7: Removing inner cannula for cleaning.

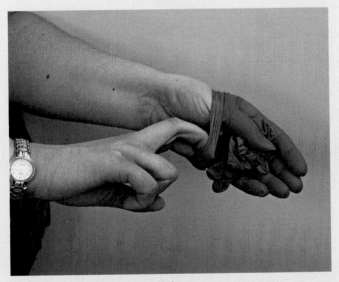

Action 7: Removing contaminated gloves.

8. Clean the inner cannula:
   a. Don sterile gloves.
   b. Remove inner cannula from soaking solution. Moisten brush or pipe cleaners in saline and insert into tube, using back-and-forth motion.
   c. Agitate cannula in saline solution. Remove and tap against inner surface of basin.
   d. Place on sterile gauze pad.

a. Sterile gloves maintain surgical asepsis.
b. Movement of brush creates friction and helps remove accumulated secretions.

c. Saline rinses inner cannula. Tapping tube against basin removes excess saline in inner tube.
d. Placing on sterile gauze maintains sterility and frees both hands for suctioning.

continues

Providing Tracheostomy Care (continued)

ACTION

RATIONALE

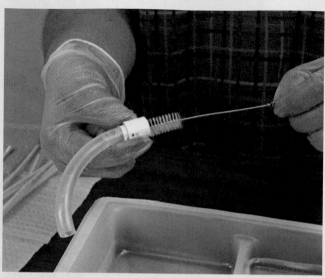

Action 8b: Using brush to clean inner cannula.

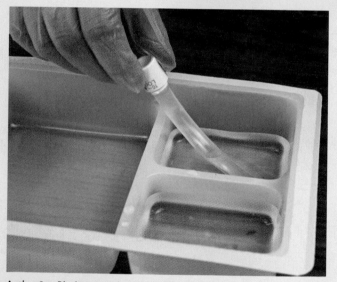

Action 8c: Rinsing cannula using an agitating motion.

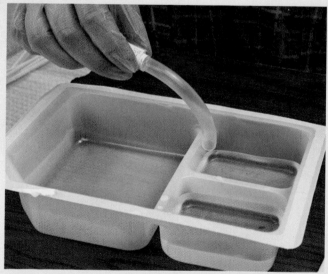

Action 8c: Tapping cannula to remove excessive moisture.

9. **Suction outer cannula using sterile technique if necessary.**

10. Replace inner cannula into outer cannula. Turn lock clockwise and check that inner cannula is secure. Reapply oxygen source if needed.

Replacing a Disposable Inner Cannula

11. Release lock. Gently remove inner cannula and place in disposal bag. Discard gloves and don sterile ones to insert new cannula. Replace with appropriately sized new cannula. Engage lock on inner cannula.

Suctioning removes any remaining secretions.

Clockwise motion secures inner cannula in place.

Disposable cannulas, although more costly, ensure that airway is clean and patent.

continues

Providing Tracheostomy Care (continued)

ACTION   **RATIONALE**

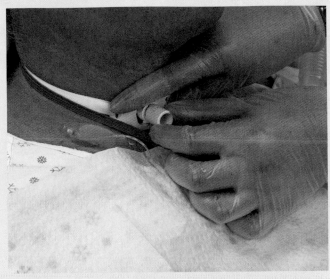

Action 10: Replacing inner cannula.

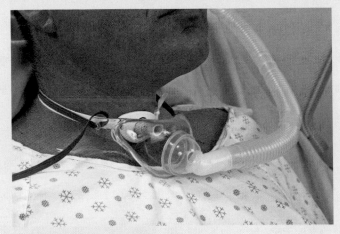

Action 10: Reapplying oxygen source.

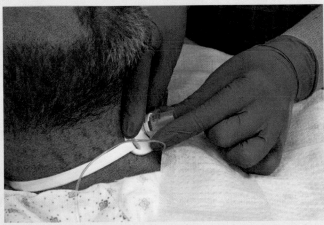

Action 11: Releasing lock on inner cannula.

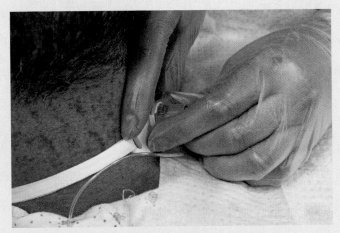

Action 11: Locking new inner cannula in place.

Applying Clean Dressing and Tape

12. Dip cotton-tipped applicator in sterile saline and clean stoma under faceplate. **Use each applicator only once, moving from stoma site outward.**

13. If secretions prove difficult to remove, apply diluted 1/2 strength hydrogen peroxide to area around stoma, faceplate, and outer cannula. Rinse area with saline.

14. Pat skin gently with dry 4″ × 4″ gauze.

15. Slide commercially prepared tracheostomy dressing or prefolded non-cotton-filled 4″ × 4″ dressing under faceplate.

Saline is nonirritating to tissue. Cleansing from stoma outward and using each applicator only once promotes aseptic technique.

Hydrogen peroxide may cause tissue damage and needs to be removed from skin and surrounding area.

Gauze removes excess moisture.

Lint or fiber from cotton-filled gauze pad can be aspirated into the trachea and cause irritation.

continues

ACTION   **RATIONALE**

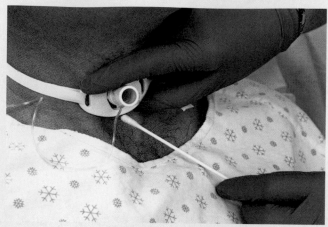

Action 12: Cleaning with cotton-tipped applicators under faceplate.

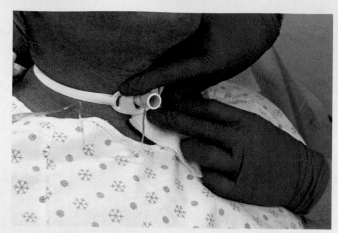

Action 14: Patting skin around stoma gently.

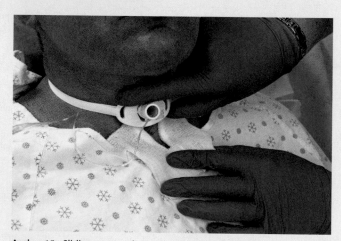

Action 15: Sliding new tracheostomy dressing under faceplate.

16. Change the tracheostomy tape:

   a. **Leave soiled tape in place until new one is applied.**

   a. Leaving tape in place ensures that tracheostomy will not be expelled if patient coughs or moves.

   b. Cut piece of tape that is twice the neck circumference plus 4″ (10 cm). Trim ends of tape on the diagonal.

   b. This action provides for secure attachment with knot in front at neckplate. Diagonal cut facilitates insertion of tape into openings on faceplate.

   c. Insert one end of tape through faceplate opening alongside old tape. Pull through until both ends are even.

   c. Doing so provides attachment for one side of faceplate.

   d. Slide both tapes under patient's neck and insert one end through remaining opening on other side of faceplate. Pull snugly and tie ends in double square knot. Check that patient can flex neck comfortably.

   d. A secure tape prevents accidental expulsion of the tracheostomy tube. Allowing one finger breadth under tape permits neck flexion that is comfortable and ensures that tape will not compromise circulation to the area.

   e. Carefully remove old tape. Reapply oxygen source if necessary.

   e. New tape provides for secure attachment.

continues

SKILL 14-17 — Providing Tracheostomy Care (continued)

ACTION	RATIONALE

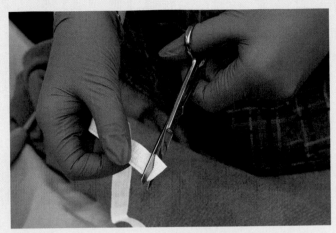

Action 16b: Cutting twill tape.

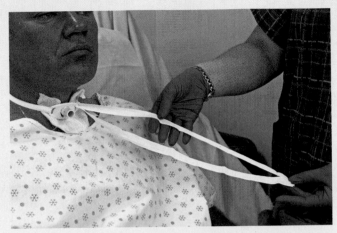

Action 16c: Pulling tape through alongside old tape.

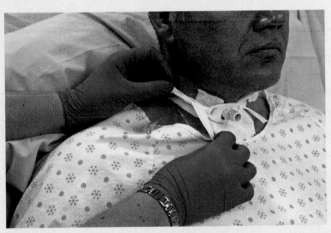

Action 16d: Tying ends with a double square knot.

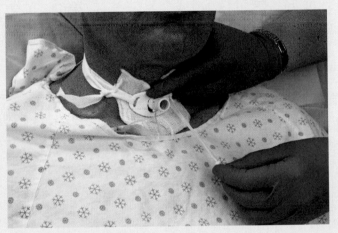

Action 16e: Removing old ties.

17. Remove gloves and discard. Perform hand hygiene. Assess patient's respirations. Document assessments and completion of procedure.

Assessment and accurate documentation provide for comprehensive care.

> 9/26/06   1300   Trach care completed; lung sounds clear in all lobes; respirations even/ unlabored; site without erythema or edema; small amount of thick yellow secretions noted at site.—C. Bausler, RN

Action 17: Documentation.

EVALUATION

The expected outcome is met when the patient exhibits a clean, dry tracheostomy site that is free of redness, irritation, or drainage and the patient demonstrates respiratory status within acceptable parameters, including bilaterally clear and equal lung sounds and oxygen saturation level >93%. In addition, the patient verbalizes that site is free of pain and exhibits no evidence of skin breakdown on the posterior portion of the neck.

continues

Providing Tracheostomy Care (continued)

Unexpected Situations and Associated Interventions

- *Patient coughs hard enough to dislodge tracheostomy:* Spare tracheostomy and obturator should be kept at bedside. Insert obturator into tracheostomy and reinsert tracheostomy into stoma. Remove obturator. Secure ties and auscultate lung sounds. Palpate for any subcutaneous emphysema.
- *Outer cannula is removed for cleaning, but when you attempt to reinsert it, it will not fit into the opening:* Spare tracheostomy at bedside is generally one size smaller than tracheostomy tube in place to account for discrepancies such as this.
- *On palpating around insertion site, you note a moderate amount of subcutaneous emphysema in tissue:* Assess for dislodgement of the tracheostomy tube. If the tube becomes displaced, a buildup of air in the subcutaneous portion of the skin is likely. Notify physician if the subcutaneous emphysema is a change in the status of the tracheostomy.

Home Care Considerations

- The patient and home caregiver should be instructed on how to perform tracheostomy care. The nurse should observe a return demonstration and provide feedback.
- Clean rather than sterile technique can be used in the home setting.
- Sterile saline can be made by mixing 1 teaspoon of table salt in 1 quart of water and boiling for 15 minutes. The solution is cooled and stored in a clean, dry container. Saline is discarded at the end of each day to prevent growth of bacteria.
- The patient who is performing self-care should use a mirror to view the steps in the procedure.

Retaping an Endotracheal Tube

Patients who have an endotracheal tube are at a higher risk for skin breakdown due to the securing of the endotracheal tube, compounded by the chance for increased secretions. The endotracheal tube should be retaped every 24 hours to prevent skin breakdown and to ensure that the tube is properly secured. Retaping an endotracheal tube requires two people. There are other ways of securing an endotracheal tube besides tape. To secure with another device, follow the manufacturer's recommendations. One example of taping an endotracheal tube is provided below, but this skill might be performed differently in your institution; always refer to specific agency policy.

Equipment

- Assistant (nurse or respiratory therapist)
- Portable or wall suction unit with tubing
- Sterile suction catheter with Y-port
- 1″ tape (cloth or silk)
- Disposable gloves
- Sterile suctioning kit
- Oral suction catheter
- Two 3-mL syringes or tongue blade
- Scissors
- Washcloth
- Benzoin (optional)
- Towel
- Razor (optional)
- Shaving cream (optional)
- Sterile saline or water
- Hand-held pressure gauge

continues

<table>
<tr><td>SKILL
14-18</td><td>Retaping an Endotracheal Tube (continued)</td></tr>
</table>

ASSESSMENT

Assess endotracheal tube length. The tube has markings on the side to ensure it is not moved during the retaping. Assess lung sounds to obtain a baseline. Ensure that the lung sounds are still heard throughout the lobes. Assess oxygen saturation level. If the tube is dislodged, the oxygen saturation level may change. Assess the chest for symmetrical rise and fall during respiration. If the tube is dislodged, the rise and fall of the chest will change. Assess patient's need for pain medication or sedation. The patient should be calm, free of pain, and relaxed during the retaping so that he or she does not move and cause an accidental extubation.

NURSING DIAGNOSIS

Determine the related factors for the nursing diagnosis based on the patient's current status. Appropriate nursing diagnoses may include:

- Ineffective Airway Clearance
- Risk for Impaired Skin Integrity
- Risk for Aspiration
- Impaired Oral Mucous Membrane
- Risk for Infection
- Risk for Injury

OUTCOME IDENTIFICATION AND PLANNING

The expected outcome to achieve when retaping an endotracheal tube is that the tube remains in place with bilaterally equal and clear lung sounds. Other outcomes may include: the patient demonstrates understanding about the reason for the endotracheal tube; skin remains intact; oxygen saturation remains >95%; chest rises symmetrically; and airway remains clear.

IMPLEMENTATION

ACTION	RATIONALE
1. Explain procedure to patient. Reassure patient that you will interrupt procedure if he or she indicates respiratory difficulty. **Administer pain medication or sedation before attempting to retape endotracheal tube.**	Explanation facilitates cooperation and provides reassurance for patient. Any procedure that compromises respiration is frightening for the patient. Retaping the endotracheal tube can stimulate coughing, which is painful for patients with surgical incisions.
2. Gather equipment and provide privacy for patient.	This provides for an organized approach.
3. Perform hand hygiene.	Hand hygiene deters spread of microorganisms.
4. Suction patient as described in Skill 14-16.	This decreases the likelihood of patient coughing during the retaping of the endotracheal tube. If the patient coughs, the tube may become dislodged.
5. Cut tape. Use enough tape to go around patient's neck to the mouth plus 8″.	Extra length is needed so that tape can be wrapped around the endotracheal tube.
6. Cut another piece of tape long enough to reach from one jaw around the back of the neck to the other jaw. Match the tapes' adhesive sides together in the center of the longer piece of tape.	This prevents the tape from sticking to the patient's hair and the back of the neck.
7. Take one 3-mL syringe or tongue blade and wrap the sticky tape around the syringe until the nonsticky area is reached. Do this for the other side as well.	This helps the nurse or respiratory therapist to manage the tape without it sticking to the sheets or the patient's hair.
8. Take one of the 3-mL syringes or tongue blade and pass it under the patient's neck so that there is a 3-mL syringe on either side of the patient's head.	This makes the tape easy to access when retaping the tube.
9. Don disposable gloves. Have assistant don gloves as well.	Gloves protect hands from exposure to pathogens.
10. **Provide oral care, including suctioning the oral cavity.**	This helps to decrease secretions in the oral cavity and pharynx region.

continues

SKILL 14-18   Retaping an Endotracheal Tube (continued)

ACTION	RATIONALE
11. Begin to unwrap old tape from around the endotracheal tube. After one side is unwrapped, have assistant hold tube to offer stabilization. Instruct assistant to hold tube as close to the lips or nares as possible.	Assistant should hold tube to prevent accidental extubation. Holding tube as close to lips or nares as possible prevents accidental dislodgement of tube.
12. **After tape is removed, have assistant gently and slowly move endotracheal tube (if orally intubated) to the other side of the mouth. Assess mouth for any skin breakdown. Before applying new tape, make sure that markings on endotracheal tube are at same spot as when retaping began.**	The endotracheal tube may cause pressure ulcers if left in the same place over time. By moving the tube, the risk for pressure ulcers is reduced.
13. Remove old tape from cheeks and side of face. Clean area to remove old tape and benzoin. If patient is male, consider shaving cheeks. Pat cheeks dry with a 4″ × 4″ gauze.	To prevent skin breakdown, remove old adhesive. Shaving helps to decrease pain when tape is removed. Cheeks must be dry before new tape is applied to ensure that it sticks. If patient has a large amount of oral secretions, consider applying benzoin across the cheek where the tape will be placed.

Action 11: Ensuring endotracheal tube is stabilized and remove old tape.

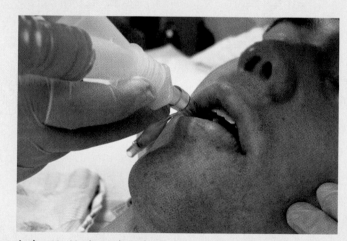

Action 12: Moving endotracheal tube to other side of mouth.

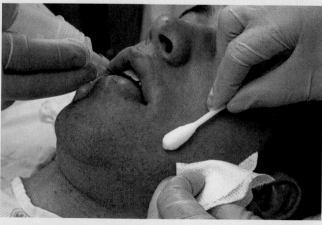

Action 13: Cleaning cheeks at site of tape.

continues

ACTION	RATIONALE
14. Consider applying benzoin. Unroll one side of the tape. Ensure that nonsticky part of tape remains behind patient's neck while pulling firmly on the tape. **Place adhesive portion of tape snugly against patient's cheek.** Split the tape in half from the end to the corner of the mouth.	The tape should be snug to the side of the patient's face to prevent accidental extubation. Benzoin helps tape remain secure even if saturated with oral secretions.
15. Wrap the top half-piece of split tape around the tube in one direction (such as over and around the tube) and then secure it across the upper lip. Wrap the bottom half-piece of split tape around the endotracheal tube in the opposite direction (such as below and around the tube) and secure the tape beneath the lower lip. Fold over tab on end of tape.	By placing one piece of tape on the lip and the other piece of tape on the tube, the tube remains secure. Tab makes tape removal easier.
16. Unwrap second piece of tape. Split to corner of the mouth. Reversing the order, place bottom piece of tape on the top lip (such as over and around the tube). Wrap top piece of tape in the opposite manner (such as below and around the tube) and secure to the lower lip. Fold over tab on end of tape.	Alternating the placement of the top and bottom pieces of tape provides more anchorage for the tube. Wrapping the tape in an alternating manner ensures that the tape will not accidentally be unwound.

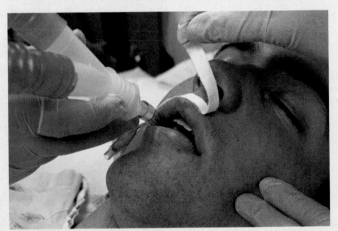

Action 15: Putting new tape in place.

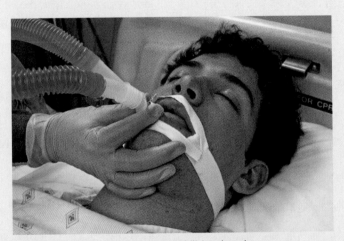

Action 16: Ensuring tape is securely stabilizing the tube.

17. **Auscultate lung sounds. Assess for cyanosis, oxygen saturation, chest symmetry, and stability of endotracheal tube. Again check to ensure that the tube is at the correct depth.**	If tube has been moved from original place, the lung sounds may change as well as oxygen saturation and chest symmetry. The tube should be stable and should not move with each respiration cycle.
18. **If endotracheal tube is cuffed, check pressure of balloon by attaching a hand-held pressure gauge to the pilot balloon of the endotracheal tube.**	The pressure of a balloon on an endotracheal tube is normally at least 20 cm H_2O to prevent aspiration and less than 25 cm H_2O to prevent trauma to the trachea.
19. Remove gloves and perform hand hygiene.	Hand hygiene deters the spread of microorganisms.
20. Document the procedure, including the depth of the endotracheal tube from teeth or lips; amount, consistency, and color of secretions suctioned; presence of any pressure ulcers; lung sounds; oxygen saturation; skin color; cuff pressure; and chest symmetry.	Documentation of nursing measures used helps assess, evaluate, and coordinate care.

continues

SKILL 14-18   Retaping an Endotracheal Tube (continued)

ACTION

RATIONALE

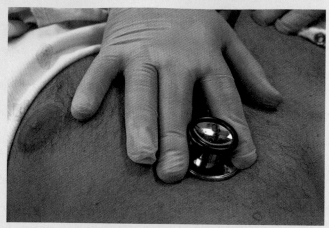

Action 17: Auscultating lung sounds.

> 9/27/06   1305   Endotracheal tube tape changed; tube remains 12 cm at lips; suctioned for tenacious, yellow secretions, copious in amount; 2-cm pressure ulcer noted on left side of tongue. Tube moved to right side of mouth; lung sounds clear and equal after retaping; pulse oximeter remains 98% on 35% FiO_2; skin pink; cuff pressure 22 cmH_2O; chest rises symmetrically.—C. Bausler, RN

Action 20: Documentation.

EVALUATION

The expected outcome is met when the endotracheal tube tape is changed without dislodgement or a depth change of the tube; lung sounds remain equal; no pressure ulcers are noted; airway remains clear; oxygen saturation remains >95%; chest rises symmetrically; skin remains acyanotic; and cuff pressure is maintained at 20 to 25 cm H_2O.

Unexpected Situations and Associated Interventions

- *Patient is accidentally extubated during tape change:* Stay with patient. Instruct assistant to notify physician. Assess patient's vital signs, ability to breathe without assistance, and oxygen saturation. Be ready to deliver assisted breaths with a bag-valve mask (Skill 14-21) or administer oxygen. Anticipate the need for reintubation.
- *Tube depth changes during retaping:* Tube depth should be maintained at the same level unless otherwise ordered by the physician. Remove tape around tube, adjust tube to ordered depth, and reapply tape.
- *Air leak (air escaping around the balloon) is heard on inspiration cycle of ventilator:* Auscultate lung sounds and check depth of endotracheal tube to ensure that it has not dislodged. Obtain hand-held pressure gauge and check pressure. Air may need to be added to balloon to prevent air leak. If pressure is already 25 cm H_2O, physician may need to be contacted before adding more air to balloon. Sometimes a change in the patient's position will resolve air leaks.
- *Patient is biting on endotracheal tube:* Obtain a bite block. With the help of an assistant, place the bite block around the endotracheal tube or in patient's mouth. If ordered, consider sedating the patient.
- *Depth of endotracheal tube changes with respiratory cycle:* Remove old tape. Repeat taping of the endotracheal tube, ensuring that tape is snug against patient's face.
- *Patient has trauma to face that prevents the use of tape when securing the endotracheal tube:* You may need to obtain an endotracheal tube securement device. There are various types on the market; check with your institution for availability.
- *Lung sounds are greater on one side:* Check the depth of the endotracheal tube. If the tube has been advanced, the lung sounds will appear greater on the side on which the tube is further down. Remove tape and move tube so that it is properly placed. If the depth has not changed, assess patient's oxygen saturation, skin color, and respiratory rate. Notify physician. Anticipate the need for a chest x-ray.

continues

Retaping an Endotracheal Tube (continued)

- *Pressure ulcer is noted in the mouth or nares (if patient is intubated via nares):* If the ulcer is painful, you may obtain an order for a topical numbing medication such as lidocaine viscous jelly. Apply topically with cotton-tipped applicator. Keep area clean by performing more frequent oral or nasal care. Ensure that tubing is not pulling on endotracheal tube, thus applying pressure on the patient's skin.
- *Pilot balloon is accidentally cut while caring for endotracheal tube:* Notify physician. Obtain a 22-gauge catheter and thread it into the pilot balloon tubing, being careful not to puncture the tubing with the needle, below the cut. Remove the needle from the catheter and apply a stopcock or needleless Luer-Lok to the catheter. If air is needed to reinflate the balloon, a syringe can be attached to the stopcock or Luer-Lok so that air may be added. Anticipate the need for a tube change.

Special Considerations

- Bag-valve mask, oxygen, and suction equipment should be kept at the bedside of a patient with an endotracheal tube at all times.

Suctioning an Endotracheal Tube

Open System

Some consider open system suctioning to be the most efficient way to suction the endotracheal tube, arguing that there are no limitations to the movement of the suction catheter while suctioning. However, an open system may be unknowingly contaminated by the nurse before insertion. In addition, with the open system, the patient must be removed from the ventilator during suctioning.

Equipment

- Suction kit or
  - Suction catheter
  - Sterile gloves
  - Basin for sterile saline or water
- Portable or wall suction unit with tubing
- Sterile suction catheter with Y-port of appropriate size
- Goggles or safety glasses and disposable gloves
- Manual resuscitation bag with oxygen
- Towel or sterile drape (optional)
- Assistant (optional)

ASSESSMENT

Assess patient's lung sounds. If patient needs to be suctioned, lung sounds will frequently be diminished or coarse, and wheezing may be present. Assess oxygen saturation level. If patient needs to be suctioned, the oxygen saturation level may be decreased. Assess for cough. Frequently patients will cough due to stimulation from the excess secretions. Also assess for pain. If patient has had abdominal surgery or other procedures, pain medication should be administered before suctioning. Assess respirations. Patients may become tachypneic if they need to be suctioned. Assess patient for signs of respiratory distress such as nasal flaring, retractions, or grunting.

continues

NURSING DIAGNOSIS	Determine the related factors for the nursing diagnosis based on the patient's current status. Appropriate nursing diagnoses may include: • Ineffective Airway Clearance • Risk for Aspiration • Risk for Infection • Impaired Gas Exchange
OUTCOME IDENTIFICATION AND PLANNING	The expected outcome to achieve when suctioning the endotracheal tube is that the patient will maintain a patent airway. Other outcomes that may be appropriate include the following: the oxygenation saturation level will increase; respirations may decrease; and the patient will exhibit no signs of respiratory distress such as retractions, nasal flaring, or grunting.

IMPLEMENTATION

ACTION	RATIONALE
1. Explain procedure to patient. Reassure patient that you will interrupt procedure if he or she indicates respiratory difficulty. **For postoperative patient, administer pain medication before suctioning.**	Explanation facilitates cooperation and provides reassurance for patient. Any procedure that compromises respiration is frightening for the patient. Suctioning stimulates coughing, which is painful for patients with surgical incisions.
2. Gather equipment and provide privacy for patient.	This provides for organized approach to task.
3. Perform hand hygiene.	Hand hygiene deters spread of microorganisms.
4. Assist patient to semi-Fowler's or Fowler's position.	Sitting position helps patient to cough and breathe more easily. This position also uses gravity to aid in the insertion of catheter.
5. **Turn suction to appropriate pressure.**	Negative pressure must be at safe level, or damage to tracheal mucosa may occur.
6. Place clean towel (if used) across patient's chest. Don goggles, mask, and gown, if necessary.	Towel protects patient and bed linens. Protective equipment prevents contamination of caregiver's mucous membranes.
7. Open sterile kit or set up equipment and prepare to suction:	
a. Place sterile drape, if available, across patient's chest.	a. Drape protects patient and bed linens.
b. Open sterile container and place on bedside table or overbed table without contaminating inner surface. Pour sterile saline into it.	b. This maintains sterile setup.
c. **Hyperoxygenate patient using manual resuscitation bag (may be easier to have assistant deliver breaths) or sigh mechanism on ventilator.**	c. This prevents hypoxemia, which can occur during suctioning.
d. **Don sterile gloves or one sterile glove on dominant hand and clean glove on nondominant hand.**	d. Gloves maintain sterility of procedure and protect nurse from microorganisms.
e. Connect sterile suction catheter to suction tubing that is held with unsterile gloved hand.	e. Sterile technique helps prevent introduction of organisms into the respiratory tract.
8. **Keeping catheter wrapped around sterile hand, remove ventilator from endotracheal tube with nonsterile hand.**	Wrapping the catheter around the sterile hand prevents contamination of the catheter.
9. **Hyperoxygenate or hyperventilate patient with manual resuscitation bag three to five times between suctionings.** Keeping the catheter sterile, gently insert the catheter into the endotracheal tube, advancing until patient begins to cough or resistance is met. **Do not occlude Y-port when inserting catheter.**	Hyperoxygenating or hyperventilating patient before suctioning helps to decrease the effects of oxygen removal during suctioning. The catheter is inserted far enough if the patient begins to cough. Suctioning when inserting the catheter can cause trauma to the mucosa and removes oxygen from the respiratory tract.

continues

SKILL 14-19 | **Suctioning an Endotracheal Tube** (continued)

ACTION

RATIONALE

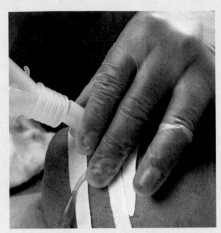

Action 8: Removing ventilator from endotracheal tube to suction.

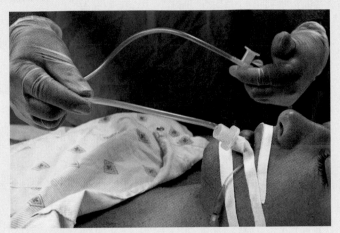

Action 9: Inserting suction catheter into endotracheal tube.

10. **Apply intermittent suction by occluding Y-port with thumb of unsterile gloved hand. Gently rotate catheter with thumb and index finger of sterile gloved hand as catheter is being withdrawn. Do not suction for more than 10 seconds.**

11. Flush catheter with saline and repeat suctioning as needed and according to patient's tolerance. **Allow patient to rest at least 1 minute between suctionings, and replace oxygen delivery setup if necessary. Limit number of suctionings to three. Reconnect to the ventilator and hyperoxygenate or hyperventilate patient with manual resuscitation bag three to five times between suctionings.**

Turning the catheter while withdrawing it helps clean surfaces of respiratory tract and prevents injury to tracheal mucosa. Suctioning for longer than 10 seconds may result in hypoxia. Hyperoxygenation and hyperventilation reoxygenate the lungs.

Flushing cleans and clears catheter and lubricates it for next insertion. Allowing time interval and replacing oxygen delivery setup helps compensate for hypoxia induced by the suctioning. Irritation from multiple suctionings results in an increased amount of secretions.

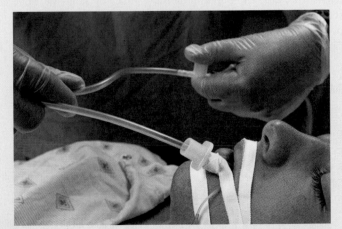

Action 10: Pulling suction catheter back with finger on thumb.

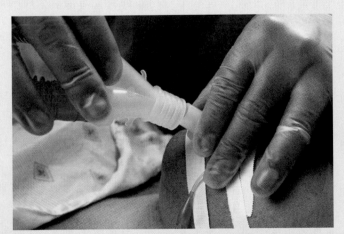

Action 11: Reconnecting ventilator tubing to endotracheal tube.

continues

ACTION	RATIONALE
12. When procedure is completed, turn off suction and disconnect catheter from suction tubing. Remove gloves inside out and dispose of gloves, catheter, and container with solution in proper receptacle.	Disposing of catheter inside of gloves deters the spread of pathogens.
13. Suction the oral cavity and perform oral hygiene.	Suctioning of the oral cavity removes secretions that may be stagnant in the mouth and pharynx, reducing the risk for infection. Oral hygiene offers comfort to the patient.
14. Perform hand hygiene.	This prevents transmission of microorganisms.
15. Adjust patient's position. Auscultate chest to evaluate breath sounds.	Auscultation helps determine whether respiratory passageways have been cleared of secretions.
16. Record the time of suctioning and the nature and amount of secretions. Also note the character of patient's respirations before and after suctioning.	This provides accurate documentation and provides for comprehensive care.

9/1/06   1850   Lung sounds coarse lower lobes, wheezes upper lobes bilaterally. Respirations 24 breaths per minute. Intercostal retractions noted. Closed endotracheal tube suction completed with 12F catheter. Small amount of thin, white secretions obtained. Specimen for culture collected and sent. After suctioning lung sounds clear in all lobes, respirations 18 breaths per minute, no intercostal retractions noted.—C. Bausler, RN

Action 16: Documentation.

Closed System

Closed system suction may be used routinely or when a patient must be frequently and quickly suctioned due to an excess of secretions, depending on the policies of the institution. Closed system suctioning is thought to decrease the risk for contamination by the nurse since everything is self-contained. One drawback is thought to be the hindrance of the sheath when rotating the suction catheter upon removal.

Equipment	• Portable or wall suction unit with tubing • Closed suction device appropriate for size of patient • 3-mL or 5-mL saline dosette
ASSESSMENT	Assess patient's lung sounds. If patient needs to be suctioned, lung sounds will frequently be diminished or coarse. Wheezing may also be present. Assess oxygen saturation level. If patient needs to be suctioned, the oxygen saturation may be decreased. Assess for cough. Frequently patients cough due to the stimulation from the excess secretions. Assess for pain. If patient has had abdominal surgery or other procedures, pain medication should be administered before suctioning. Assess respirations. Patients may become tachypneic if they need to be suctioned. Assess patient for signs of respiratory distress such as nasal flaring, retractions, or grunting.

continues

SKILL
14-19

Suctioning an Endotracheal Tube (continued)

NURSING DIAGNOSIS

Determine the related factors for the nursing diagnosis based on the patient's current status. Appropriate nursing diagnoses may include:

- Ineffective Airway Clearance
- Risk for Aspiration
- Risk for Infection
- Impaired Gas Exchange

OUTCOME IDENTIFICATION AND PLANNING

The expected outcome to achieve when suctioning the endotracheal tube is that the patient will demonstrate a patent airway. Other outcomes that may be appropriate include the following: the oxygenation saturation level will increase and the patient will exhibit no signs of respiratory distress such as retractions, nasal flaring, or grunting.

IMPLEMENTATION

ACTION	RATIONALE
1. Explain procedure to patient. Reassure patient that you will interrupt procedure if he or she indicates respiratory difficulty. **Administer pain medication before suctioning a postoperative patient.**	Explanation facilitates cooperation and provides reassurance for patient. Any procedure that compromises respiration is frightening for the patient. Suctioning stimulates coughing, which is painful for patients with surgical incisions.
2. Gather equipment and provide privacy for patient.	This provides for organized approach to task.
3. Perform hand hygiene.	Hand hygiene deters spread of microorganisms.
4. Assist patient to semi-Fowler's or Fowler's position.	Sitting position helps patient to cough and breathe more easily. This position also uses gravity to aid in the insertion of catheter. If closed system suction device is already in place, proceed to Action 11.
To use a closed suction device:	
5. Open sterile package of closed suction device. **Make sure that the device remains sterile.**	The device must remain sterile to prevent a nosocomial infection.
6. Don sterile gloves.	Gloves deter the spread of microorganisms.
7. Using nondominant hand, disconnect ventilator from endotracheal tube. **Place ventilator tubing so that the inside of the tubing remains sterile.**	This provides access to the endotracheal tube while keeping one hand sterile. The inside of the ventilator tubing should remain sterile to prevent a nosocomial infection.
8. **Using dominant hand and keeping device sterile, connect the closed suctioning device so that the suctioning catheter is parallel with the endotracheal tube.** Attach suction tubing to suction catheter (do not need to remain sterile for this step).	Keeping the device sterile decreases the risk for a nosocomial infection.
9. **Keeping the inside of the ventilator tubing sterile, attach ventilator tubing to port perpendicular to the endotracheal tube.**	The inside of the ventilator tubing must remain sterile to prevent a nosocomial infection. By connecting the ventilator tubing to the port, the patient does not need to be disconnected from the ventilator to be suctioned.
10. **Turn suction to appropriate pressure.**	Negative pressure must be at safe level, or damage to tracheal mucosa may occur.
11. Pop top off sterile normal saline dosette. Open plug to port by suction catheter and insert saline dosette.	The saline will help to clean the catheter between suctioning.
12. **Hyperoxygenate or hyperventilate by using the sigh button on the ventilator before suctioning.** Turn safety cap on suction button of catheter so that button is easily depressed.	Hyperoxygenating or hyperventilating before suctioning helps to decrease the effects of oxygen removal during suctioning. The safety button is to keep the patient from accidentally depressing the button and decreasing the oxygen saturation.

continues

SKILL 14-19   Suctioning an Endotracheal Tube (continued)

ACTION

13. Grasp suction catheter through protective sheath, about 6″ (15 cm) from the endotracheal tube. Gently insert the catheter into the endotracheal tube. Release the catheter while holding onto the protective sheath. Return sheath to original place. **Grasp catheter through sheath and repeat procedure, advancing until patient begins to cough. Do not occlude Y-port when inserting catheter.**

14. **Apply intermittent suction by depressing the suction button with thumb of nondominant hand. Gently rotate catheter with thumb and index finger of dominant hand as catheter is being withdrawn. Do not suction for more than 10 seconds. Hyperoxygenate or hyperventilate with sigh button on ventilator as ordered.**

15. Once catheter is withdrawn back into sheath, depress the suction button while gently squeezing the normal saline dosette until catheter is clean. **Allow patient to rest at least 1 minute between suctioning, and replace oxygen delivery setup if necessary. Limit number of suctionings to three.**

RATIONALE

The sheath keeps the suction catheter sterile. The catheter is inserted far enough if the patient begins to cough. Suctioning when inserting the catheter can cause trauma to mucosa and removes oxygen from the respiratory tract.

Turning the catheter while withdrawing it helps clean surfaces of respiratory tract and prevents injury to tracheal mucosa. Suctioning for longer than 10 seconds may result in hypoxia. Hyperoxygenation and hyperventilation reoxygenate the lungs.

Flushing cleans and clears catheter and lubricates it for next insertion. Allowing time interval and replacing oxygen delivery setup help compensate for hypoxia induced by the suctioning. Irritation from multiple suctioning results in an increased amount of secretions.

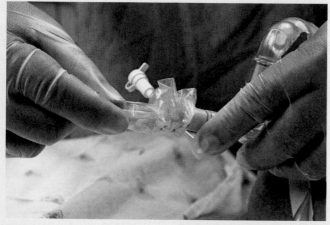

Action 13: Inserting catheter through sheath and into catheter.

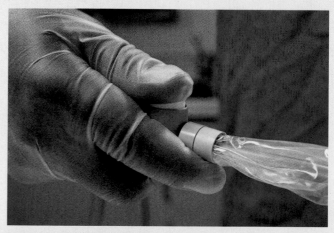

Action 14: Pushing on suction button.

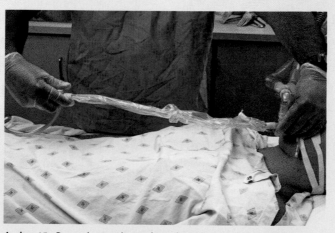

Action 15: Removing suction catheter by pulling back into sheath.

continues

Suctioning an Endotracheal Tube (continued)

ACTION	RATIONALE
16. When procedure is completed, ensure that catheter is withdrawn into sheath, and turn safety button. Remove normal saline dosette and apply cap to port.	By turning safety button, the suction is blocked at the catheter so the suction cannot remove oxygen from the endotracheal tube.
17. Suction the oral cavity and perform oral hygiene.	Suctioning of the oral cavity removes secretions that may be stagnant in the mouth and pharynx, reducing the risk for infection. Oral hygiene offers comfort to the patient.
18. Perform hand hygiene.	This prevents transmission of microorganisms.
19. Adjust patient's position. Auscultate chest to evaluate breath sounds.	Auscultation helps determine whether respiratory passageways have been cleared of secretions.
20. Record the time of suctioning and the nature and amount of secretions. Also note the character of patient's respirations before and after suctioning.	This provides accurate documentation and provides for comprehensive care.

EVALUATION

The expected outcome is met when the patient's airway is clear and patent and oxygen saturation levels are within acceptable parameters. In addition, the patient exhibits no signs of respiratory distress such as nasal flaring, grunting, or retractions.

Unexpected Situations and Associated Interventions

- *Catheter or sterile glove is contaminated:* Reconnect patient to ventilator. Discard gloves and suction catheter. Gather supplies and begin procedure again.
- *Patient is extubated during suctioning:* Remain with patient. Call for help to notify the physician. Assess patient's vital signs, ability to breathe without assistance, and oxygen saturation. Be ready to deliver assisted breaths with a bag-valve mask (Skill 14-18) or administer oxygen. Anticipate the need for reintubation.
- *Oxygen saturation level decreases after suctioning:* Hyperoxygenate patient. Auscultate lung sounds. If lung sounds are absent over one lobe, alert staff to notify physician. Remain with patient. Patient may have pneumothorax. Anticipate an order for a stat chest x-ray and chest tube placement.
- *When suctioning, you notice small yellow plugs in the secretions:* Assess patient's hydration status as well as the humidification on the ventilator. These mucous plugs may cause a ventilation-perfusion mismatch if not resolved. Patient may need more humidification.
- *When suctioning, your eye becomes contaminated with respiratory secretions:* After attending to patient, perform hand hygiene and flush eye with large amount of sterile water. Contact employee health or house supervisor immediately for further treatment.
- *Patient develops signs of intolerance to suctioning: oxygen saturation level decreases and remains low after hyperoxygenating, patient becomes cyanotic, or patient becomes bradycardic:* Stop suctioning. Auscultate lung sounds. Consider hyperventilating patient with manual resuscitation device. Remain with patient. Alert staff to notify physician.

Collecting a Sputum Specimen by Suctioning (Endotracheal Tube)

Sputum cultures may be ordered to determine the source of an infection in the pulmonary system. Due to the increased risk of infection related to the introduction of an artificial airway into the respiratory tract, frequent samples of sputum may be sent for culture to determine the types of infection that may be present.

Equipment

- Suction kit or
  - Suction catheter
  - Sterile gloves
  - Basin for sterile saline or water
- Portable or wall suction unit with tubing
- Sterile suction catheter with Y-port of appropriate size
- Goggles or safety glasses
- Manual resuscitation bag with oxygen
- Towel or sterile drape (optional)

ASSESSMENT

Assess patient's lung sounds. In patients who need to be suctioned, lung sounds are frequently diminished or coarse; wheezing may also be present. Assess patient's oxygen saturation level; it may be decreased if the patient needs to be suctioned. Assess for cough. Frequently patients cough due to the stimulation from the excess secretions. Assess for pain. If the patient has had abdominal surgery or other procedures, pain medication should be administered before suctioning. Assess respirations. Patients may become tachypneic if they need to be suctioned. Assess patient for signs of respiratory distress such as nasal flaring, retractions, or grunting.

NURSING DIAGNOSIS

Determine the related factors for the nursing diagnosis based on the patient's current status. Appropriate nursing diagnoses may include:

- Ineffective Airway Clearance
- Risk for Aspiration
- Risk for Infection

Many other nursing diagnoses may require the use of this skill.

OUTCOME IDENTIFICATION AND PLANNING

The expected outcome to achieve when suctioning the endotracheal tube to gain a sputum specimen is that a specimen will be obtained while airway patency is maintained. Other outcomes that may be appropriate include the following: oxygenation saturation level will improve; respiratory status will remain within acceptable parameters; and patient will exhibit no signs of respiratory distress such as retractions, nasal flaring, or grunting.

IMPLEMENTATION

ACTION	RATIONALE
1. Explain procedure to patient. Reassure patient that you will interrupt procedure if he or she indicates respiratory difficulty. **In postoperative patient, administer pain medication before suctioning.**	Explanation facilitates cooperation and provides reassurance for patient. Any procedure that compromises respiration is frightening for the patient. Suctioning stimulates coughing, which is painful for patients with surgical incisions.
2. Gather equipment and provide privacy for patient.	This provides for organized approach to task.
3. Perform hand hygiene.	Hand hygiene deters spread of microorganisms.
4. Assist patient to semi-Fowler's or Fowler's position.	Sitting position helps patient to cough and breathe more easily. This position also uses gravity to aid in the insertion of catheter.
5. Connect specimen container to suction tubing. **Turn suction to appropriate pressure.**	Negative pressure must be at safe level, or damage to tracheal mucosa may occur.

continues

SKILL 14-20   Collecting a Sputum Specimen by Suctioning (Endotracheal Tube) (continued)

ACTION	RATIONALE
6. Place clean towel, if used, across patient's chest. Don goggles, mask, and gown if necessary.	Towel protects patient and bed linens. Wearing protective equipment prevents contamination of the caregiver's mucous membranes.
7. Open sterile kit or set up equipment and prepare to suction:	
a. Place sterile drape, if available, across patient's chest.	a. Drape protects patient and bed linens.
b. Open sterile container and place on bedside table or overbed table without contaminating inner surface. Pour sterile saline into it.	b. This maintains sterile setup.
c. **Hyperoxygenate patient using manual resuscitation bag (may be easier if assistant delivers breaths with bag) or sigh mechanism on ventilator.**	c. This prevents hypoxemia, which can occur during suctioning.
d. **Don sterile gloves or one sterile glove on dominant hand and clean glove on nondominant hand.**	d. Gloves maintain sterility of procedure and protect the nurse from microorganisms.
e. Connect sterile suction catheter to specimen container, which is held with unsterile gloved hand.	e. Sterile technique helps prevent introduction of organisms into the respiratory tract.
8. Keeping catheter wrapped around sterile hand, remove ventilator from endotracheal tube with nonsterile hand.	Wrapping the catheter around the sterile hand prevents contamination of the catheter.
9. **Hyperoxygenate or hyperventilate with manual resuscitation bag three to five times between suctionings. Keeping the catheter sterile, gently insert it into the endotracheal tube, advancing until resistance is met or patient begins to cough. Do not occlude Y-port when inserting catheter.**	Hyperoxygenating or hyperventilating before suctioning helps to decrease the effects of oxygen removal during suctioning. The catheter is inserted far enough if resistance is met or the patient begins to cough. Suctioning when inserting catheter can cause trauma to mucosa and removes oxygen from the respiratory tract.
10. **Apply intermittent suction by occluding Y-port with thumb of unsterile gloved hand. Gently rotate catheter with thumb and index finger of sterile gloved hand as catheter is being withdrawn. Do not suction for more than 10 seconds. Reconnect to ventilator and hyperoxygenate or hyperventilate with manual resuscitation bag three to five times between suctionings.**	Turning the catheter while withdrawing it helps clean surfaces of respiratory tract and prevents injury to tracheal mucosa. Suctioning for longer than 10 seconds may result in hypoxia. Hyperoxygenation and hyperventilation reoxygenate the lungs.
11. Repeat suctioning as needed and according to patient's tolerance. If 1 to 2 mL of sputum has been obtained, disconnect specimen container and connect suction tubing to the suction catheter. The catheter may then be flushed with normal saline before suctioning again. If <1 mL has been collected, suction patient again before flushing catheter with normal saline. If secretions are extremely thick or tenacious, the catheter may flushed with a small amount (1 to 2 mL) of sterile normal saline. **Allow patient to rest at least 1 minute between suctioning, and replace oxygen delivery setup if necessary. Limit number of suctionings to three.**	Flushing cleans and clears catheter and lubricates it for next insertion, but it may thin the specimen so that an adequate culture and sensitivity cannot be performed. Allowing a time interval and replacing the oxygen delivery setup helps compensate for hypoxia induced by the suctioning. Irritation from multiple suctionings results in an increased amount of secretions.
12. When procedure is completed, turn off suction and disconnect catheter from suction tubing. Remove gloves inside out and dispose of gloves, catheter, and container with solution in proper receptacle.	Disposing of catheter inside of gloves deters the spread of pathogens.

continues

SKILL 14-20   Collecting a Sputum Specimen by Suctioning (Endotracheal Tube) (continued)

ACTION	RATIONALE

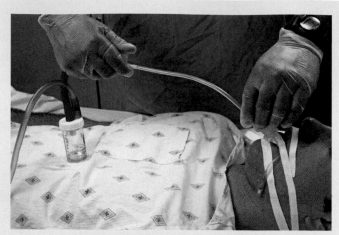

Action 11: Specimen trapped between suction tubing and suction catheter.

ACTION	RATIONALE
13. Suction the oral cavity and perform oral hygiene.	Suctioning of the oral cavity removes secretions that may be stagnant in the mouth and pharynx, reducing the risk for infection. Oral hygiene offers comfort to the patient.
14. Perform hand hygiene.	This prevents transmission of microorganisms.
15. Adjust patient's position. Auscultate chest to evaluate breath sounds.	Auscultation helps determine whether respiratory passageways have been cleared of secretions.
16. Label container with patient's name, time specimen was collected, any antibiotics administered within the past 24 hours, route of collection, and any other information required by institutional policy.	This helps the laboratory to log the specimen correctly.
17. Record the time of suctioning, specimen sent, and the nature and amount of secretions. Also note the character of patient's respirations before and after suctioning. Note on the laboratory request form any antibiotics administered in the past 24 hours.	This provides accurate documentation and promotes comprehensive care.

EVALUATION   The expected outcome is met when a specimen is obtained in a sterile manner and sent to the laboratory as soon as possible. The patient exhibits an oxygen saturation level within acceptable parameters and a patent airway and remains free of any signs and symptoms of respiratory distress.

Unexpected Situations and Associated Interventions

- *Large amount of saline is needed to flush secretions into container:* Anticipate the need to repeat the culture if the specimen is inadequate.
- *Specimen was supposed to be obtained before initiation of antibiotics, but due to an error the antibiotics were administered before obtaining the specimen:* Obtain specimen. Notify physician and laboratory of error.

SKILL 14-21   Using a Bag and Mask

If the patient is not breathing with an adequate rate and depth, or if the patient has lost the respiratory drive, a bag and mask may be used to deliver oxygen until the patient is resuscitated or can be intubated with an endotracheal tube. Bag and mask devices are frequently referred to as Ambu bags ("air mask bag unit") or BVMs ("bag-valve-mask" device). The bags come in infant, pediatric, and adult size. The bag consists of a oxygen reservoir (commonly referred to as the tail), oxygen tubing, the bag itself, a one-way valve to prevent secretions from entering the bag, an exhalation port, an elbow so that the bag can lie across the patient's chest, and a mask.

Equipment

- Bag-valve-mask device
- Oxygen source
- Disposable gloves
- Safety glasses or goggles (optional)

ASSESSMENT

Assess the patient's respiratory effort and drive. If the patient is breathing <10 breaths per minute, is breathing too shallowly, or is not breathing at all, assistance with a BVM may be needed. Assess the oxygen saturation level. Patients who have decreased respiratory effort and drive may also have a decreased oxygen saturation level. Assess the heart rate and rhythm. Bradycardia may occur with a decreased oxygen saturation level, leading to a cardiac dysrhythmia. Many times the use of a BVM is a crisis situation.

NURSING DIAGNOSIS

Determine the related factors for the nursing diagnosis based on the patient's current status. Appropriate nursing diagnoses may include:

- Ineffective Breathing Pattern
- Impaired Gas Exchange
- Decreased Cardiac Output
- Risk for Aspiration

Many other nursing diagnoses may require the use of this skill.

OUTCOME IDENTIFICATION AND PLANNING

The expected outcome to achieve when using a bag and mask is that the patient will exhibit signs and symptoms of adequate oxygen saturation. Other outcomes that may be appropriate include the following: patient will receive adequate volume of respirations with BVM; patient will maintain normal sinus rhythm.

IMPLEMENTATION

ACTION	RATIONALE
1. Perform hand hygiene (if not crisis situation). Don disposable gloves. Put on goggles or safety glasses.	Hand hygiene deters the spread of microorganisms. Gloves and goggles protect the nurse from pathogens.
2. **Ensure that the mask is connected to the bag device, the oxygen tubing is connected to the oxygen source, and the oxygen is turned on.** This may be done through visualization or by listening to the open end of the reservoir or tail: if air is heard flowing, the oxygen is attached and on.	Expected results may not be accomplished if the oxygen is not attached and on.
3. If possible, get behind head of bed and remove headboard. **Slightly hyperextend patient's neck (unless contraindicated). If unable to hyperextend, use jaw thrust maneuver to open airway.**	Standing at head of bed makes positioning easier when obtaining seal of mask to face. Hyperextending the neck opens the airway.

continues

ACTION   **RATIONALE**

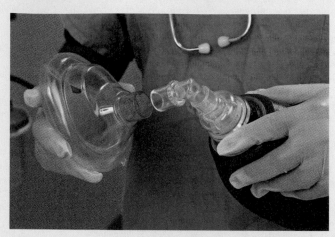

Action 2: Connecting mask to bag-valve device.

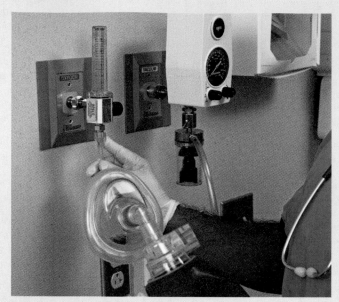

Action 2: Connecting oxygen tubing on bag to oxygen source.

4. Place mask over patient's face with opening over oral cavity. If mask is teardrop-shaped, the narrow portion should be placed over the bridge of the nose.

This helps ensure an adequate seal so that oxygen may be forced into the lungs.

5. **With dominant hand, place three fingers on mandible, keeping head slightly hyperextended. Place thumb and one finger in C position around the mask, pressing hard enough to form a seal around patient's face.**

This helps ensure an adequate seal is formed so that oxygen may be forced into the lungs.

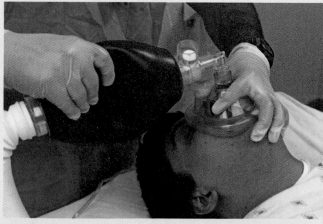

Action 5: Creating a seal between mask and patient's face.

6. **Using nondominant hand, gently and slowly (over 2 to 3 seconds) squeeze the bag, watching chest for symmetrical rise.** If two people are available, one person should maintain a seal on the mask with two hands while the other squeezes the bag to deliver the ventilation and oxygenation.

Volume of air needed is based on patient's size. Enough has been delivered if chest is rising. If air is introduced rapidly, it may enter the stomach.

continues

Using a Bag and Mask (continued)

ACTION	RATIONALE
7. Continue delivering breaths until patient's drive returns or until patient is intubated.	Once patient's airway has been stabilized or patient is breathing on own, bag-mask delivery can be stopped.
8. Remove gloves and perform hand hygiene.	Hand hygiene deters the spread of microorganisms.
9. Document the incident, including patient's respiratory effort prior to initiation of bag-mask breaths; lung sounds; oxygen saturation; chest symmetry; and resolution of incident (ie, intubation or patient's respiratory drive returns).	This provides accurate documentation and promotes comprehensive care.

9/1/06 2015   Patient arrived to emergency department with respiratory rate of 4 breaths per minute; respirations shallow; manual breaths delivered using adult bag with mask and 100% oxygen, oxygen saturation increased from 78% to 100% after 8 breaths delivered; Dr. Alsup at bedside; patient sedated with 5 mg midazolam prior to intubation with 7.5 oral endotracheal tube, taped 10 cm at lips; lung sounds clear and equal all lobes; see graphics for ventilator settings. Nasogastric tube placed via R naris to low intermittent suction, small amount of dark green drainage noted, chest x-ray obtained.—C. Bausler, RN

Action 9: Documentation.

EVALUATION

The expected outcome is met when the patient demonstrates pale pink skin color and nail beds without evidence of cyanosis, an oxygen saturation level greater than 95%, and normal sinus rhythm. In addition, the patient maintains a patent airway and exhibits spontaneous respirations.

Unexpected Situations and Associated Interventions

- *Breaths become increasingly difficult to deliver due to resistance:* Obtain order for placement of naso- or orogastric tube to remove air from the stomach (many institutions have policies that allow placement of a gastric tube during resuscitation). If air is delivered too fast, it may be introduced into the stomach. When the stomach fills with air, it decreases the space available for the lungs to inflate.
- *Chest is not rising when breaths are delivered, and resistance is felt:* Reposition the head or perform the jaw thrust maneuver. If the chest is not rising at all and resistance is being met, the tongue or another object is most likely obstructing the airway. If repositioning does not resolve the effort, consider performing the Heimlich maneuver.
- *Chest is rising asymmetrically:* Instruct assistant to listen to lung sounds bilaterally. Patient may need a chest tube placed due to pneumothorax. Anticipate the need for chest tube placement.
- *Oxygen saturation decreases from 100% to 80%:* Assess whether chest is rising. If chest is rising asymmetrically, the patient may have a pneumothorax. Anticipate the need for a chest tube. Check oxygen tubing. Someone may have stepped on the tubing, either kinking the tubing or pulling the tubing from the oxygen device.
- *Patient becomes hypocapnic:* Decrease the volume or amount of breaths delivered during a minute.
- *A seal cannot be formed around the patient's face, and a large amount of air is escaping around mask:* Assess face and mask. Is the mask the correct size for the patient? If the mask size is correct, reposition fingers, or have a second person hold the mask while you compress the bag.

■ Developing Critical Thinking Skills

1. Scott Mingus has a mediastinal chest tube in place after thoracic surgery. The chest tube had been draining 20 to 30 mL of serosanguineous fluid every hour. Suddenly, the chest tube output is 110 mL and the drainage is bright red. What should the nurse do?
2. Saranam Srivastava has a right-sided chest tube inserted due to a pneumothorax after a car accident. The water seal chamber is noted to be continuously bubbling. What should the nurse do?
3. Paula Cunningham needs to be suctioned but begins to vomit during suctioning. What should the nurse do?

Bibliography

Blazys, D. (2000). Clinical nurses forum. Teaching suctioning. *Journal of Emergency Nursing, 26*(6), 584.

Carroll, P. (2001). How to intervene before asthma turns deadly. *RN, 64*(4), 52–60.

Carroll, P. (2002). A guide to mobile chest drains. *RN, 65*(5), 56–62.

Dixon, B., & Tasota, F. (2003). Inadvertent tracheal decannulation. *Nursing, 33*(1), 96.

Gattoni, L., Tognoni, G., Pesenti, A., et al. (2001). Effect of prone positioning on the survival of patients with acute respiratory failure. *New England Journal of Medicine, 345*(8), 568–573.

Lazzara, D. (2002). Eliminate the air of mystery from chest tubes. *Nursing, 32*(6), 36–43.

Little, C. (2000). Manual ventilation. *Nursing, 30*(3), 50–51.

Martin, B., Llewellyn, J., Faut-Callahan, M., & Meyer, P. (2000). The use of telemetric oximetry in the clinical setting. *MedSurg Nursing, 9*(2), 71–76.

McConnell, E. (2000). Suctioning a tracheostomy tube. *Nursing, 30*(1), 80.

McConnell, E. (2002). Providing tracheostomy care. *Nursing, 32*(1), 17.

McConnell, E. (2002). Teaching your patient to use a metered-dose inhaler. *Nursing, 32*(2), 73.

McConnell, E. (2002). Using an automated external defibrillator. *Nursing, 32*(10), 18.

Mehta, M. (2003). Assessing respiratory status. *Nursing, 33*(2), 54–56.

Miracle, V. (2002). Action stat: Asthma attack. *Nursing, 32*(11), 104.

North American Nursing Diagnosis Association. (2003). *NANDA nursing diagnoses: Definitions and classification, 2003–2004.* Philadelphia: Author.

Seay, S., Gay, S., & Strauss, M. (2002). Tracheostomy emergencies: Correcting accidental decannulation or displaced tracheostomy tube. *American Journal of Nursing, 102*(3), 59–63.

Smeltzer, S., & Bare, B. (2004). *Brunner and Suddarth's textbook of medical–surgical nursing* (10th ed.). Philadelphia: Lippincott Williams & Wilkins.

Tate, J., & Tasota, F. (2000). Using pulse oximetry. *Nursing, 30*(9), 30.

Togger, D., & Brenner, P. (2001). Metered dose inhalers. *American Journal of Nursing, 101*(10), 26–32.

Wong, D., Hockenberry, M., Wilson, D., et al. (2001). *Wong's essentials of pediatric nursing* (6th ed.). St. Louis: Mosby.

Fluid, Electrolyte, and Acid–Base Balance

Chapter 15

Focusing on Patient Care

This chapter will help you develop some of the skills related to fluid, electrolyte, and acid–base balance necessary to care for the following patients:

Simon Lawrence, age 3, has been admitted to the pediatric floor with dehydration after vomiting for 2 days. He needs intravenous fluids to become rehydrated.

Melissa Cohen, age 32, was just involved in a motor vehicle crash. She has lost a large amount of blood and needs a blood transfusion.

Jack Tracy, age 67, is undergoing chemotherapy. He is to be discharged and needs his port deaccessed.

Learning Outcomes

After studying this chapter the reader should be able to:

1. Start an IV infusion
2. Change IV solution and tubing
3. Monitor an IV site and infusion
4. Change an IV dressing
5. Cap a primary line for intermittent use
6. Administer a blood transfusion
7. Change a PICC line dressing
8. Access an implanted port
9. Deaccess an implanted port
10. Draw blood from a central venous access device

Key Terms

acid: substance containing a hydrogen ion that can be liberated or released

acidosis: condition characterized by a proportionate excess of hydrogen ions in the extracellular fluid; pH falls below 7.35

active transport: movement of ions or molecules across cell membranes, usually against a pressure gradient and with the expenditure of metabolic energy

agglutinin: antibody that causes a clumping of specific antigens

alkalosis: condition characterized by a proportionate lack of hydrogen ions in the extracellular fluid concentration; pH exceeds 7.45

anion: ion that carries a negative electric charge

antibody: immunoglobulin produced by the body in response to a specific antigen

antigen: foreign material capable of inducing a specific immune response

continues

Key Terms (continued)

autologous transfusion: a blood transfusion donated by the patient in anticipation that he or she may need the transfusion during a hospital stay

base: substance that can accept or trap a hydrogen ion; synonym for alkali

buffer: substance that prevents body fluid from becoming overly acid or alkaline

cation: ion that carries a positive electric charge

colloid osmotic pressure: pressure exerted by plasma proteins on permeable membranes in the body; synonym for oncotic pressure

crossmatching: determining the compatibility of two blood specimens

dehydration: decreased water volume

diffusion: tendency of solutes to move freely throughout a solvent from an area of higher concentration to an area of lower concentration until equilibrium is established

edema: accumulation of fluid in body tissues

electrolyte: substance capable of breaking into ions and developing an electric charge when dissolved in solution

filtration: passage of a fluid through a permeable membrane whose spaces do not allow certain solutes to pass; passage is from an area of higher pressure to one of lower pressure

hydrostatic pressure: force exerted by a fluid against the container wall

hypertonic: having a greater concentration than the solution with which it is being compared

hypervolemia: excess of blood volume

hypotonic: having a lesser concentration than the solution with which it is being compared

hypovolemia: deficiency of blood volume

ion: atom or molecule carrying an electric charge in solution

isotonic: having about the same concentration as the solution with which it is being compared

osmolarity: the concentration of particles in a solution, or a solution's pulling power

osmosis: passage of a solvent through a semipermeable membrane from an area of lesser concentration to an area of greater concentration until equilibrium is established

overhydration: increased water volume

pH: expression of hydrogen ion concentration and resulting acidity of a substance

solute: substance dissolved in a solution

solvent: liquid holding a substance in solution

typing: determining a person's blood type (A, B, AB, or O)

Because fluid is the main constituent of the body, the body's fluid balance is very important. Body fluid contains water (50% to 60% of the human body by weight is water) and other dissolved substances in the form of electrolytes, nonelectrolytes, and gases. The balance, or homeostasis, of water and dissolved substances is maintained through the functions of almost every organ of the body. Nurses routinely care for patients with serious and even life-threatening fluid, electrolyte, and acid–base disturbances. One of nursing's most important roles is the prevention of these disturbances in high-risk populations, such as infants, older people, and patients with cardiac and renal disorders.

This chapter discusses the skills needed to care for patients with fluid, electrolyte, and acid–base balance needs. Please look over the summary figures, tables, and boxes in the beginning of this chapter for a quick review of critical knowledge to assist you in understanding the skills related to fluid, electrolyte, and acid–base balance.

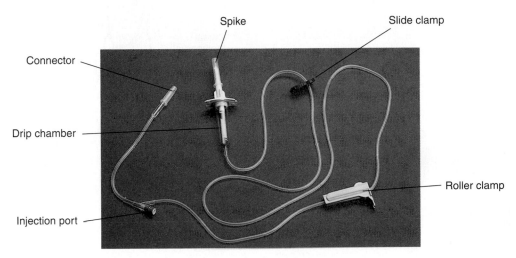

FIGURE 15-1 Basic administration set for intravenous therapy.

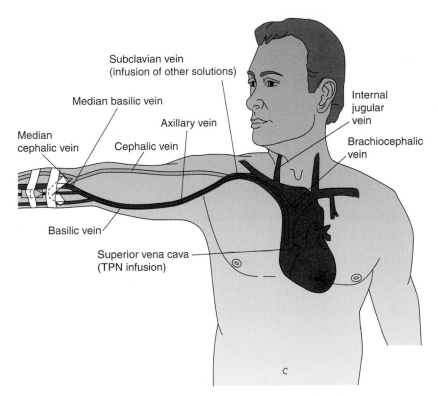

FIGURE 15-2 Placement of peripherally inserted central catheter (PICC).

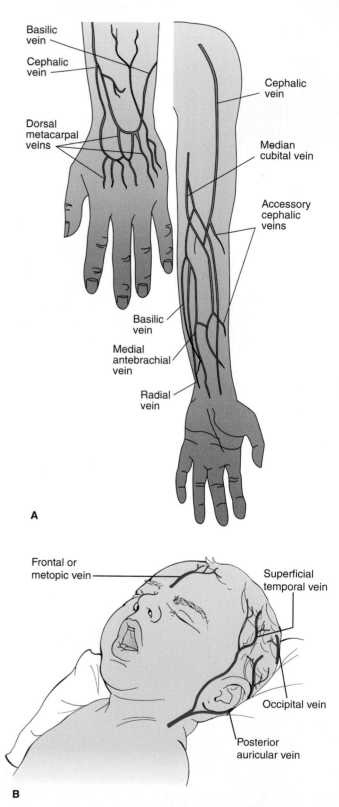

A

B

FIGURE 15-4 Infusion sites. (**A**) Ventral and dorsal aspects of lower arm and hand. (**B**) Scalp vein sites.

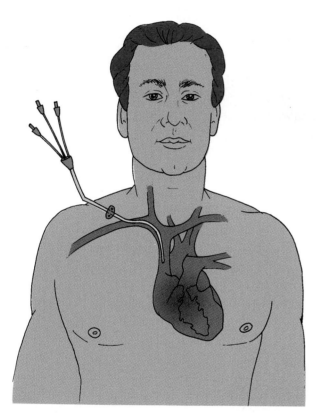

FIGURE 15-3 Placement of triple-lumen nontunneled percutaneous central venous catheter.

TABLE 15-1 Balance of Fluid Intake and Output in a Healthy State

Fluid Intake (mL)

Ingested water	1,300
Ingested food	1,000
Metabolic oxidation	300
Total	*2,600*

Fluid Output (mL)

Kidneys	1,500
Skin	
Insensible loss	200–400
Sensible loss	300–500
Lungs	400
Gastrointestinal	100
Total	*2,500–2,900*

TABLE 15-2 Complications Associated With Intravenous Infusions

Complication/Cause	Signs and Symptoms	Nursing Considerations

Infiltration: the escape of fluid into the subcutaneous tissue
  Dislodged needle
  Penetrated vessel wall
	Swelling, pallor, coldness, or pain around the infusion site; significant decrease in the flow rate	Check the infusion site several times per shift for symptoms.
		Discontinue the infusion if symptoms occur.
		Restart the infusion at a different site.
		Limit the movement of the extremity with the IV.

Sepsis: microorganisms invade the bloodstream through the catheter insertion site
  Poor insertion technique
  Multilumen catheters
  Long-term catheter insertion
  Frequent dressing changes
	Red and tender insertion site
	Fever, malaise, other vital sign changes
		Assess catheter site daily.
		Notify physician immediately if any signs of infection.
		Follow agency protocol for culture of drainage.
		Use scrupulous aseptic technique when starting an infusion.

Phlebitis: an inflammation of a vein
  Mechanical trauma from needle or catheter
  Chemical trauma from solution
  Septic (due to contamination)
	Local, acute tenderness; redness, warmth, and slight edema of the vein above the insertion site	Discontinue the infusion immediately.
		Apply warm, moist compresses to the affected site.
		Avoid further use of the vein.
		Restart the infusion in another vein.

Thrombus: a blood clot Tissue trauma from needle or catheter	Symptoms similar to phlebitis IV fluid flow may cease if clot obstructs needle	Stop the infusion immediately. Apply warm compresses as ordered by the physician. Restart the IV at another site. *Do not rub or massage the affected area.*
Speed shock: the body's reaction to a substance that is injected into the circulatory system too rapidly Too rapid a rate of fluid infusion into circulation	Pounding headache, fainting, rapid pulse rate, apprehension, chills, back pains, and dyspnea	If symptoms develop, discontinue the infusion immediately. Report symptoms of speed shock to the physician immediately. Monitor vital signs if symptoms develop. Use the proper IV tubing. A microdrip (60 gtt/mL) should be used on all pediatric patients. Carefully monitor the rate of fluid flow. Check the rate frequently for accuracy. A time tape is useful for this purpose.
Fluid overload: the condition caused when too large a volume of fluid infuses into the circulatory system Too large a volume of fluid infused into circulation	Engorged neck veins, increased blood pressure, and difficulty in breathing (dyspnea)	If symptoms develop, slow the rate of infusion. Notify the physician immediately. Monitor vital signs. Carefully monitor the rate of fluid flow. Check the rate frequently for accuracy.
Air embolus: air in the circulatory system Break in the IV system above the heart level allowing air in the circulatory system as a bolus	Respiratory distress Increased heart rate Cyanosis Decreased blood pressure Change in level of consciousness	Pinch off catheter or secure system to prevent entry of air. Place patient on left side in Trendelenburg position. Call for immediate assistance. Monitor vital signs and pulse oximetry.

TABLE 15-3 Blood Products

Blood Product	Filter	Rate of Administration	ABO Compatibility	Double-Checked by 2 People
Packed red blood cells	Yes	1 unit over 2–3 hours; no longer than 4 hours	Yes	Yes
Platelets	Yes (in provided tubing)	As fast as patient can tolerate	No	Yes
Cryoprecipitate	No	IV push over 3 minutes	Recommended	Yes
Fresh-frozen plasma	No	200 mL/hr	Yes	Yes
Albumin	In tubing provided	1–10 mL/min (5%) 0.2–0.4 cc/min (25%)	No	No

TABLE 15-4 Transfusion Reactions

Reaction	Signs and Symptoms	Nursing Activity
Allergic reaction: allergy to transfused blood	Hives, itching Anaphylaxis	• Stop transfusion immediately and keep vein open with normal saline. • Notify physician stat. • Administer antihistamine parenterally as necessary.
Febrile reaction: fever develops during infusion	Fever and chills Headache Malaise	• Stop transfusion immediately and keep vein open with normal saline. • Notify physician. • Treat symptoms.
Hemolytic transfusion reaction: incompatibility of blood product	Immediate onset Facial flushing Fever, chills Headache Low back pain Shock	• Stop infusion immediately and keep vein open with normal saline. • Notify physician stat. • Obtain blood samples from site. • Obtain first voided urine. • Treat shock if present. • Send unit, tubing, and filter to lab. • Draw blood sample for serologic testing and send urine specimen to the lab.
Circulatory overload: too much blood administered	Dyspnea Dry cough Pulmonary edema	• Slow or stop infusion. • Monitor vital signs. • Notify physician. • Place in upright position with feet dependent.
Bacterial reaction: bacteria present in blood	Fever Hypertension Dry, flushed skin Abdominal pain	• Stop infusion immediately. • Obtain culture of patient's blood and return blood bag to lab. • Monitor vital signs. • Notify physician. • Administer antibiotics stat.

BOX 15-1 Regulating IV Flow Rate

Follow agency's guidelines to determine if infusion should be administered by electronic pump or by gravity.

- Check physician's order for IV solution.
- Check patency of IV line and needle.
- Verify drop factor (number of drops in 1 mL) of the equipment in use.
- Calculate the flow rate:
  EXAMPLE—Administer 1000 mL D5W over 10 hours (set delivers 60 gtt/1 mL).

a. Standard formula

$$gtt/min = \frac{volume\ (mL) \times drop\ factor\ (gtt/mL)}{time\ (in\ minutes)}$$

$$gtt/min = \frac{1000\ mL \times 60}{600\ (60\ min \times 10\ h)}$$

$$= \frac{60,000}{600}$$

$$= 100\ gtt/min$$

b. Short formula using milliliters per hour

$$gtt/min = \frac{milliliters\ per\ hour \times drop\ factor\ (gtt/mL)}{time\ (60\ min)}$$

Find milliliters per hour by dividing 1000 mL by 10 hours:

$$\frac{1000}{10} = 100\ mL/hr$$

$$gtt/min = \frac{100\ mL \times 60}{60\ min}$$

$$= \frac{6,000}{60}$$

$$= 100\ gtt/min$$

c. Dimensional analysis

$$gtt/min = \frac{gtt}{mL} \times \frac{mL}{hr} \times \frac{hr}{min}$$

$$gtt/min = \frac{60\ gtt}{1\ mL} \times \frac{1000\ mL}{10\ hr} \times \frac{1\ hr}{60\ min}$$

$$= \frac{60,000\ gtt}{600\ min}$$

$$= 100\ gtt/min$$

- Count drops per minute in drip chamber (number of gtt/15 sec interval × 4 = gtt/min). Hold watch beside drip chamber.
- Adjust IV clamp as needed and recount drops per minute.
- Mark IV container according to agency policy and manufacturer's recommendations. Use a time tape or label if indicated to measure amount to be infused at timed intervals.
- Monitor IV flow rate at frequent intervals. Document patient's response to infusion at prescribed rate.

SKILL
15-1

Starting an Intravenous Infusion

Administering and monitoring IV fluids is an essential part of routine patient care. Physicians often order IV therapy to prevent or correct problems in fluid and electrolyte balance. For IV therapy to be administered, an IV must be inserted.

Equipment

- IV solution
- Towel or disposable pad
- Nonallergenic tape
- IV infusion set
- Gauze or transparent dressing (according to agency policy)
- Electronic infusion device (if ordered)
- IV tubing
- Tourniquet
- Time tape or label (for IV container)
- Armboard (if needed)
- Cleansing swabs (alcohol, povidone-iodine, or chlorhexidine)
- Site protector or tube-shaped elastic netting (optional)
- Disposable gloves
- IV pole
- Anesthetic (numbing) cream (if ordered)
- Lidocaine injection (if ordered)
- 1-mL syringe (for lidocaine)
- IV catheter (over the needle, Angiocath) or butterfly needle

continues

SKILL 15-1   Starting an Intravenous Infusion (continued)

ASSESSMENT

Assess arms and hands for potential sites for initiating the IV. The site should not be over a joint: placing it over a joint would mean the IV would be occluded every time the patient moves the extremity. Inspect the area, looking for a vein that is straight in an area approximately 5 cm long. Determine the type of IV catheter to use. Ascertain which extremity is the patient's dominant arm, and try to use the nondominant arm for the patient's comfort. Auscultate the lungs to establish a baseline for future comparison. Review any recent laboratory values or diagnostic test results.

NURSING DIAGNOSIS

Determine the related factors for the nursing diagnosis based on the patient's current status. Appropriate nursing diagnoses may include:

- Deficient Fluid Volume
- Impaired Skin Integrity
- Risk for Injury
- Anxiety

Many other nursing diagnoses may require the use of this skill.

OUTCOME IDENTIFICATION AND PLANNING

The expected outcome to achieve when starting IV therapy is that the IV catheter is inserted on the first attempt. Also, the patient experiences minimal trauma and the IV solution flows freely without any indications of complications.

IMPLEMENTATION

ACTION	RATIONALE
1. Gather all equipment and bring to bedside. Check IV solution and medication additives against physician's order.	Having equipment available saves time and facilitates accomplishment of task. Checking the order ensures that the patient receives the ordered IV solution and medication.
2. Explain the need for the IV and procedure to patient.	Explanation allays anxiety.
3. Perform hand hygiene. If using an anesthetic (numbing) cream, apply cream to a few potential insertion sites.	Hand hygiene deters the spread of microorganisms. Anesthetic (numbing) cream decreases the amount of pain felt at the insertion site. Some of the numbing creams take up to an hour to become effective.
4. Prepare IV solution and tubing:	
a. **Maintain aseptic technique when opening sterile packages and IV solution.**	a. Asepsis is essential for preventing the spread of microorganisms.
b. Clamp tubing, uncap spike, and insert into entry site on bag as manufacturer directs.	b. This punctures the seal in the IV bag.
c. Squeeze drip chamber and allow it to fill at least halfway.	c. Suction causes fluid to move into drip chamber and prevents air from moving down the tubing.
d. Remove cap at end of tubing, release clamp, and allow fluid to move through tubing. **Allow fluid to flow until all air bubbles have disappeared.** Close clamp and recap end of tubing, maintaining sterility of setup.	d. This removes air from tubing; in larger amounts, air can act as an embolus.
e. If an electronic device is to be used, follow manufacturer's instructions for inserting tubing and setting infusion rate.	e. This ensures correct flow rate and proper use of equipment.
f. Apply label if medication was added to container (pharmacy may have added medication and applied label). Label tubing with date and time that tubing was hung.	f. This provides for administration of correct solution with prescribed medication or additive.
g. Place time-tape on container and hang IV on pole.	g. This permits immediate evaluation of IV according to schedule.

continues

Starting an Intravenous Infusion (continued)

ACTION

RATIONALE

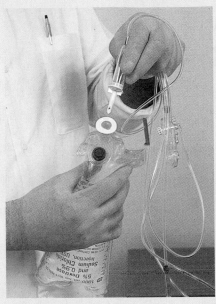

Action 4b: Insert spike into IV bag.

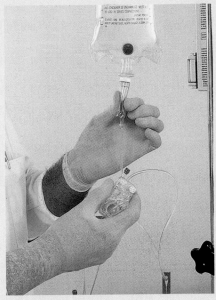

Action 4c: Squeeze drip chamber.

5. Place patient in low Fowler's position in bed. Place protective towel or pad under patient's arm.

6. **Select an appropriate site and palpate accessible veins.**

7. If the site is hairy and agency policy permits, clip a 2″ area around the intended site of entry.

8. Apply a tourniquet 5″ to 6″ above the venipuncture site to obstruct venous blood flow and distend the vein. Direct the ends of the tourniquet away from the site of entry. Make sure the radial pulse is still present.

The supine position permits either arm to be used and allows for good body alignment.

The use of an appropriate site decreases discomfort for the patient and reduces the risk for damage to body tissues.

Hair can harbor microorganisms.

Interrupting the blood flow to the heart causes the vein to distend. Interrupting the arterial flow impedes venous filling. Distended veins are easy to see, palpate, and enter. The end of the tourniquet could contaminate the area of injection if directed toward the site of entry.

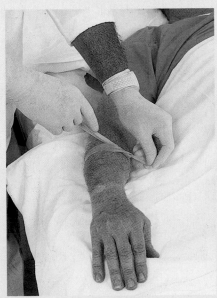

Action 8: Apply tourniquet.

continues

SKILL 15-1 Starting an Intravenous Infusion (continued)

ACTION	RATIONALE
9. Ask patient to open and close fist. Observe and palpate for a suitable vein. Try the following techniques if a vein cannot be felt:	Contracting the muscles of the forearm forces blood into the veins, thereby distending them further.
a. Release tourniquet and have patient lower arm below heart level to fill the veins. Reapply tourniquet and gently tap over intended vein to help distend it.	a. Lowering the arm below heart level, tapping the vein, and applying warmth help distend veins by filling them with blood.
b. Remove tourniquet and place warm moist compresses over intended vein for 10 to 15 minutes.	b. Warm moist compresses help dilate veins.
10. Don clean gloves.	Gloves protect against transmission of HIV and other blood-borne infections.
11. If using intradermal lidocaine, cleanse insertion site with alcohol using a circular motion. Inject a small amount (0.2 to 0.3 mL) of lidocaine into the area. If numbing cream was used, wipe cream off insertion site. **Cleanse site with an antiseptic solution (alcohol swab) followed by antimicrobial solution (povidone-iodine) according to agency policy. Use a circular motion to move from the center outward for several inches.**	The lidocaine numbs the skin and makes the insertion less painful. Cleansing that begins at the site of entry and moves outward in a circular motion carries organisms away from the site of entry. Organisms on the skin can be introduced into the tissues or the bloodstream with the needle.
12. Use the nondominant hand, placed about 1″ or 2″ below entry site, to hold the skin taut against the vein. **Avoid touching the prepared site.**	Pressure on the vein and surrounding tissues helps prevent movement of the vein as the needle or catheter is being inserted. The needle entry site and catheter must remain free of contamination from unsterile hands.
13. Enter the skin gently, holding the catheter by the hub in your dominant hand, bevel side up, at a 10- to 30-degree angle. Catheter may be inserted from directly over the vein or the side of the vein. While following the course of the vein, advance the needle or catheter into the vein. A sensation of "give" can be felt when the needle enters the vein.	This allows needle or catheter to enter vein with minimal trauma and deters passage of the needle through the vein.
14. When blood returns through the lumen of the needle or the flashback chamber of the catheter, advance either device ⅛″ to ¼″ farther into the vein. A catheter needs to be advanced until the hub is at the venipuncture site, but the exact technique depends on the type of device used.	The tourniquet causes increased venous pressure, resulting in automatic backflow. Placing the catheter well into the vein helps to prevent dislodgement.
15. Release the tourniquet. Quickly remove the protective cap from the IV tubing and attach the tubing to the catheter or needle. Stabilize the catheter or needle with your nondominant hand.	Bleeding is minimized and the patency of the vein is maintained if the connection is made smoothly between the catheter and tubing.
16. Start the flow of solution promptly by releasing the clamp on the tubing. Examine the tissue around the entry site for signs of infiltration.	Blood clots form readily if IV flow is not maintained. If catheter accidentally slips out of vein, solution will accumulate and infiltrate into surrounding tissue.
17. Secure the catheter with narrow nonallergenic tape (½″) placed sticky side up under the hub and crossed over the top of the hub.	The smooth structure of the vein does not offer resistance to the movement of the catheter. The weight of the tubing is sufficient to pull it out of the vein if it is not well anchored. Nonallergenic tape is less likely to tear fragile skin.

continues

Starting an Intravenous Infusion (continued)

ACTION

18. **Place sterile dressing over venipuncture site.** Agency policy may direct nurse to use gauze dressing or transparent dressing. Apply tape to dressing if necessary. Loop the tubing near the site of entry, and anchor to dressing.

19. Mark the date, time, site, and type and size of catheter used for the infusion on the tape anchoring the tubing.

RATIONALE

Transparent dressing allows easy visualization of site but may place patient at increased risk for infection. Gauze dressing absorbs drainage and may have a decreased infection rate. Discussion continues about effectiveness of various types of dressings.

Other personnel working with the infusion will know what type of device is being used, the site, and when it was inserted.

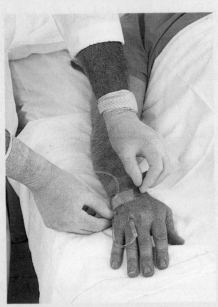

Action 17: Secure the catheter.

20. Remove all equipment and dispose of properly. Remove gloves and perform hand hygiene.

21. Anchor arm to an armboard for support if necessary, or apply a site protector or tube-shaped mesh netting over the insertion site.

22. Adjust the rate of solution flow according to the amount prescribed, or follow manufacturer's directions for adjusting flow rate on infusion pump.

23. Document procedure and patient's response. Chart time, site, device used, and solution.

24. Return to check flow rate and observe for infiltration 30 minutes after starting infusion.

Hand hygiene deters the spread of microorganisms.

An armboard or site protector helps to prevent the position of the catheter in the vein from changing.

The physician prescribes the rate of flow.

This provides accurate documentation and ensures continuity of care.

This documents patient's response to infusion.

11/02/06 0830   20G IV started in L hand. Dressing applied. Site without redness, drainage, or edema. D51/2 NS with 20 mEq KCl begun at 110 mL/hr. Patient instructed to call with any pain or swelling.—S. Barnes, RN

Action 23: Documentation.

continues

SKILL 15-1   Starting an Intravenous Infusion (continued)

EVALUATION

The expected outcome is met when the IV is started on the first attempt and fluid flows easily into the vein without any signs of edema, infiltration, or pain. The patient verbalizes minimal complaints related to insertion and demonstrates understanding of the reasons for the IV.

Unexpected Situations and Associated Interventions

- *Fluid does not easily flow into the vein:* Attempt to flush the IV with 3 mL of saline in a syringe. Check IV connector to ensure that clamp is fully open. If fluid still does not flow easily, or if resistance is met while flushing, the IV may be against a valve and may need to be restarted in a different location.
- *Fluid does not flow easily into the vein, and the skin around the insertion site is edematous and cool to the touch:* IV has infiltrated. Don gloves and remove catheter. Pressure may need to be held with a sterile gauze pad. Apply a Band-Aid over insertion site and restart IV in a new location.
- *A small hematoma is forming at the site while you are inserting the catheter:* The vein is "blowing": a small hole has been made in the vein and blood is leaking out into the tissues. Remove and discard the catheter and choose an alternate insertion site.
- *Fluids are leaking around the insertion site:* Change dressing on IV. If site continues to leak, remove IV to decrease risk of infection, and restart it in a new location.
- *IV infusion set becomes disconnected from IV:* Discard IV tubing to prevent infection. Attempt to flush IV with 3 mL of normal saline. If the IV is still patent without any signs of infiltration, the site may still be used.
- *IV catheter is partially pulled out of insertion site:* Do not reinsert the catheter. Whether the IV is salvageable depends on how much of the catheter remains in the vein. If this catheter is not removed, it should be monitored closely for signs of infiltration.

Infant and Child Considerations

- Scalp and feet can be used as alternate insertion sites. Palpate any scalp sites before insertion to ensure that an artery is not being used.
- Hand insertion sites should not be the first choice for children because nerve endings are very close to the surface of the skin, and it is more painful. Once the child can walk, do not use the feet as insertion sites.
- Do not replace peripheral catheters in children unless clinically indicated (Centers for Disease Control and Prevention, 2002).
- Catheter can be inserted with bevel side down if veins are blowing using the bevel-up technique.

Older Adult Considerations

- Avoid using vigorous friction and too much alcohol at the insertion site. Both can traumatize fragile skin and veins in the elderly.
- To decrease the risk for trauma to the vessel, experienced nurses may omit use of a tourniquet if the patient has prominent but especially fragile veins.

Changing IV Solution and Tubing

Because fluid infusions sometimes involve multiple bags or bottles of fluid, a nursing responsibility in managing IV therapy is to monitor the fluid levels and to replace the fluid containers as needed. Keep the following in mind:

- If more than one container of solution is ordered, check agency policy to make sure additional containers can be attached to the existing tubing.
- As one bag is infusing, prepare the next bag so it is ready for a change when <50 mL of fluid remains in the original container.
- Always check the practitioner's order for the fluids.

Before switching the containers, check the date and time of the infusion administration set to ensure it does not need to be replaced also.

Equipment

For solution change:

- IV solution as ordered by physician
- Sterile dressing and antiseptic solutions (according to agency policy)

For tubing change:

- Administration set
- Sterile gauze
- Timing tape for label

ASSESSMENT

Check the IV infusion. Observe the infusion solution and the label, confirming that it is the correct solution ordered. Inspect the rate of flow, checking the drip chamber and timing the drops if it is a gravity infusion or checking the settings of an infusion pump if used.

Inspect the IV site. The dressing should be intact, adhering to the skin on all edges. Check to see if there are any leaks or fluid under or around the dressing. Inspect the tissue around the IV entry site for swelling, pain, coolness, or pallor. These are signs of fluid infiltration into the tissue around the IV catheter. Also inspect the site for redness, swelling, heat, or pain: these signs might indicate the development of phlebitis or an inflammation of the blood vessel at the site. Auscultate lung sounds and review the results of any laboratory or diagnostic test results.

NURSING DIAGNOSIS

Determine the related factors for the nursing diagnosis based on the patient's current status. An appropriate nursing diagnosis is Risk for Injury. Other nursing diagnoses that may be appropriate include:

- Risk for Infection
- Deficient Fluid Volume

Many other nursing diagnoses also may require the use of this skill.

OUTCOME IDENTIFICATION AND PLANNING

The expected outcome to achieve when changing IV solution and tubing is that the patient experiences minimal to no trauma when solution and tubing is changed. In addition, the IV infusion continues without interruption.

IMPLEMENTATION

ACTION	RATIONALE
1. Gather all equipment and bring to bedside. Check IV solution and medication additives against physician's order.	Having equipment available saves time and facilitates accomplishment of task. Checking ensures that patient receives the ordered IV solution and medication.
2. Explain procedure and reason for change to patient.	Explanation allays anxiety.
3. Perform hand hygiene.	Hand hygiene deters the spread of microorganisms.

continues

SKILL 15-2   Changing IV Solution and Tubing (continued)

ACTION	RATIONALE

To Change IV Solution

4. Carefully remove protective cover from new solution container and expose bag entry site.

   This maintains sterility of IV solution.

5. **Close clamp on tubing.**

   Clamping stops the flow of IV fluid during solution change.

6. Lift container off IV pole and invert it. **Quickly remove the spike from the old IV container, being careful not to contaminate it.**

   This maintains sterility of IV setup.

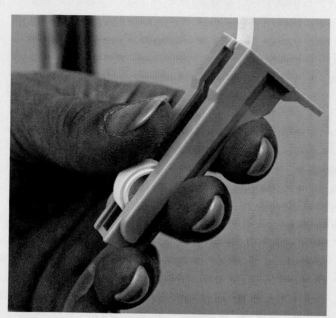

Action 5: Clamp the tubing on administration set.

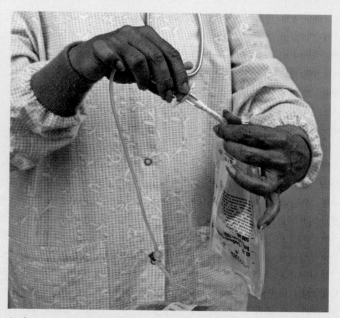

Action 6: Invert the solution bag and remove the spike.

7. Steady new container and insert spike. Hang on IV pole.

   This allows for uninterrupted flow of new solution.

8. Reopen clamp, check the drip chamber of the administration set on tubing, and adjust flow.

   Opening clamp regulates flow rate into drip chamber.

9. Label container according to agency policy. Record on intake and output record and document on chart according to agency policy. Discard used equipment properly. Perform hand hygiene.

   This ensures accurate continuation and administration of correct IV solution. Hand hygiene deters the spread of microorganisms.

To Change IV Tubing and Solution

10. Follow Actions 1 through 4.

    This maintains sterility of IV setup. Once clamp is closed, the bag can be spiked without loss of solution.

11. Open the administration set and close clamp on new tubing. Remove protective covering from infusion spike. Using sterile technique, insert the spike into the entry port of the new container.

    These actions create a system for infusing the new solution.

continues

Changing IV Solution and Tubing (continued)

ACTION	RATIONALE

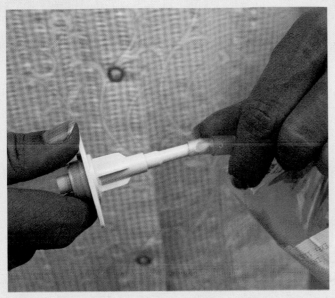

Action 7: Spike the new solution bag.

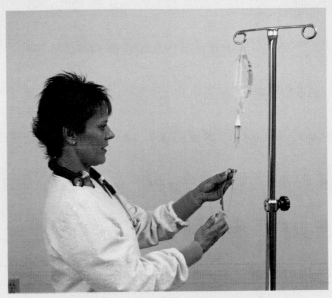

Action 8: Reopen the clamp and adjust the flow rate.

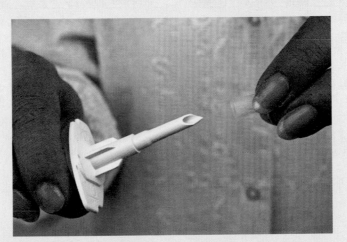

Action 11: Remove protective cap from tubing.

12. Hang IV container on pole and squeeze drip chamber to fill at least halfway.

Gravity and suction cause fluid to move into drip chamber.

13. Remove cap at end of tubing, release clamp, and allow fluid to move through tubing until all air bubbles have disappeared. Close clamp, attach adapter or connector (if necessary) to the end of the tubing, and recap end of tubing.

This removes air from tubing; in larger amounts, air can act as an embolus. Recapping maintains the sterility of the setup.

continues

ACTION   **RATIONALE**

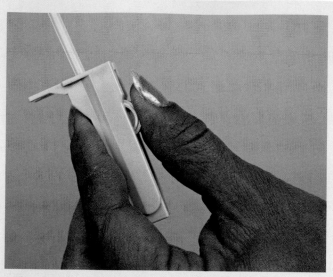

Action 13: Release clamp to allow IV fluid through tubing.

To Change Tubing on a Short Extension Set

14. Close the clamp on the existing IV tubing. Also close the clamp on the short extension tubing connected to the IV catheter in the patient's arm.

A short closed tubing set (extension set) with an injection port and closure clamp between the catheter or angiocath hub and the tubing reduces the risk for blood exposure. Clamping the existing IV tubing prevents leakage of fluid. Clamping the tubing on the extension set prevents introduction of air into the line.

15. Remove the current infusion tubing from the resealable cap on the short extension IV tubing. Using an alcohol wipe, swab the resealable cap and insert the new IV tubing into the cap. Proceed to Action 22.

Cleansing the port reduces the risk for contamination.

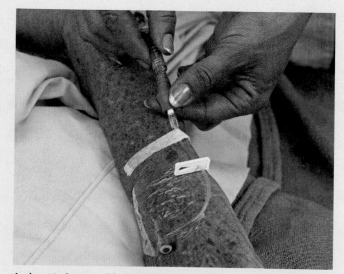

Action 15: Remove old administration set tubing.

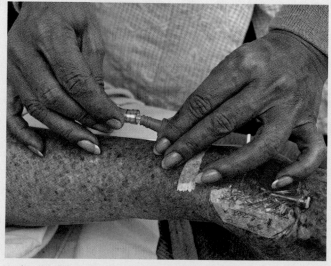

Action 15: Insert new IV tubing into extension tubing.

continues

Changing IV Solution and Tubing (continued)

ACTION	RATIONALE
To Change Tubing Connected Directly Into the Hub of the IV Access Catheter	
16. Follow Actions 10 through 13.	
17. Loosen tape at IV insertion site. Don clean gloves. **Carefully remove dressing and tape.**	Removing dressing provides access to needle hub necessary for tubing change. Using gloves is necessary with contact with the patient's blood is possible, such as when in close proximity to the IV insertion site. This prevents transmission of HIV and other blood-borne infections.
18. Place sterile gauze square under catheter hub.	Gauze absorbs any leakage when tubing is disconnected from catheter.
19. Place new IV tubing close to IV site and slightly loosen protective cap.	This facilitates removal of cap and attachment to needle hub.
20. Clamp old IV tubing. **Steady the needle hub with non-dominant hand until change is completed.** Remove tubing with dominant hand using a twisting motion.	This stabilizes the catheter and prevents dislodgement.
21. Set old tubing aside. **While maintaining sterility, carefully remove the covering or cap from the new administration set and insert sterile end of tubing into catheter hub. Twist to secure it; tape connection if necessary.** Remove gauze square from under needle hub. Remove soiled gloves.	This maintains sterility of IV setup.
22. Open the clamp on the IV tubing and check the flow.	Opening clamp allows solution to flow to patient.
23. Reapply sterile dressing to site or tape catheter to patient according to agency protocol (see Skill 15-4).	This deters entry of microorganisms at site.
24. **Regulate IV flow according to physician's order.**	This ensures that patient receives IV solution at prescribed rate.
25. **Label IV tubing with date, time, and your initials. Label container and record procedure according to agency policy.** Discard used equipment properly and perform hand hygiene.	This documents IV tubing change. Hand hygiene deters the spread of microorganisms.
26. Record patient's response to IV infusion.	This ensures accurate documentation of patient's response.

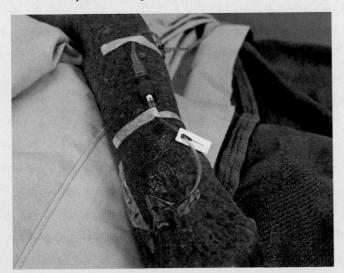

Action 23: Clamp open on new tubing, with short extension tubing taped in place.

11/3/06   1015   IV fluid changed from
D51/2 NS with 20 mEq KCl/L to D5 0.9NS with
20 mEq KCl/L. IV site pink, warm, and dry, no
drainage noted.—S. Barnes, RN

Action 26: Documentation.

continues

SKILL 15-2 Changing IV Solution and Tubing (continued)

EVALUATION

The expected outcome is achieved when the IV solution and tubing is changed without interrupting the ordered infusion therapy and the patient experiences minimal to no trauma when solution and tubing is changed.

Unexpected Situations and Associated Interventions

- *Infusion does not flow or flow rate changes after bag and tubing is changed:* Make sure that the flow clamp is open and the drip chamber is approximately half-full. Check the IV site for possible problems with the catheter, such as bending; inspect the IV site for signs and symptoms of complications. Readjust the flow rate.
- *After attaching new IV tubing, you note air bubbles in the tubing:* If the bubbles are above the roller clamp, you can easily remove them by closing the roller clamp, stretching the tubing downward, and tapping the tubing with your finger so the bubbles rise to the drip chamber. If there is a larger amount of air in the tubing, swab the medication port on the tubing below the air with alcohol, allow it to dry, then insert a needle and syringe into the port below the air. Using the syringe, aspirate the air from the tubing. Remember that air bubbles in the tubing can be reduced if the tubing is primed slowly with fluid instead of allowing a wide-open flow of the solution.

SKILL 15-3 Monitoring an IV Site and Infusion

The nurse is responsible for monitoring the infusion rate and the IV site. This is routinely done as part of the initial patient assessment at the beginning of a work shift, then at periodic intervals throughout the day. Monitoring the infusion rate is a very important part of the patient's overall management. Another responsibility involves checking the IV site for possible complications. IV sites are checked at specific intervals and each time an IV medication is given, as dictated by the institution's policies. It is common to check IV sites every hour, but be familiar with the requirements of your institution.

Equipment

- None needed

ASSESSMENT

Inspect the infusion solution and the label. Confirm it is the solution ordered. Assess the current rate of flow by timing the drops if it is a gravity infusion or verifying the settings on the infusion control device. Look at the tubing for anything that might clamp or interfere with the flow of solution. Inspect the IV site. The dressing should be intact, adhering to the skin on all edges. Auscultate the patient's lung sounds and assess urinary output, comparing it with fluid intake. Assess the patient's knowledge of IV complications.

NURSING DIAGNOSIS

Determine the related factors for the nursing diagnosis based on the patient's current status. Appropriate nursing diagnoses may include:

- Excess Fluid Volume
- Deficient Fluid Volume
- Risk for Infection
- Risk for Injury

In addition, many other nursing diagnoses also may require the use of this skill.

OUTCOME IDENTIFICATION AND PLANNING

The expected outcome to be met when monitoring the IV infusion and site is that the patient remains free from injury and demonstrates signs and symptoms of fluid balance.

continues

Monitoring an IV Site and Infusion (continued)

IMPLEMENTATION
ACTION

1. **Monitor IV infusion several times a shift. More frequent checks may be necessary if medication is being infused:**

   a. Check physician's order for IV solution.

   b. Check drip chamber and time drops if IV is not regulated by an infusion control device.

   c. Check tubing for anything that might interfere with flow. Be sure that clamp is in the open position. **Observe dressing for leakage of IV solution.**

   d. Observe settings, alarm, and indicator lights on infusion control device if one is being used.

2. **Inspect site for swelling, pain, coolness, or pallor, which may indicate infiltration. This necessitates removing IV and restarting at another site.**

3. **Inspect site for redness, swelling, heat, and pain, which may indicate phlebitis. IV will need to be discontinued and restarted at another site. Notify physician if you suspect phlebitis.**

4. **Check for local or systemic manifestations that indicate an infection is present at the site. IV should be discontinued and physician notified. Be careful not to disconnect IV tubing when putting on patient's hospital gown.**

RATIONALE

This promotes safe administration of IV fluids and medication. Too rapid administration of medications can result in the development of speed shock.

   a. This ensures that the correct solution is being given at the correct rate and in the proper sequence with the correct medications.

   b. This ensures that flow rate is correct.

   c. Any kink or pressure on tubing may interfere with flow. Leakage may occur at the connection of the tubing with the hub of needle or catheter and allow for loss of IV solution.

   d. Observation ensures that infusion control device is functioning and that alarm is in "on" position.

Catheter may become dislodged from vein, and IV solution may flow into subcutaneous tissue.

Chemical irritation or mechanical trauma causes injury to the vein and can lead to phlebitis.

Poor aseptic technique may allow bacteria to enter the needle or catheter insertion site or tubing connection.

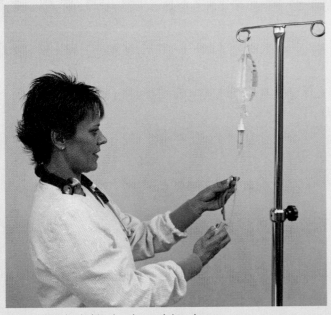

Action 1b: Check drip chamber and time drops.

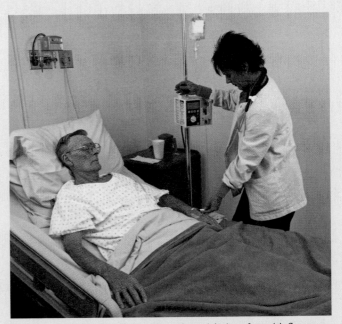

Action 1c: Check tubing for anything that might interfere with flow rate.

continues

SKILL 15-3   Monitoring an IV Site and Infusion (continued)

ACTION

RATIONALE

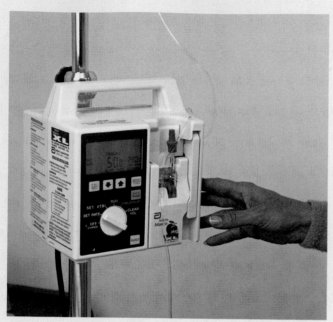

Action 1d: Check the settings of the infusion device.

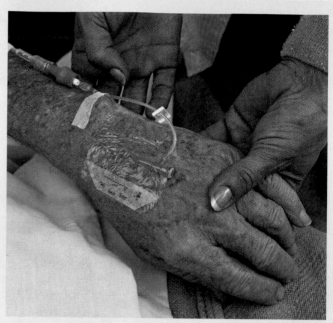

Action 2: Inspect IV site.

5. Be alert for additional complications of IV therapy.

   a. **Circulatory overload can result in signs of cardiac failure and pulmonary edema. Monitor intake and output during IV therapy.**

   b. Bleeding at the site is most likely to occur when the IV is discontinued.

6. **If possible, instruct patient to call for assistance if any discomfort is noted at site, solution container is nearly empty, flow has changed in any way, or pump alarm sounds.**

7. Document IV infusion, any complications of therapy, and patient's reaction to therapy.

a. Infusing too much IV solution results in an increased volume of circulating fluid.

b. Bleeding may be caused by anticoagulant medication.

This facilitates cooperation of patient and safe administration of IV solution.

This provides accurate documentation and ensures continuity of care.

> 11/6/06   1020   IV site pink, warm, and dry. D50.9NS with 20 mEq KCl/L continues to infuse at 110 mL/hr. Patient instructed to call nurse with any swelling or pain.
> —S. Barnes, RN

Action 7: Documentation.

EVALUATION

The expected outcome is achieved when the patient remains free of injury (specifically, complications related to IV therapy) and exhibits an IV site that is pink, warm, dry, and pain-free. The IV solution infuses at the prescribed flow rate.

continues

Monitoring an IV Site and Infusion (continued)

Unexpected Situations and Associated Interventions

- *Patient's lung sounds were previously clear, but now some crackles in the bases are auscultated:* Notify physician immediately. The patient may be exhibiting signs of fluid overload. Be prepared to tell the physician what the past intake and output totals were.
- *IV is not flowing as easily as it previously had:* If there is no medication in the IV, open the clamp and see if the IV is patent (you may also flush with 3 mL of normal saline). If the IV does not flow with the clamp open, check all other clamps on the tubing and check tubing for any kinking. If the IV is over a joint, reposition the extremity and see if this helps the flow. An armboard may need to be applied. If the IV is painful or you meet resistance when attempting to flush, discontinue the IV and restart in another place.

Changing an IV Dressing

The IV site is a potential entry point for microorganisms into the bloodstream. To prevent this, sealed IV dressings are used to occlude the site and prevent complications. Whenever these dressings need to be changed, it is important to observe meticulous technique to minimize the possibility of contamination. As always, the institution's policies determine the type of dressing used and when these dressing are changed. IV site dressing changes often coincide with IV site rotations. However, dressing changes might be required more often, based on your nursing assessment and judgment. Any IV dressing that is damp, loosened, or soiled should be changed immediately.

Equipment

- Sterile gauze (2 × 2 or 4 × 4) or transparent occlusive dressing
- Povidone-iodine (Betadine) swabs
- Adhesive remover (optional)
- Alcohol swabs
- Tape
- Clean gloves
- Towel or disposable pad
- Masks for nurse and patient (optional)

ASSESSMENT

Assess IV site, looking for any drainage, redness, leakage, or other indications that the dressing needs to be changed. Also assess the patient's need to keep IV. If patient does not need IV, discuss with physician the possibility of discontinuing it. Ask the patient about any allergies, specifically to iodine.

NURSING DIAGNOSIS

Determine the related factors for the nursing diagnosis based on the patient's current status. An appropriate nursing diagnosis is Risk for Infection. Many other nursing diagnoses also may require the use of this skill.

OUTCOME IDENTIFICATION AND PLANNING

The expected outcome to achieve when changing an IV dressing is that the patient will exhibit an IV site that is clean, dry, and without evidence of any signs and symptoms of infection. In addition, the dressing will be clean, dry, and intact.

**SKILL
15-4**   **Changing an IV Dressing** (continued)

IMPLEMENTATION

ACTION	RATIONALE

For a Peripheral IV Insertion Site

1. Assess the need for dressing change.

   Agency policy determines interval for dressing change (every 24 to 72 hours). **The presence of moisture or a nonadhering dressing increases the risk for bacterial contamination at the site.**

2. Gather equipment and bring to bedside.

   Having equipment available saves time and facilitates the performance of the task.

3. Explain procedure to patient.

   Explanation allays anxiety.

4. **Perform hand hygiene. Don clean gloves.**

   Hand hygiene deters the spread of microorganisms. Gloves prevent transmission of HIV and other blood-borne infections.

5. Place towel or disposable pad under the arm with the IV site. **Carefully remove old dressing, but leave tape that anchors the IV needle or catheter in place.** Discard properly.

   This prevents IV needle or catheter from becoming dislodged.

6. **Inspect IV site for presence of inflammation or infiltration. Discontinue and relocate IV if noted.**

   Inflammation or infiltration causes trauma to tissues and necessitates removal of the IV needle or catheter.

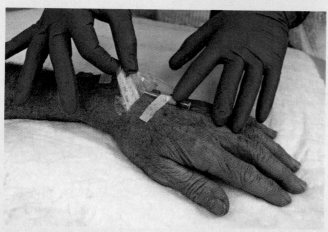

Action 5: Remove the old dressing.

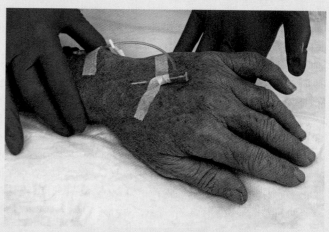

Action 6: Inspect the site.

7. Loosen and gently remove tape, being careful to steady catheter with one hand. Use adhesive remover if necessary.

   Tape stabilizes needle and prevents it from becoming dislodged.

8. **Cleanse the entry site with an alcohol swab using a circular motion, moving from the center outward. Allow to dry. Follow with povidone-iodine swab using the same process.**

   Cleaning in a circular motion while moving outward carries organisms away from the entry site. Use of antiseptic solutions reduces the number of microorganisms on the skin surface.

9. Reapply tape strip to needle or catheter at entry site.

   Tape anchors needle or catheter to prevent dislodgement.

10. Apply sterile gauze or transparent polyurethane dressing over entry site. Remove gloves and perform hand hygiene.

    Dressing protects site and deters contamination with microorganisms. Hand hygiene deters the spread of microorganisms.

continues

ACTION   **RATIONALE**

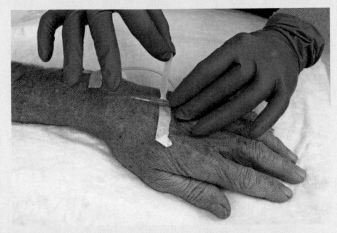

Action 7: Loosen tape while stabilizing the catheter.

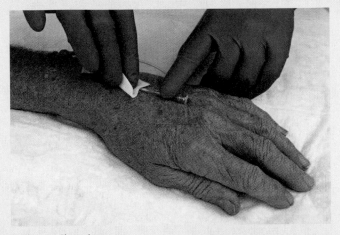

Action 8: Clean site.

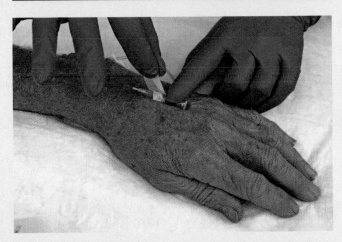

Action 9: Reapply a tape strip.

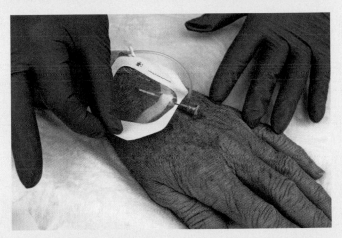

Action 10: Apply a new dressing.

11. **Secure IV tubing with additional tape if necessary. Label dressing with date, time of change, and initials. Check that IV flow is accurate and system is patent.** Document findings.

Labeling and documentation ensure communication about IV dressing change.

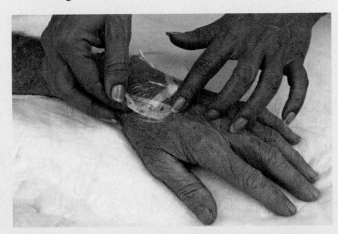

Action 11: Label the dressing.

11/15/06   1120   Dressing change to IV site in L hand complete. Site without erythema, edema, or drainage. 0.9 NS infusing at 75 mL/hr. Patient instructed to call nurse with any pain, swelling, or questions.
—S. Barnes, RN

Action 11: Documentation.

continues

SKILL 15-4   Changing an IV Dressing (continued)

ACTION	RATIONALE
For a Central Venous Access Device	
12. Follow Actions 1 through 5.	
13. Remove gloves and wash hands thoroughly. Open dressing kit using sterile technique. **If agency requires, nurse and patient should put on a mask.**	Unclean hands and improper technique are potential sources for infecting a central venous access device. Most facilities have all sterile dressing supplies gathered in a single unit.
14. **Put on sterile gloves.**	Use of gloves maintains surgical asepsis.
15. Cleanse the site according to agency policy, such as with alcohol swabs, moving in a circular fashion from the insertion site outward (1.5" to 2" area). Allow to dry.	The alcohol kills *Staphylococcus aureus* and *S. epidermidis,* the most common causes of central line infections.
16. Follow alcohol cleansing with povidone-iodine swabs, using the same technique. **Allow to dry.**	Povidone-iodine kills fungi, which are responsible for 25% of central line infections.
17. Reapply sterile dressing or securement device according to agency policy. Secure tubing or lumens to prevent tugging on insertion site.	Dressing prevents contamination of the IV catheter and protects insertion site.
18. Note date, time of dressing change, size of catheter, and initials on tape or dressing.	Labeling documents that dressing change occurred.
19. Discard equipment properly and perform hand hygiene.	Hand hygiene protects against spread of microorganisms.
20. Record patient's response to dressing change and observation of site.	This provides accurate documentation and ensures continuity of care.

EVALUATION   The expected outcome is met when the patient remains free of any signs and symptoms of infection at the IV site. In addition, the IV dressing is clean, dry, and intact.

Unexpected Situations and Associated Interventions
- *Patient complains that IV site feels "funny" and hurts:* Observe IV site for redness, edema, and warmth. If present, clamp the tubing to stop the solution flow, remove the catheter, and apply a gauze dressing. Notify physician and start a new IV at a different site.

Capping a Primary Line for Intermittent Use

Sometimes a continuous infusion of IV solution is no longer needed, but the patient still needs an access for the administration of medications or periodic fluid infusions. An IV line can then be capped, leaving the site as an access point for intermittent or emergency use. Basically, a capped line consists of the IV catheter connected to a short length of extension tubing sealed with a cap. Some facilities put the resealable cap directly into the IV catheter hub. Because there are different ways to cap an IV line, review your agency's policies. Capped lines are flushed at periodic intervals with normal saline or heparin to keep the IV catheter patent and to prevent clots from forming in the catheter.

Equipment

- Lock device
- Clean gloves
- 4″ × 4″ gauze pad
- Normal saline or heparin flush prepared in a syringe (1 to 3 mL) according to agency policy
- Alcohol wipe
- Tape
- Extension tubing (optional)

ASSESSMENT

Assess IV insertion site, noting color, temperature, and drainage. Verify the physician's orders to ensure that continuous infusions are no longer necessary.

NURSING DIAGNOSIS

Determine the related factors for the nursing diagnosis based on the patient's current status. Appropriate nursing diagnoses may include Risk for Infection and Risk for Injury. Many other nursing diagnoses also may require the use of this skill.

OUTCOME IDENTIFICATION AND PLANNING

The expected outcome to achieve when capping a primary IV line is that the patient will remain free of injury and any signs and symptoms of infection. In addition, the capped IV device will remain patent.

IMPLEMENTATION

ACTION	RATIONALE
1. Gather equipment and verify physician's order. Fill lock or adapter device with normal saline or heparin flush according to agency policy. Recap syringe for use in Action 10.	Having equipment available saves time and facilitates the task. Checking the order ensures that the procedure has been ordered by the physician. Flushing maintains patency of lock and tubing.
2. Explain procedure to patient.	Explanation allays anxiety.
3. Perform hand hygiene.	Hand hygiene deters the spread of microorganisms.
4. Assess the IV site.	Complications such as infiltration or phlebitis necessitate discontinuation of the IV infusion at that site.
5. **Clamp off primary IV tubing.**	Clamping prevents inadvertent blood loss when IV and tubing are disconnected.
When Extension Tubing Is Present	
6. Don clean gloves according to hospital policy. Clamp the extension tubing if a clamp is present. Remove the primary IV tubing from the extension set and attach the lock or adapter device. Cleanse the cap of the lock of adapter device with an alcohol swab.	Clamping prevents air from entering the line. Cleaning the cap reduces the risk for contamination.
7. Unclamp the extension set and insert a saline or heparin flush syringe into the cap and flush the line according to agency policy. Reclamp the extension tubing and remove the syringe.	Flushing maintains patency of the IV line.
8. Use tape to secure the extension tubing. Proceed to Action 18.	

continues

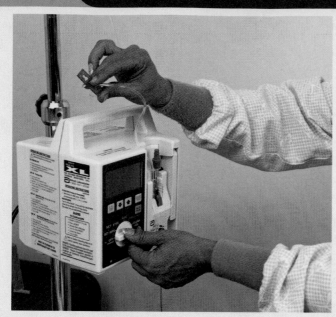

Action 5: Clamp off the primary line.

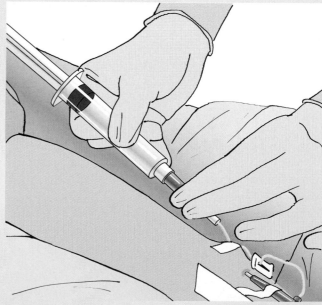

Action 6: Remove IV tubing.

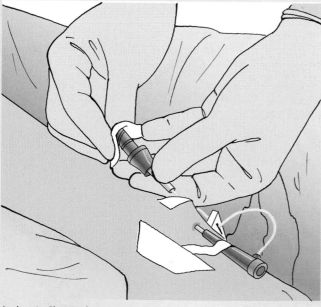

Action 6: Cleanse the cap.

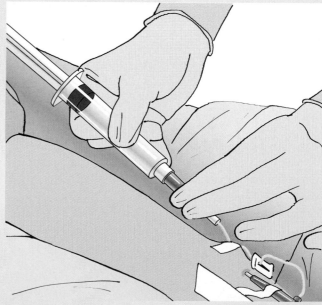

Action 7: Flush the line.

ACTION	RATIONALE
When Connecting Directly to the Hub of the IV Access Catheter	
9. Follow Actions 1 through 5.	These actions prepare the patient and nurse and reduce the risk for contamination.
10. Prime the lock of adapter device and extension set (if one is to be attached to the device) with normal saline. Clamp the extension set if one is being used.	Priming the equipment prevents air from being introduced into the IV line when connected. Sometimes a short extension tubing is used to connect the lock or adapter device directly to the catheter hub, reducing the risk for blood exposure.

continues

SKILL 15-5

Capping a Primary Line for Intermittent Use (continued)

ACTION	RATIONALE
11. Don clean gloves.	Gloves protect the nurse from contact with the patient's blood.
12. Place gauze 4 × 4 sponge underneath IV connection hub between IV catheter and tubing.	Gauze absorbs any blood leakage when IV and tubing are disconnected.
13. **Stabilize hub of IV catheter with nondominant hand. Use dominant hand to quickly twist and disconnect IV tubing from the catheter. Discard it. Attach the primed lock or adapter device (or adapter device and extension set) to the IV catheter hub.**	This maintains sterility of IV setup.
14. **Cleanse cap with an alcohol wipe and unclamp the extension set (if used).**	Cleansing removes surface bacteria at the heparin lock entry site.
15. Insert the syringe with blunt cannula or standard syringe and gently flush with saline or heparin flush as per agency policy. Remove syringe carefully and reclamp the extension tubing (if used).	This maintains patency of the IV access line. Clinical evidence has demonstrated that a saline flush is as effective as heparin for peripheral IVs, avoids the adverse effects of heparin, is less expensive, and prevents drug incompatibilities. **Some institutions recommend a positive pressure flush. To do this, clamp the connecting tubing as you are flushing the IV.**
16. Remove gloves and dispose of them appropriately.	Proper disposal of soiled gloves reduces the risk for infection transmission.
17. Tape lock or adapter device (and extension tubing if used).	Tape secures the lock or device in the proper position.
18. Perform hand hygiene and ensure the patient is comfortable.	Hand hygiene deters the spread of microorganisms.
19. Chart on IV administration record or medication Kardex per institutional policy.	Accurate documentation is necessary to prevent error.

11/12/06 IV fluids discontinued, IV flushes easily; site pink, warm, and dry without drainage; converted to saline lock.
—S. Barnes, RN

Action 19: Documentation.

EVALUATION

The expected outcome is met when the IV catheter flushes easily, indicating patency, and the patient exhibits an IV site that is pink, warm, and dry without any drainage.

Unexpected Situations and Associated Interventions

- *IV site leaks fluid whenever flushed:* To prevent infection, remove this IV and restart it in another location.
- *IV does not flush easily:* Check insertion site. The catheter may be blocked or clotted due to a kinked catheter at the insertion site. If the catheter has pulled out a short distance, do not reinsert it: it is no longer sterile. The catheter will most likely need to be removed and started in a new location.

SKILL 15-6 Administering a Blood Transfusion

A blood transfusion is the infusion of whole blood or a blood component such as plasma, red blood cells, or platelets into a patient's venous circulation. Before a patient can receive blood, his or her blood must be typed to ensure that he or she receives compatible blood. Otherwise, clumping and hemolysis of the red blood cells result, and death can occur.

Equipment

- Blood product
- Blood administration set (tubing with in-line filter and Y for saline administration)
- 0.9% normal saline
- IV pole
- IV catheter (20 gauge or larger)
- Disposable gloves
- Tape

ASSESSMENT

Obtain a baseline assessment of the patient, including heart and lung sounds and urinary output. Review the most recent laboratory values. Ask the patient about any previous transfusions, including the number he or she has had and any reactions experienced during a transfusion. Inspect the IV insertion site and check the type of solution being given.

NURSING DIAGNOSIS

Determine the related factors for the nursing diagnosis based on the patient's current status. Appropriate nursing diagnoses may include:

- Risk for Injury
- Deficient Fluid Volume
- Ineffective Peripheral Tissue Perfusion
- Decreased Cardiac Output

IMPLEMENTATION

ACTION	RATIONALE
1. Determine whether patient knows reason for transfusion. Ask if the patient has had a transfusion or a transfusion reaction in the past.	This directs teaching before beginning transfusion.
2. Explain to patient what will happen. Check for signed consent for transfusion if required by agency. Advise patient to report any chills, itching, rash, or unusual symptoms. If the physician has ordered any premedication, administer it now.	Explanation provides reassurance and facilitates cooperation. Any reaction to the transfusion necessitates stopping the transfusion immediately.
3. Perform hand hygiene and put on clean gloves.	Hand hygiene deters the spread of microorganisms. Gloves protect against accidental exposure to the patient's blood.
4. **Hang container of 0.9% normal saline with blood administration set to initiate IV infusion and follow administration of blood.**	Dextrose may lead to clumping of red blood cells and hemolysis. The filter in the blood administration set removes particulate material formed during storage of blood.
5. Start IV with 18 or 19 gauge catheter if not already present (see Skill 15-1). Keep IV open by starting flow of normal saline.	A large-bore needle or catheter is necessary for the infusion of blood products. The lumen must be large enough not to cause damage to red blood cells. IV should be started before obtaining blood in case the procedure takes longer than 30 minutes.
6. Obtain blood product from blood bank according to agency policy.	Blood must be stored at a carefully controlled temperature (4°C).

continues

ACTION

7. **Complete identification and checks as required by agency:**
   a. **Identification number**
   b. **Blood group and type**
   c. **Expiration date**
   d. **Patient's name**
   e. **Inspect blood for clots.**

8. **Take baseline set of vital signs before beginning transfusion.**

9. Start infusion of the blood product:
   a. Prime in-line filter with blood.
   b. **Start administration slowly (no more than 25 to 50 mL for the first 15 minutes). Stay with the patient for the first 5 to 15 minutes of transfusion.**
   c. **Check vital signs at least every 15 minutes for the first half-hour. Follow institution's recommendations for taking vital signs during the remainder of the transfusion.**
   d. Observe patient for flushing, dyspnea, itching, hives, or rash.
   e. Never warm blood in a microwave. Use a blood warming device, if indicated or ordered, especially with rapid transfusions through a CVP catheter.

RATIONALE

Most states/agencies require two registered nurses to verify information: unit numbers match; ABO group and Rh type are the same; expiration date (after 35 days, red blood cells begin to deteriorate). Blood is never administered to a patient without an identification band. If clots are present, blood should be returned to blood bank.

Any change in vital signs during the transfusion may indicate a reaction.

a. Priming is necessary for blood to flow properly.
b. Transfusion reactions typically occur during this period, and a slow rate will minimize the volume of red blood cells infused.
c. If there have been no adverse effects during this time, the infusion rate is increased. If complications occur, they can be observed and the transfusion can be stopped immediately.
d. These symptoms may be early indication of a transfusion reaction.
e. Rapid administration of cold blood can result in cardiac arrhythmias.

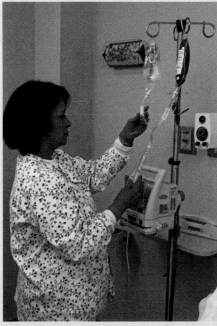

Action 9a: Prime in-line filter.

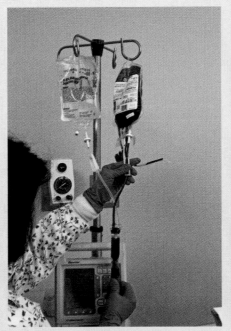

Action 9b: Start transfusion slowly.

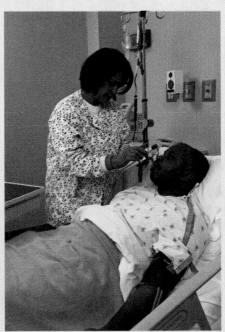

Action 9c: Assess vital signs.

continues

ACTION	RATIONALE
10. Maintain the prescribed flow rate as ordered or as deemed appropriate based on the patient's overall condition, keeping in mind the outer limits for safe administration. **Assess frequently for transfusion reaction. Stop blood transfusion if you suspect a reaction. Quickly replace the blood tubing with new tubing and 0.9% sodium chloride. Notify physician and blood bank.**	Rate must be carefully controlled, and patient's reaction must be monitored frequently. If a transfusion reaction is suspected, the blood must be stopped. Do not infuse the normal saline through the blood tubing because you would be allowing more of the blood into the patient's body, which could complicate a reaction.
11. When transfusion is complete, clamp off blood and begin to infuse 0.9% normal saline.	Saline prevents hemolysis of red blood cells and clears remainder of blood in IV line.
12. Record administration of blood and patient's reaction as ordered by agency. Return blood transfusion bag to blood bank according to agency policy.	This provides for accurate documentation of patient's response to the transfusion.

EVALUATION

The expected outcome is met when the patient receives the blood transfusion without any evidence of a transfusion reaction or complication. The patient exhibits signs and symptoms of fluid balance, improved cardiac output, and enhanced peripheral tissue perfusion.

Unexpected Situations and Associated Interventions

- *Patient is becoming febrile but is exhibiting no other signs of a transfusion reaction:* Notify physician. The physician may have you pause the blood transfusion and medicate the patient with acetaminophen and an antihistamine before resuming the transfusion. If this is ordered, flush the IV with 3 mL of normal saline while waiting so that the IV remains patent.
- *Patient reports shortness of breath, and on auscultation you note crackles bilaterally in the bases:* Notify physician. The physician may order a dose of a diuretic or may have you slow the infusion.
- *Patient is febrile, tachycardic, and complaining of back pain:* Patient is having a transfusion reaction. Stop the transfusion immediately. Obtain new IV tubing with 0.9% sodium chloride. Notify physician and blood bank. Send blood unit, tubing, and filter to the lab.
- *Blood is not infusing quickly enough:* Adjust the rate with the clamp. If this does not work, try flushing the IV with 3 mL of saline.

Special Considerations

- Electronic infusion devices may be used to maintain the prescribed rate but must be specifically designed for use with blood transfusions.

Home Care Considerations

- Home care agencies evaluate patients who are candidates for a blood transfusion at home.
- Home transfusion is not appropriate for patients who are actively bleeding, require more than 4 hours for the transfusion, or recently had a reaction to a blood transfusion. Written consent must be obtained from the patient and the physician.
- The nurse transports the blood product to the patient's home in a special cooler. The nurse and the patient's caregiver check the serial number and other identification information together.

Changing a PICC Line Dressing

When caring for a patient with a PICC line, you must use sterile technique to prevent infection. Dressings are placed at the insertion site to occlude the site and prevent the introduction of microorganisms into the bloodstream. Scrupulous care of the site is required to control contamination. Agency policy generally determines the type of dressing used and the intervals for dressing change, but any dressing that is damp, loosened, or soiled should be changed immediately.

Equipment

- Sterile tape or Steri-Strips
- Sterile semipermeable transparent dressing (or gauze dressing)
- Several 2 × 2s
- Sterile towel or drape
- Sterile povidone-iodine and alcohol swab sticks (three each)
- Masks (two)
- Clean gloves
- Sterile gloves
- Sterile skin protectant pad
- PICC injection caps

ASSESSMENT

Inspect the insertion site closely for any color change, drainage, swelling, or pain. Ask the patient about any complaints at the insertion site.

NURSING DIAGNOSIS

Determine the related factors for the nursing diagnosis based on the patient's current status. An appropriate nursing diagnosis is Risk for Infection. Many other nursing diagnoses also may require the use of this skill.

OUTCOME IDENTIFICATION AND PLANNING

The expected outcome to achieve when changing a PICC line dressing is that the patient will remain free of any signs and symptoms of infection. The site will be clean and dry, with an intact dressing.

IMPLEMENTATION

ACTION	RATIONALE
1. Gather equipment and verify physician's order (often this will be a standing protocol).	Having equipment available saves time and facilitates the task. Checking the order ensures that the procedure has been ordered by the physician.
2. Explain procedure to patient.	Explanation allays anxiety.
3. Perform hand hygiene.	Hand hygiene deters the spread of microorganisms. Unclean hands and improper technique are potential sources for infecting a central venous access device.
4. **If agency requires, apply a mask and have patient also put on a mask.** Don clean gloves. Set up sterile field on area to be used. Have patient place the arm in the middle of the sterile field. Open dressing kit using sterile technique and place on sterile towel.	Masks help to deter the spread of microorganisms. Gloves prevent transmission of HIV and other blood-borne infections. Sterile towel gives the nurse a large clean area to work on. Most facilities have all sterile dressing supplies gathered in a single unit.
5. Assess PICC insertion site through old dressing. Remove old dressing by lifting it distally and then working proximally. Remove and dispose of gloves properly. Put on sterile gloves.	When assessing PICC insertion site, note how PICC is secured. Most PICC lines are not sutured in but rather taped and are easy to dislodge when changing dressings.
6. Starting at insertion site and continuing in a circle, wipe off any old blood or drainage with a sterile alcohol wipe. **Clean according to agency policy, such as with alcohol swab sticks: One at a time, move in a circular fashion from the insertion site outward (2″ to 3″ area). Allow to dry.**	The alcohol kills *Staphylococcus aureus* and *S. epidermidis*, the most common causes of central line infections.

continues

ACTION

7. Follow alcohol cleansing with povidone-iodine swabs, using the same technique. **Allow to dry.** If needed, you can then apply the skin protectant pad to this area, working from the insertion site out. Allow to dry.

RATIONALE

Povidone-iodine kills fungi, which are responsible for 25% of central line infections.

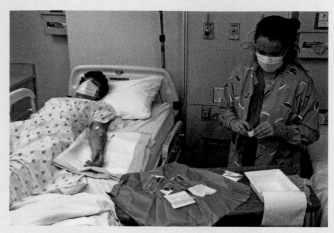

Action 4: Set up sterile field in preparation for dressing change.

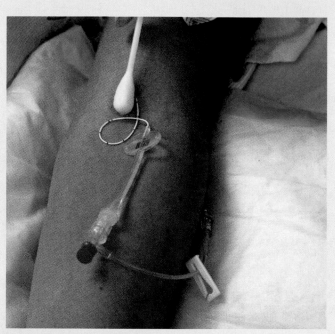

Action 6: Clean site with alcohol swab using circular motion.

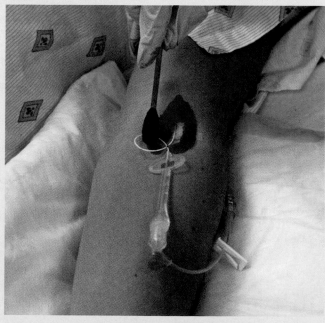

Action 7: Clean site with povidone–iodine swab using circular motion.

continues

ACTION	RATIONALE
8. **Reapply sterile dressing or securement device according to agency policy.** Secure tubing or lumens to prevent tugging on insertion site.	Dressing prevents contamination of the IV catheter and protects insertion site.
9. **Clamp all lines of the PICC and remove injection caps. Cleanse the catheter ends with alcohol and then apply new injection caps. Tape the distal ends down securely.**	The catheter ends should be cleaned and injection caps changed to prevent infection. The distal ends are secured to prevent the catheter from becoming dislodged.
10. Note date, time of dressing change, size of catheter, and initials on tape or dressing.	Data documents that dressing change occurred.

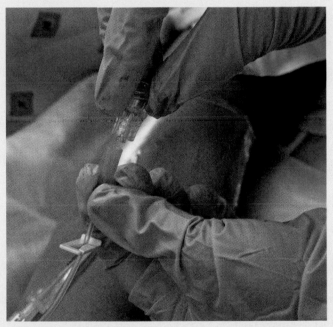

Action 9: Apply new injection cap.

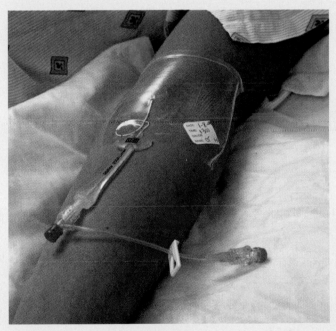

Action 10: Note date, time, size of catheter, and initials on dressing.

11. Discard equipment properly and perform hand hygiene.	Hand hygiene protects against spread of microorganisms.
12. Record patient's response to dressing change and observation of site.	This provides accurate documentation and ensures continuity of care.

EVALUATION   The expected outcome is met when the dressing is changed without any complications, including dislodgement of the PICC. The patient exhibits an insertion site that is clean and dry without redness or swelling. Dressing is clean, dry, and intact.

Unexpected Situations and Associated Interventions

- *While dressing is being changed, PICC is inadvertently dislodged.* If PICC is not all the way out, notify physician. The physician will most likely want a chest x-ray to determine where the end of the PICC line is. Before the chest x-ray, reapply a dressing so that the PICC is not further dislodged.
- *When the dressing is removed, purulent drainage is noted at the insertion site:* Swab the drainage with a culture swab, clean the area, reapply a dressing, and then notify the physician. This prevents the PICC line from being open to air and unprotected while you are notifying the physician. If the physician does not want the culture, you can dispose of the culture kit.

Accessing an Implanted Port

Totally implantable access devices allow long-term access without having a catheter protrude from the skin. The system includes the subcutaneous injection port and a catheter, which is usually inserted into the superior vena cava. When venous access is desired, the location of the injection port must be palpated. The system is accessed with a noncoring needle. Patency is maintained by periodic flushing. The length and gauge of the needle used to access the port should be selected based on the patient's anatomy and anticipated infusion requirements. In general, a ¾″ 20-gauge needle is most frequently used. If the patient has a significant amount of subcutaneous tissue, a longer length (1″ or 1.5″) may be selected. A larger gauge (19-gauge) is preferred for administration of blood products.

Equipment	• Sterile dressing kit • Huber needle • Vial of sodium chloride • Blunt needles (two) • 10-mL syringes (two) • Needleless injection cap • Sterile gauze 2 × 2 (optional) • Vial of heparin (as indicated by agency policy)
ASSESSMENT	Inspect the skin over port, looking for any swelling, redness, or drainage. Also assess site over port for any pain or tenderness. Review the patient's history for the length of time the port has been in place.
NURSING DIAGNOSIS	Determine the related factors for the nursing diagnosis based on the patient's current status. An appropriate nursing diagnosis is Risk for Infection. Many other nursing diagnoses, such as Acute Pain, Risk for Injury, and Deficient Knowledge also may require the use of this skill.
OUTCOME IDENTIFICATION AND PLANNING	The expected outcome to achieve when accessing an implanted port is that the port is accessed with minimal to no discomfort to the patient. The patient experiences no trauma to the site.

IMPLEMENTATION

ACTION	RATIONALE
1. Gather equipment and verify physician's order (many times this will be a standing protocol).	Having equipment available saves time and facilitates the task. Checking the order ensures that the procedure has been ordered by the physician.
2. Explain procedure to patient.	Explanation allays anxiety.
3. Perform hand hygiene.	Hand hygiene deters the spread of microorganisms. Unclean hands and improper technique are potential sources for infecting a central venous access device.
4. Raise bed to comfortable working height.	Raising the bed helps reduce strain on the nurse's back.
5. Attach the blunt needles to the 10-mL syringes. Withdraw 10 mL of sodium chloride from the vial (see Chap. 5 for more information).	

continues

SKILL 15-8   Accessing an Implanted Port (continued)

ACTION	RATIONALE
6. Connect the intermittent injection cap to the extension tubing on the Huber needle. Attach the 10-mL syringe to the intermittent injection cap and flush the needle with tubing. Clamp the tubing. Remove the syringe from the injection cap.	The needles and tubing must be free of air so that patient does not experience an air embolus.
7. If transparent dressing is in place, don clean gloves and gently pull it back, beginning with edges and proceeding around the edge of the dressing. Once dressing is removed, gently pull straight back on needle. Discard in appropriate receptacle and remove gloves.	Gently pulling the edges of the dressing will be less traumatic to the patient.
8. **Open the kit using sterile technique. Don the mask and the first pair of sterile gloves. Set up your sterile field.** If port is not accessed, proceed to Action 9.	Improper technique is a potential source for infecting a central venous device.
9. **Cleanse according to agency policy. For example, using the alcohol swab sticks, cleanse in a circular fashion from the insertion site outward (2″ to 3″ area). Use each swab once and discard. Allow site to dry.**	The alcohol kills *Staphylococcus aureus* and *S. epidermidis*, the most common causes of central line infections.
10. Follow alcohol cleansing with povidone-iodine swabs, using the same technique. **Allow to dry.**	Povidone-iodine kills fungi, which are responsible for 25% of central line infections.
11. **Locate the port septum by palpation.** With your non-dominant hand, hold the port stable, keeping the skin taut but without touching the port side.	The edges of the port must be palpated so that the needle can be inserted into the center of the port. Hold the port with your nondominant hand so that you can stick the port with your dominant hand.

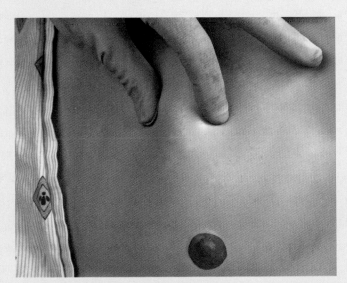

Action 11: Stabilize port with nondominant hand.

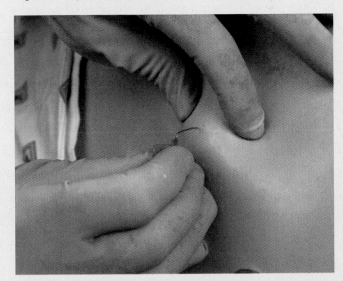

Action 12: Prepare to push needle into port.

12. Visualize the center of the port. **Push the Huber needle (non-coring 90-degree) to the skin into the portal septum until it hits the back of the port septum.**	To infuse fluids properly, the needle must be located in the middle of the port and inserted to the back of the port.
13. Cleanse the injection cap with alcohol and insert the syringe with normal saline.	The alcohol kills *Staphylococcus aureus* and *S. epidermidis*, the most common causes of central line infections.

continues

ACTION	RATIONALE

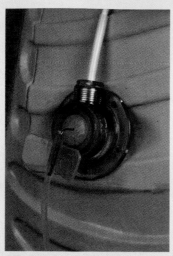

Action 12: Huber needle in place.

14. **Open the clamp and push down on the syringe plunger, flushing the device with 3 to 5 mL of saline, while observing for fluid leak or infiltration. It should flush easily, without resistance.**

If needle is not inserted correctly, fluid will leak into tissue, causing the tissue to swell and producing signs of infiltration. Flushing without resistance is also a sign that the needle is inserted into the correct place.

15. Pull back on the syringe plunger to aspirate for blood return. Aspirate only a few milliliters of blood; do not allow blood to enter syringe.

The ability to withdraw blood is a sign that the port is patent. Not allowing blood to enter the syringe ensures that the needle will be flushed with pure saline.

16. Flush with the remainder of saline in syringe.

This ensures that the port will remain patent.

17. Clamp the tubing, remove the syringe, and attach the heparin-filled syringe (if appropriate for the institution). Clamp the tubing while maintaining positive pressure on the syringe barrel at the end of the flush.

Heparin ensures patency of the port. Flushing with positive pressure prevents blood from back-flowing into the port and clamping it off.

18. Remove the syringe. **If space exists between the skin and the needle, place a sterile folded 2 × 2 in the space to support the needle.** If using a "Gripper" needle, remove the gripper portion from the needle by squeezing the sides together and lifting off the needle while holding the needle securely to the port with the other hand.

The 2 × 2 helps keep the needle from moving.

19. Apply tape or Steri-Strips in a starlike pattern over the needle to secure it.

The tape will help prevent the needle from accidentally pulling out.

20. Cover the entire needle and port with the transparent dressing, leaving the ports of the extension tubing uncovered for easy access.

Dressing prevents contamination of the IV catheter and protects insertion site.

21. Remove gloves and discard. Perform hand hygiene.

Hand hygiene deters the spread of microorganisms.

22. Label the dressing with the date, time, size needle used, and your initials, according to agency policy.

This documents IV tubing change.

continues

ACTION	RATIONALE
23. Document procedure, including time, date, type and location of port, condition of skin at site, size needle used, presence of blood return, and any difficulties encountered.	This provides accurate documentation and ensures continuity of care.

> 11/22/06 1245 Implanted port R subclavian, old dressing removed, no drainage, swelling, or redness noted; 20G 3/4 Huber needle used to access port. Flushes easily with good blood return. Pt instructed to call nurse with any swelling, pain, or leaking.—S. Barnes

Action 23: Documentation.

EVALUATION

The expected outcome is met when the port can be accessed without difficulty or pain, and the patient remains free of signs and symptoms of infection or trauma.

Unexpected Situations and Associated Interventions

- *Port begins to swell when flushing with saline:* Stop flushing. Gently push on syringe and slowly begin to flush again. The needle may have become dislodged from the septum of the port. If the swelling continues, stop flushing and notify physician.
- *Port does not flush:* Check clamp to make sure tubing is open. Gently push down on needle and again try to flush. Ask the patient to perform a Valsalva maneuver. Try having the patient change position or place the affected arm over the head, or try raising or lowering the head of the bed. If the port still does not flush, notify physician.
- *Port flushes but does not draw blood:* Notify physician. Anticipate an order for a thrombolytic.

Special Considerations

- Groshong devices do not require the use of heparin for flushing.
- Some institutions call for a power flush (rapidly pushing the flush in small amounts).
- Implanted ports need to be accessed every 4 to 6 weeks (according to agency policy) to be flushed.

SKILL 15-9   Deaccessing an Implanted Port

When an implanted port will not be used for a period of time, such as when a patient is being discharged, the port can be deaccessed. Deaccessing a port involves removing the noncoring needle from the port.

Equipment

- Clean gloves
- Syringe filled with 10 mL saline
- Syringe filled with 5 mL heparin (100 u/mL or institution's recommendations)
- Sterile gauze sponge
- Alcohol wipe
- Band-Aid

ASSESSMENT

Inspect the insertion site, looking for any swelling, redness, or drainage. Also assess site over port for any pain or tenderness. Review the patient's history for the length of time the port and noncoring needle have been in place.

NURSING DIAGNOSIS

Determine the related factors for the nursing diagnosis based on the patient's current status. An appropriate nursing diagnosis is Risk for Injury. Many other nursing diagnoses, such as Acute Pain and Deficient Knowledge, also may require the use of this skill.

OUTCOME IDENTIFICATION AND PLANNING

The expected outcome to achieve when deaccessing an implanted port is that the needle is removed with minimal to no discomfort to the patient. The patient experiences no trauma to the site.

IMPLEMENTATION

ACTION	RATIONALE
1. Gather equipment and verify physician's order (many times this will be a standing protocol).	Having equipment available saves time and facilitates the task. Checking the order ensures that the procedure has been ordered by the physician.
2. Explain procedure to patient.	Explanation allays anxiety.
3. Perform hand hygiene.	Hand hygiene deters the spread of microorganisms. Unclean hands and improper technique are potential sources for infecting a central venous access device.
4. Raise bed to comfortable working height.	Raising the bed helps to reduce strain on the nurse's back.
5. Don gloves.	Gloves prevent the transmission of HIV and other blood-borne diseases.
6. Gently pull back transparent dressing, beginning with edges and proceeding around the edge of the dressing. Carefully remove all the tape that is securing the needle in place.	Gently pulling the edges of the dressing is less traumatic to the patient.
7. Clean the injection cap and insert the saline-filled syringe. **Unclamp the catheter's extension tubing and begin to flush with a minimum of 10 mL normal saline.**	It is important to flush all substances out of the well of the implanted port, because it will be inactive for several weeks.
8. **Remove the syringe and insert the heparin-filled syringe, flushing with 5 mL heparin (100 u/mL or agency's policy). Clamp the extension tubing while maintaining positive pressure on the barrel of the syringe. Remove the syringe.**	Since the catheter will be inactive for several weeks, the heparin prevents clots from forming.

continues

SKILL 15-9   Deaccessing an Implanted Port (continued)

ACTION	RATIONALE
9. Secure the port on either side with the fingers of your nondominant hand. Grasp the needle/wings with the fingers of your dominant hand. Firmly and smoothly, pull the needle straight up at a 90-degree angle from the skin to remove it from the septum.	By grasping the port, the port is held in place while the needle is removed.

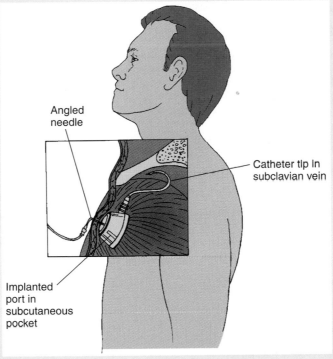

Angled needle

Catheter tip in subclavian vein

Implanted port in subcutaneous pocket

Action 9: An implanted port with the tip in the subclavian vein and non-coring needle inserted and dressing removed.

ACTION	RATIONALE
10. Apply gentle pressure with the gauze to the insertion site. A Band-Aid may be applied over the port if any oozing occurs.	A small amount of blood may form from the needlestick.
11. Remove gloves and place bed in the lowest position. Make sure that the patient is comfortable before you leave the room.	Placing the bed in the lowest position helps to prevent the patient from falling when trying to get out of bed.
12. Perform hand hygiene.	Hand hygiene deters the spread of microorganisms.
13. Document the date and time of deaccessing, the appearance of the site, ability to flush, and medication used to flush.	This provides accurate documentation and ensures continuity of care.

11/13/06   1020   Implanted port flushed without resistance using 10 mL of saline and 5 mL of heparin. Positive pressure maintained. No hematoma noted. Site without redness, swelling, drainage, or heat.—S. Barnes, RN

Action 13: Documentation.

continues

SKILL 15-9 Deaccessing an Implanted Port (continued)

EVALUATION	The expected outcome is met when the port flushes easily, the needle is removed, and the site is clean, dry, and without evidence of redness, irritation, or warmth.

Unexpected Situations and Associated Interventions	• *Port does not flush:* Check clamp to make sure tubing is open. Gently push down on needle and again try to flush. Ask patient to perform a Valsalva maneuver. Have patient change position or place the affected arm over the head, and raise or lower the head of the bed. If the port still does not flush, notify physician. • *Site does not stop bleeding:* Continue to hold pressure. If the patient is neutropenic due to medications, pressure may need to be applied for a slightly longer duration.
Special Considerations	• Groshong devices do not require heparin. • Some institutions call for a power flush (rapidly pushing the flush in small amounts).

SKILL 15-10 Drawing Blood from a Central Venous Access Device (CVAD)

In patients who have undergone repeated venipunctures or those who have chronic conditions or acute illness, it may be difficult to obtain blood samples from peripheral veins, and CVADs may be used instead. The skill presented here is a generic one. Policies for drawing blood samples vary between institutions, so check the procedures for your agency.

Equipment	• Clean gloves • Mask • Eye protection • 20-mL syringe with needleless cannula • 10-mL syringes with needleless cannula • Needleless injection cap • Alcohol wipes • Vial of normal saline • Heparin solution for flushing (if ordered) • Vacutainer sleeve with needleless cannula • Appropriate tubes and specimen labels • Additional 5-mL tube for discard
ASSESSMENT	Assess insertion site of catheter, noting any drainage, swelling, redness, or pain. Check all lumens to determine what fluids are infusing and which port should be used.
NURSING DIAGNOSIS	Determine the related factors for the nursing diagnosis based on the patient's current status. Appropriate nursing diagnoses may include Risk for Infection and Risk for Injury. Many other nursing diagnoses also may require the use of this skill.
OUTCOME IDENTIFICATION AND PLANNING	The expected outcome to achieve when obtaining a blood specimen from a CVAD is that a specimen will be collected without injury to the patient. In addition, the CVAD will remain patent.

continues

IMPLEMENTATION

ACTION	RATIONALE
1. Gather equipment and verify physician's order (many times this will be a standing protocol).	Having equipment available saves time and facilitates the task. Checking the order ensures that the procedure has been ordered by the physician.
2. Explain procedure to patient.	Explanation allays anxiety.
3. Perform hand hygiene.	Hand hygiene deters the spread of microorganisms. Unclean hands and improper technique are potential sources for infecting a CVAD.
4. Raise bed to comfortable working height.	Raising the bed helps to reduce strain on the nurse's back.
5. Don gloves, mask, and protective eyewear.	Gloves and protective eyewear prevent the transmission of HIV and other blood-borne diseases. Masks prevent the transmission of bacteria.
6. **If IV fluids are infusing through the CVAD, stop the flow of fluids. Depending on facility policy, it could be for up to 1 minute for standard IV fluids or up to 5 minutes for total parenteral nutrition, heparin, or any other solutions that may alter lab results.**	The well of the port must be empty of the medication before drawing blood, or the test results may be inaccurate.
7. Position patient for easy access to the CVAD, draping if necessary to expose only the CVAD site.	Draping the patient provides for modesty.
8. **If more than one lumen is present, draw blood samples from the proximal lumen if possible.**	Using the same port for each blood draw maintains consistency. This also decreases contamination risks of other ports.

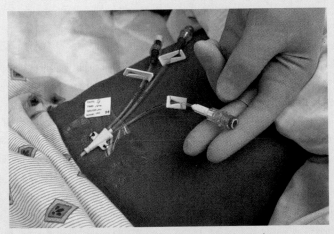

Action 8: Locate the proximal lumen on a multilumen catheter.

9. Cleanse the injection cap with alcohol and allow to air dry.	The alcohol kills *Staphylococcus aureus* and *S. epidermidis*, the most common causes of central line infections.
10. If blood is not being drawn with needless Vacutainer, skip to Action 17. Place the Vacutainer adapter with the needleless cannula into the injection cap.	By attaching the Vacutainer directly to the central line, the chance of a needlestick is decreased.
11. Insert the discard tube into the Vacutainer and snap it into place. Fill the tube; 5 mL is the minimum for discard. Remove the discard tube from the sleeve and quickly insert and fill the desired collecting tubes.	This prevents any IV fluid from skewing results.

continues

SKILL 15-10   Drawing Blood from a Central Venous Access Device (CVAD) (continued)

ACTION	RATIONALE
12. When the last tube of blood is obtained, remove the tube from the sleeve. Remove the Vacutainer cannula from the injection cap.	The blood has been obtained and now the lumen is ready to be flushed.
13. **Flush the lumen.** If the lumen is not going to be used at present, flush with the appropriate saline, then heparin flush (if heparin is agency policy). If IV fluids are to be resumed, flush the lumen with 10 mL normal saline and resume IV fluids. Dispose of equipment appropriately.	Flushing the lumen ensures that it remains patent. Some agencies routinely flush with heparin.
14. Remove gloves and **place bed in lowest position.** Make sure the patient is comfortable before you leave the room.	Lowering the bed helps to decrease the risk for a patient fall.
15. Label specimen tubes according to facility policy.	Labeling ensures that the correct results are given to the right patient.
16. Document the procedure according to agency policy and send the specimen to the lab.	This provides accurate documentation and ensures continuity of care.
17. If a Vacutainer is not used, clamp the lumen and insert a 10-mL syringe with a needleless cannula into the injection cap of the lumen. Unclamp the lumen and withdraw 5 mL of blood for discard. Clamp the lumen and remove the syringe and discard.	Drawing off sufficient waste prevents the lab testing from being skewed by the IV fluid or flush left in the tubing.
18. Insert a 10- or 20-mL syringe with a needleless cannula into the injection cap, unclamp the lumen, and withdraw the blood needed for the studies. The total amount will depend on the amount needed for the ordered tests.	This provides the blood needed for the testing.
19. Clamp the lumen and remove the syringe. Connect a blunt-ended needle to the syringe. Place blood in the appropriate tubes.	Blunt-ended needles help to prevent needlestick injuries. Place blood in purple and blue tubes first, since these tests cannot have any blood clots in them.
20. **Clean the port and then flush the lumen with the appropriate saline, then heparin flush, according to facility policy.**	Flushing ensures the patency of the lumen.
21. Dispose of equipment appropriately. Remove gloves. Place bed in lowest position.	Lowering the bed helps to decrease the risk of a patient fall.
22. Label specimen tubes according to facility policy.	Labeling ensures that the correct results are given to the right patient.
23. Document according to agency policy and send the specimen to the lab.	This provides accurate documentation and ensures continuity of care.

11/1/06   0910   Complete blood count and
potassium level drawn via proximal lumen.
Lumen flushes easily. Physician notified of lab
results. No orders received.—S. Barnes, RN

Action 23: Documentation.

continues

<table>
<tr><td>

**SKILL
15-10**

</td><td>

Drawing Blood from a Central Venous Access Device (CVAD) (continued)

</td></tr>
</table>

EVALUATION

The expected outcome is met when the blood specimens are obtained without incident. The patient remains free of injury and the catheter remains patent.

Unexpected Situations and Associated Interventions

- *Lumen flushes easily but does not draw blood:* Use alternate lumen for blood draw. Notify physician. An antithrombolytic may be placed in lumen to prevent any fibrin or clot formation from blocking lumen.
- *Lab results come back unexpectedly skewed:* Some of the IV fluids may have been sent with the sample. Notify physician and redraw sample.
- *After you attach one of the collection tubes to the Vacutainer connected to a CVAD, the blood flow into the tube becomes sluggish or stops:* Try a new collection tube. Some of the tubes are defective and have inadequate negative pressure. If after attaching a new collection tube the flow does not improve, try clamping the tubing and removing the tube and Vacutainer. Then flush the lumen with 5 mL saline solution, redraw your waste, and attempt to finish collecting the required blood samples. Ask the patient to change position, cough, and put his or her hands over the head. If still unsuccessful, clamp the tubing, remove the Vacutainer and collection tube, flush the lumen according to policy, and clamp the tubing. Notify the physician.

Special Considerations

- Groshong catheters do not require flushing with heparin because of their unique construction.
- Follow this procedure for drawing blood from a heplock, except you might need to place a tourniquet 4–6 inches above the IV site to facilitate blood removal.

■ Developing Critical Thinking Skills

1. Simon Lawrence's mother is asking about the risks associated with IV placement. What would you tell her about the risks associated with IV placement and rehydration?
2. During the first 7 minutes of Melissa Cohen's transfusion of packed red blood cells, she reports a headache and low back pain. When you assess her, you find that she has a temperature of 38.5°C and she is shivering. What actions would be most appropriate at this time?
3. Mr. Tracy asks about care of his new implanted port. What are some topics you should discuss with him before he is discharged?

Bibliography

Adrogue, H., & Madias, N. (2000). Primary care: Hyponatremia. *New England Journal of Medicine, 342*(21), 1581–1589.

Bennett, J. (2000). Dehydration: Hazards and benefits. *Geriatric Nursing, 21*(2), 84–87.

Castialione, V. (2000). Hyperkalemia. *American Journal of Nursing, 100*(1), 55–56.

CDC website: http://www.cdc.gov/ncidod/dvbid/westnile/qa/transfusion.htm

Centers for Disease Control and Prevention (2002). Guidelines for the prevention of intravascular catheter-related infections. *Morbidity and Mortality Weekly Report, 51,*(RR10), 1–32.

Chang, L., Tsai, J., Huang, S., & Shih, C. (2003). Evaluation of infectious complications of the implantable venous access system in a general oncologic population. *American Journal of Infection Control, 31*(1), 34–39.

Dobson, P. (2001). A model for home infusion therapy initiation and maintenance. *Journal of Infusion Nursing, 24*(6), 385–394.

Ellenberger, A. (2002). How to change a PICC dressing. *Nursing, 32*(2), 50–52.

Fabian, B. (2000). Intravenous complication: Infiltration. *Journal of IV Nursing, 23*(4), 229–231.

Fitzpatrick, L. (2002). When to administer modified blood products. *Nursing, 32*(5), 36–42.

LaRue, G., & Farnsworth, P. (2000). Silicone catheter fracture secondary to stress events and a dressing technique to reduce those events. *Journal of IV Nursing, 23*(2), 89–98.

Maag, M. (2001). An online ABG learning activity. *CIN Plus, 4*(1), 1, 4–5.

Macklin, D. (2000). Removing PICC. *American Journal of Nursing, 100*(1), 52–54.

McConnell, E. (2000). Do's & don'ts: Infusing packed RBCs. *Nursing, 30*(2), 17.

McConnell, E. (2001). Do's & don'ts: Administering total parenteral nutrition. *Nursing, 31*(11), 17.

Metheny, N. (2000). *Fluid and electrolyte balance: Nursing considerations* (4th ed.). Philadelphia: Lippincott Williams & Wilkins.

Millam, D., & Hadaway, L. (2000). On the road to successful IV starts. *Nursing, 30*(4), 34–38.

Millam, D., & Hadaway, L. (2000). From container to cannula: Trends in IV therapy. *Nursing, 30*(4), 39–48.

Miller, R. (2002). Blood component therapy. *Urologic Nursing, 22*(5), 331–339.

Moreau, N. (2002). IV rounds: How to remove a PICC with ease. *Nursing, 32*(5), 30.

Newell-Stokes, V., Broughton, S., Guiliano, K., & Stetler, C. (2001). Developing an evidence-based procedure: Maintenance of central venous catheters. *Clinical Nurse Specialist, 15*(5), 199–204.

North American Nursing Diagnosis Association. (2003). *NANDA nursing diagnoses: Definitions and classification, 2003–2004.* Philadelphia: Author.

O'Grady, N., Alexander, M., Dellinger, E., et al. (2002). Guidelines for the prevention of intravascular catheter-related infections. *American Journal of Infection Control, 30*(8), 476–489.

Orr, M. (2002). The peripherally inserted central catheter: What are the current indications for its use? *Nutrition in Clinical Practice, 17*(2), 99–104.

Satarawala, R. (2000). Confronting the legal perils of IV therapy. *Nursing, 30*(8), 44–48.

Skokal, W. (2000). IV push at home? *RN, 63*(10), 26–30.

Smeltzer, S., & Bare, B. (2004). *Brunner and Suddarth's textbook of medical–surgical nursing* (10th ed.). Philadelphia: Lippincott Williams & Wilkins.

White, S. (2001). Peripheral intravenous therapy-related phlebitis rates in an adult population. *Journal of IV Nursing, 24*(1), 19–24.

Young, J. (2000). Transfusion reaction. *Nursing, 30*(12), 33.

Zerwekh, J. (2003). End-of-life hydration: benefit or burden? *Nursing, 33*(2).

Cardiovascular Care

This chapter will help you develop some of the skills related to cardiovascular care necessary to care for the following patients:

Coby Pruder, age 40, is to undergo an electrocardiogram as part of his physical examination. Although he considers himself healthy, he is nervous.

Harry Stebbings, age 67, is admitted to the emergency department for chest pain and cardiac monitoring.

Ann Kribell, age 54, is admitted to the intensive care unit for heart failure and cardiac monitoring. She needs to have an arterial blood gas drawn.

Learning Outcomes

After studying this chapter, the reader should be able to:

1. Obtain a 12-lead ECG
2. Apply a cardiac monitor
3. Obtain an arterial blood sample from an arterial line
4. Remove arterial and femoral lines
5. Perform cardiopulmonary resuscitation (CPR)
6. Perform emergency defibrillation (asynchronous)
7. Use an external pacemaker

Key Terms

Allen's test: an assessment determining the adequacy of the ulnar artery prior to accessing the radial artery for an arterial blood gas

arterial blood gas (ABG): a laboratory test that evaluates the oxygen, carbon dioxide, bicarbonate, and pH of an arterial blood sample, determining metabolic or respiratory alkalosis or acidosis

cardiac arrest: sudden cessation of functional circulation of the heart (pulse), such as asystole or defibrillation, typically caused by the occlusion of one or more of the coronary arteries. Electrical activity may still be occurring and seen on the cardiac monitor, as in electromechanical disassociation.

cardiac monitoring: visualization and monitoring of the cardiac electrical activity stimulating the heartbeat

cardiopulmonary resuscitation (CPR): revival after apparent death by manually pumping the heart through the sternum and forcing oxygen into the lungs using mouth-to-mouth or rescue breathing

cardioversion: conversion of a pathologic cardiac rhythm to normal sinus rhythm through low doses of electricity, using a device that applies synchronized countershocks to the heart

defibrillation: stopping fibrillation of the heart by using an electrical device that applies countershocks to the heart through electrodes on the chest wall. This countershock is given in an attempt to allow the heart's normal pacemaker to take over.

electrocardiogram (ECG/EKG): graphing of the electrical activity of the heart

The heart is an organ at the "heart" of the circulatory system. It provides the propulsive force (heartbeat) for circulating the blood through the vascular system. This four-chamber muscle pumps 2 to 3 ounces of blood into the arteries with each heartbeat. The pressure exerted is equal to lifting 80 pounds at 1 foot per minute. The heart averages 72 beats a minute or 38 million beats a year.

Assessment of heart function commonly involves noninvasive techniques such as auscultation, palpation, and sometimes percussion. Pulse rate, strength, and rhythm; blood pressure; skin color; and level of consciousness are additional basic and important indicators of the heart's effectiveness. Noninvasive heart monitoring involves electrocardiography and cardiac monitoring. Arterial blood gases (ABGs) are used to measure the oxygen level and pH of the blood, providing information about a patient's acid–base balance. Should the heart stop pumping, it can be manually pumped via cardiopulmonary resuscitation (CPR) until electrical defibrillation and additional medical support arrives.

Invasive techniques such as pulmonary artery monitoring, Swan-Ganz catheterization, cardiac output determination, and cardiac support via an external pacemaker or intraaortic balloon pump (IABP) typically are used by trained critical care personnel to provide additional monitoring and support. These techniques are beyond the scope of this text.

This chapter will cover selected noninvasive skills to assist the nurse in providing cardiovascular care. Please look over the summary boxes and figures at the beginning of this chapter for a quick review of critical knowledge to assist you in understanding the skills related to cardiovascular care.

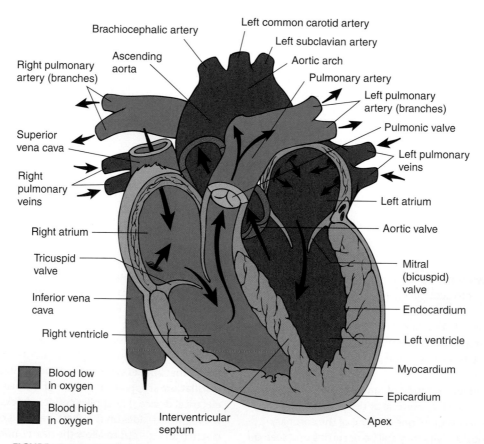

FIGURE 16-1 Cardiac anatomy.

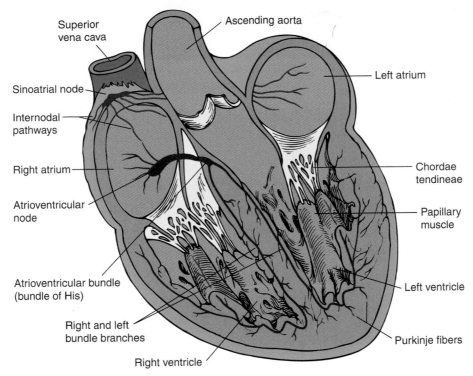

FIGURE 16-2 Cardiac conduction system.

Superior vena cava

Sinoatrial node

Internodal pathways

Right atrium

Atrioventricular node

Atrioventricular bundle (bundle of His)

Right and left bundle branches

Right ventricle

Ascending aorta

Left atrium

Chordae tendineae

Papillary muscle

Left ventricle

Purkinje fibers

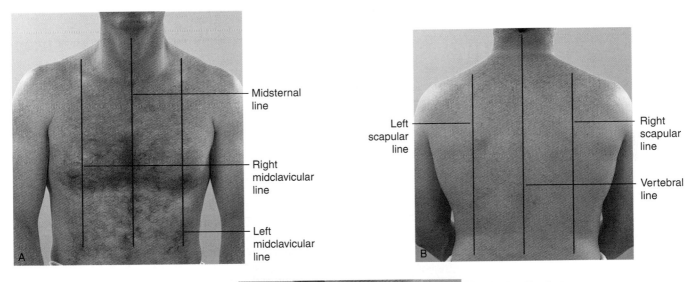

Midsternal line

Right midclavicular line

Left midclavicular line

Left scapular line

Right scapular line

Vertebral line

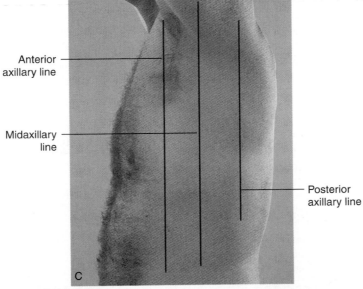

Anterior axillary line

Midaxillary line

Posterior axillary line

FIGURE 16-3 Cardiac landmarks: Reference lines. (**A**) Anterior chest. (**B**) Posterior chest. (**C**) Lateral chest.

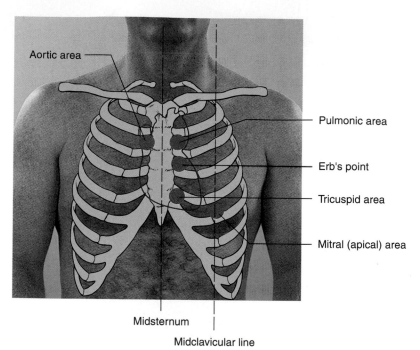

Aortic area

Pulmonic area

Erb's point

Tricuspid area

Mitral (apical) area

Midsternum

Midclavicular line

FIGURE 16-4 Cardiac landmarks: Auscultation areas.

BOX 16-1 **ECG Complex**

The ECG complex consists of five waveforms labeled with the letters P, Q, R, S, and T. In addition, sometimes a U wave appears.

- **P wave:** Represents atrial depolarization (conduction of the electrical impulse through the atria); the first component of ECG waveform
- **PR interval:** Tracks the atrial impulse from the atria through the AV node, bundle of His, and right and left bundle branches; measures from the beginning of the P wave to the beginning of the QRS complex.
- **QRS complex:** Follows the P wave and represents depolarization of the ventricles (the time it takes for the impulse to travel through the bundle branches to the Purkinje fibers) or impulse conduction. The Q wave appears as the first negative deflection in the QRS complex, the R wave as

the first positive deflection. The S wave appears as the second negative deflection or the first negative deflection after the R wave.

- **ST segment:** Represents the end of ventricular conduction or depolarization and the beginning of ventricular recovery or repolarization; the J point marks the end of the QRS complex and the beginning of the ST segment.
- **T wave:** Represents ventricular recovery or repolarization
- **QT interval:** Measures ventricular depolarization and repolarization; varies with the heart rate (i.e., the faster the heart rate, the shorter the QT interval); extends from the beginning of the QRS complex to the end of the T wave.
- **U wave:** Represents the recovery period of the Purkinje fibers or ventricular conduction fibers; not present on every rhythm strip.

BOX 16-2 **Rhythm Strip Interpretation**

1. Determine the rhythm.
2. Determine the rate.
3. Evaluate the P wave.
4. Determine the duration of the PR interval.
5. Determine the duration of the QRS complex.
6. Evaluate the T waves.
7. Determine the duration of the QT interval.
8. Evaluate any other components.

BOX 16-3 Electrical Therapy Devices

In addition to defibrillation, electrical therapy may be delivered via the following devices:

- *Implantable cardioverter-defibrillator* (ICD) is a sophisticated device that automatically discharges an electric current when it senses ventricular tachyarrhythmias. Patients with a history of ventricular fibrillation may be candidates for this type of device.
- *Automated external defibrillator* (AED) is a device equipped with a microcomputer that senses and analyzes a patient's heart rhythm at the push of a button. Then it audibly or visually prompts the onlooker or rescuer to deliver a shock. Commonly used to meet the need for early defibrillation, currently considered the most effective treatment for ventricular fibrillation. Instruction in using the AED is required as part of Basic Life Support (BLS) and Advanced Cardiac Life Support (ACLS) training. Some facilities now require an AED in every non-critical care unit. Law enforcement and firefighting personnel are trained to perform early defibril-

lation. AEDs are becoming more common in such public places as shopping malls, sports stadiums, and airplanes.

- *Synchronized cardioversion* is the treatment of choice for arrhythmias that do not respond to vagal maneuvers or drug therapy, such as atrial tachycardia, atrial flutter, atrial fibrillation, and symptomatic ventricular tachycardia. Cardioversion is performed similarly to defibrillation but is synchronized with the heart rhythm and uses fewer joules. Cardioversion works by delivering an electric charge to the myocardium at the peak of the R wave. This causes immediate depolarization, interrupting reentry circuits and allowing the sinoatrial node to resume control. Synchronizing the electric charge with the R wave ensures the current will not be delivered on the vulnerable T wave and thus disrupt repolarization. It is usually performed in a critical care area, in the presence of a physician, an anesthesiologist, and emergency equipment. The patient is premedicated with pain medicine.

SKILL 16-1

Obtaining an ECG

One of the most valuable and frequently used diagnostic tools, electrocardiography (ECG) measures the heart's electrical activity; the data are graphed as waveforms. Impulses moving through the heart's conduction system create electric currents that can be monitored on the body's surface. Electrodes attached to the skin can detect these electric currents and transmit them to an instrument that produces a record (the electrocardiogram) of cardiac activity.

ECG can be used to identify myocardial ischemia and infarction, rhythm and conduction disturbances, chamber enlargement, electrolyte imbalances, and drug toxicity.

The standard 12-lead ECG uses a series of electrodes placed on the extremities and the chest wall to assess the heart from 12 different views. The 12 leads consist of three standard bipolar limb leads (designated I, II, III), three unipolar augmented leads (aV_R, aV_L, aV_F), and six unipolar precordial leads (V_1 to V_6). The limb leads and augmented leads show the heart from the frontal plane. The precordial leads show the heart from the horizontal plane.

The ECG device measures and averages the differences between the electrical potential of the electrode sites for each lead and graphs them over time, creating the standard ECG complex, called PQRST. Variations of standard ECGs include exercise ECG (stress ECG) and ambulatory ECG (Holter monitoring).

Today, ECG is typically accomplished using a multichannel method. All electrodes are attached to the patient at once and the machine prints a simultaneous view of all leads.

Equipment
- ECG machine
- Recording paper
- Disposable pregelled electrodes
- 4×4 gauze pads

continues

Obtaining an ECG (continued)

ASSESSMENT

Review the patient's medical record and plan of care for information about the patient's need for ECG. Assess the patient's cardiac status, including heart rate, blood pressure, and auscultation of heart sounds. If the patient is already connected to a cardiac monitor, remove the electrodes to accommodate the precordial leads and minimize electrical interference on the ECG tracing. Keep the patient away from objects that might cause electrical interference, such as equipment, fixtures, and power cords. Inspect the patient's chest for areas of irritation, breakdown, or excessive hair that might interfere with electrode placement.

NURSING DIAGNOSIS

Determine the related factors for the nursing diagnoses based on the patient's current status. Appropriate nursing diagnoses may include:

- Decreased Cardiac Output
- Excess Fluid Volume
- Acute Pain
- Deficient Knowledge
- Ineffective Health Maintenance
- Activity Intolerance
- Anxiety

Many other nursing diagnoses may require the use of this skill.

OUTCOME IDENTIFICATION AND PLANNING

The expected outcome to achieve is that a cardiac electrical tracing is obtained without any complications. Other appropriate outcomes may include: the patient displays an increased understanding about the ECG and reduced anxiety.

IMPLEMENTATION

ACTION	RATIONALE
1. Place the ECG machine close to the patient's bed, and plug the power cord into the wall outlet.	Having equipment available saves time and facilitates accomplishment of task.
2. Perform hand hygiene. Check the patient's identification.	Hand hygiene deters the spread of microorganisms. Verification of the patient's identity validates that the correct procedure is being done on the correct patient.
3. As you set up the machine to record a 12-lead ECG, explain the procedure to the patient. Tell the patient that the test records the heart's electrical activity and it may be repeated at certain intervals. Emphasize that no electrical current will enter his or her body. Tell the patient the test typically takes about 5 minutes.	Explanation helps allay anxiety and facilitates compliance.
4. Have the patient lie supine in the center of the bed with the arms at the sides. Raise the head of the bed if necessary to promote comfort. Expose the patient's arms and legs, and drape appropriately. Encourage the patient to relax the arms and legs. If the bed is too narrow, place the patient's hands under the buttocks to prevent muscle tension. Also use this technique if the patient is shivering or trembling. Make sure the feet do not touch the bed's footboard.	This helps increase patient comfort and will produce a better tracing. Having the arms and legs relaxed minimizes muscle trembling, which can cause electrical interference.
5. Select flat, fleshy areas on which to place the electrodes. Avoid muscular and bony areas. If the patient has an amputated limb, choose a site on the stump.	Tissue conducts the current more effectively than bone, producing a better tracing.
6. If an area is excessively hairy, clip the hair. Clean excess oil or other substances from the skin.	Oils and excess hair interfere with electrode contact.

continues

Obtaining an ECG (continued)

ACTION

RATIONALE

7. Apply the electrode paste or gel or the disposable electrodes to the patient's wrists and to the medial aspects of the ankles. If using paste or gel, rub it into the skin. If using disposable electrodes, peel off the contact paper and apply the electrodes directly to the prepared site, as recommended by the manufacturer. **Position disposable electrodes on the legs with the lead connection pointing superiorly.**

Paste or gel facilitates contact and enhances tracing. Having the lead connection pointing superiorly guarantees the best connection to the lead wire.

8. If using paste or gel, secure electrodes promptly after you apply the conductive medium. **Never use alcohol or acetone pads in place of the electrode paste or gel.**

This prevents drying of the medium, which could impair ECG quality. Acetone and alcohol impair electrode contact with the skin and diminish the transmission of electrical impulses.

9. Connect the limb lead wires to the electrodes. The tip of each lead wire is lettered and color-coded for easy identification. The white or RA leadwire goes to the right arm; the green or RL lead wire to the right leg; the red or LL lead wire to the left leg; the black or LA lead wire to the left arm; and the brown or V_1 to V_6 lead wires to the chest. Make sure the metal parts of the electrodes are clean and bright.

Dirty or corroded electrodes prevent a good electrical connection.

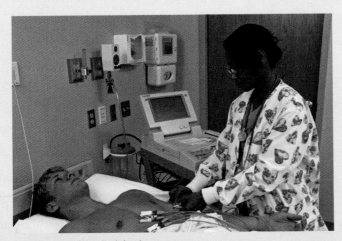

Action 9: Applying limb lead.

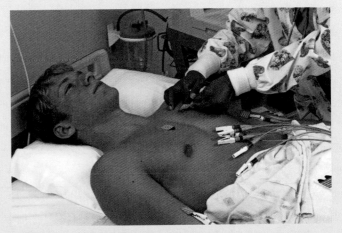

Action 10: Applying chest lead.

10. Expose the patient's chest. Put a small amount of electrode gel or paste on a disposable electrode at each electrode position. Position chest electrodes as follows:
    - V_1: Fourth intercostal space at right sternal border
    - V_2: Fourth intercostal space at left sternal border
    - V_3: Halfway between V_2 and V_4
    - V_4: Fifth intercostal space at midclavicular line
    - V_5: Fifth intercostal space at anterior axillary line (halfway between V_4 and V_6)
    - V_6: Fifth intercostal space at midaxillary line, level with V_4

Proper lead placement is necessary for accurate test results.

continues

SKILL
16-1   **Obtaining an ECG** (continued)

ACTION

RATIONALE

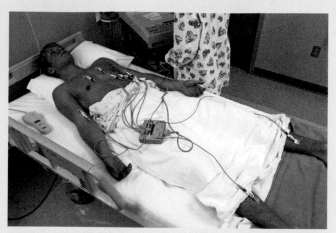

Action 10: Completed application of 12-lead ECG.

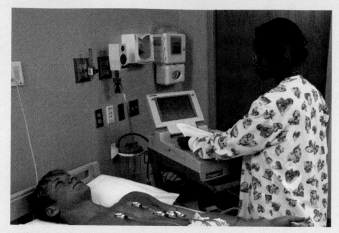

Action 14: Observing tracing quality.

11. Make sure the paper speed selector is set to the standard 25 m/second and that the machine is set to full voltage.

12. If necessary, enter the appropriate patient identification data.

13. Ask the patient to relax and breathe normally. **Tell him or her to lie still and not to talk while you record the ECG.**

14. Press the AUTO button. Observe the tracing quality. The machine will record all 12 leads automatically, recording three consecutive leads simultaneously. Some machines have a display screen so you can preview waveforms before the machine records them on paper. Adjust waveform if necessary. If any part of the waveform extends beyond the paper when you record the ECG, adjust the normal standardization to half-standardization and repeat. Note this adjustment on the ECG strip, because this will need to be considered in interpreting the results.

15. When the machine finishes recording the 12-lead ECG, remove the electrodes and clean the patient's skin.

16. After disconnecting the lead wires from the electrodes, dispose of or clean the electrodes, as indicated.

17. Label the ECG recording with the patient's name, room number, and facility identification number, if this was not done by the machine. Also record the date and time as well as any appropriate clinical information on the ECG. Document the test's date and time as well as significant responses by the patient in the medical record.

The machine will record a normal standardization mark—a square that is the height of two large squares or 10 small squares on the recording paper.

This allows for proper identification of the ECG strip.

Lying still and not talking produces a better tracing.

Observation of tracing quality allows for adjustments to be made if necessary. Notation of adjustments ensures accurate interpretation of results.

Removal and cleaning promote patient comfort.

Proper disposal deters the spread of microorganisms. Proper cleaning after use ensures that the machine will be ready for next use.

Documentation provides communication and promotes continuity of care.

continues

EVALUATION

The expected outcome is achieved when a quality ECG reading is obtained without any undue patient anxiety or complications or injury. In addition, the patient states the reason for the ECG.

Unexpected Situations and Associated Interventions

- *An artifact appears on the tracing:* An artifact may be due to loose electrodes or patient movement. Reassess electrode connections and ask the patient to lie extremely still.
- *Minimal complexes are seen:* This may be due to extreme bradycardia. Run longer strips.
- *A wandering baseline is noted, and respirations distort the recording:* Ask the patient to hold his or her breath briefly to reduce baseline wander in the tracing.

Special Considerations

- For female patients, place the electrodes below the breast tissue. In a large-breasted woman, you may need to displace the breast tissue laterally.
- Small areas of hair on the patient's chest or extremities may be trimmed, but this usually is not necessary.
- If the patient's skin is exceptionally oily, scaly, or diaphoretic, rub the electrode site with a dry 4 × 4 gauze or alcohol pad before applying the electrode to help reduce interference in the tracing.
- If the patient has a pacemaker, you can perform an ECG with or without a magnet, according to the physician's orders. Note the presence of a pacemaker and the use of the magnet on the strip.

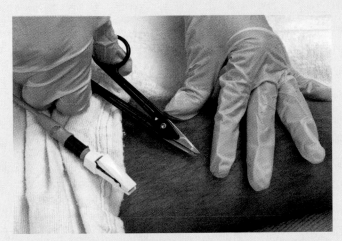

Special considerations: Trimming leg hair.

SKILL 16-2   Applying a Cardiac Monitor

Because it allows continuous observation of the heart's electrical activity, cardiac monitoring is used for patients with conduction disturbances and for those at risk for life-threatening arrhythmias. Like other forms of electrocardiography (ECG), cardiac monitoring uses electrodes placed on the patient's chest to transmit electrical signals that are converted into a tracing of cardiac rhythm on an oscilloscope.

Two types of monitoring may be performed: hardwire or telemetry. In hardwire monitoring, the patient is connected to a monitor at the bedside. The rhythm display appears at the bedside but may also be transmitted to a console at a remote location. Telemetry uses a small transmitter connected to the ambulatory patient to send electrical signals to another location, where they are displayed on a monitor screen. Battery-powered and portable, telemetry frees the patient from cumbersome wires and cables and lets him or her be comfortably mobile and safely isolated from the electrical leakage and accidental shock occasionally associated with hardwire monitoring. Telemetry is especially useful for monitoring arrhythmias that occur during sleep, rest, exercise, or stressful situations.

Regardless of the type, cardiac monitors can display the patient's heart rate and rhythm, produce a printed record of cardiac rhythm, and sound an alarm if the heart rate exceeds or falls below specified limits. Monitors also recognize and count abnormal heartbeats as well as changes. For example, ST segment monitoring helps detect myocardial ischemia, electrolyte imbalance, coronary artery spasm, and hypoxic events. The ST-segment represents early ventricular repolarization, and any changes in this waveform component reflect alterations in myocardial oxygenation. Any monitoring lead that views an ischemic heart region will reveal ST-segment changes. The monitor's software establishes a template of the patient's normal QRST pattern from the selected leads; then the monitor displays ST-segment changes. Some monitors display such changes continuously, while other monitors do this only on command.

Equipment
- Lead wires
- Pregelled electrodes (number varies from three to five)
- Alcohol pads
- Gauze pads
- Patient cable for cardiac monitor
- Transmitter, transmitter pouch, and telemetry battery pack for telemetry

ASSESSMENT

Review the patient's medical record and plan of care for information about the patient's need for cardiac monitoring. Assess the patient's cardiac status, including heart rate, blood pressure, and auscultation of heart sounds. Inspect the patient's chest for areas of irritation, breakdown, or excessive hair that might interfere with electrode placement. Electrode sites must be dry, with minimal hair. The patient may be sitting or supine, in a bed or chair.

NURSING DIAGNOSIS

Determine the related factors for the nursing diagnoses based on the patient's current status. Appropriate nursing diagnoses may include:
- Decreased Cardiac Output
- Acute Pain
- Deficient Knowledge
- Fear
- Anxiety (related to unknown procedure)

Many other nursing diagnoses may require the use of this skill.

continues

Applying a Cardiac Monitor (continued)

OUTCOME IDENTIFICATION AND PLANNING

The expected outcome to achieve when performing cardiac monitoring is that a clear waveform, free from artifact, is displayed on the cardiac monitor. Other appropriate outcomes may include: the patient displays understanding of the reason for monitoring, and the patient shows reduced anxiety and fear.

IMPLEMENTATION

ACTION	RATIONALE

1. Gather all equipment and bring it to the bedside.
 	
   a. Plug the cardiac monitor into an electrical outlet and turn it on to warm up the unit while preparing the equipment and the patient. For telemetry monitoring, insert a new battery into the transmitter. Match the poles on the battery with the polar markings on the transmitter case. Press the button at the top of the unit, test the battery's charge, and test the unit to ensure that the battery is operational.
 	
   b. Insert the cable into the appropriate socket in the monitor.
 	
   c. Connect the lead wires to the cable. In some systems, the lead wires are permanently secured to the cable. Each lead wire should indicate the location for attachment to the patient: right arm (RA), left arm (LA), right leg (RL), left leg (LL), and ground (C or V). These markings should appear on the lead wire (if it is permanently connected) or at the connection of the lead wires and cable to the patient. For telemetry, if the lead wires are not permanently affixed to the telemetry unit, attach them securely. If they must be attached individually, connect each one to the correct outlet.
 	
   d. Then connect an electrode to each of the lead wires, carefully checking that each lead wire is in its correct outlet.
	Having equipment available saves time and facilitates accomplishment of task. Proper setup ensures proper functioning

2. Explain the procedure to the patient and provide privacy.	This helps allay anxiety and promotes compliance.
3. Perform hand hygiene.	Hand hygiene deters the spread of microorganisms.
4. Expose the chest and determine electrode positions, based on which system and leads are being used. If necessary, clip the hair from an area about 10 cm in diameter around each electrode site. Clean the area with an alcohol pad and dry it completely to remove skin secretions that may interfere with electrode function.	These actions allow for better adhesion of the electrode and thus better conduction.
5. Remove the backing from the pregelled electrode. Check the gel for moistness. If the gel is dry, discard it and replace it with a fresh electrode. **Apply the electrode to the site and press firmly to ensure a tight seal.** Repeat with the remaining electrodes to complete the three-lead or five-lead system.	Gel acts as a conduit and must be moist and secured tightly.

continues

ACTION

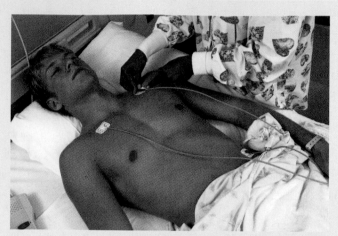

Action 5: Applying the electrodes for three-lead monitoring system.

RATIONALE

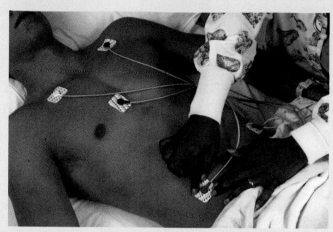

Action 5: Applying electrodes for five-lead monitoring system.

6. When all the electrodes are in place, check waveform for clarity, position, and size. **To verify that the monitor is detecting each beat, compare the digital heart rate display with a palpated or auscultated count of the patient's heart rate.** If necessary, use the gain control to adjust the size of the rhythm tracing, and use the position control to adjust the waveform position on the monitor.

This ensures accuracy of reading.

7. Set the upper and lower limits of the heart rate alarm, based on unit policy. Turn the alarm on.

Setting the alarm allows for audible notification if the heart rate is beyond limits.

8. For telemetry, place the transmitter in the pouch. Tie the pouch strings around the patient's neck and waist, making sure that the pouch fits snugly without causing discomfort. If no pouch is available, place the transmitter in the patient's bathrobe pocket.

Patient comfort lends to compliance.

9. To obtain a rhythm strip, press the RECORD key either at the bedside for monitoring or at the central station for telemetry. Label the strip with the patient's name and room number, date, time, and rhythm identification. Place the rhythm strip in the appropriate location in the patient's chart. Analyze strip as appropriate.

A rhythm strip provides a baseline.

10. Record the date and time that monitoring begins and the monitoring lead used in the medical record. Document a rhythm strip at least every 8 hours and with any changes in the patient's condition (or as stated by your facility's policy). Label the rhythm strip with the patient's name and room number, date, and time.

Documentation provides communication and promotes continuity of care.

EVALUATION   The expected outcome is achieved when the cardiac monitoring waveform displays the patient's cardiac rhythm, with a waveform that is detecting each beat and is appropriate for clarity, position, and size. In addition, the patient demonstrates no undue anxiety and remains free of complications or injury.

continues

SKILL
16-2   **Applying a Cardiac Monitor** (continued)

Unexpected Situations and Associated Interventions

- *False high-rate alarm sounds:* Assess for monitor that is interpreting large T waves as QRS complexes, thus doubling the rate, or skeletal muscle activity. Reposition electrodes to a lead where the QRS complexes are taller than the T waves, and place electrodes away from major muscle masses.
- *False low-rate alarm sounds:* Assess for a shift in the electrical axis due to patient movement, making QRS complexes too small to register; low amplitude of QRS; or poor contact between skin and electrode. Reapply electrodes. Set gain so that the height of complex is greater than 1 millivolt.
- *Low amplitude:* Assess for gain dial set too low; poor contact between skin and electrodes; dried gel; broken or loose lead wires; poor connection between patient and monitor; or malfunctioning monitor. Check connections on all lead wires and monitoring cable. Replace electrodes as necessary. Reapply electrodes, if required.
- *Wandering baseline:* Assess for poor position or contact between electrodes and skin, or thoracic movement with respirations. Reposition or replace electrodes.
- *Artifact (waveform interference):* Assess for patient movement, improperly applied electrodes, or static electricity. Attach all electrical equipment to a common ground. Check plugs to make sure prongs are not loose.
- *Skin excoriation under electrodes:* Assess for allergic reaction to electrode adhesive or electrodes being left on the skin too long. Remove electrodes and apply hypoallergenic electrodes and hypoallergenic tape or remove electrode, clean site, and reapply electrode at new site.

Special Considerations

- Make sure all electrical equipment and outlets are grounded to avoid electric shock and interference (artifacts). Also ensure that the patient is clean and dry to prevent electric shock.
- Avoid opening the electrode packages until just before using to prevent the gel from drying out.
- Avoid placing the electrodes on bony prominences, hairy locations, areas where defibrillator pads will be placed, or areas for chest compression.
- If the patient's skin is very oily, scaly, or diaphoretic, rub the electrode site with a dry 4 × 4 gauze pad before applying the electrode to help reduce interference in the tracing. Have the patient breathe normally during the procedure. If respirations distort the recording, ask the patient to hold his or her breath briefly to reduce baseline wander in the tracing.
- Assess skin integrity and reposition the electrodes every 24 hours or as necessary.
- If the patient is being monitored by telemetry, show him or her how the transmitter works. If applicable, identify the button that will produce a recording of the ECG at the central station. Instruct the patient to push the button whenever symptoms occur; this causes the central console to print a rhythm strip. Also, advise patient to notify nurse immediately. Tell the patient to remove the transmitter during showering or bathing, but stress that he or she should let you know the unit is being removed.

SKILL 16-3 Obtaining an Arterial Blood Sample From an Arterial Line

Obtaining an arterial blood sample requires percutaneous puncture of the brachial, radial, or femoral artery (see Chapter 14). However, a blood sample can also be obtained from an arterial line. When collected, the sample can be analyzed to determine arterial blood gas (ABG) values. The inserted arterial line may be an open or closed system.

Equipment

- ABG kit, or the following:
  - Syringe specific for drawing blood for ABG analysis
  - 20G 1¼″ needle
  - 22G 1″ needle
  - 1 mL ampule of aqueous heparin (1:1000)
- Gloves
- 5 mL syringe, 10 mL syringe
- Alcohol or povidone–iodine pad
- 2 × 2 gauze pads
- Rubber cap for syringe hub or rubber stopper for needle
- Ice-filled plastic bag or cup
- Label
- Laboratory request form

Many healthcare facilities use a commercial ABG kit that contains everything you need to perform this procedure, except an adhesive bandage and ice. If your facility does not use such a kit, obtain a sterile syringe specially made for drawing blood for ABG values, and use a clean emesis basin or Styrofoam cup filled win ice instead of the plastic bag to transport the sample to the laboratory.

ASSESSMENT

Review the patient's medical record and plan of care for information about the patient's need for an ABG. Assess the patient's cardiac status, including heart rate, blood pressure, and auscultation of heart sounds. Also assess the patient's respiratory status, including respiratory rate, excursion, lung sounds, and use of oxygen if ordered. Check the potency and functioning of the arterial line. Assess the patient's understanding about the need for specimen collection. Ask the patient if he or she has ever felt faint, sweaty, or nauseated when having blood drawn.

NURSING DIAGNOSIS

Determine the related factors for the nursing diagnoses based on the patient's current status. Appropriate nursing diagnoses may include:

- Impaired Gas Exchange
- Decreased Cardiac Output
- Ineffective Airway Clearance
- Acute Pain
- Risk for Injury
- Excess Fluid Volume
- Anxiety
- Fear

In addition, many other nursing diagnoses also may require the use of this skill.

OUTCOME IDENTIFICATION AND PLANNING

The expected outcome to achieve when obtaining an ABG is that a specimen is obtained with minimal discomfort and anxiety and without injury to the patient. In addition, the patient demonstrates understanding about the need for specimen collection.

continues

IMPLEMENTATION

ACTION	RATIONALE
1. Assemble equipment. Label the syringe clearly with the patient's name and room number, the physician's name, the date and time of collection, and the initials of the person performing the ABG. If it is not already done, heparinize the syringe and needle (see Skill 14-6).	Having equipment available saves time and facilitates accomplishment of task. Heparinizing the syringe and needle prevents the sample from clotting.
2. Check the patient's identification. Tell the patient you need to collect an arterial blood sample, and explain the procedure. Tell the patient the specimen will be obtained from the arterial line.	Checking the patient's identification validates the correct patient and procedure. Explanation helps allay anxiety and promotes cooperation.
3. Perform hand hygiene and put on gloves.	Hand hygiene and gloving deter the spread of microorganisms.

Obtaining an Arterial Blood Sample From an Open System

ACTION	RATIONALE
4. Assemble the equipment, taking care not to contaminate the dead-end cap, stopcock, and syringes. Turn off or temporarily silence the monitor alarms, depending on your facility's policy (some facilities require that alarms be left on).	The integrity of the system is being altered, which will cause the system to sound an alarm.
5. Locate the stopcock nearest the patient. Open a sterile 4 × 4 gauze pad. Remove the dead-end cap from the stopcock, and place it on the gauze pad.	This will allow access while not contaminating the cap.
6. Attach a syringe and obtain the discard sample into the syringe. Follow your facility's policy on how much discard blood to collect. In most cases, you will withdraw 5 to 10 mL through a 5- or 10-mL syringe.	This sample is discarded because it is diluted with flush solution.
7. Turn the stopcock off to the flush solution. Slowly retract the syringe to withdraw the discarded sample. Then turn the stopcock halfway back to the open position to close the system in all directions. **If you feel resistance, reposition the affected extremity and check the insertion site for obvious problems (such as catheter kinking).** After correcting the problem, resume blood withdrawal.	Turning the stopcock off maintains the integrity of the system.
8. Remove the discard syringe and dispose of the blood in the syringe, observing standard precautions.	Diluted blood still poses a risk for infection transmission.
9. Place the syringe for the laboratory sample in the stopcock, turn the stopcock off to the flush solution, and slowly withdraw the required amount of blood. For each additional sample required, repeat this procedure. If the physician has ordered coagulation tests, obtain blood for this sample from the final syringe.	Turning the stopcock off to the flush solution prevents dilution from the flush device.

continues

SKILL 16-3   Obtaining an Arterial Blood Sample From an Arterial Line (continued)

ACTION	RATIONALE
10. After obtaining blood for the final sample, turn the stopcock off to the syringe and remove the syringe. Activate the fast-flush release (pigtail). Then turn off the stopcock to the patient, and repeat the fast flush to clear the stopcock port.	The fast-flush release will clear the tubing and then the stopcock port.

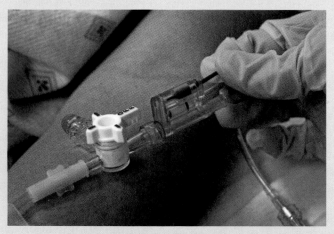

Action 10: Repeating fast flush to clear stopcock port.

11. Turn the stopcock off to the stopcock port, and replace the dead-end cap. Reactivate the monitor alarms. Attach needles to the filled syringes and transfer the blood samples to the appropriate containers, labeling them according to facility policy. Send all samples to the laboratory with appropriate documentation.	Reactivating the system ensures proper functioning.
12. Check the monitor for return of the arterial waveform and pressure reading.	This ensures proper functioning and integrity of the system.

Obtaining an Arterial Blood Sample From a Closed System

13. Assemble the equipment, maintaining aseptic technique. Locate the closed-system reservoir and blood sampling site. Deactivate or temporarily silence monitor alarms (some facilities require that alarms be left on).	The integrity of the system is being altered, causing the system to sound an alarm.
14. Clean the sampling site with an alcohol swab.	Cleaning the sampling site prevents contamination with microorganisms.
15. Holding the reservoir upright, grasp the flexures and slowly fill the reservoir with blood over a 3- to 5-second period. **If you feel resistance, reposition the affected extremity and check the catheter site for obvious problems (such as kinking).** Then resume blood withdrawal.	This blood serves as discard blood.

continues

ACTION	RATIONALE
16. Turn the one-way valve off to the reservoir by turning the handle perpendicular to the tubing. Using a syringe with attached cannula, insert the cannula into the sampling site. (Make sure the plunger is depressed to the bottom of the syringe barrel.) Slowly fill the syringe. Then grasp the cannula near the sampling site and remove the syringe and cannula as one unit. Repeat the procedure as needed to fill the required number of syringes. If the physician has ordered coagulation tests, obtain blood for those tests from the final syringe.	Turning the one-way valve off prevents dilution of the sample with flush solution.
17. After filling the syringes, turn the one-way valve to its original position, parallel to the tubing. Now smoothly and evenly push down on the plunger until the flexures lock in place in the fully closed position and all fluid has been reinfused. The fluid should be reinfused over a 3- to 5-second period. Then activate the fast-flush release.	Repositioning the stopcock clears blood from the tubing and reservoir.
18. Clean the sampling site with an alcohol swab. Reactivate the monitor alarms. Using the blood transfer unit, transfer blood samples to the appropriate Vacutainers, labeling them according to facility policy. Send all samples to the laboratory with appropriate documentation.	Reactivating the system ensures proper functioning. Collection is completed.
19. Follow Actions 11 and 12 for an open system.	These actions ensure proper functioning.
20. Remove gloves and perform hand hygiene.	Proper glove disposal and hand hygiene deter the spread of microorganisms.
21. Document the time when the sample was obtained, patient's temperature, arterial puncture site, amount of time pressure was applied to the site to control bleeding, and type and amount of oxygen therapy, if any, the patient was receiving.	Documentation provides communication and promotes continuity of care.

EVALUATION   The expected outcome is achieved when the specimen is collected without any undue patient anxiety or complications. In addition, the patient is able to state the reason for the arterial sample and remains free of injury.

Unexpected Situations and Associated Interventions

- *The specimen obtained is dark:* Dark blood means a vein may have been accessed, or the blood may be poorly oxygenated. Ensure that the line from which you are obtaining the specimen is indeed an arterial line. Also, check the patient's oxygen saturation level to evaluate for possible hypoxemia. Make sure that the artery was punctured before sending the specimen to the laboratory.
- *When retracting the syringe for the discarded sample, you feel resistance.* Reposition the affected extremity and check the insertion site for obvious problems (such as catheter kinking). Then attempt to obtain the sample to be discarded. If resistance is still felt, notify the physician.

continues

SKILL 16-3 Obtaining an Arterial Blood Sample From an Arterial Line (continued)

- *After obtaining the specimen and reactivating the arterial pressure monitoring system, no waveform is noted.* Check the stopcock to make sure that it is open to the patient and recheck all connections and components of the system to ensure proper set up. If necessary, rebalance the transducer or replace the system as necessary. Additionally, suspect a clotter catheter tip. If agency policy permits, attempt to aspirate the close with a syringe and if successful, flush the line. However, do not attempt to flush the line if the clot cannot be aspirated. Notify the physician.

Special Considerations

- If the patient is receiving oxygen, make sure that this therapy has been underway for at least 15 minutes before collecting an arterial blood sample. Indicate on the laboratory request slip the amount and type of oxygen therapy the patient is receiving. Also note the patient's current temperature, most recent hemoglobin level, and current respiratory rate. If the patient is receiving mechanical ventilation, note the fraction of inspired oxygen and tidal volume.
- If the patient is not receiving oxygen, indicate that he or she is breathing room air.
- If the patient has just received a nebulizer treatment, wait about 20 minutes before collecting the sample.

Removing Arterial and Femoral Lines

Arterial and femoral lines are used for more intensive and continuous cardiac monitoring and intraarterial access. Once the lines are no longer necessary or have become ineffective, they will need to be removed. Consult facility policy to determine whether you are permitted to perform this procedure.

Equipment

- Gloves
- Gown
- Mask
- Protective eyewear
- Two sterile 4 × 4 gauze pads
- Sheet protector
- Sterile suture removal set
- Dressing
- Alcohol pads
- Hypoallergenic tape
- For femoral line: small sandbag (wrapped in towel or pillowcase)

ASSESSMENT

Review the patient's medical record and plan of care for information about discontinuation of the arterial line. Assess the patient's coagulation status, including laboratory studies, to reduce the risk of complications secondary to impaired clotting ability. Assess the patient's understanding of the procedure. Inspect the site for leakage, bleeding, or hematoma.

NURSING DIAGNOSIS

Determine the related factors for the nursing diagnoses based on the patient's current status. Appropriate nursing diagnoses may include:

- Risk for Injury
- Impaired Skin Integrity
- Risk for Infection
- Anxiety

Many other nursing diagnoses also may require the use of this skill.

OUTCOME IDENTIFICATION AND PLANNING

The expected outcome to achieve when removing an arterial or femoral line is that the line is removed intact and without injury to the patient. In addition, the site remains clean and dry without evidence of infection.

IMPLEMENTATION

ACTION	RATIONALE
1. Explain the procedure to the patient.	This helps allay anxiety and promotes patient cooperation.
2. Assemble all equipment. Perform hand hygiene. Observe standard precautions, including gloves and personal protective equipment.	Hand hygiene deters the spread of microorganisms. Proper infection control precautions reduce the risk for disease transmission.
3. Turn off the monitor alarms and then turn off the flow clamp to the flush solution. Carefully remove the dressing over the insertion site. Remove any sutures using the suture removal kit; make sure all sutures have been removed.	These measures help prepare for withdrawal of line.
4. **Withdraw the catheter using a gentle, steady motion. Keep the catheter parallel to the artery during withdrawal.**	Using a gentle, steady motion parallel to the artery reduces the risk for traumatic injury.

continues

ACTION	RATIONALE
5. **Immediately after withdrawing the catheter, apply pressure to the site with a sterile 4 × 4 gauze pad. Maintain pressure for at least 10 minutes (longer if bleeding or oozing persists).** Apply additional pressure to a femoral site or if the patient has coagulopathy or is receiving anticoagulants.	If sufficient pressure is not applied, a large, painful hematoma may form.
6. Cover the site with an appropriate dressing and secure the dressing with tape. If stipulated by facility policy, make a pressure dressing for a femoral site by folding four sterile 4 × 4 gauze pads in half, and apply the dressing. Cover the dressing with a tight adhesive bandage, and then cover the femoral bandage with a sandbag. Maintain the patient on bed rest for 6 hours with the sandbag in place.	Sufficient pressure is needed to prevent continued bleeding and hematoma formation.
7. Remove and properly dispose of gloves and personal protective equipment. Perform hand hygiene.	Proper removal and disposal of equipment and hand hygiene deter the spread of microorganisms.
8. Observe the site for bleeding. Assess circulation in the extremity distal to the site by evaluating color, pulses, and sensation. Repeat this assessment every 15 minutes for the first 4 hours, every 30 minutes for the next 2 hours, then hourly for the next 6 hours.	Continued assessment allows for early detection and prompt intervention should problems arise.
9. Document the time the line was removed, how long pressure was applied, peripheral circulation, appearance of site, type of dressing applied, and the timed assessments.	Documentation provides communication and promotes continuity of care.

EVALUATION   The expected outcome is met when the patient exhibits an arterial or femoral line site that is clean and dry without evidence of injury or infection. In addition, the patient demonstrates intact peripheral circulation and verbalizes a reduction in anxiety.

Unexpected Situations and Associated Interventions
- *You note fresh blood on the site dressing:* Apply pressure. If bleeding continues, notify the physician.
- *The patient has a history of peripheral vascular disease:* Assess the peripheral circulation for changes; if necessary, apply slightly decreased pressure at the insertion site.

Special Considerations
- If the physician has ordered a culture of the catheter tip (to diagnose a suspected infection), gently place the catheter tip on a 4×4 sterile gauze pad. When the bleeding is under control, hold the catheter over the sterile container. Using sterile scissors, cut the tip so it falls into the sterile container. Label the specimen and send it to the laboratory.

**SKILL
16-5**

Performing Cardiopulmonary Resuscitation (CPR)

Cardiopulmonary resuscitation (CPR), also known as basic life support, is used in the absence of spontaneous respirations and heartbeat to preserve heart and brain function while waiting for defibrillation. It is a combination of "mouth-to-mouth" or rescue breathing, which supplies oxygen to the lungs, and chest compressions, which manually pump the heart to circulate blood to the body systems.

Equipment
- Personal protective equipment such as a face shield or one-way valve mask preferable
- Ambu-bag and oxygen, if possible

ASSESSMENT

Assess the patient's vital parameters and determine the patient's level of responsiveness. Check for partial or complete airway obstruction.

NURSING DIAGNOSIS

Determine the related factors for the nursing diagnoses based on the patient's current status. Appropriate nursing diagnoses may include:
- Decreased Cardiac Output
- Ineffective Airway Clearance
- Impaired Gas Exchange
- Inability to Sustain Spontaneous Ventilation
- Ineffective Tissue Perfusion
- Risk for Aspiration
- Risk for Injury

Many other nursing diagnoses may require the use of this skill.

OUTCOME IDENTIFICATION AND PLANNING

The expected outcome to achieve when performing CPR is that the patient's heart and lungs maintain adequate function to sustain life. Another appropriate outcome may be that the patient experiences no signs and symptoms of injury.

IMPLEMENTATION

ACTION	RATIONALE
1. Assess responsiveness; call for help and pull call bell if patient is not responsive.	Assessing responsiveness prevents starting CPR on a conscious victim. Calling for help and pulling the call bell help provide a rapid response.
2. Position the patient supine on his or her back and use the head tilt–chin lift maneuver to open the airway.	This maneuver may be enough to open the airway and promote spontaneous respirations.
3. Look, listen, and feel for air exchange.	These techniques provide information about the patient's breathing and the need for rescue breathing.
4. If no spontaneous breathing is noted, pinch the nose while sealing the patient's mouth with the face shield or one-way valve mask (mouth and nose with Ambu bag), if available. If not available, seal mouth with your mouth.	Sealing the patient's mouth prevents air from escaping. Devices such as masks reduce the risk for transmission of infections.
5. Instill two breaths, each lasting 2 seconds. Take a deep breath after providing each breath.	Breathing into the patient provides oxygen to the patient's lungs. Taking a deep breath after providing each breath allows time for the patient's chest to expand and relax and prevents gastric distention.

continues

ACTION

RATIONALE

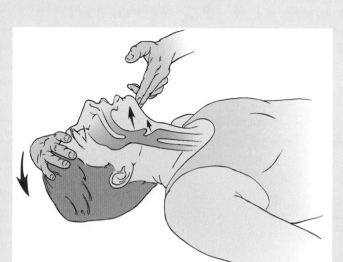

Action 2: Using the head tilt–chin lift method to open the airway.

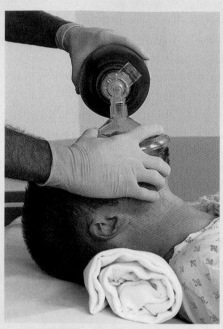

Action 4: Using hand-held resuscitation mask.
(Photo © B. Proud.)

6. If you are unable to ventilate or the chest does not rise during ventilation, reposition the patient's head and reattempt to ventilate. Place the patient in the recovery position if breathing resumes. If you still cannot ventilate, perform a blind finger sweep and attempt five abdominal thrusts to remove the obstruction. Repeat finger sweep and attempt to ventilate. Repeat this cycle as necessary.

Inability to ventilate indicates that the airway may still be obstructed. Abdominal thrusts help to move the obstruction.

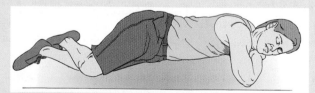

Action 6: Patient placed in the recovery position.

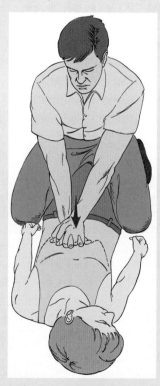

Action 6: Attempting to clear an obstruction in an unconscious patient.

continues

SKILL 16-5 — Performing Cardiopulmonary Resuscitation (CPR) (continued)

ACTION

RATIONALE

7. Check the carotid pulse and listen for spontaneous breathing.

Pulse assessment indicates cardiac function.

8. If there is no pulse, place a backboard under the patient (often the footboard of the patient's bed). Position the heel of one hand approximately 2 fingerbreadths above the xiphoid process directly over the sternum; then place the other hand directly on top of the first hand, keeping fingers above the chest.

A backboard provides a firm surface on which to apply compressions. Proper hand positioning ensures that the force of compressions is on the sternum, thereby reducing the risk of rib fracture, lung puncture, or liver laceration.

9. Perform 15 chest compressions at a rate 100 per minute, counting "one and two and" up to 15, keeping elbows locked, arms straight, and shoulders directly over the hands.

Chest compressions manually pump the heart to circulate blood through the circulatory system.

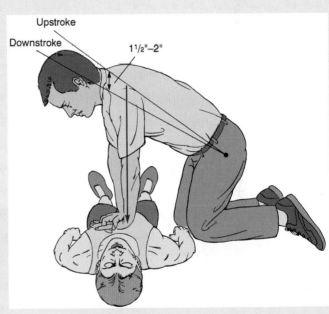

Upstroke

Downstroke

1½"–2"

Action 9: Using correct body alignment for chest compressions.

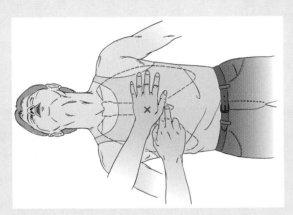

Action 8: Using correct hand placement for chest compressions.

10. Give two rescue breaths after each set of 15 compressions. Do four complete cycles of 15 compressions and two ventilations.

Breathing and compressions simulate lung and heart function, providing oxygen and circulation.

11. Reassess breathing and pulse after each set of four compression/breathing cycles.

Reassessment determines the need for continued CPR.

12. Continue CPR until the patient resumes spontaneous breathing and pulse, medical help arrives, or you are too exhausted to continue.

Once started, CPR must continue until one of these three conditions is met. In a hospital setting, help should arrive within a few minutes.

13. Document the time you discovered the patient unresponsive and started CPR. Continued intervention, such as by the code team, is typically documented on a code form, which identifies the actions and drugs provided during the code. Provide a summary of these events in the patient's medical record.

Documentation provides communication and promotes continuity of care.

continues

Performing Cardiopulmonary Resuscitation (CPR) (continued)

EVALUATION

The expected outcome is met when the patient exhibits functioning of the heart and lungs by resuming spontaneous breathing and heart contraction, without complications, or maintains heart and lung function by healthcare interventions.

Unexpected Situations and Associated Interventions

- *When performing chest compression, you hear something crack:* Most commonly this sound indicates cracking of the ribs. Recheck your hand position. Then continue with gentle but firm chest compressions.
- *You come upon a patient lying on the floor:* Determine the patient's level of responsiveness. If the patient is unresponsive, quickly clear an area, call for assistance, and begin CPR.

Special Considerations

- For a choking conscious patient, perform the Heimlich maneuver until the obstruction is removed. If the patient is obese or pregnant, use chest thrusts.
- Perform CPR in the same manner if the patient is pregnant or obese.
- If you cannot completely seal the patient's mouth for reasons such as oral trauma, perform mouth-to-nose breathing. If the patient has a tracheostomy, provide ventilations through the tracheostomy instead of the mouth.

Infant and Child Considerations

- If the victim is under 8 years of age, use the heel of one hand to provide chest compressions and compress to a depth of 1″ to 1.5″.
- For an infant under 1 year of age, use two or three fingers placed in the midline one finger-breadth below the nipple line and compress 0.5″ to 1″.
- To open the airway of a child, place one hand on the child's forehead and gently lift the chin with the other hand (called the sniffing position in infants).
- If available, use a one-way valve mask over the child's nose and mouth when performing CPR.

Performing Emergency Defibrillation (Asynchronous)

Electrical therapy is used to quickly terminate or control potentially lethal arrhythmias. Electrical therapy can be administered by defibrillation, cardioversion, or a pacemaker.

Defibrillation delivers large amounts of electric current to a patient over brief periods of time. It is the standard treatment for ventricular fibrillation (VF) and is also used to treat ventricular tachycardia (VT), in which the patient has no pulse. The goal is to temporarily depolarize the irregularly beating heart and allow more coordinated contractile activity to resume. It does so by completely depolarizing the myocardium, producing a momentary asystole. This provides an opportunity for the natural pacemaker centers of the heart to resume normal activity. The electrode paddles delivering the current may be placed on the patient's chest or, during cardiac surgery, directly on the myocardium. Because ventricular fibrillation leads to death if not corrected, the success of defibrillation depends on early recognition and quick treatment of this arrhythmia.

Equipment

- Defibrillator (monophasic or biphasic)
- External paddles (or internal paddles sterilized for cardiac surgery)
- Conductive medium pads
- Electrocardiogram (ECG) monitor with recorder (often part of the defibrillator)
- Oxygen therapy equipment

continues

Performing Emergency Defibrillation (Asynchronous) (continued)

- Hand-held resuscitation bag
- Airway equipment
- Emergency pacing equipment
- Emergency cardiac medications

ASSESSMENT

Assess the patient to determine unresponsiveness and absent pulse. Call for help and perform cardiopulmonary resuscitation (CPR) until the defibrillator and other emergency equipment arrive.

NURSING DIAGNOSIS

Determine the related factors for the nursing diagnoses based on the patient's current status. Appropriate nursing diagnoses may include:

- Decreased Cardiac Output
- Impaired Gas Exchange
- Ineffective Peripheral Tissue Perfusion
- Risk for Injury

Many other nursing diagnoses may require the use of this skill.

OUTCOME IDENTIFICATION AND PLANNING

The expected outcome to achieve when performing defibrillation is that the patient establishes a spontaneous heart rate to sustain perfusion to the vital organs with minimal complications.

IMPLEMENTATION

ACTION	RATIONALE
1. Assess the patient to determine if a pulse is present. Call for help and perform cardiopulmonary resuscitation (CPR) until the defibrillator and other emergency equipment arrive.	Initiating CPR preserves heart and brain function while awaiting defibrillation.
2. If the defibrillator has "quick-look" capability, place the paddles on the patient's chest. Otherwise, connect the monitoring leads of the defibrillator to the patient and assess the cardiac rhythm.	Connecting the monitor leads to the patient allows for a quick view of the cardiac rhythm.
3. Expose the patient's chest, and apply conductive pads at the paddle placement positions. For anterolateral placement, place one paddle to the right of the upper sternum, just below the right clavicle, and the other over the fifth or sixth intercostal space at the left anterior axillary line. For anteroposterior placement, place the anterior paddle directly over the heart at the precordium, to the left of the lower sternal border. Place the flat posterior paddle under the patient's body beneath the heart and immediately below the scapulae (but not under the vertebral column).	This placement ensures that the electrical stimulus needs to travel only a short distance to the heart.

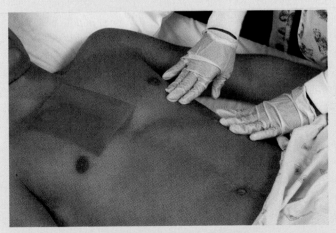

Action 3: Placing defibrillator pads on patient's chest.

continues

SKILL 16-6   Performing Emergency Defibrillation (Asynchronous) (continued)

ACTION	RATIONALE

ACTION

4. Turn on the defibrillator.

   a. If performing external defibrillation, set the energy level for 200 joules for an adult patient when using monophasic defibrillator. Use clinically appropriate energy levels for biphasic defibrillators.

   b. Charge the paddles by pressing the charge buttons, which are located either on the machine or on the paddles themselves.

   c. **Place the paddles over the conductive pads and press firmly against the patient's chest, using 25 lb (11 kg) of pressure.**

RATIONALE

Charging and placement prepare for defibrillation.

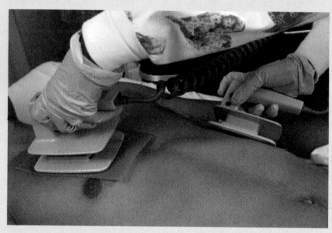

Action 4c: Placing paddles on patient's chest.

5. Reassess the cardiac rhythm.

6. If the patient remains in VF or pulseless VT, **instruct all personnel to stand clear of the patient and the bed, including yourself.**

7. Discharge the current by pressing both paddle charge buttons simultaneously.

8. Leaving the paddles in position on the patient's chest, reassess the cardiac rhythm and have someone else assess the pulse.

9. If necessary, prepare to defibrillate a second time.

   a. **Instruct someone to reset the energy level on the defibrillator to 200 to 300 joules or the biphasic energy equivalent.**

   b. Announce that you are preparing to defibrillate and follow the procedure described above.

10. Reassess the patient.

The rhythm may have changed during preparation.

Standing clear of the bed and patient helps prevent electrical shocks to personnel.

Pressing the charge buttons discharges the electric current for defibrillation.

Reassessment provides information about the return of perfusion and facilitates stacking of shocks.

Additional shocking may be needed to stimulate the heart.

Reassessment is necessary to determine whether perfusion has returned and to evaluate the effectiveness of treatment.

continues

ACTION	RATIONALE
11. **If defibrillation is again necessary, instruct someone to reset the energy level to 360 joules or biphasic energy equivalent.** Then follow the same procedure as before for a total of three shocks.	Stacking shocks facilitates the return to a perfusing rhythm.
12. If the patient still has no pulse after three initial defibrillations: a. Resume CPR. b. Give supplemental oxygen. c. Begin administering appropriate medications such as epinephrine. d. Consider possible causes for failure of the rhythm to convert, such as acidosis or hypoxia.	Advanced cardiac life support is necessary in an attempt to stimulate the heart.
13. If defibrillation restores a normal rhythm: a. Check the central and peripheral pulses and obtain a blood pressure reading, heart rate, and respiratory rate. b. Assess the patient's level of consciousness, cardiac rhythm, breath sounds, skin color, and urine output. c. Obtain baseline arterial blood gas levels and a 12-lead ECG. d. Provide supplemental oxygen, ventilation, and medications as needed. e. Check the chest for electrical burns and treat them, as ordered, with corticosteroid or lanolin-based creams. f. Prepare the defibrillator for immediate reuse.	The patient will need continuous monitoring to prevent further problems. Continuous monitoring helps provide for early detection and prompt intervention should additional problems arise.
14. Document the procedure, including the patient's ECG rhythms both before and after defibrillation; the number of times defibrillation was performed; the voltage used during each attempt; whether a pulse returned; the dosage, route, and time of drug administration; whether CPR was used; how the airway was maintained; and the patient's outcome.	Documentation provides communication and promotes continuity of care.

EVALUATION

The expected outcome is met when the patient demonstrates a stable heart rate and rhythm that sustains perfusion of the vital organs. In addition, the patient remains free of complications.

Unexpected Situations and Associated Interventions

- *The patient develops a skin burn at the site of the pad placement:* In most cases, an insufficient amount of conductive medium is the cause. Prepare to treat the burn area as ordered, such as with corticosteroid or lanolin-based creams.

Special Considerations

- Defibrillation can cause accidental electric shock to those providing care.
- Defibrillators vary from one manufacturer to the next, so familiarize yourself with your facility's equipment. Defibrillator operation should be checked at least every 8 hours, and after each use.
- Defibrillation can be affected by several factors, including paddle size and placement, condition of the patient's myocardium, duration of the arrhythmia, chest resistance, and the number of countershocks.

SKILL 16-7   Using an External (Transcutaneous) Pacemaker

A temporary pacemaker consists of an external, battery-powered pulse generator and a lead or electrode system to electrically stimulate heartbeat. In a life-threatening situation, when time is critical, a transcutaneous pacemaker is the best choice. This device works by sending an electrical impulse from the pulse generator to the patient's heart by way of two electrodes, which are placed on the front and back of the patient's chest. This stimulates the heart's pacemaker. Transcutaneous pacing is quick and effective but is used only until the physician can institute transvenous pacing.

Equipment
- Transcutaneous pacing generator
- Transcutaneous pacing electrodes
- Cardiac monitor

ASSESSMENT

Review the patient's medical record and plan of care for information about the patient's need for pacing. Monitor heart rate, respiratory rate, level of consciousness, and skin color. If pulselessness returns, begin CPR.

NURSING DIAGNOSIS

Determine the related factors for the nursing diagnoses based on the patient's current status. An appropriate nursing diagnosis is Decreased Cardiac Output. Many other nursing diagnoses also may require the use of this skill.

OUTCOME IDENTIFICATION AND PLANNING

The expected outcome to achieve when using an external pacemaker is that the patient demonstrates an adequate heart rate that is capable of sustaining perfusion.

IMPLEMENTATION

ACTION	RATIONALE
1. If patient is responsive, explain the procedure to the patient and perform hand hygiene.	External pacemakers are typically used with unconscious patients because most alert patients cannot tolerate the uncomfortable sensations produced by the high energy levels needed to pace externally. If responsive, the patient will most likely be sedated. Hand hygiene deters the spread of microorganisms.
2. If necessary, clip the hair over the areas of electrode placement. **However, do not shave the area.**	If you nick the skin, the current from the pulse generator could cause discomfort.
3. Attach monitoring electrodes to the patient in the lead I, II, and III positions. Do this even if the patient is already on telemetry monitoring. If you select the lead II position, adjust the LL (left leg) electrode placement to accommodate the anterior pacing electrode and the patient's anatomy.	Connecting the telemetry electrodes to the pacemaker is required.

4. Prepare the equipment.
 	
  a. Put the patient cable into the ECG input connection on the front of the pacing generator. Set the selector switch to the MONITOR ON position.
 	
  b. Note the ECG waveform on the monitor. Adjust the R-wave beeper volume to a suitable level and activate the alarm by pressing the ALARM ON button. Set the alarm for 10 to 20 beats lower and 20 to 30 beats higher than the intrinsic rate.
 	
  c. Press the START/STOP button for a printout of the waveform.
	These actions ensure that the equipment is functioning properly.

continues

Using an External (Transcutaneous) Pacemaker (continued)

ACTION	RATIONALE

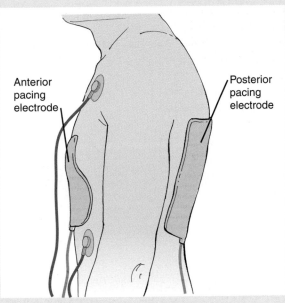

Actions 5 and 6: Transcutaneous pacemaker pads in place.

5. Apply the two pacing electrodes. Make sure the patient's skin is clean and dry to ensure good skin contact. Pull the protective strip from the posterior electrode (marked BACK) and apply the electrode on the left side of the back, just below the scapula and to the left of the spine.

This placement ensures that the electrical stimulus must travel only a short distance to the heart.

6. Apply the anterior pacing electrode (marked FRONT), which has two protective strips: one covering the gelled area and one covering the outer rim. Expose the gelled area and apply it to the skin in the anterior position, to the left side of the precordium in the usual V_2 to V_5 position. Move this electrode around to get the best waveform. Then expose the electrode's outer rim and firmly press it to the skin.

This placement ensures that the electrical stimulus must travel only a short distance to the heart.

7. Prepare to pace the heart.

This sets the pacing threshold.

   a. After making sure the energy output in milliamperes (mA) is on 0, connect the electrode cable to the monitor output cable.

   b. Check the waveform, looking for a tall QRS complex in lead II.

   c. Check the selector switch to PACER ON. **Tell the patient he or she may feel a thumping or twitching sensation. Reassure the patient you will provide medication if the discomfort is intolerable.**

continues

SKILL 16-7   Using an External (Transcutaneous) Pacemaker (continued)

ACTION	RATIONALE

d. Set the rate dial to 10 to 20 beats higher than the intrinsic rhythm. Look for pacer artifact or spikes, which will appear as you increase the rate. If the patient does not have an intrinsic rhythm, set the rate at 60.

e. **Slowly increase the amount of energy delivered to the heart by adjusting the OUTPUT mA dial. Do this until capture is achieved: you will see a pacer spike followed by a widened QRS complex that resembles a premature ventricular contraction.**

8. Increase output by 10%. **Do not go higher because of the increased risk of discomfort to the patient.**

Increasing the output ensures consistent capture. With full capture, the patient's heart rate should be approximately the same as the pacemaker rate set on the machine. The usual pacing threshold is 40 to 80 mA.

9. Document the reason for pacemaker use, time that pacing began, electrode locations, pacemaker settings, patient's response to the procedure and to temporary pacing, complications, and nursing actions taken. **If possible, obtain a rhythm strip before, during, and after pacemaker placement; any time that pacemaker settings are changed; and whenever the patient receives treatment because of a complication due to the pacemaker.**

Documentation provides communication and promotes continuity of care.

10. Assess the patient's vital signs, skin color, level of consciousness, and peripheral pulses.

Assessment helps determine the effectiveness of the paced rhythm.

11. Perform a 12-lead ECG and perform additional ECGs daily or with clinical changes.

ECG monitoring provides a baseline for further evaluation.

12. Continually monitor the ECG readings, noting capture, sensing, rate, intrinsic beats, and competition of paced and intrinsic rhythms. If the pacemaker is sensing correctly, the sense indicator on the pulse generator should flash with each beat.

Continuous monitoring helps evaluate the patient's condition and determine the effectiveness of therapy.

EVALUATION   The expected outcome is met with the capture of at least the minimal set heart rate, with minimal patient complications.

Unexpected Situations and Associated Interventions

- *Failure to pace:* This happens when the pacemaker either doesn't fire or fires too often. The pulse generator may not be working properly, or it may not be conducting the impulse to the patient. If the pacing or sensing indicator flashes, check the connections to the cable and the position of the pacing electrode in the patient (by X-ray). The cable may have come loose, or the electrode may have been dislodged, pulled out, or broken. If the pulse generator is turned on but the indicators still aren't flashing, change the battery. If that does not help, use a different pulse generator. Check the settings if the pacemaker is firing too rapidly. If they are correct, or if altering them (according to your facility's policy or the physician's order) does not help, change the pulse generator.

continues

- *Failure to capture:* Here, you see pacemaker spikes but the heart is not responding. This may be caused by changes in the pacing threshold from ischemia, an electrolyte imbalance (high or low potassium or magnesium levels), acidosis, an adverse reaction to a medication, a perforated ventricle, fibrosis, or the position of the electrode. If the patient's condition has changed, notify the physician and ask him or her for new settings. If pacemaker settings have been altered by the patient (or family members), return them to their correct positions and then make sure the face of the pacemaker is covered with a plastic shield. Tell the patient and family members not to touch the dials. If the heart is not responding, try any or all of these suggestions:
  - Carefully check all connections, making sure they are placed properly and securely.
  - Increase the milliamperes slowly (according to your facility's policy or the physician's order).
  - Turn the patient on his or her left side, then on the right side (if turning to the left did not help).
  - Schedule an anteroposterior or lateral chest x-ray to determine the position of the electrode.
- *Failure to sense intrinsic beats:* This could cause ventricular tachycardia or ventricular fibrillation if the pacemaker fires on the vulnerable T wave. This could be caused by the pacemaker sensing an external stimulus as a QRS complex, which could lead to asystole, or by the pacemaker not being sensitive enough, which means it could fire anywhere within the cardiac cycle. If the pacing is undersensing, turn the sensitivity control completely to the right. If it is oversensing, turn it slightly to the left. If the pacemaker is not functioning correctly, change the battery or the pulse generator. Remove items in the room causing electromechanical interference (e.g., razors, radios, cautery devices). Check the ground wires on the bed and other equipment for obvious damage. Unplug each piece and see if the interference stops. When you locate the cause, notify the staff engineer and ask him or her to check it. If the pacemaker is still firing on the T wave and all else has failed, turn off the pacemaker and notify the physician. Make sure atropine is available in case the patient's heart rate drops. Be prepared to call a code and institute cardiopulmonary resuscitation if necessary.

Special Considerations

- If the patient needs emergency defibrillation, make sure the pacemaker can withstand the procedure. If you are unsure, disconnect the pulse generator to avoid damage.
- Do not place the electrodes over a bony area, because bone conducts current poorly.
- With a female patient, place the anterior electrodes under the patient's breast but not over her diaphragm.
- Do not use electrical equipment that is not grounded, such as telephones, electric shaver, television, or lamps; otherwise, the patient may experience microshock.

■ Developing Critical Thinking Skills

1. Coby Pruder becomes visibly anxious when you bring in the ECG machine and begin to open the supplies. What could you do to help alleviate his anxiety?
2. You go in to assess Harry Stebbings and find him unresponsive. How should you respond?
3. Prior to obtaining the ABG on Ann Kribell, you perform the Allen's test on her left arm. After releasing the pressure on the ulnar artery, you observe that her left hand remains quite pale. What should you do?

Bibliography

American Heart Association. (August 2000). Guidelines 2000 for Cardiopulmonary Resuscitation and Emergency Cardiovascular Care: International Consensus on Science. *Circulation, 102*(8 Suppl), 1–384.

American Heart Association. (2001). *ACLS Provider Manual.*

Asselin, M. E., & Cullen, H. A. (February 2002). A new beat for BLS and ACLS guidelines. *Nursing Management, 33*(2).

Dries, D. J., & Sample, M. A. (March 2002). Recent advances in emergency life support. *Nursing Clinics of North America, 37*(10), 1–10.

Freeman, J. J., & Hedges, C. H. (June 2003). Cardiac arrest: The effect on the brain. *American Journal of Nursing, 103*(6), 50–55.

Lynn-McHale, D. J., & Carlson, K. K. (2001). *Procedure manual for critical care* (4th ed.). Philadelphia: W. B. Saunders.

Mair, M. (August 2003). Monophasic and biphasic defibrillators. *American Journal of Nursing, 103*(8), 58–60.

Mastering ACLS (2002). Springhouse, PA: Springhouse Corp.

Nursing procedures made incredibly easy (2002). Springhouse, PA: Springhouse Corp.

Skillbuilders: Expert ECG interpretation (2003). Philadelphia: Lippincott Williams & Wilkins.

Weber, J., & Kelley, J. (2003). *Health assessment in nursing* (2nd ed.). Philadelphia: Lippincott Williams & Wilkins.

Neurological Care

This chapter will help you develop some of the skills related to neurological care necessary to care for the following patients:

Nikki Gladstone is a neonate born at 32 weeks' gestation. She has just received an external ventriculostomy to relieve hydrocephalus.

Yuka Chong, age 16, has received spinal rods to resolve her scoliosis and is to be "logrolled."

Aleta Jackson, age 68, was involved in a head-on collision. She is complaining that the cervical collar is beginning to hurt her neck.

Learning Outcomes

After studying this chapter, the reader should be able to:

1. Care for an external ventriculostomy device
2. Care for a fiberoptic intracranial catheter
3. Apply a two-piece cervical collar
4. Logroll a patient

Key Terms

cerebral perfusion pressure (CPP): a way of calculating cerebral blood flow; the formula is MAP (mean arterial pressure) minus ICP (intracranial pressure) equals CPP; normal CPP for an adult is 80 to 100 mm Hg

consciousness: the degree of wakefulness or ability to be aroused

intracranial pressure (ICP): pressure within the cranial vault; normal ICP is less than 15 mm Hg

ventriculostomy: a catheter inserted through a hole made in the skull into the ventricular system of the brain; can be used to monitor ICP and or drain cerebrospinal fluid

Many patients experience injury to the head, neck, or spinal column. In addition, numerous disorders, such as infections and tumors, can affect the brain and spinal cord, interfering with neurological function. Specialized devices may be used to monitor and control intracranial pressure. Meticulous care is needed after injury or trauma to ensure that further injury does not occur.

This chapter will cover skills to assist the nurse in providing neurological care. Please look over the summary figure, table, and box at the beginning of this chapter for a quick review of critical knowledge to assist you in understanding the skills related to neurological care.

TABLE 17-1 Glasgow Coma Scale

Component	Response	Score
Eye opening	Spontaneous	4
	To verbal command	3
	To pain	2
	No response	1
Motor response	To verbal command	6
	To localized pain	5
	Flexes/withdraws	4
	Flexes abnormally	3
	Extends abnormally	2
	No response	1
Verbal response	Oriented/talks	5
	Disoriented/talks	4
	Inappropriate words	3
	Incomprehensible sounds	2
	No response	1

BOX 17-1 Interpreting ICP Waveforms

Three waveforms—A, B, and C—are used to monitor intracranial pressure (ICP). A waves are an ominous sign of intracranial decompensation and poor compliance. B waves correlate with changes in respiration, and C waves correlate with changes in arterial pressure.

Normal Waveform

A normal ICP waveform typically shows a steep upward systolic slope followed by a downward diastolic slope with a dicrotic notch. In most cases, this waveform occurs continuously and indicates an ICP between 0 and 15 mm Hg—normal pressure.

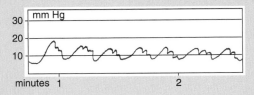

A Waves

The most clinically significant ICP waveforms are A waves, which may reach elevations of 50 to 100 mm Hg, persist for 5 to 20 minutes, then drop sharply—signaling exhaustion of the brain's compliance mechanisms. A waves may come and go, spiking from temporary rises in thoracic pressure or from a condition that increases ICP beyond the brain's compliance limits. Such activities as sustained coughing or straining during defecation can cause temporary elevations in thoracic pressure.

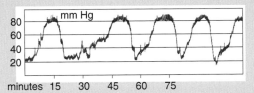

B Waves

B waves, which appear sharp and rhythmic with a sawtooth pattern, occur every 11/2 to 2 minutes and may reach elevations of 50 mm Hg. Their clinical significance isn't clear, but the waves correlate with respiratory changes and may occur more frequently with decreasing compensation. Because B waves sometimes precede A waves, notify the doctor if B waves occur frequently.

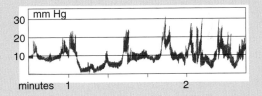

C Waves

Like B waves, C waves are rapid and rhythmic, but they aren't as sharp. Clinically insignificant, they may fluctuate with respirations or systemic blood pressure changes.

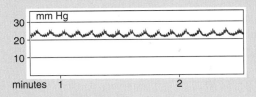

BOX 17-2 Signs and Symptoms of Increased Intracranial Pressure

- Change in level of consciousness, including:
  - Lethargy
  - Stupor
  - Coma
  - Confusion
  - Restlessness
  - Irritability
- Hypoactive reflexes
- Slowed response time
- Ataxia
- Aphasia
- Slowed speech
- Progressively severe headache
- Nausea and vomiting (usually projectile vomiting)
- Seizures
- Changes in pupil size; unequal pupils
- Slowed or lack of pupillary response to light
- Widening of pulse pressure
- Respiratory pattern changes
- Leakage of clear yellow or pinkish fluid from ear or nose

SKILL 17-1   Caring for an External Ventriculostomy (Intraventricular Catheter–Fluid-Filled System)

An external ventriculostomy is an example of an intraventricular catheter that uses a fluid-filled system. This device is inserted through a hole in the skull into the ventricle(s) of the brain. The ventriculostomy can be used to measure the ICP, to drain cerebrospinal fluid (CSF), such as removing excess fluid associated with hydrocephalus, or to decrease the volume in the cranial vault, thereby decreasing the ICP.

Equipment
- Flashlight
- Ventriculostomy setup

ASSESSMENT

Assess the color of the fluid draining from the ventriculostomy. Normal CSF is clear or straw-colored. Cloudy CSF may suggest an infection. Red or pink CSF may indicate bleeding. Assess vital signs, because changes in vital signs can reflect a neurological problem. Assess the patient's pain level. The patient may be experiencing pain at the ventriculostomy insertion site.

Assess the patient's level of consciousness. If the patient is awake, assess for his or her orientation to person, place, and time. If the patient's level of consciousness is decreased, note the patient's ability to respond and be aroused. Inspect pupil size and response to light. Pupils should be equal and round and should react to light bilaterally. Any changes in level of consciousness or pupillary response may suggest a neurological problem. If the patient can move the extremities, assess strength of hands and feet (see Chapter 2 for detailed instructions on assessing muscle strength). A change in strength or a difference in strength on one side compared to the other may indicate a neurological problem.

NURSING DIAGNOSIS

Determine the related factors for the nursing diagnoses based on the patient's current status. Appropriate nursing diagnoses may include:
- Risk for Injury
- Risk for Infection
- Pain

Other nursing diagnoses may include:
- Activity Intolerance
- Risk for Latex Allergy Response
- Risk for Aspiration

OUTCOME IDENTIFICATION AND PLANNING

The expected outcome to achieve when caring for a ventriculostomy is that the patient maintains normal intracranial and cerebral perfusion pressures. Other outcomes that may be appropriate include: patient is free from infection; patient is free from pain; and patient understands the need for the ventriculostomy.

IMPLEMENTATION

ACTION	RATIONALE
1. Explain procedure to patient. Review physician's order for specific information about parameters.	Explanation relieves anxiety and facilitates cooperation. The nurse needs to know the most recent order for the height of the ventriculostomy. If the physician's order states that the ventriculostomy is to be at 10 cm, this means the patient's ICP must rise above 10 cm before the ventriculostomy will drain CSF.
2. Perform hand hygiene; apply gloves if indicated.	Hand hygiene and gloving deter the spread of microorganisms.
3. Assess patient for any changes in neurological status.	Patients with ventriculostomies are at risk for problems with the neurological system.

continues

Caring for an External Ventriculostomy (Intraventricular Catheter–Fluid-Filled System) (continued)

ACTION	RATIONALE
4. **Assess the height of the ventriculostomy by ensuring that the stopcock is at the level of the foramen of Monro (outer canthus of the eye).** Adjust the height of the system if needed. **Move the drip chamber to the ordered height.** Assess the amount of CSF in the drip chamber if the ventriculostomy is draining.	For measurements to be accurate, the stopcock must be at the level of the outer canthus of the eye (this correlates well with the location of the foramen of Monro, which is the actual level for measurements). If the ventriculostomy is used just to measure the ICP and not to drain CSF, the stopcock will be turned off to the drip chamber. If the ventriculostomy is to drain CSF, the nurse must turn the stopcock off to the drip chamber. After the ICP value is obtained, remember to turn the stopcock back off to the transducer so that CSF is allowed to drain.
5. **Zero the transducer.** Turn stopcock off to the patient. Remove the cap from the transducer, being careful not to touch the end of the cap. Press and hold the calibration button on the monitor until the monitor beeps. Return the cap to the transducer. **Turn the stopcock off to the drip chamber to obtain an ICP reading. After obtaining the reading, turn the stopcock off to the transducer.**	The readings would not be considered accurate if the transducer had not been recently zeroed. If the stopcock is not turned off to the patient, when opened to room air, CSF will flow out of the stopcock. The end of the cap must remain sterile to prevent an infection. The stopcock must be off to the drip chamber to obtain an ICP and off to the transducer to drain CSF.
6. **Move the ventriculostomy to prevent too much drainage, too little drainage, or inaccurate ICP readings.**	If the patient's head is lower than the ventriculostomy, the drainage of CSF will slow or stop. If the patient's head is higher than the ventriculostomy, the drainage of CSF will increase. Any ICP readings taken when the ventriculostomy is not level with the outer canthus of the eye would be inaccurate.

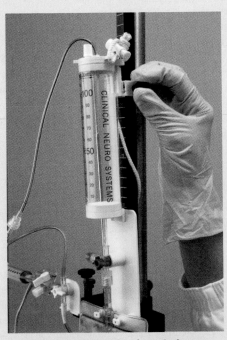

Action 4: Adjusting height of ventriculostomy.

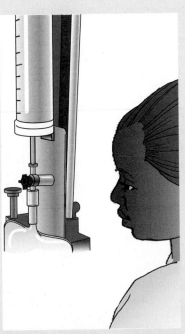

Action 4: Ensuring stopcock is level with outer canthus of the eye.

continues

Caring for an External Ventriculostomy
(Intraventricular Catheter–Fluid-Filled System) (continued)

ACTION   **RATIONALE**

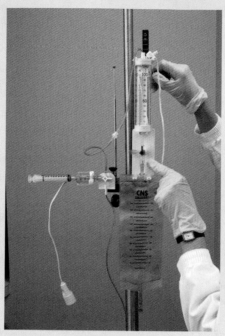

Action 4: Moving drip chamber.

7. Care for the insertion site according to the institution's policy. Assess the site for any signs of infection, such as purulent drainage, redness, or warmth.

Site care varies, possibly ranging from leaving the site open to air to applying antibiotic ointment and gauze.

8. Perform hand hygiene.

Hand hygiene deters the spread of microorganisms.

9. Document the following information: amount and color of CSF; ICP; CPP; pupil status; motor strength bilaterally; orientation to time, person, and place; level of consciousness; vital signs; pain; appearance of insertion site; and height of ventriculostomy.

Documentation ensures continuity of care and provides an ongoing assessment record.

11/2/06   External ventriculostomy zeroed; transducer level with outer canthus of eye, drip chamber 10 cm; draining cloudy, straw-colored CSF (12 cc), physician notified of clarity. Strong equal grip bilaterally. Patient awake, alert, and oriented to person, place, and time. Pupils equal round and reactive to light 6/4 bilaterally. See graphics for vital signs. Patient denies pain. ICP 10 mm Hg, CPP 83 mm Hg. Ventriculostomy insertion site with small amount of serosanguineous drainage; open to air.
—B. Traudes, RN

Action 9: Documentation.

continues

SKILL 17-1   Caring for an External Ventriculostomy (Intraventricular Catheter–Fluid-Filled System) (continued)

EVALUATION

The expected outcome is met when the patient demonstrates a CPP above 80 mm Hg and an ICP below 15 mm Hg; remains free from infection; understands the need for the ventriculostomy; and reports no pain.

Unexpected Situations and Associated Interventions

- *CSF stops draining:* Assess for any kinks or narrowing of tubing. Assess that all connections on the tubing are well connected and that CSF is not leaking anywhere from the tubing. Assess the height of the system and the height of the drip chamber. If the system is too high, the CSF drainage will taper off. Assess for any liquid on the sheets around the patient's head. If the ventriculostomy has become clogged, the CSF may begin to leak around the insertion site. Assess the patency of the ventriculostomy catheter. Raise and lower the system. If the ventriculostomy catheter is patent, the fluid in the tube will tidal or rise and fall with the position change. If CSF still is not draining or if you believe that tube is clogged, notify the physician. The tube may need to be flushed sterilely to ensure patency.
- *The amount of CSF drainage increases:* Assess the height of the system and the height of the drip chamber. If the system is too low, the amount of CSF drainage will increase. If CSF continues to drain at an increased amount, notify the physician. The height of the drip chamber may need to be increased.
- *CSF has changed from clear to cloudy:* Notify the physician immediately. This can signify an infection, and antibiotics may need to be started.
- *CSF has changed from straw-colored to pink-tinged or serosanguineous:* Notify the physician immediately. This can signify bleeding in the ventricles of the brain.
- *Catheter is accidentally dislodged:* Notify the physician immediately. Don sterile gloves and cover the insertion site with sterile gauze. Monitor for color and amount of CSF if draining from site.

SKILL 17-2   Caring for a Fiberoptic Intracranial Catheter

Fiber optic catheters can monitor the ICP and CPP. Newer fiberoptic catheters can also drain CSF. Fiberoptic catheters can be inserted into the ventricle, subarachnoid space, subdural space, or brain parenchyma or under a bone flap.

Equipment

- None needed

ASSESSMENT

Perform a neurological assessment. Assess the patient's level of consciousness. If the patient is awake, assess the patient's orientation to person, place, and time. If the patient's level of consciousness is decreased, note the patient's ability to respond and be aroused. Inspect pupil size and response to light. Pupils should be equal and round and should react to light bilaterally. Any changes in level of consciousness or pupillary response may suggest a neurological problem. If the patient can move the extremities, assess strength of hands and feet (see Chapter 2 for detailed instructions on assessing muscle strength). A change in strength or a difference in strength on one side compared to the other may indicate a neurological problem.

Assess vital signs, because changes in vital signs can reflect a neurological problem. Assess the patient's pain level. The patient may be experiencing pain at the fiberoptic catheter insertion site.

continues

SKILL 17-2   Caring for a Fiberoptic Intracranial Catheter (continued)

NURSING DIAGNOSIS	Determine the related factors for the nursing diagnoses based on the patient's current status. Appropriate nursing diagnoses may include: • Risk for Infection • Risk for Injury • Pain • Ineffective Protection Many other nursing diagnoses also may require the use of this skill.
OUTCOME IDENTIFICATION AND PLANNING	The expected outcome to achieve when caring for a fiberoptic intracranial catheter is that the patient exhibits normal intracranial and cerebral perfusion pressures. Other outcomes that may be appropriate include: patient is free from infection and injury; patient experiences minimal to no pain; and patient demonstrates understanding about the need for the catheter and monitoring.

IMPLEMENTATION

ACTION	RATIONALE
1. Explain procedure to patient. Review physician's order.	Explanation relieves anxiety and facilitates cooperation. Nurse needs to know the most recent order for acceptable ICP and CPP values.
2. Perform hand hygiene.	Hand hygiene deters the spread of microorganisms.
3. Assess patient for any changes in neurological status.	Patients with intracranial catheters are at risk for problems with the neurological system.
4. Assess insertion site for redness, drainage, or warmth.	The insertion site may become infected. Routine inspections are necessary to note and treat any signs of infection quickly.
5. **Assess ICP, MAP, and CPP at least hourly. Note ICP waveforms as shown on the monitor. Notify the physician if A or B waves are present.**	CPP equals MAP minus ICP. By monitoring every hour, the nurse can note and report subtle changes. ICP waveforms (see Fig. 17-1) should be noted at least every hour. C waves are insignificant. B waves commonly signal increasing ICP, with the brain still compensating for the higher ICP. A waves must be treated immediately. A waves are ominous and indicate a rise in the ICP with a decrease in the brain's ability to compensate.
6. Perform hand hygiene.	Hand hygiene deters the spread of microorganisms.
7. Document the following information: ICP; CPP; pupil status; motor strength bilaterally; orientation to time, person, and place; level of consciousness; vital signs; pain; appearance of insertion site.	Documentation ensures continuity of care and provides an ongoing assessment record.

11/2/06   1710   Patient sedated; disoriented and combative when awake. Pupils equal round and reactive to light 6/4 bilaterally. See graphics for vital signs. ICP 22 mm Hg, CPP 61 mm Hg; physician notified. Dopamine drip increased to 8 mcg/kg/min. Insertion site with small amount of serosanguineous drainage; site open to air.—B. Traudes, RN

Action 7: Documentation.

continues

SKILL 17-2	**Caring for a Fiberoptic Intracranial Catheter** (continued)

ACTION	RATIONALE

EVALUATION

The expected outcomes are met when the patient maintains a CPP above 80 mm Hg and an ICP below 15 mm Hg, remains free from infection or injury, and demonstrates an understanding about the need for monitoring.

Unexpected Situations and Associated Interventions

- *Fiberoptic catheter is accidentally dislodged:* Notify the physician immediately. Don sterile gloves and cover the site with sterile gauze. Observe for any CSF leakage from site.
- *Waveforms are not changing with procedures known to cause an increase in the ICP (suctioning):* Fiberoptic catheter may be damaged. Check the manufacturer's instructions for troubleshooting. Notify the physician.
- *CSF is leaking from insertion site:* Notify the physician. CSF is a prime medium for bacteria, and leakage can lead to an infection. Follow your institution's policy. Some institutions may have the nurse apply a sterile dressing around the insertion site; others may have the nurse cleanse the area more frequently.

SKILL 17-3	**Applying a Two-Piece Cervical Collar**

Patients suspected of having injuries to the cervical spine must be immobilized with a cervical collar to prevent further damage to the spinal cord. A cervical collar maintains the neck in a straight line, with the chin slightly elevated and tucked in. Care must be taken when applying the collar not to hyperflex or hyperextend the patient's neck.

Equipment

- Nonsterile gloves
- Tape measure
- Cervical collar of appropriate size
- Washcloth
- Soap
- Towel

ASSESSMENT

Assess for a patent airway. If airway is occluded, try repositioning using the jaw thrust–chin lift method, which helps open the airway without moving the patient's neck. Inspect and palpate the cervical spine area for tenderness, swelling, deformities, or crepitus. Do not ask the patient to move the neck if a cervical spinal cord injury is suspected. Assess the patient's level of consciousness and ability to follow commands to determine any neurological dysfunction. If the patient is able to follow commands, instruct him or her not to move the head or neck. If another person is available to help, have him or her stabilize the cervical spine by holding the patient's head firmly on either side of the head directly above the ears.

NURSING DIAGNOSIS

Determine the related factors for the nursing diagnoses based on the patient's current status. Appropriate nursing diagnoses may include:

- Risk for Injury
- Acute Pain
- Risk for Aspiration
- Ineffective Breathing Pattern

continues

SKILL
17-3   **Applying a Two-Piece Cervical Collar** (continued)

OUTCOME IDENTIFICATION AND PLANNING

The expected outcome to achieve when applying a two-piece cervical collar is that the patient's cervical spine is immobilized, preventing further injury to the spinal cord. Other outcomes that may be acceptable include: patient maintains head and neck without movement; patient experiences minimal to no pain; and patient demonstrates an understanding about the need for immobilization.

IMPLEMENTATION

ACTION	RATIONALE
1. Explain procedure to patient. Review physician's order.	Explanation relieves anxiety and facilitates cooperation. Checking the order ensures that the proper intervention is being implemented.
2. Perform hand hygiene and put on nonsterile gloves.	Hand hygiene and gloving deter the spread of microorganisms.
3. Assess patient for any changes in neurological status.	Patients with cervical spine fractures are at risk for problems with the neurological system.
4. Gently cleanse the face and neck with a mild soap and water. If the patient has experienced trauma, inspect the area for broken glass or other material that could cut the patient or the nurse. Pat the area dry.	Blood, glass, leaves, and twigs may be present on the patient's neck. The area should be clean prior to placing the cervical collar to prevent skin breakdown.
5. With a second person stabilizing the cervical spine, measure from the bottom of the chin to the top of the sternum, and measure around the neck. Match these height and circumference measurements to the manufacturer's recommended size chart.	To immobilize the cervical spine and to prevent skin breakdown under the collar, the correct size of collar should be placed.
6. Slide the flattened collar under the patient's head. **The center of the collar should line up with the center of the patient's neck. Do not allow the patient's head to move when passing the collar under the head.**	The person stabilizing the cervical spine should prevent the head from moving to prevent further damage to the cervical spine. Placing the collar in the center ensures that the neck is straight in alignment.
7. Place the front of the collar centered over the chin, while ensuring that the chin area fits snugly in the recess. Be sure that the front half of the collar overlaps the back half. Secure Velcro straps on both sides.	The collar should fit snugly to prevent the patient from moving the neck and causing further damage to the cervical spine. Velcro will help hold the collar securely in place.
8. **Check the skin under the cervical collar at least every 4 hours for any signs of skin breakdown.** Remove the top half of the collar daily and cleanse the skin under the collar. **When the collar is removed, have a second person immobilize the cervical spine.**	Skin breakdown may occur under the cervical collar if the skin is not inspected and cleansed.
9. Remove gloves and perform hand hygiene.	Hand hygiene deters the spread of microorganisms.
10. Document condition of skin under the cervical collar, patient's level of consciousness, and patient's pain level.	Documentation ensures continuity of care and provides an ongoing assessment record.

11/22/06   Patient arrived on unit; cervical spine immobilized; medium cervical collar applied. Skin pink, warm, and dry. 3-cm laceration noted on R anterior side of neck. Wound cleansed and antibiotic ointment applied. Patient instructed to refrain from moving without assistance; call bell placed in right hand.
—B. Traudes, RN

Action 10: Documentation.

continues

Applying a Two-Piece Cervical Collar (continued)

ACTION	RATIONALE

EVALUATION

The expected outcomes are met when the patient's cervical spine is immobilized without further injury. The patient verbalizes minimal to no pain and demonstrates an understanding of the rationale for cervical spine immobilization.

Unexpected Situations and Associated Interventions

- *The height and neck circumference measurements are between two sizes:* Start with the smaller size. If the collar is too large, the neck may not be immobilized.
- *Skin breakdown is noted on the shoulder, neck, or ear:* Apply a protective dressing over the area and continue to assess for further skin breakdown.
- *Patient complains that the collar is "choking" him:* If not contraindicated, place the patient in the reverse Trendelenburg position to see if this helps. Assess the tightness of the cervical collar; you should be able to slide at least one finger under the collar.
- *Patient is able to move head from side to side with cervical collar on:* Tighten the cervical collar if possible. If the collar is as tight as possible, apply a collar one size smaller and evaluate for a better fit.

Logrolling a Patient

The "logrolling" technique is a maneuver that involves moving the patient's body as one unit so that the spine is not twisted or bent. This technique is commonly used to reposition patients who have had spinal or back surgery or who have suffered back or neck injuries. If the patient is being logrolled due to a neck injury, do not use a fluffy pillow under the patient's head. However, the patient may need a bath blanket or small pillow under the head to keep the spinal column straight. The neck should remain straight.

Equipment

- At least one other person to help
- Small pillow for between the legs
- Wedge pillow or two pillows for behind the patient's back

ASSESSMENT

Assess the patient's neurological status by testing strength in the extremities, asking about paresthesia, and assessing for pain. If the patient is complaining of pain, consider medicating the patient prior to repositioning.

NURSING DIAGNOSIS

Determine the related factors for the nursing diagnoses based on the patient's current status. Appropriate nursing diagnoses may include:

- Risk for Injury
- Acute Pain
- Impaired Physical Mobility
- Risk for Impaired Skin Integrity

OUTCOME IDENTIFICATION AND PLANNING

The expected outcome to achieve when logrolling a patient is that the patient's spine remains in proper alignment, thereby reducing the risk for injury. Other outcomes may include: patient verbalizes relief of pain; patient maintains joint mobility; and patient remains free of skin breakdown.

continues

SKILL 17-4   Logrolling a Patient (continued)

IMPLEMENTATION

ACTION	RATIONALE
1. Explain procedure to patient. Review physician's order.	Explanation relieves anxiety and facilitates cooperation. Reviewing the physician's order helps to ensure that the proper action is implemented.
2. Perform hand hygiene.	Hand hygiene deters the spread of microorganisms.
3. Stand on one side of the bed and have one or two assistants stand on the opposite side of the bed. Place the bed in flat position. Raise the bed so that it is level with your hips. Place a small pillow between the patient's knees.	Using two or more people to turn the patient helps ensure that the spinal column will remain in straight alignment. Raising the bed reduces the strain placed on the nurse's back. A pillow placed between the knees helps keep the spinal column aligned.
4. If the patient can move the arms, ask the patient to cross the arms on the chest. Roll or fanfold the drawsheet and grasp it (you and the assistants). On the count of 3, gently slide the patient to the side of the bed opposite to that which the patient will be turned. Make sure the sheet is straightened and wrinkle free. Roll the drawsheet on the side from which the patient is being turned.	Crossing arms across the chest keeps the arms out of the way while rolling the patient. This also encourages patient not to help by pulling on the side rails. Moving the patient to the side opposite to that which the patient will be turned prevents the patient from being uncomfortably close to the side rail. If the patient is large, more assistants may be needed to prevent injury to the patient. Drawsheet should be wrinkle free to prevent skin breakdown. Rolling the drawsheet strengthens the sheet and helps the nurse hold onto the sheet.
5. Grasp the drawsheet at hip and shoulder level; have assistants on the opposite side grasp the drawsheet above and below your area. On a predetermined signal, begin to turn the patient in one smooth motion.	The patient's spine should not twist during the turn. The spine should move as one unit.

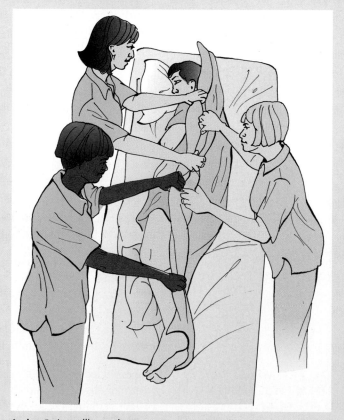

Action 5: Logrolling patient.

continues

SKILL 17-4 | Logrolling a Patient (continued)

ACTION	RATIONALE
6. **Once the patient has been turned, place a wedge or two pillows behind the patient so that he or she remains on the side and the spine is in a straight line.**	The pillows or wedge provide support and ensure continued spinal alignment after turning.
7. Have an assistant gently ease the patient back onto the pillows or wedge in one fluid movement.	The patient should not be jerked. The spine should not twist while easing the patient to the pillows.
8. **Stand at the foot of the bed and assess the spinal column. It should be straight, without any twisting or bending.** Ensure that the call bell and telephone are within reach. Replace covers. Lower bed height.	The nurse ensures that the patient's back is not twisted or bent. Lowering the bed ensures patient safety.
9. Perform hand hygiene.	Hand hygiene deters the spread of microorganisms.
10. Document the condition of skin on the patient's back; if any wounds or dressings are present, describe them; document the patient's pain level.	Documentation ensures continuity of care and provides an ongoing assessment record.

> 11/15/06 1120   *Patient logrolled with 2-person assist. Placed on left side. Patient pushed PCA button prior to turning. Dressing over middle of back from base of neck to lumbar region is clean, dry, and intact; no redness noted on back or buttocks.*—B. Traudes, RN

Action 10: Documentation.

EVALUATION

The expected outcome is met when the patient remains free of injury after turning and exhibits proper spinal alignment in the side-lying position. Other expected outcomes are met when the patient states that pain was minimal on turning; the patient demonstrates adequate joint mobility; and the patient exhibits no signs and symptoms of skin breakdown.

■ Developing Critical Thinking Skills

1. Mr. and Mrs. Gladstone are going to hold Nikki for the first time since the placement of the ventriculostomy. What steps should you take when placing the infant in her mother's arms?
2. Yuka Chong had spinal surgery yesterday and is to be logrolled every 2 hours. The nurse caring for Yuka had her push her patient-controlled analgesia button 10 minutes prior to turning. When you go to turn Yuka and change her bed linens, you find that Yuka's dressing has a small saturated spot that has soiled the sheet. What should you do?
3. Aleta Jackson, age 68, was involved in a head-on collision. She has begun to complain that the cervical collar is hurting her neck. What should you do?

Bibliography

Brodie, M. J., et al. (2001). *Epilepsy: Fast facts* (2nd ed.). Oxford, England: Health Press Limited.
Critical care challenges: Disorders, treatments, and procedures. (2003). Philadelphia: Lippincott Williams & Wilkins.
Crowley, L. V. (2001). *An introduction to human disease: Pathology and pathophysiology correlations* (5th ed.). Sudbury, MA.: Jones and Bartlett Publishers.

Elkin, M. K., et al. (2004). *Nursing interventions and clinical skills* (3rd ed.). St. Louis: Mosby.

Gupta, A. K. (2002). Monitoring the injured brain in the intensive care unit. *Journal of Post-Graduate Medicine, 48*(3), 218–225.

Hickey, J. V. (2003). *The clinical practice of neurological and neurosurgical nursing* (5th ed.). Philadelphia: Lippincott Williams & Wilkins.

Kingsley, R. E. (2000). *Concise text of neuroscience* (2nd ed.). Philadelphia: Lippincott Williams & Wilkins.

Lower, J. (2002). Facing neuro assessment fearlessly. *Nursing, 32*(2), 58–64.

Lynn-McHale, D., & Carlson, K. K. (2001). *AACN procedure manual for critical care* (4th ed.). Philadelphia: W. B. Saunders.

March, K. (2000). Intracranial pressure monitoring and assessing intracranial compliance in brain injury. *Critical Care Nursing Clinics of North America, 12*(4): 429–436.

Nursing procedures and protocols. (2003). Philadelphia: Lippincott Williams & Wilkins.

Porth, C. (2002). *Pathophysiology: Concepts of altered health states* (6th ed.). Philadelphia: Lippincott Williams & Wilkins.

Shoemaker, W., et al. (2002). *Procedures and monitoring for the critically ill.* Philadelphia: W. B. Saunders.

Sirven, J., & Malamut, B. (2002). *Clinical neurology of the older adult.* Philadelphia: Lippincott Williams & Wilkins.

Smeltzer, S. C., & Bare, B. G. (2004). *Brunner and Suddarth's textbook of medical-surgical nursing* (10th ed.). Philadelphia: Lippincott Williams & Wilkins.

Taylor, C., Lillis, C., & LeMone, P. (2005). *Fundamentals of nursing: The Art & Science of Nursing Care* (5th ed.). Philadelphia: Lippincott Williams & Wilkins

Integrated Case Studies

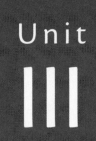

These case studies are designed to focus on integrating concepts. They are not meant to be all-inclusive. The critical thinking questions should guide your discussions of related issues. The discussion within the integrated nursing care section represents possible nursing care solutions to problems; you may find other solutions that are equally acceptable.

Basic Case Studies

Case Study
Abigail Cantonelli

Abigail Cantonelli, age 80, injured her left knee and wrist when she fell on an icy sidewalk. She has been on your orthopedic and neurologic unit for several days. She has an extended history of cardiomyopathy, for which she receives furosemide (Lasix). Her vital signs are stable and she rates her pain as a 2 on a scale of 1 to 10 (10 = worst pain). Since Mrs. Cantonelli has an increased risk of falling, her physician has ordered physical therapy and cane-walking instructions before discharge. Although the physical therapy staff has already initiated the cane-walking instructions, you will need to ambulate Mrs. Cantonelli with her cane during your shift. While you are ambulating down the hall, she says, "Oh, dear! I feel dizzy." She begins to lose her balance and falls toward you.

Medical Orders

Physical therapy for cane-walking instruction
Ambulate every shift with cane assistance
Lasix 20 mg PO q AM

KCl 10 mEq PO qd
Lortab 5 one tab PO q 4–6 hours prn pain

Critical Thinking Questions

- Identify Mrs. Cantonelli's risk factors for falling.

- Describe the actions you would implement when Mrs. Cantonelli begins to fall.

- Considering these risk factors, what special assessments and precautions should you implement before ambulating her? While ambulating her?

(continued)

Case Study
Abigail Cantonelli
(Continued)

Integrated Nursing Care

Concepts

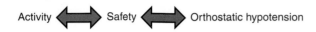

Activity ⟷ Safety ⟷ Orthostatic hypotension

Falls are the leading cause of accidental death in people over age 79. Because of Mrs. Cantonelli's age, past history of falls, and impaired mobility, she continues to be at risk for falls. Her weakness and pain from her injuries also contribute to this risk. In addition, she is taking Lortab for pain and Lasix, which is a diuretic. These medications contribute to an increased risk for falling and subsequent injury (Taylor et al., 2005).

Before ambulating Mrs. Cantonelli, you could implement several assessments and precautions to prevent orthostatic hypotension. Have her sit on the side of the bed for a few minutes and make sure she does not feel dizzy, weak, or lightheaded (see Chapter 9). Since she has a history of cardiomyopathy, assess for shortness of breath and chest pain. If she cannot tolerate sitting up on the side of the bed without having these symptoms, then she will not tolerate standing up or ambulating. Assess her pain level immediately before ambulation. If you have to medicate her for pain, then wait until the pain medicine has had time to take effect before ambulating. Since she is weaker on her left side, assess strength on her right side to ensure she will be able to support her weight with the cane (see Chapter 9). If she has difficulty maintaining her balance, consider using a special safety belt before she begins to ambulate with the cane (some institutions require the use of a safety belt).

While Mrs. Cantonelli is ambulating with her cane, observe her closely. Assess her technique with the cane. Observe for symptoms such as dizziness, chest pain, and shortness of breath. As she continues ambulating, evaluate how she tolerates this activity. Before she is discharged from the hospital, assess her self-confidence as well as her overall ability to use the cane.

When Mrs. Cantonelli begins to fall, it is important to protect her while also protecting yourself. As you feel her start to fall, maintain a wide base of support and place her weight against your body. You can then gently and slowly guide her down toward the floor (see Chapter 9). Assess her orientation and stay with her while waiting for help from another nurse. Take her vital signs to determine if there is a change from baseline. Thoroughly explore other factors that may have contributed to her fall, and plan interventions that will prevent future falls. If Mrs. Cantonelli continues to have problems with falling, a walker may need to be considered.

Case Study
Tiffany Jones

Tiffany Jones, age 17, is scheduled to undergo an ovarian cyst biopsy under local anesthesia. She has been NPO since midnight. Her ID bracelet is on and her consent form is signed. Her mother is in the waiting room. You are to provide her preoperative care. You place an IV in her left hand without difficulty. The next procedure is to insert an indwelling urinary (Foley) catheter. You set up the sterile field between her legs. As you clean the urinary meatus, Tiffany keeps drawing her legs closer together. When you remind her, she opens her legs and says, "Sorry, I didn't mean to move." As you place the catheter at the opening of the urinary meatus, Tiffany is startled and slams her knees together. When she opens her knees, the catheter appears to be inserted, but there is no urine flowing.

Medical Orders

IVF: D5 1/2 NS @ 50 mL/hr
Foley catheter to straight drainage

Critical Thinking Questions

• Where is the urinary catheter, and should you advance the catheter further?

• How do you determine whether the catheter and the sterile field are still sterile?

(continued)

Case Study
Tiffany Jones (Continued)

- How could you have set up a more stable sterile field?

- Describe methods of responding to Tiffany's nervousness.

- Identify issues that are of concern to patients before surgery.

Integrated Nursing Care

Concepts

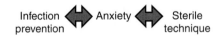

Infection prevention ⬌ Anxiety ⬌ Sterile technique

The female urethra is short, only about 1.5″ to 2.5″ long. If the catheter is advanced that far and no urine is flowing, the catheter may be in the vagina. Do not remove the catheter; it will serve as a guide to locate the urethral opening, which is just above the vagina (see Chapter 12). You would not advance the catheter further even if it were in the urethra, because it is probable that when Tiffany closed her legs, the catheter came into contact with her skin and is no longer sterile. Advancing a nonsterile catheter into the urethra would increase her risk for developing a urinary tract infection. Since you are not certain whether her legs touched the sterile field, the sterile field is also no longer considered sterile (see Chapter 12).

You will need to obtain another complete catheter insertion kit. Cover Tiffany and verify that she understands your plans. As you set up the new kit, place it on the bedside table, not between her legs, to prevent accidental contamination (see Chapter 12).

Teenagers are generally uncomfortable with urinary catheterization because in this procedure, the nurse must look at and touch a very private area. Teenage girls may have "nervous legs": as you touch their inner thighs or labia, the knees slam shut almost involuntarily. Such an invasion of privacy is traumatic at an age when girls are easily embarrassed. Have a second nurse or a relative attend to the teenager. The nurse or relative can distract and soothe the teen, minimizing the unpleasantness of the experience, and can also keep a "reminder" hand on Tiffany's open knee to help you maintain sterility.

Like most preoperative patients, Tiffany has several reasons to feel nervous. She is facing surgery, an unknown and anxiety-producing experience. The preoperative procedures, such as IV insertion and urinary catheterization, are unpleasant and uncomfortable. There are several strategies you can implement to reduce preoperative patients' anxiety. Have a familiar person stay with the patient. Tell the patient your name. Clearly explain procedures, and provide instructions to the patient before you begin. Instructions should include the rationale and the length of time the procedure will take. For urinary catheterization, the patient may also want to know how long he or she will have the catheter in place. Emphasize to the patient that it is all right to ask questions. Describe how the procedure will feel to the patient—for example, "when I clean you, it will feel cold and wet." Keep your voice calm and very matter-of-fact throughout the procedure (see Chapter 6).

Case Study
James White

James White is a patient with an exacerbation of COPD on your medical-surgical unit. You need to obtain his vital signs per the MD order and give him a bath. His vital signs at 8 a.m. were as follows: temperature, 98.4°F; pulse, 86 beats/minute and regular; respirations, 18/minute; blood pressure, 130/68 mm Hg. The physical therapist who is working with this patient on conditioning therapy has just brought him back from his exercises. You notice that his breathing is labored, with audible expiratory wheezes. While you are obtaining his oral temperature and vital signs, you continue to hear audible expiratory wheezing. His vital signs now are as follows: temperature, 96.8°F; pulse, 106 beats/minute and irregular; respirations, 26/minute; blood pressure, 140/74 mm Hg.

Medical Orders

Daily physical therapy for conditioning
Vital signs q 4 hr

Oxygen at 2 L via nasal prongs prn for pulse oximetry <90%
Oxygen saturation levels via pulse oximeter every shift and prn

Critical Thinking Questions

- Did you take the second set of vital signs at the most appropriate time? Why or why not?

- Describe the timing and type of bath you think Mr. White requires and the degree of assistance he will need. Explain your rationale.

- How have Mr. White's exercises affected the accuracy of his vital signs?

- What would be your course of action in response to his labored breathing?

(continued)

Case Study
James White (Continued)

Integrated Nursing Care

Concepts

Vital signs ⟷ Oxygenation ⟷ Activity

Always compare vital signs with the baseline before making further clinical decisions (see Chapter 1). As you compare the previous vital signs with the ones you just obtained, you notice that Mr. White's pulse rate, respiratory rate, and blood pressure are elevated. Your assessment of his pulse also indicates that his pulse is now irregular. Mr. White has just experienced a significant increase in activity, and waiting until he has "caught his breath" would be more appropriate in order to obtain a resting set of vital signs.

What does the very low temperature indicate? Remember that you continued to hear Mr. White's heavy breathing while obtaining the remainder of the vital signs. Mr. White could not keep his lips pursed in a seal around the thermometer, and this often gives an inaccurate temperature. Mouth breathing and respiratory distress are contraindications for obtaining an oral temperature. As a nurse, you are responsible for determining the most appropriate site to obtain the temperature (see Skill 1-1).

Does Mr. White's elevated respiratory rate and noisy breathing indicate respiratory distress or a need for oxygen? Obtain an oxygen saturation level via pulse oximetry; an order already exists for this intervention. If the oxygen saturation level is satisfactory for Mr. White, then you can be confident his body is compensating for the increased oxygen demand. Allow him to rest, with the head of his bed elevated, and retake his vital signs in 15 to 30 minutes. Take vital signs as often as the patient's condition warrants. If Mr. White's oxygen saturation and vital signs continue to deviate from baseline after a rest period, notify the physician (see Chapter 1).

A bath represents another increase in activity. Mr. White needs time to recover from the exercises before attempting the bath. He should be able to sit in a chair and, in fact, will breathe more comfortably sitting up than lying down. Having him lie flat could make him decompensate, so you should not perform occupied bed-making. If encouraged to sit up, he will probably be able to complete much of his bath by himself.

Case Study
Naomi Bell

Naomi Bell, age 90, was admitted to the hospital yesterday after experiencing chest pain. She wears a hearing aid in her left ear. In report you were told that she is "confused" and "doesn't answer questions appropriately." Her night vital signs were as follows: temperature, 98.0°F; pulse, 52 beats/minute; respirations, 18/minute; blood pressure, 132/86 mm Hg. She is due for her AM medications. As you give Mrs. Bell her medications and state their purpose, she points to the Lanoxin and says, "Honey, I don't take that pill."

Medical Orders

Lanoxin 0.125 mg PO q AM
Lasix 20 mg PO q AM
KCl 10 mEq PO q AM

ECASA 1 tab PO qd
Pepcid 20 mg PO BID
Captopril 50 mg PO TID

Critical Thinking Questions

- How would you respond to Mrs. Bell's statement, "Honey, I don't take that pill"?

- Suggest ways in which you can confirm you are giving Mrs. Bell the correct medications.

(continued)

Case Study
Naomi Bell (Continued)

- Identify the medications that require assessment prior to administration.

- How would you determine Mrs. Bell's level of confusion?

- Describe factors that can contribute to inappropriate answers, and identify nursing actions to diminish these factors.

Integrated Nursing Care

Concepts

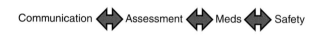

When patients question you regarding their medications, listen to them. Questions like this should send a "red flag" to the nurse. Often patients are familiar with what they normally take and can alert you that this may not be the right medication. Do not insist that Mrs. Bell take the Lanoxin until you confirm the accuracy of the order. In this case, it could be that Mrs. Bell just didn't hear what you said. Always confirm what patients say to you by restating it back to them. It could also be that she is more familiar with this drug's other name, which is digoxin.

To give medications safely, there are many safety checks you can use. Some measures include researching the drug before giving it and double-checking all of the five "rights." Compare the Kardex to the physician's order. If the order still remains unclear to you, call the physician to clarify it (see Chapter 5).

Some medications require assessment before you administer them to the patient. In this case, Mrs. Bell takes four medications that will require assessment prior to administration. Lanoxin, Lasix, and captopril will affect pulse and blood pressure. In addition, laboratory test results should be available on KCl and digoxin levels. If Mrs. Bell has a low pulse rate, low blood pressure, or a toxic laboratory value, you will not administer these medications and will notify the physician (see Chapter 5).

Sometimes elderly patients become confused in the hospital; this is known as "sundowner syndrome." However, do not assume this is always the case. The nurse who gave you report may have assumed that Mrs. Bell's inappropriate answers were due to confusion, when in fact they may be related to Mrs. Bell's hearing problem. When patients with hearing impairment are admitted to the hospital, encourage them to wear their hearing aids and help them check their batteries to ensure they are working. If you are still unclear whether Mrs. Bell is confused, perform a standard mental status examination used by your institution. This will establish a baseline assessment of her mental status that you can use to individualize her nursing plan of care.

If you determine she is confused, assess the source of confusion. Given Mrs. Bell's cardiac condition, assess her respiratory status and oxygen saturation level via pulse oximetry to determine whether she is experiencing hypoxia or ischemia. If the cause is physiologic, notify the physician immediately. Another source contributing to confusion could be isolation caused by hearing loss. One way to reduce possible confusion for Mrs. Bell is to improve communication. Ensure that her hearing aid battery is operating and that the unit is placed correctly. Other ways to improve communication include talking to her at eye level, facing her directly when speaking, or even speaking into her "good" ear. If Mrs. Bell's vision is better than her hearing, you can also give her pertinent information in writing.

Case Study
John Willis

You are a nursing student in your first semester of nursing school and your second week of clinical. You are asked to take care of John Willis, a man with suspected tuberculosis (TB) and a positive culture of methicillin-resistant *Staphylococcus aureus* (MRSA) in his sputum. You tell your clinical instructor you are scared of catching TB and MRSA, but your instructor explains that since you have reviewed this subject in lab, you are ready to take care of this patient. When you go to your patient's room, you see the isolation cart containing the infection control precaution supplies outside the room, with the hospital's policy and procedure posted for precautions to use for TB and MRSA. You see there are individual masks in plastic bags with different people's names on them, as well as masks with protective eye shields. You remember hearing something in lab about wearing a specially fitted mask when implementing these precautions. You find your instructor, who is very busy consulting with a physician and a student about an emergent patient situation. You interrupt your nursing instructor and say, "I don't have a mask to care for my patient." Your instructor snaps at you, saying, "Just go take care of your patient." You think it is your duty to care for this patient, so you gown and glove and "borrow" a mask from one of the bags. You go into your patient's room to take his vital signs and obtain a sputum specimen. The patient coughs frequently and is able to expectorate the sputum specimen. Upon leaving the room, you place the mask in your pocket and then assist the staff nurse with obtaining vital signs on other patients.

Medical Orders

Airborne precautions
Contact precautions
Sputum specimen for C&S
Vital signs q shift

Critical Thinking Questions

- Compare the mode of transmission for TB and MRSA.

- Identify the appropriate protective equipment needed to care for a patient with TB and a patient with MRSA.

- What can occur if you place the mask in your pocket and then enter other patient rooms?

- What may have led to the nursing instructor's snapping?

- Describe another way in which you could have approached this situation.

(continued)

Case Study
John Willis (Continued)

Integrated Nursing Care

Concepts

Safety ⟷ Isolation ⟷ Communication

TB transmission occurs through airborne respiratory droplets. MRSA transmission can occur through contact with contaminated blood or body fluids. MRSA can be spread by direct or indirect contact. In this case, MRSA could be transmitted indirectly by coming into contact with any soiled items, such as the mask (CDC, 2003, p. 3).

Agencies will require the use of gowns, gloves, and masks when caring for patients with TB and MRSA. Unique to the airborne precautions needed for TB is the use of specially fitted masks called high-efficiency particulate air (HEPA) masks that prevent the inspiration of airborne microorganisms (see Chapter 4). There are also disposable masks available, but they usually require fit-testing as well. If a fit-tested mask is required by your agency, you would either need to be fit-tested for a mask (often done by employee health) or reassigned to another patient. In addition, to protect yourself whenever there is the potential for contamination to your eyes, such as coughing, you should wear goggles or a mask with a face shield (Taylor et al., 2005). Institutions vary greatly in their supplies. If you place an MRSA-contaminated mask in your pocket and then enter other rooms to provide care,

the potential for transmitting a nosocomial infection is high. It is always your responsibility, even as a student, to follow the policy and procedure of the agency where you are placed for clinical.

Hospitals are stressful places, even for nursing instructors. Understanding when and how to confront others will serve you well in nursing. In this situation, waiting for the instructor to resolve the emergency before confronting him would have been the ideal situation. Since there was no urgency to obtain the vital signs and sputum specimen, they could have waited until the instructor was more available. With time and experience, you will learn to prioritize what is urgent and what can wait.

If you meet with an angry response when trying to communicate, learn to develop a "tough skin." Nurses are sometimes on the receiving end of anger, even when the anger is not directed at them. It is a learned skill to stay calm in the face of anger and understand it is not a personal attack. Your goal in communicating about patients is to acquire the information you need in order to provide the best care possible. While waiting for the instructor, you could get your "ducks in a row"—that is, obtain as much information as possible. Background research and knowledge are powerful tools. Examples of resources you can access include the hospital policy and procedure manual, the infection control nurse, and experienced staff members. Then when your instructor is available, you can share this information with him to plan your care for that day.

Case Study
Claudia Tran

Claudia Tran, age 84, has been on your skilled nursing floor for several weeks following a CVA. She had previously been a resident of a long-term care facility. Her neuro checks and vital signs are unchanged from her baseline admission. Her CVA has impaired her ability to chew and swallow. She has left-sided weakness with flaccidity of her left hand. She is emaciated and her skin is very fragile. She has reddened areas on her coccyx, heels, and elbows. She is receiving weekly vitamin B_{12} injections for pernicious anemia. Over the past week, Mrs. Tran has become increasingly confused and incontinent. Because of this, soft wrist restraints have been ordered. She has a nasogastric tube for tube feedings, which she receives every 8 hours. During your shift, Mrs. Tran is due for a tube feeding. You check the residual and it is approximately 380 mL.

Medical Orders

Soft wrist restraints for safety
Vitamin B_{12} injection 1,000 mcg IM weekly

Nasogastric tube feedings q 8 hr
Physical therapy daily, passive and active ROM as tolerated

Critical Thinking Questions

- Considering Mrs. Tran's condition, what special safety measures should be implemented with her restraints?

- What are the risks of falling for this patient?

(continued)

Case Study
Claudia Tran (Continued)

- Identify the risks associated with tube feeding for this patient.

- Identify appropriate sites for the vitamin B$_{12}$ injections in Mrs. Tran. Develop a schedule of rotating sites for this injection.

- Identify risk factors and preventive measures for Mrs. Tran's skin breakdown.

Integrated Nursing Care

Concepts

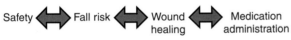

Safety ⟷ Fall risk ⟷ Wound healing ⟷ Medication administration

Soft wrist restraints should be used only as a last resort after all other measures have failed. Other measures could include placing her bed in a low position, having a family member sit with her, and placing her in a room near the nurses' station. Restraints must be used only with a physician's order, and you must follow strict guidelines to protect the patient. Since Mrs. Tran already has skin breakdown, pad the restraints and make sure they are the correct size. An additional safety measure would be performing frequent neurovascular checks, such as checking warmth, sensation, and capillary refill. Most agencies require releasing restraints at specified frequencies. This will improve the circulation to her extremities, reduce the chance of skin breakdown, and give you an opportunity to assess the site. Mrs. Tran has left-sided weakness; therefore, applying a restraint on her flaccid arm could cause harm and is not needed (see Chapter 3).

Mrs. Tran has many risk factors for skin breakdown, including immobilization, malnutrition, altered mental status, age, incontinence, and positioning for tube feedings. To reduce these risk factors and prevent further skin breakdown will require a multifaceted approach. Placing Mrs. Tran on a turning schedule is essential. She could benefit from a special type of mattress, such as an air mattress. Implementing a physical therapy program of passive ROM exercises would

be helpful. A nutritional consult would be of utmost importance to ensure she will receive adequate protein, as well as other vitamins and minerals essential for skin integrity.

What skin breakdown complications could result from immobilization and incontinence? You and the doctor could consider the risks versus benefits of placement of a urinary retention catheter for Mrs. Tran. A noninvasive way to reduce the chance of recurrent incontinence is to offer Mrs. Tran a bedpan at regular intervals.

Since Mrs. Tran is confused and in a restraint, her risk for falling is high. Her bed should be in a low position at all times and her call light within reach. Frequently check on patients such as Mrs. Tran to decrease isolation and provide orientation.

Mrs. Tran is receiving tube feedings and has an excessive residual. She is at increased risk for aspiration of tube feedings into her lungs if positioned supine. To decrease the risk for aspiration, check the residual amount before every feeding. In this situation, Mrs. Tran's residual was over 300 mL. Therefore, her head should remain elevated, her tube feeding will be held, and her physician should be contacted as soon as possible (see Chapter 11).

When giving Mrs. Tran vitamin B$_{12}$ injections, use larger muscles and rotate sites. Implement the rotation schedule for this injection in her plan of care. This is particularly important since Mrs. Tran is emaciated and does not have good muscle mass. Avoid areas that are reddened or have palpable nodules and scars. Since vitamin B$_{12}$ injections can be irritating, inject the medication slowly to minimize pain, trauma, and discomfort (see Chapter 5).

Case Study
Joe LeRoy

Joe LeRoy, age 60, was brought in by his daughter and admitted to your small rural hospital. He has had the stomach flu at home for several days and is suffering from dehydration. He has right-sided hemiplegia due to a CVA 3 years ago. Mr. LeRoy has been remaining in bed during his hospital stay due to extreme weakness and fatigue. You received report on your seven patients. From report, you note that Mr. LeRoy continues to have frequent liquid stools (averaging about three or four times/shift). The doctor has ordered a stool sample for culture and sensitivity. When entering his room, you notice his sheets are very dirty and he has a body odor.

Medical Orders

IVF: D5 1/2 NS IV at 125 mL/hr
Stool sample for C&S
VS q shift

Critical Thinking Questions

- Develop your priorities and rationales for the following nursing care for Mr. LeRoy:
  - Changing his sheets

  - Completing the AM assessment

  - Obtaining vital signs

  - Collecting the sample

  - Giving a bath

- What considerations should be taken into account when collecting the stool sample?

- Are there any assessments that you would want to pay particular attention to during your nursing care?

- Describe how your attitude and nonverbal behavior could affect Mr. LeRoy's hospital experience.

(continued)

Case Study
Joe LeRoy (Continued)

Integrated Nursing Care

Concepts

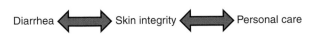

Diarrhea ⟷ Skin integrity ⟷ Personal care

Prioritizing care is a difficult but important skill for all nurses. Determine whether Mr. LeRoy can provide his own AM care, although this is unlikely due to his hemiplegia and weakness. If you need to assist him with his personal care, determine the needs of your other patients before beginning this task. Before leaving Mr. LeRoy, let him know your plan and the time he can expect to have assistance with his bath. Another alternative is letting a nursing assistant (if you have one on your unit) know of Mr. LeRoy's need for a bath and linen change. On your initial assessment of Mr. LeRoy, cover any very obviously dirty areas of his sheets with a blue waterproof pad or a clean sheet. You could also offer him a wet, warm washcloth and a dry towel for initial cleaning while you are completing his assessment. You should also inform him of the need for a stool specimen.

If your floor has no nursing aide, return to his room after your other patient assessments are complete. An experienced nurse would first obtain the warm stool sample, give the bath, and then change his linens. This sequence saves time and energy for both the nurse and the patient, because when giving an occupied bath or assisting a patient on a bedpan, you can easily soil the linens.

While wearing gloves, collect and send the stool specimen promptly to the laboratory. Specimens should be sent while still warm, as the microorganisms present at body temperature may die when the specimen temperature changes, and this would produce a false-negative result (see Chapter 13).

During your assessment, pay particular attention to his skin. Mr. LeRoy is at risk for pressure ulcers due to his age, diarrhea, altered nutrition, and immobility. Have Mr. LeRoy turn over so that you can inspect his back and bony prominences, the most likely areas for skin breakdown. If you notice any skin breakdown, notify the physician so that treatment can begin promptly.

A nurse's nonverbal behavior can have a dramatic impact on a patient's hospital experience. This may just be another day at work for you, but for a patient, spending time in the hospital is a significant life event. Projecting a cheerful attitude and providing nonjudgmental care help a patient cope with hospitalization. You may be offended by Mr. LeRoy's body odor and the smell of his stool, but as a nurse you will need to learn strategies to manage strong odors and make sure that your facial expressions or body language do not convey discomfort or disgust.

Case Study
Kate Townsend

Kate Townsend, a 70-year-old patient with COPD, has just returned to your medical-surgical unit from surgery for excision of a nonmalignant polyp. She has a midline abdominal transverse incision secured with sutures and covered with a dry sterile dressing. She has a right peripheral IV with D5 1/2 NS @ 75 mL/hr. She has a history of long-term steroid use for her COPD. She has a nasogastric tube in her right naris, which is clamped at this time. The physician orders oxygen 2 L via nasal cannula. This is your first semester, fourth week in nursing school, and the nurse asks you to place the patient on oxygen. When you attempt to place the cannula in the patient's naris with the NG tube, you think it is uncomfortable and a little odd. For comfort, you decide to place a simple oxygen mask on Mrs. Townsend instead. Her vital signs are as follows: temperature, 99.6°F; pulse, 76 beats/minute; respirations, 24 breaths/minute; blood pressure, 110/70 mm Hg.

Medical Orders

NG clamped
MSO₄ 2–4 mg q 4–6 hr prn pain
IVF: D5 1/2 NS @ 75 mL/hr

Incentive spirometry prn
Oxygen 2 L via nasal cannula

Critical Thinking Questions

- What is the difference between oxygen given in a nasal cannula and that given via a simple oxygen mask?

- What comfort measures would you want to provide for Mrs. Townsend?

(continued)

Case Study
Kate Townsend (Continued)

- What is a complication that could occur with Mrs. Townsend when changing her to a simple oxygen mask?

- Considering Mrs. Townsend's chronic lung disease, what are the complications that can occur, and what nursing interventions could decrease these complications?

- Develop a discharge plan for Mrs. Townsend.

Integrated Nursing Care

Concepts

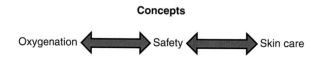

Oxygenation ⟷ Safety ⟷ Skin care

Several delivery systems exist to provide oxygen to patients, and they deliver varying amounts of oxygen. Oxygen delivered via a nasal cannula set at 2 L would deliver about 28% oxygen, whereas oxygen delivered in a simple mask could deliver 40% to 60% oxygen, depending on the flow meter setting (see Chapter 14). Oxygen is considered a medicine, so it is not a nursing order but a medical order. Nurses are not allowed to change oxygen delivery systems or the oxygen concentration without a physician's order.

For people without chronic lung disease, breathing is driven by the buildup of carbon dioxide levels in the blood (hypercapnia). The drive to breathe for patients with COPD is a lack of oxygen (hypoxia). Because of this, increasing oxygen levels in patients with COPD will, in fact, make them stop breathing. Therefore, when changing Mrs. Townsend for comfort reasons from the nasal cannula to the mask, you could have increased her oxygen anywhere from 12% to 32%, and even a small increase in oxygen has the potential to stop her breathing. Although it is not entirely comfortable to have a NG tube, much less another tube in the naris, it is not unusual for this to occur. Both will fit with some manipulation by the nurse.

Patients with chronic lung disease are at increased risk after surgery for pulmonary complications, including atelectasis and pneumonia. General anesthesia alters all of the muscles involved in breathing and clearing the airway. COPD is a restrictive lung disease, meaning that the patient's lungs lose their elasticity and become less compliant. For Mrs. Townsend, this combination of underlying disease and the effects of surgery results in a decreased ability to mobilize secretions, which could lead to atelectasis and possibly pneumonia. Mrs. Townsend may be experiencing atelectasis due to her temperature of 99.6°F. Other signs of atelectasis would be decreased breath sounds in the lung bases, shortness of breath, increased respiratory rate, and decreased oxygen saturation of pulse oximetry. Without nursing intervention, atelectasis could lead to pneumonia. Measures to facilitate lung expansion and mobilization of secretions will minimize atelectasis. These nursing measures include elevation of the head of her bed, deep-breathing exercises, incentive spirometry, adequate pain control, and early ambulation.

Long-term steroid use can make the skin very fragile, increase the potential for skin breakdown, and delay wound healing. To prevent this, observe the skin under her NG and oxygen cannula tubing. The pressure of the tubes on her face and behind her ears could cause a break in skin integrity. Repositioning the tape that is holding the NG tube may make it more comfortable. If needed, you may need to "pad" the skin under the cannula tubing with hydrocolloids, especially if the skin becomes reddened. There are many commercial products to hold oxygen nasal cannulas, as well as NG tubes, which may also increase her comfort.

Discharge plans for Mrs. Townsend would need to address both her underlying lung disease as well as her recent intestinal surgery. Patient education should focus on measures that enable Mrs. Townsend to improve her lung compliance and increase her oxygenation. Incentive spirometry and a daily activity schedule will be imperative. Due to her prolonged use of steroids, she may also have delayed wound healing at her incision site. Patient education should address optimal nutrition and prevention of infection. Before discharge, validate Mrs. Townsend's knowledge of measures to prevent pulmonary and wound complications.

Case Study
Tula Stillwater

Tula Stillwater is a 36-year-old Native American who has had diabetes since age 26. She weighs 218 lb. She is gravida 1 para 1 and delivered a 9 lb, 6 oz boy via cesarean section 3 days ago. She has a transverse abdominal incision with staples and reports tenderness on the right side of the incision but acute pain on the left side of the incision. Her 8 a.m. vital signs are as follows: temperature, 101.6°F; pulse 76 beats/min; respirations, 18 per minute; blood pressure, 134/78 mm Hg. Her blood sugar before breakfast is 185 mg/dL; her blood sugars on previous days had ranged from 90 to 124 mg/dL.

On your assessment, you find her incision is open to air and the staples are intact. The incision is well approximated and without erythema on the right side. However, the left side of the incision is pulling apart and is edematous and warm to the touch, with a scant amount of purulent drainage.

Medical Orders

VS q 4 hr
FSBS AC & QHS
Regular insulin per sliding scale

Standing order: Remove staples before discharge.
Standing order: Discharge on third day if stable.

Critical Thinking Questions

- What is your interpretation of her vital signs? Who should be notified and when?

- How would you determine whether Mrs. Stillwater meets the criteria for discharge?

- What is the relationship between Mrs. Stillwater's diabetes and her postsurgical condition?

- What factors affect her staple removal?

- How should you respond to her FSBS?

- What nursing interventions would you foresee performing?

- Describe the timing and the technique for administering her insulin.

(continued)

Case Study
Tula Stillwater (Continued)

Integrated Nursing Care

Concepts

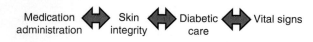

Medication administration ⟷ Skin integrity ⟷ Diabetic care ⟷ Vital signs

Mrs. Stillwater's vital signs should alert you to a potential complication. She may have an infection related to her incision, as evidenced by her increased temperature and her subjective report of acute pain at the incision. Her blood pressure could be a result of her pain, but it should be compared to her baseline and monitored. You inspected the incision carefully for signs of infection. Her physician needs to be notified immediately of this potential complication.

Wound healing may be impaired in people with diabetes, so any patient with diabetes requires vigilant wound assessment. Additionally, the stress of surgery usually results in increased blood sugar levels. Mrs. Stillwater's FSBS is elevated from her baseline, another symptom of a possible infection. When you see a dramatic increase in blood sugar in a patient with diabetes, consider the possible etiologies.

Despite the urgency of this new complication of wound infection, Mrs. Stillwater should receive her insulin and breakfast as she usually would. Administer her insulin in a subcutaneous site; she can help you identify the site where she should receive her insulin. Patients who are accustomed to managing their diabetes at home will have preferences when in the hospital, and these preferences should be honored.

Many women who have had cesarean sections are discharged on the third day. One of the expected outcomes for discharge would include being free of infection. Mrs. Stillwater is not free of infection: she has pain at her incision site, a fever, and an elevated FSBS. When you notify the physician of these symptoms, she orders a complete blood count, a wound culture, incision site care, and cancellation of the discharge.

Given the delayed discharge and impaired wound healing, you would not want to remove the staples from this incision because removing the staples at this time could place Mrs. Stillwater at risk for dehiscence. Another factor affecting the risk for dehiscence and impaired wound healing is Mrs. Stillwater's increased subcutaneous fat (Taylor et al., 2005).

Did you foresee obtaining a complete blood count and a wound culture and performing incision site care? Did you also anticipate that this patient should not be discharged nor have her staples removed? In addition, although her physiologic care is very important, you will also need to relieve anxiety related to this infection and acknowledge her disappointment that she cannot go home today.

Intermediate Case Studies

Olivia Greenbaum is a 9-month-old infant admitted with respiratory syncytial virus (RSV). She was born prematurely at 30 weeks' gestation. Her complications at birth included respiratory distress syndrome (RDS), suspected sepsis ×1, and formula intolerance. She was discharged home after 5 weeks on soy-based formula. This is her first hospitalization since her birth. Olivia is Mr. and Mrs. Greenbaum's only child, and they are very anxious. Mrs. Greenbaum is her primary care provider.

Olivia is receiving supplemental humidified oxygen administered via oxygen tent at 40%. She is very fussy and is not tolerating separation from her mother well. She has a peripheral IV inserted in her right hand; it is infusing D5 $\frac{1}{4}$ NS at 20 mL/hr. It is covered with a sock puppet. She is wearing a T-shirt and a disposable diaper. She is quite active within the crib. Her previous vital signs were as follows: temperature, 36.4°C ax; pulse, 84 beats/min; respirations, 38/minute; blood pressure, 94/58 mm Hg.

Mrs. Greenbaum spent the night and is currently sleeping in the recliner in Olivia's room. You enter the room and observe Olivia sleeping. She is pale with circumoral cyanosis. Her respiratory rate is 40/minute with an audible expiratory wheeze. Her heart rate on the monitor is 86 bpm; her pulse rate is 62 bpm. The pulse oximeter is currently showing an oxygen saturation level of 68%, and the alarm is turned off.

Medical Orders

VS q 4 hr
O_2 via tent at 40%
Continuous pulse oximetry when quiet; may obtain q hr intermittent pulse oximeter readings when active
IVF: D5 1/4 NS @ 20 mL/hr

Encourage coughing.
Maintain O_2 saturation 93% to 97%. Adjust O_2 in increments of 2% up to a max of 50%.
Isomil 6–8 oz q 4 hr when awake
HR/resp. monitor

Critical Thinking Questions

- What is your first priority after observing Olivia sleeping?

- Should you increase the oxygen being administered?

- What is your interpretation of her vital signs and oxygen saturation?

- Give examples of how to manage thermoregulation within an oxygen tent.

(continued)

Case Study
Olivia Greenbaum
(Continued)

- Identify factors that affect the accuracy of the oxygen saturation reading.

- How frequently should Olivia's IV site be assessed? What is the function of the sock puppet?

- How do you encourage coughing in a 9-month-old baby?

Integrated Nursing Care

Concepts

Oxygenation ⬄ Hypothermia ⬄ Infant care

Your first priority is to establish whether Olivia is hypoxic. You noted a rapid respiratory rate and circumoral cyanosis, both potential symptoms of hypoxia. The pulse oximeter heart rate does not match the cardiac monitor heart rate. Gently, without disturbing Olivia, you begin to reattach the pulse oximeter.

Your preliminary assessment is that the pulse oximeter is not accurately assessing her oxygenation. You are able to hold the probe to her toe and get a reading of 95%. Olivia begins to wake up. Take her apical heart rate, which is the most reliable site for infants and small children (see Chapter 1). Compare her apical pulse rate to the heart rate on the pulse oximeter as well as the heart rate on the cardiac monitor. Nurses must always verify that the equipment is accurately reflecting the patient's status. Next, you take her temperature, which is 36.2°C. The humidified oxygen is also cooling Olivia, making her hands, feet, and lips appear cold, blue, and dusky (see Chapter 14).

Once Olivia is awake, she will not tolerate having the pulse oximeter probe on her toe and keeps pulling it off. You will need to check the oxygen saturation intermittently. Your next priority is to warm her up. When children become chilled, they have increased energy ex-penditure. When infants are stressed beyond aerobic metabolism, they use anaerobic metabolism. This produces lactic acid, which increases the acidity of the blood, exacerbating respiratory distress. Urge her mother to bring in more clothes and to layer her clothes to keep Olivia thermoregulated within the humidified tent. You do not need to increase the oxygen level; what at first looked like hypoxia is in fact hypothermia!

The accuracy of a pulse oximetry reading is affected by several factors, including patient perfusion and peripheral vasoconstriction. Other factors that prevent the detection of oxygen saturation may be as simple as nail polish or artificial nails (see Chapter 14).

Encouraging coughing in an infant is accomplished either through crying or laughing. If the infant is periodically crying vigorously, that is sufficient. You can try tickling or playing peek-a-boo to get a 1-year-old to laugh. Crying and laughing require deep breaths and will cause a patient to cough, thus promoting airway clearance.

Check this patient's IV site every hour to ensure there are no signs of infiltration. The sock puppet is one way to disguise the IV site dressing while leaving it accessible for examination. If a young child can see the IV site dressing, he or she will often persist in trying to remove the tape and dressing despite all your efforts. If you cover the site, the child will not remember it is there. Piaget's theory of cognitive development includes the concept of object permanence (Taylor et al., 2005). At 9 months old, a child cannot imagine what he or she cannot see—in other words, what is out of sight is out of mind.

Case Study
Victoria Holly

Victoria Holly, age 68, is newly admitted to the hospital due to anemia and severe dehydration. To treat the dehydration she has an IV of D5 1/2 NS infusing into the right hand. To treat the anemia, she has a heparin lock in her left arm to be used for blood administration only. She recently received 2 units of packed red blood cells. You have MD orders to draw a complete blood count and a CMP. Mrs. Holly also has an ileostomy, which she has managed for several years on her own. Upon your initial physical assessment of Mrs. Holly, you find her vital signs are as follows: temperature, 97.2°F; pulse, 96 beats/minute; respirations, 18/minute; blood pressure, 88/50 mm Hg. Her skin is "tenting" and you cannot palpate her peripheral pulses. Her lips are dry and cracked. The skin around her stoma site is bright red and open in areas. You notice that her ostomy pouch was cut much larger than the stoma site. She reports she is very tired and "lacks energy." Her family informs you that she has always been a very independent person but in the last couple of months she just "hasn't been herself."

Medical Orders

IVF: D5 1/2 NS IV @ 125 mL/hr
Daily weights

Strict I&O
CBC and CMP stat

Critical Thinking Questions

- Identify appropriate sites and equipment needed to draw the blood.

- Describe how you would assess Mrs. Holly's peripheral circulation.

- What concerns you about Mrs. Holly's present condition in relationship to performing her ADLs independently?

- What is alarming about her ileostomy? Identify possible explanations for the stoma's condition.

- What are measurable physical parameters you can use to determine whether fluid replacement therapy and blood administration are sufficient?

- Develop a discharge teaching plan for Mrs. Holly related to her ostomy care.

Integrated Nursing Care

Concepts

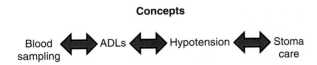

Blood sampling ⬌ ADLs ⬌ Hypotension ⬌ Stoma care

You cannot draw blood specimens from a dedicated line such as the one Mrs. Holly has for blood administration. You also cannot obtain the specimen from above the IV in her right hand because the specimen will be diluted with the D5 1/2 NS solution and will, thus, be inaccurate. You should not stick her again because she already has a usable IV in her right hand. You can draw her CBC and CMP by briefly stopping and flushing the IV fluid (per hospital policy), then drawing the blood sample. Some hospital laboratories require a "waste" sample be drawn before obtaining the actual samples; check your hospital laboratory's policy regarding drawing blood specimens from IV infusions. You will also

(continued)

Case Study
Victoria Holly (Continued)

need to flush the IV afterwards per hospital policy and restart the infusion. Equipment you will need to draw the blood includes syringes, needles, alcohol swabs, the hospital's IV flush solution, laboratory tubes, gloves, and a tourniquet.

Mrs. Holly's vital signs are disconcerting because her blood pressure is low. Because of her hypotension, ADLs may unduly tax her. Until you see a positive change in her vital signs, you should provide assistance with her ADLs (see Chapter 7). In addition, Mrs. Holly has an IV in each arm. It would be difficult for her to care for the ostomy while attempting to keep the IV sites free from infection.

One outcome to anticipate with Mrs. Holly would be an increase in blood pressure. Other outcomes include palpable peripheral pulses and normal skin turgor. Subjectively, Mrs. Holly should report that she has an increase in energy. Her family may also comment that she is becoming more "like herself." Sometimes healthcare workers make judgments about elderly people, thinking that they are always tired. Since the healthcare workers are often unfamiliar with their patients' normal conditions, comments made by family members can often be very helpful in determining progress. This is especially true if your patient cannot communicate. Objectively, one outcome would be that Mrs. Holly becomes more active in her own care.

When a patient has no peripheral pulses, you must investigate further. Never ignore the absence of pulses, as this could signal a life-threatening condition. Have another nurse check the pulses, or you can use a Doppler. Upon checking Mrs. Holly's pulses with a Doppler device, you were able to hear them and marked them with an "x" to facilitate future assessments. In your initial assessment, you were not surprised that Mrs. Holly's pulses were nonpalpable, as she has a very low circulating volume (see Chapter 1).

Mrs. Holly's ileostomy site is very red and excoriated. You are alarmed, as this could place her at risk for infection; the physician will need to be notified. Do not assume that a physician has seen the excoriation around the ostomy site. If the patient came into the hospital with more pressing matters such as decreased blood pressure, the physician may not have observed the ileostomy. Sometimes it is only the nurse who completes a thorough head-to-toe assessment. Mrs. Holly may lack knowledge about the appropriate method for cutting stoma patches. You suspect that she may be cutting the patches such that they are leaving skin exposed to the liquid stool, which is then causing the excoriation (see Chapter 13).

One area you should investigate is Mrs. Holly's ability to care for the ostomy before she came to the hospital. It is possible that her skin around the stoma site has looked like this for a period of time. Before her hospital discharge, evaluate her knowledge through return demonstration to ensure that she can care for the stoma and can identify possible family resources. She may benefit from a home health referral to ensure she is caring for her stoma properly.

Case Study
Tula Stillwater

It is now day 5 in the hospital for Mrs. Stillwater. She has developed a staphylococcal infection in her cesarean section incision. This is the second time you have cared for this patient. You are familiar with her diabetic status, baseline vital signs, and routine postpartum care. She is currently receiving an IV antibiotic. Her vital signs are as follows: temperature, 99.2°F; pulse, 74 beats/min; respirations, 18/minute; blood pressure, 130/80 mm Hg. Her FSBS before breakfast is 120 mg/dL.

You learned in report that her incision is intact and healing on the right side, but the far left side of her incision is being packed with iodoform strips, requiring about half a bottle to fill the wound. The open part of the incision is approximately 1″ long, 0.5″ wide, and 1″ deep. This part of her incision is draining copious amounts of foul-smelling, yellow to green purulent drainage. The incision is very painful. Mrs. Stillwater reports her pain at a 6 on a scale of 1 to 10 (10 = worst) before her pain medication is administered.

Mrs. Stillwater's 5-day-old boy is now bottle-feeding regularly. He is taking 3 oz of Similac with Iron every 4 hours. Mrs. Stillwater is eager to assume the majority of his care.

Medical Orders

IV lock; flush q shift and prn
Vancomycin 1.0 g IV q 12 hr
Sterile dressing change with iodoform packing q shift
Irrigate wound with NS with dressing change
FSBS q ac and q hs
Regular insulin per s.s.
VS q 4 hr
Lortab 7.5 mg, 1 to 2 tabs q 4 to 6 hr prn pain

Case Study
Tula Stillwater (Continued)

Critical Thinking Questions

- How will you plan her dressing change, and what equipment will you need?

- How will you organize your nursing care to provide uninterrupted time for Mrs. Stillwater to care for her 5-day-old son?

- Describe your assessment and interventions for this wound.

- What techniques can you show Mrs. Stillwater to improve her mobility and ability to hold and care for her infant?

- Identify factors that will promote wound healing in Mrs. Stillwater.

- Describe the procedure you will use to administer the IV antibiotic.

Integrated Nursing Care

Concepts

Pain ⟷ Infection ⟷ Wound healing ⟷ Mother/baby care

Mrs. Stillwater's dressing change will be stressful and uncomfortable. To manage the pain, the dressing change should be performed after she has taken her pain medication and you have allowed enough time for it to be effective. Given her diabetic status, she should be allowed to eat her breakfast and receive her insulin before you begin her dressing change. Mrs. Stillwater's focus is probably on her son. Encourage her to give him his morning bottle and to be satisfied that he is comfortable before you begin the dressing change.

Review Chapter 8 to develop the list of equipment you will need for the dressing change. You will need to set up a sterile field and stringently maintain the sterility of the dressing change. Mrs. Stillwater can be positioned supine and rotated slightly to her left to promote drainage of the wound during irrigation.

Your assessment of the wound will include the size, the presence of granulation tissue, a description of the drainage, wound color, the presence of edema and erythema, and temperature (see Chapter 7). Note the condition of the skin at the wound edges as well as the skin where the wound dressing is taped. Look for changes in the condition of the wound and note how Mrs. Stillwater is tolerating the dressing change. If she will be taught to care for this wound and perform the dressing changes at home, instruction and return demonstration would become part of her discharge planning.

For Mrs. Stillwater's wound to heal, the infection must be resolved and the wound edges will need to become approximated. To optimize wound healing, Mrs. Stillwater will need a diet high in protein and minerals. You may need to obtain a nutritional consultation (Taylor et al., 2005).

The care of her infant son is a priority for Mrs. Stillwater. Cluster your nursing care such as wound dressings, vital signs, and medication administration to allow her sufficient time to provide care for her son.

Make sure Mrs. Stillwater knows how to use a splint, such as a pillow, across her abdomen to give support to her abdominal musculature when moving or coughing. Spending time in a comfortable chair will be preferable to getting in and out of bed. Assess that Mrs. Stillwater is

(continued)

Case Study
Tula Stillwater (Continued)

using the "football hold" to feed and comfort her son. The advantage of this position is that the infant does not rest on the mother's abdomen. Mrs. Stillwater should have several pillows available to provide support for her arms when holding her infant.

To give the IV antibiotic, assess the IV site for patency, flush the IV per hospital policy prior to administration, administer the antibiotics according to the manufacturer's instructions, and then flush the heparin lock after the antibiotic is infused.

Case Study
Jason Brown

Jason Brown is a 21-year-old college football player. It is the second postop day following surgical repair of a fracture of his right tibia and fibula. He has sutures over the anterior knee and lateral malleolus and a posterior splint on the right leg. He continues to report considerable pain. His vital signs at midnight were as follows 98.3°F; pulse, 58 beats/min; respirations, 12/minute; blood pressure 118/70 mm Hg. He reported his pain as a 3 on a scale of 1 of 10 (10 = worst) at about 10 p.m. He has a peripheral IV in his left forearm infusing D5 1/2 NS as a keep-vein-open (TKO) rate. He is using a PCA pump for pain relief. The nursing care for the morning includes routine a.m. care, cast care, and a trip to PT. You are on the day shift. Shortly after morning report, the unit clerk catches you and says, "Jason says he needs a nurse. He is in terrible pain."

You enter the room. Jason is pale and diaphoretic. His sheets are damp with some wet spots. He says, "My leg hurts. It really hurts." You ask him to rate his pain, and he answers, "At least an 8. I've been pushing my pain pump but I'm still in pain." His IV site looks okay. You say, "I'm going to find out why it is hurting. I need to get your vital signs first." His vital signs now are as follows: temperature, 98.9°F; pulse, 72 beats/min; respirations, 20/minute; blood pressure, 124/78 mm Hg.

Medical Orders

VS q 4 hr
IVF: D5 1/2 NS TKO
Ambien 5 mg q HS

PCA—MSO$_4$ 1 mg q 6 min lock, max 40 mg in 4 hr
Physical therapy for weight-bearing as tolerated

Critical Thinking Questions

- What is the significance of the changes in Jason's vital signs?

- What interventions for Jason's pain must occur immediately before administering nursing care and PT?

- How do you assess the following:
  - Infection versus inflammation?

  - Neurovascular compromise?

  - IV patency?

(continued)

Case Study
Jason Brown (Continued)

Integrated Nursing Care

Concepts

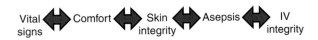

Vital signs ◆▶ Comfort ◆▶ Skin integrity ◆▶ Asepsis ◆▶ IV integrity

Always compare vital signs to a comparable baseline and the previous vital signs (see Chapter 1). While Jason's temperature is elevated slightly, it has not increased dramatically, as it would be with an infection. His respiratory rate and pulse rate were quite low at midnight. Since he is a young, healthy athlete, his resting pulse rate may be lower than what is often considered as the norm. You notice that his resting pulse rates on the night shift have been running from 56 to 60 beats/min. Another factor contributing to his decreased pulse rate is the effect of the Ambien that he took at 9 p.m. to help him sleep. Therefore, while his morning respiratory rate and pulse rate are still within normal range, they represent a significant increase from his resting baseline. These are objective assessments supporting his assertion of increased pain.

One reason for an increase in pain with any postsurgical patient is the possibility of infection. Quickly assess all surgical incision sites and observe for redness, swelling, or a foul odor (Chapter 8). Due to short hospital stays, signs and symptoms of infection do not usually appear until after the patient is discharged (Taylor et al., 2005).

In addition to infection, Jason is at risk for neurovascular compromise because of the trauma to his right leg as well as from the splint and dressing. Assess for neurovascular compromise and perform cast care (see Chapter 9). Jason's fracture has been placed in a splint rather than a cast, which is a more current surgical practice, but nurses still refer to the care of the affected extremity as "cast care." Determine whether there are any signs of compartment syndrome (see Chapter 9). You need no additional equipment for this assessment, and it should take very little time; do this immediately.

Upon assessment, you find that Jason's foot and leg are pink and warm with 2+ pulses, no edema, full sensation, motion, and capillary refill measuring less than 3 seconds. The incision sites show no redness, swelling, drainage, or foul odor.

Another possible reason for his pain is that his IV may no longer be patent and, therefore, he would not be receiving any pain medication. You remember the wet spots on the bed as you begin systematically checking each of the IV administration-set connections. Your assessment of the IV site shows no swelling, and he reports no pain at the site. Your next check should be from the IV site to the IV tubing. You find that the connection of the IV tubing to the IV insertion catheter is loose and leaking. Determine whether the IV site is still patent (see Chapter 15). If the IV is still patent, replace the IV tubing (see Chapter 5). Check the medication in the PCA pump to ensure it is the correct medication. Most agencies will require that you check the PCA history to determine the amount of medication used as well as the amount remaining (see Chapter 10).

Contact the physician to explain that the PCA pain medication was infusing onto the sheets, and obtain an order for an appropriate bolus dose so that Jason can obtain immediate pain relief. After 30 minutes, obtain another set of vital signs and perform a pain assessment. Document the evaluation of your interventions. Jason's pain will need to be controlled before initiating additional nursing care. Coordinating with PT to reschedule his therapy until his pain is resolved is a nursing responsibility.

Case Study
Kent Clark

Kent Clark, age 29, was admitted 24 hours ago for observation related to a suspected closed head injury following a motor vehicle accident (MVA). Mr. Clark's baseline vital signs are stable. He has a cervical collar and is scheduled to undergo a MRI to determine if he has a cervical spine injury. The physician has asked you to reduce his activity until cervical spinal injuries are ruled out.

Currently, Mr. Clark is awake, alert, and oriented (AAO ×3); his pupils are equally round and reactive to light and accommodation (PERRLA). He moves all four extremities bilaterally. His head is elevated 30 degrees to minimize increased intracranial pressure (ICP) and edema. A peripheral IV in his right arm is infusing D5 1/2 NS at 20 mL/hr.

Just before you are scheduled to take him to Special Procedures, Mr. Clark becomes restless and anxious. During the neuro check you notice that his right pupil is sluggish. Although he denies pain, he says, "I don't care what the doctors say. I am not going to stay in this bed any longer!" When you call the physician, he orders Valium 5 mg IV push. However, as you give the IV push medication to Mr. Clark, you notice a cloudy substance forming in the IV line and he reports a slight burning at his IV insertion site.

(continued)

Case Study
Kent Clark (Continued)

Medical Orders

Bedrest
HOB elevated 30 degrees
Cervical collar

IVF: D5 1/2 NS at 20 mL/hr
Neuro checks q 2 hr
Valium 5 mg IV push now

Critical Thinking Questions

- What clinical symptoms alert you that Mr. Clark's condition is changing, and what additional assessments will you do?

- Identify the source of the pain at the IV insertion site and the cloudy substance in the IV tubing.

- Describe special positioning and transfer techniques to be followed for Mr. Clark.

- What could you have done to prevent these complications, and how will you intervene now?

- How will you handle Mr. Clark's anger and prevent him from getting out of bed?

Integrated Nursing Care

Concepts

Neuro assessment ⟷ IV push ⟷ Safety

In a patient with a closed head injury, bleeding or swelling may occur within the confines of the skull, leading to increased ICP. This increased ICP could cause extensive brain damage. Mr. Clark became increasingly restless and anxious, which could be a subtle sign of increased ICP. Even slow bleeding inside the cranium can cause changes. When you observe a change, immediately complete a neuro assessment to determine if there are further neurologic alterations. When Mr. Clark became restless, you found that his right pupil was more sluggish to light than the left, which is another sign of in-

creased ICP. Complete neuro checks as often as his condition warrants, and immediately report subtle changes in neuro checks to the physician. Meticulous documentation of baseline neuro checks and subsequent assessments is important to detect subtle neurologic changes (see Chapter 17).

Cervical spinal injuries can vary in severity, and even hairline fractures can become unstable if the patient is not positioned and transferred correctly. Mr. Clark has a cervical collar and the physician has asked you to minimize his movement. If you need to turn Mr. Clark, keep his head lowered and then logroll him as a unit without flexing or turning his neck. Obtain help from additional staff so that you can stabilize his head, neck, and torso in straight alignment while he is being turned (Taylor et al., 2005). When Mr. Clark is transferred from the bed to a stretcher, use a drawsheet to gently and carefully move him as a unit. Even though he has

(continued)

Case Study
Kent Clark (Continued)

a cervical collar, do not assume that it is safe for him to sit up further in the bed or get up and move around.

Mr. Clark is angry and wants to get out of bed. Restraints would be the least desirable option for him. At this time, placing restraints on him could increase his agitation and make him feel more trapped, and this could increase his ICP (see Chapter 3). For Mr. Clark, careful pharmacologic sedation may be a better option. The physician has ordered Valium to reduce his agitation and anxiety. Another possible intervention is to help Mr. Clark feel more in control of his environment. This could be as simple as having a family member stay with him, and checking on his needs frequently.

Pain at the IV site could mean that the IV is not patent. Carefully observe the IV site for any signs of phlebitis or infiltration before and while giving the IV push. If you determine that Mr. Clark's IV has a good blood return and is not infiltrated, the burning sensation at his IV site may be from the Valium administration. Valium as well as other medications can be irritating. Give the medication and the flush that follows at a slower rate. If not contraindicated, some medications can also be diluted if ordered (Karch, 2004).

The most probable cause for the cloudy appearance in Mr. Clark's IV line is precipitation of the drug due to chemical incompatibility of the Valium and the IV fluid of D5 1/2 NS. When giving any medication through an IV line, you must know whether the drug and IV solution are chemically compatible (see Chapter 5). When IV drugs are not compatible, a reaction immediately occurs that may not be visible to the eye but nevertheless can be dangerous. To prevent this, flush the IV line before and after medication administration per institution policy. Since a precipitate has already formed, clamp the tubing off closest to Mr. Clark and make sure that the cloudy substance does not reach him (see Chapter 5). Some hospitals require discontinuing the IV and restarting another IV with new IV tubing; other hospitals require changing only the IV tubing. If signs of incompatibility occur, notify the physician and continue to assess Mr. Clark's need for further medication.

Case Study
Lucille Howard

Lucille Howard, age 78, is in the hospital for a severe urinary tract infection (UTI). She has a history of urinary retention and UTIs. She is overweight, has a history of heart failure, and is allergic to many medications, including several antibiotics. Twenty-four hours ago she had severe nausea and vomiting and was ordered nothing by mouth (NPO). She has an IV catheter inserted in her left arm, infusing D5 1/2 NS @ 75 mL/hr. Mrs. Howard just had a triple-lumen urinary retention catheter inserted for continuous bladder irrigation with amphotericin B. The catheter was inserted at 6:30 a.m. and your shift started at 6:45 a.m. During your shift, you notice that she begins to have some coarse audible breath sounds and difficulty breathing. She reports pain in her abdomen.

Medical Orders

Amphotericin B 50 mg in 1,000 mL sterile H_2O irrigating in bladder at 40 mL/hr for 5 days
Strict I&O

IVF: D5 1/2 NS @ 75 mL/hr
NPO

Critical Thinking Questions

- What are possible causes of Mrs. Howard's current symptoms?

- What actions will you take?

- How would you identify the source of her current symptoms?

(continued)

Case Study
Lucille Howard (Continued)

Integrated Nursing Care

Concepts

Fluid overload ⟷ Allergic reactions ⟷ I & Os

There are several potential causes for Mrs. Howard's symptoms. In light of her drug sensitivities, she may be allergic to the amphotericin B. Allergic responses can include difficulty breathing as well as itching and a rash. Another source of her symptoms could be related to her heart problems. People with heart problems can easily become overloaded with fluid. Symptoms of fluid overload, a common problem for patients with heart failure, include crackles, abnormal heart sounds, and possibly edema. A final possibility is that her catheter is placed incorrectly in the vagina rather than the bladder.

To determine the cause of Mrs. Howard's symptoms, you need to perform several assessments. First, auscultate her heart and lung sounds and palpate her abdomen. Also assess for a rash on her skin, and ask her if she has any itching. If her heart and lung sounds are normal but her lower abdomen is hard, check for the position of the catheter. Sometimes it is difficult to tell if the catheter is in the right position just by looking, especially if the area around the catheter is swollen or if your patient is overweight. You can also check inputs to see if they match outputs. Currently, Mrs. Howard is getting 75 mL/hr of IV fluid and 40 mL/hr of the amphotericin B irrigant. She should be putting out in her urine at least 70 mL/hr: the hourly output of the urinary irrigant (40 cc) plus the least amount of urine you would expect to see in an hour (30 mL). If the catheter is in the correct place and her overall input is higher than the output, you are placing Mrs. Howard at risk for overload. If the catheter is not in the correct place, then you are giving her a vaginal irrigation and not the bladder irrigation that is ordered (see Chapter 12).

If Mrs. Howard is having an allergic reaction, stop the irrigant immediately, follow anaphylactic protocol, and notify the physician. If she is beginning to have problems with fluid overload due to her heart problems, reduce the IV rate to TKO, stop the irrigant, and notify the physician for further orders. If you discover that the catheter was not placed correctly, stop the irrigant, leave the catheter in place, and obtain another catheter kit. Insert the new triple-lumen urinary retention catheter into the urinary meatus and then remove the other catheter. Begin your irrigations once the new catheter is in place, and notify the physician. Continue to monitor Mrs. Howard until you are certain she is stabilized and her symptoms have resolved.

Case Study
Janice Romero

Janice Romero, age 24, has recently been diagnosed with acute lymphocytic leukemia (ALL). To provide long-term venous access, she was admitted to have an implanted port placed. She had a 21-gauge peripheral IV inserted in her right arm prior to surgery. After her port was placed, Mrs. Romero's physician ordered 2 units of packed red blood cells (PRBCs). Once you obtain the PRBCs from the blood bank, you note to the nursing aide that the blood seems very cold. She says, "Oh, that isn't a problem; it's just like warming up lunch." When you talk to Mrs. Romero about giving consent for the blood transfusion, she tells you that the last time she received blood she had chills and fever during the transfusion.

Medical Orders

2 units packed RBCs stat
IVF: D5 1/2 NS at 50 mL/hr

Critical Thinking Questions

- Identify the site you will use to administer blood to Mrs. Romero. Why did you choose this site?

- Describe the technique you will use to administer blood to Mrs. Romero.

(continued)

Case Study
Janice Romero (Continued)

- Identify the purposes for warming blood, and describe the safest way to warm blood.

- Considering Mrs. Romero's history and diagnosis, describe the precautions you will implement before giving her blood.

Integrated Nursing Care

Concepts

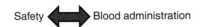

Safety ⬌ Blood administration

Before Mrs. Romero can receive blood, you must select an appropriate site (see Chapter 15). Site selection depends on the gauge of the IV and the fluid infusing in the IV. Blood must be given through a large-bore catheter to prevent red blood cell damage. Since dextrose will cause hemolysis, blood can be administered only with normal saline. For these two reasons, the optimal site for blood administration is her implanted port. Before you give her blood through the port, be certain that the port is not dedicated for other infusions, such as chemo.

Since the implanted port is new, ensure that it is working properly prior to use. Depending on your hospital policy, wear a mask and sterile gloves when accessing the port, particularly since she has leukemia and may be immunocompromised. In addition, a larger-gauge (19) Huber needle is recommended for giving blood (see Chapter 15). Check the port for patency and blood return per hospital policy. Infuse the normal saline slowly while you observe the implanted port site for signs of swelling. If the port shows any sign of infiltration, notify the physician, and choose another site to give her blood.

Some patients may need to have their blood warmed before it is administered. This includes patients who are at risk for cardiac arrhythmias, patients with unusual immune responses, as well as neonatal and pediatric patients. Various devices exist to warm blood. Do not use the microwave to warm any blood product: it coagulates the proteins of the blood and causes severe hemolysis that could be fatal. Whenever you need to warm blood, always use a blood warmer that has been approved by your institution.

Mrs. Romero's past history of chills and fever are signs of a possible transfusion reaction; thus, she is at increased risk for a transfusion reaction. Ensure that she has a signed consent form and that she fully understands her need for the blood. The physician needs to be aware of this history of a transfusion reaction. The physician may order premedication with diphenhydramine (Benadryl), acetaminophen (Tylenol), or hydrocortisone prior to blood administration to reduce the risk for developing another reaction. Stay with her for at least 15 minutes at the beginning of the transfusion. Continue to monitor her vital signs frequently per hospital policy. When you leave her room, make sure her call light is available, and instruct her to contact you if she has any unusual symptoms.

Case Study
Gwen Galloway

Mrs. Galloway, age 64, had a left-sided mastectomy and is now receiving follow-up chemotherapy for recurrent breast cancer with axillary node involvement. She has been hospitalized for 48 hours. She reports pain on her left side and under her left arm. She has a right double-lumen Hickman catheter inserted. Recent laboratory work shows a low white blood cell count of 1.8 µL and a low platelet count of 39,000/µL. She also bleeds and bruises very easily. You have to obtain vital signs and provide a.m. care. You also need to draw a complete blood count and change the dressing on her central line.

Medical Orders

VS q 4 hr
CBC now and every a.m.
Morphine sulfate (MSO$_4$) IV 6–8 mg q 2 hr and prn pain
Cefazolin sodium (Ancef) 1 g IV q 8 hr
Change central line dressing q 72 hr

(continued)

Case Study
Gwen Galloway (Continued)

Critical Thinking Questions

- What special precautions should you take while obtaining Mrs. Galloway's vital signs?

- Explain why some sites would be contraindicated when taking Mrs. Galloway's temperature.

- Describe the special precautions you would take when drawing blood from Mrs. Galloway; identify the site where you would draw the blood.

- Identify your interventions when changing Mrs. Galloway's central line dressing and the rationale for these interventions.

- Discuss the equipment used, restrictions, and concerns regarding Mrs. Galloway's personal care.

Integrated Nursing Care

Concepts

Vital signs ⬌ Bleeding risk ⬌ Infection risk

To individualize care, always assess your patient's condition and special needs. When a patient undergoes a mastectomy, she will often have lymph nodes removed from the affected side. Taking a blood pressure reading in the affected arm could interfere with circulation and harm the extremity (see Chapter 1). In Mrs. Galloway's case, her affected side is on the left, so take her blood pressure on the right side.

Mrs. Galloway has a low platelet count, which places her at risk for bleeding (see Chapter 1). In addition, her low white blood cell count places her at risk for infection and other complications. Therefore, taking a rectal temperature would be contraindicated for Mrs. Galloway. It would also be contraindicated to take a left-sided axillary temperature on Mrs. Galloway because she is still having some discomfort due to her recent mastectomy.

Given Mrs. Galloway's risk for bleeding, would sticking her be the best choice to obtain her CBC? Due to the risk for prolonged bleeding, her central line may provide the best access for a blood specimen (see Chapter 15). Determine whether her physician has restricted her central line for chemotherapy. If her central line is dedicated to chemotherapy only, obtain a blood specimen by doing a direct stick. If you needed to do a direct stick, using Mrs. Galloway's left side would be contraindicated due to the mastectomy. You will need to apply pressure to the site for a longer period of time because of her increased risk for bleeding.

When changing Mrs. Galloway's central line dressing, use strict sterile technique due to her increased risk for infection. Depending on agency policy, you may also need to place a mask on yourself and Mrs. Galloway. To prevent bleeding and bruising at the central line site, do not move or pull on the catheter as you are manipulating the central line dressing.

Several restrictions could apply when performing Mrs. Galloway's personal care. Patients at risk for bleeding should avoid shaving. Another concern is the potential for bleeding from the mucous membranes when using a hard-bristled toothbrush and dental floss. Use mouth rinses and very soft toothettes to minimize trauma (see Chapter 7).

Case Study
George Patel

George Patel, age 64, was admitted to your floor 3 days ago following surgical insertion of a tracheostomy tube. His diagnosis prior to surgery was acute upper airway obstruction. He has a left IV heparin lock. Currently, he is receiving O_2 per his trach at 40%. His pulse oximetry readings have been consistently running in the low 90s. He quickly becomes short of breath when his oxygen is interrupted during suctioning. During your shift, you will have to suction Mr. Patel as needed and provide routine trach care. You will also need to transport him with portable oxygen to radiology for his AP and lateral chest x-rays.

Medical Orders

MSO_4 2–6 mg IV q 2–4 hr prn for pain
Pulse ox q shift and prn
Trach care q shift and prn
Suction trach prn

AP and lateral chest x-rays
O_2 per trach Venturi mask at 40%
IV lock flush q shift

Critical Thinking Questions

- How would you determine when Mr. Patel needs to be suctioned?

- Describe expected outcomes when suctioning and providing trach care.

- How would you determine when Mr. Patel needs to have trach care?

- When transporting Mr. Patel to the radiology department, what precautions should you implement to ensure his safety?

Integrated Nursing Care

Concepts

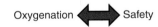

Oxygenation ⬌ Safety

To evaluate the need for suctioning, first assess Mr. Patel's respiratory status. Examine his oxygen saturation and compare it to his baseline. If his oxygen saturation is decreased from his baseline, this may be an indication that he needs to be suctioned. If you have a physician's order to hyperoxygenate, this would be the time to do so. Observe his respirations to determine if they are more labored than usual. Listen to his lung sounds for crackles or wheezes. Also, listen around his trach for gurgling. Does he have a productive cough? All of these signs and symptoms are indications that he needs to be suctioned.

To assess the need for trach care (see Chapter 14), closely examine his trach as well as the trach ties and precut gauze dressing. If it appears wet or moist, trach care would be indicated. If his trach dressing appears dry and intact, you may want to wait until later in your shift to do trach care. Suctioning and subsequent coughing will often soil the trach dressings, so experienced nurses wait until after suctioning to change the trach dressing.

(continued)

Case Study
George Patel (Continued)

Your expected outcomes when suctioning a tracheostomy include minimizing hypoxia, discomfort, and fatigue. Hypoxia may be reduced by hyperoxygenating the patient before suctioning (which must be ordered by a physician). When you suction Mr. Patel, limit the length of suction time to 10 seconds and allow him to rest before suctioning him again (see Skill 14-16). During trach care or repeat suctioning, quickly replace his oxygen source and limit the time his oxygen is interrupted. Since Mr. Patel has a "fresh" trach, it is very likely he will need to be premedicated with morphine for pain. Morphine depresses respirations, so continually assess Mr. Patel's respiratory status after administering the pain medication. In addition, adequate rest periods are needed to minimize fatigue from suctioning. Mr. Patel may require a rest period between suctioning the trach and his trach care.

The precautions you would take when transporting Mr. Patel focus on providing adequate oxygenation. First, assess Mr. Patel's oxygen saturation and respiratory status prior to transport. If indicated, suction Mr. Patel before he leaves his room. You must also check that the green portable oxygen tank is full and the label says "oxygen." Before turning off his wall oxygen, make sure the portable oxygen tank is working properly and that the equipment is ready. This avoids interruption of his oxygenation while placing him on the portable oxygen.

Advanced Case Studies

Cole McKean is a 4-year-old boy in the pediatric intensive care unit (PICU). He weighs 22 kg. He was admitted 3 days ago after nearly drowning in a neighbor's pool. He was submerged for 5 to 10 minutes. The neighbor initiated CPR and the rescue team had a heart rate established within 10 minutes of their arrival. The aspirated pool water caused a severe inflammatory response resulting in pulmonary edema. Cole is intubated with an endotracheal tube (ETT) and is on a mechanical ventilator. The past 2 days he produced copious bronchial secretions and required suctioning about every 2 hours. Today his breath sounds are clearer and he requires less frequent suctioning. He is being weaned off oxygen. The plan for today is possible extubation. An arterial line is in place in his left radial artery, infusing NS at 2 to 3 mL/hr. A PICC line with an infusion of D5 1/2 NS @ 75 mL/hr is inserted into his right arm. His heart rate, respiratory rate, and arterial waveform are being monitored. The pulse oximeter sensor is applied to his right toe. He has an indwelling urinary (Foley) catheter to gravity drainage and a nasogastric tube in place to low intermittent suction. He is receiving sedation but is opening his eyes at times and moving his extremities. He is becoming more active.

The alarm goes off on the ventilator. You look at Cole. His eyes are open and he is making crying sounds. You know when a child is properly intubated he or she cannot make sounds. You notice that his oxygen saturation level has dropped to 81% and his color is dusky. He is breathing on his own around the tube; his abdomen is rounded. You are assessing Cole's respiratory status and oxygenation when the physician comes to the bedside. The physician tells you to remove the ET tube and begin oxygen at 40% via face mask. When you place Cole on the face mask, his oxygen saturation returns to the mid-90s. The physician says, "This little fellow was ready to get rid of his tube." She orders a follow-up ABG to be drawn in 15 minutes.

Medical Orders

Continuous pulse oximetry
Maintain O$_2$ saturation 92–98%
Vent settings: 36% O$_2$, IMV 36, Pressures 26/6
VS q 1 hr
Neuro checks q 1 hr
Suction prn

Foley to gravity
I&O
NG to low intermittent suction
ABGs q 2 hr
IVF: D5 1/2 NS @ 75 mL/hr
Arterial line: NS 2–3 mL/hr

Critical Thinking Questions

- Describe your initial actions in response to a possible extubation.

- How can the technique of drawing ABGs be adapted for a pediatric patient?

(continued)

Case Study
Cole McKean (Continued)

- How will Cole's response be evaluated now that he is on an oxygen mask?

- Identify the nursing skills involved in monitoring Cole's respiratory status.

- Develop a plan of care that will allow Cole rest and sleep periods but also allow hourly assessments.

Integrated Nursing Care

Concepts

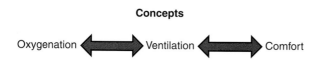

Oxygenation ⟷ Ventilation ⟷ Comfort

When a patient is intubated, the patency of this airway is a critical priority. When you hear Cole cry, you must determine if his ETT is in the proper place. Listen with your stethoscope over the lung fields and abdomen. If you do not hear ventilator-induced breath sounds over the lung fields, then the ETT is not in place. Because a child's neck is so short, it is not difficult to displace a tracheal tube into the esophagus. If this occurs, you may hear ventilator-cycled sounds in the abdomen. Signs that an ETT is not in the correct position include unstable oxygen saturation levels, cyanosis, and abdominal distention. In Cole's situation, you determine that the ETT is no longer in the lungs. All patients on mechanical ventilation must have an Ambu bag and a mask of the correct size at the bedside. Cole did not require mask-bag respirations at this time, but he has the potential for this need.

When you are evaluating Cole's response, the ABG results will guide clinical decision making regarding oxygen delivery. In Cole's case, 10 to 15 minutes after changing to the 40% oxygen mask, you draw an ABG (see Chapter 16). The results come back as follows: PaO_2, 82 mm Hg; $PaCO_2$, 46 mm Hg; pH, 7.34; HCO_3, 20 mEq/L. This ABG shows that Cole's oxygen level is acceptable and there is no indication for immediate reintubation. ABGs will continue to be drawn periodically to evaluate Cole's response to treatment.

To monitor his respiratory status, observe his work of breathing, count his respiratory rate, observe his color, and auscultate breath sounds. If he shows no significant respiratory distress and has a stable respiratory rate and clear breath sounds, he is responding well to the change in his oxygen source. In addition, continuously monitor the oxygen saturation level via pulse oximetry. Immediately report to the physician any increases or decreases in oxygen saturation.

Because children have a small total blood volume, the blood drawn back in the arterial line is usually not discarded but returned to the patient after the laboratory sample is drawn. Smaller volumes of blood are sent to the laboratory in pediatric specimen tubes. The setup for a pediatric arterial line delivers a smaller volume of fluid when the fast-flush release is activated (i.e., the pigtail is pulled).

When a patient, especially a child, is critically ill, cluster your hands-on care so that the patient will have a significant amount of sleep and rest between hourly interventions. One of the initial assessments a nurse makes in an intensive care setting is to determine that each of the monitoring devices is accurately displaying the patient's status (see Chapters 14 and 16). After you determine that the monitors accurately reflect the patient's vital signs, obtaining alternating sets of vital signs from the patient and from the monitor may be permitted, according to hospital policy. Maintain a quiet environment. Because of the noise and activity of the intensive care unit, many infant and child intensive care units dim the lights at night to create day/night cycles for the children.

Case Study
Dewayne Wallace

Dewayne Wallace, age 19, was admitted to the emergency department approximately 4 hours ago with a stab wound that he received in a knife fight while intoxicated. You are told to "pick up" Dewayne's case while his nurse attends to a new emergency. She gives you the following report: He was admitted in respiratory distress and bleeding from the stab wound. His wound is on the right side at the sixth intercostal space and is approximately 1″ in length, sutured and intact. The chest x-ray confirmed a right hemothorax, and as a result the physician inserted a chest tube. The chest tube is connected to a disposable drainage system and placed to suction at −20 cm H_2O. The chest tube is draining a small amount of dark-red blood. There has not been any new drainage for the past 2 hours.

Dewayne's most recent vital signs were as follows: temperature, 98.4°F; pulse, 88 beats/min; respirations, 24/minute; blood pressure, 112/74 mm Hg. He is receiving oxygen via face mask at 30% and is on continuous pulse oximetry. The oxygen saturation level is currently 96%. He says he feels short of breath. He does not have labored breathing and is not using accessory muscles. He reports pain at the chest tube insertion site and stab wound site. He has a patent IV infusing in his left forearm. His lab work reported a blood alcohol level of 0.12. The nurse giving report says, "Good luck with that delinquent. He says he's in pain, but I think he already drank his pain medication from a bottle."

Dewayne turns on his call light. When you approach him, you notice his breathing is labored with subclavicular retractions. The pulse oximeter reads 95%. Dewayne says, "This thing in my side really hurts."

You take another set of vital signs: temperature, 98.6°F; pulse, 90 beats/min; respirations, 37/minute; blood pressure, 118/78 mm Hg. You find the breath sounds are diminished on the right. The chest drainage tubing is in the bed without a dependent loop, and Dewayne has been lying on a segment of the tubing. You ask him to rate his pain on a scale of 1 to 10 (10 = worst), and he says, "About a 5." You ask if the medicine he got earlier helped with the pain, and he answers that he didn't get any pain medicine. When you check the chart you find that an order for hydrocodone bitartrate 5 mg/acetaminophen 500 mg (Lortab 5/500) was written about 3 hours ago, but when you look over the medication Kardex you do not see that any has been administered. You find his nurse and ask if the Lortab was given. The response you get is, "Are you kidding? If he's tough enough to drink and fight, he's tough enough for a little chest tube. He made his bed; he can just lie in it."

Medical Orders

Chest tube with drainage system to suction @ −20 cm H_2O
Oxygen at 30% via face mask
Continuous pulse oximetry

IVF: NS at 100 mL/hr
Lortab 5/500, 1 or 2 tabs q 4–6 hr PO prn pain

Critical Thinking Questions

- Which of Dewayne's needs is your first priority? Describe your assessments related to your first priority.

- How would you troubleshoot his chest tube drainage system? What could be the source of his respiratory distress?

- Describe the purpose of a chest tube drainage system for a hemothorax.

- Discuss valid reasons a nurse might not give a pain medication when there is a prn order.

(continued)

Case Study
Dewayne Wallace
(Continued)

- Discuss prejudices nurses may have that may prohibit adequate pain management.

Integrated Nursing Care

Concepts

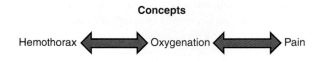

Hemothorax ⟷ Oxygenation ⟷ Pain

Your first priority is Dewayne's increased respiratory distress. While the change in oxygen saturation levels is very small, this is only because Dewayne's body is compensating for it now. Dewayne's work of breathing has dramatically changed, signaling a change in his respiratory status. Your preliminary assessment showed a respiratory rate of 37 breaths/minute, up significantly from his earlier respiratory rate of 24. When you inspected the chest you found subclavicular retractions; this indicates that Dewayne is using his intercostal muscles to breathe. When you auscultated breath sounds you found decreased air movement on the right, indicating a hemothorax.

In a hemothorax, blood collects in the pleural space and compresses a lung. The purpose of the chest tube is to evacuate the blood and allow the lung to expand fully. In Dewayne's case, the stab wound created a puncture in the pleura, allowing blood to accumulate within the pleural space. The right lung will need to be evaluated on a routine basis to make sure the blood in the pleural space has been removed so that the lung can re-expand. Any change in respiratory status may indicate a problem with the chest tube drainage system.

As you noted in this case, Dewayne has had a change in his respiratory status. Since you have completed his physical assessment, now begin inspecting the equipment. As with any equipment check, begin inspection at the patient and move to the equipment. Start your inspection at the insertion site of the chest tube. Observe the dressing to ensure it is occlusive and inspect the tubing for leaks, kinks, and dependent loops. Compare the amount of recent drainage in the drainage system to the volume of old

drainage, and check the amount of suction (see Chapter 14). In this case, Dewayne has been lying on his tubing, which would prevent it from draining properly. When you reposition Dewayne's tubing, approximately 60 mL of dark old blood flows into the drainage set. His respiratory status improves quickly. Thus, this accumulated blood in the pleural space was the source of his respiratory distress.

There are several situations in which giving a narcotic analgesic is contraindicated. During a life-saving procedure, pain is not always a priority. In this case, Dewayne did not receive pain medication before the insertion of his chest tube as he was at risk for respiratory arrest. Narcotics are also contraindicated when it is critical to assess alertness, because the narcotic might mask neurologic changes. Narcotic analgesics also are associated with the side effects of respiratory depression and vital sign changes. Patients sometimes do not receive the pain medication ordered because the nurse is worried about these side effects. Because of this, controversy exists as to whether the benefit of pain control outweighs the risk of side effects. Many hospitals have committees that can assist with these ethical decisions. A dialog among nurses, doctors, and pharmacists can result in optimal pain control with minimal side effects. Speak with the physician before independently deciding to withhold pain medication to prevent side effects.

Another reason nurses may withhold medication is their own preconception of the patient's pain and their own prejudices. Some nurses are not even aware that they have these feelings. As a nursing student, you need to understand how you will respond to patients, and you need to explore your own beliefs and prejudices. The accepted standard in nursing is that a patient defines his or her own pain and that it is the nurse's responsibility to manage it properly. Guidelines for pain management have been written by state Boards of Nursing, the U.S. Department of Health and Human Services, the World Health Organization, as well as other professional organizations.

Case Study
Robert Espinoza

Robert Espinoza, age 44, has just had exploratory abdominal surgery. The post-anesthesia recovery room (PACU) nurse calls at 2:10 p.m. to report on Mr. Espinoza and tells you he has a peripheral IV inserted in his right arm, infusing NS at 50 mL/hour. He has a midline abdominal dressing that is dry and intact with two Jackson-Pratt (JP) drains in place. He also has a nasogastric (NG) tube and an indwelling urinary (Foley) to gravity drainage. She reports that his NG tube has been checked for placement and has been draining moderate amounts of yellow-green contents. His vital signs in the PACU are as follows: temperature, 98.0°F; pulse, 86 beats/min; respirations, 16/minute; blood pressure, 134/80 mm Hg. At 2 p.m., he received 6 mg morphine sulfate (MSO$_4$) IV for a pain rating of 6 on a scale of 1 to 10 (10 = worst).

At 3 p.m., you receive Mr. Espinoza on your medical-surgical unit via stretcher by a hospital transporter. The NG tube tape that secured the NG to his nose is no longer in place. You also notice that the urinary drainage bag lying on top of his legs has a small amount of amber urine in the reservoir. While you are in his room, Mr. Espinoza says, "Hey, it feels like there's something wet under my back." His vital signs on arrival are as follows: temperature, 98.0°F; pulse, 130 beats/min; respirations, 18/minute; and blood pressure, 100/68 mmHg. His respirations are regular and unlabored and his skin color is pink. He now rates his pain as a 2 on a scale of 1 to 10 (10 = worst). Mr. Espinoza's family is anxiously waiting in the waiting room on your floor.

Medical Orders

Indwelling urinary catheter (Foley) to gravity
Strict I&O
NG to intermittent wall suction
IVF: NS @ 50 mL/hr

Routine JP drain care
Routine postop VS
MSO$_4$ 4–10 mg IV q 2–4 hr for pain

Critical Thinking Questions

- Considering Mr. Espinoza's immediate postop status, describe how you would transfer him from the stretcher to his bed.

- Prioritize, with rationales, your assessments and nursing care for Mr. Espinoza in the following areas:
  - Immediate physical assessments and interventions
  - Assessment and management of tubes
  - Pain management and comfort level
  - Care of his family

Integrated Nursing Care

Concepts

Postoperative care ⬌ Prioritization ⬌ Comfort

When transferring Mr. Espinoza to his bed, consider the following factors: minimizing his pain level, protecting his incision, and protecting the patency of his tubes. Excessive strain from moving can cause disruption and bleeding to his abdominal incision. Per hospital policy, carefully transfer him with the assistance of others. During transfer, be careful not to disrupt his tubes or dressings. Once Mr. Espinoza is in his bed, place his urinary drainage bag on the bed frame so that it hangs below the level of his bladder. This position will allow the urine to drain by gravity and decrease the possibility of a urinary tract infection (see Chapter 12).

Since Mr. Espinoza is a new postoperative patient, your first priority is to perform an assessment based on the ABC

(continued)

Case Study
Robert Espinoza (Continued)

criteria (airway, breathing, and circulation). Compare his vital signs upon arrival to his baseline vital signs. Mr. Espinoza's respiratory rate has not changed significantly from his baseline. If not contraindicated, elevate his head to facilitate deep breathing and continue to assess his airway and respiratory status (see Chapter 6).

Circulation is the next immediate priority. In Mr. Espinoza's case, his blood pressure has decreased and his heart rate has increased from his baseline in the PACU. Both of these changes could indicate decreased blood volume related to bleeding. Therefore, assess Mr. Espinoza's abdominal dressing to evaluate if it is dry and intact. Never assume that an incision is dry just because you cannot see any blood on top of the dressing. If the abdominal dressing is covered by foam tape, blood underneath the tape may not be easily visualized. Look under the patient to see if blood has trickled underneath the dressing. Mr. Espinoza said that he felt something "wet" under his back, and when turning him, you discover that there is a large puddle of bright-red blood underneath him that is caused by acute bleeding from his abdominal incision. Do not remove the abdominal dressing. You may, however, reinforce the dressing if you have a physician's order.

Identify all other possible sources of bleeding. When you assess the JP drains, note the color, amount, and consistency of blood. Assess his abdomen for signs of internal bleeding such as abdominal distention. Also check for decreased urine output, another sign indicating a possible decrease in blood volume. A urine output of less than 30 mL/hr may be a sign of hypovolemic shock. Although Mr. Espinoza is bleeding and has signs of decreased blood volume, he is not yet in hypovolemic shock. If Mr. Espinoza's blood pressure continues to drop, elevate his feet to increase venous return. Report all indications of internal and/or external bleeding to the physician. Acute postop bleeding requires surgical repair.

Your next priority is to ensure that all of his tubes are intact and working properly. One of the first tubes you want to assess for patency is his IV, particularly since he may be returning to surgery. The next tubes you want to examine are the JP drains. To maintain suction, a JP drain must be less than half full. Assess the color and other characteristics of the JP drainage (see Chapter 8). Next, assess his NG tube. Mr. Espinoza's NG tube tape is not secure, so you cannot assume that the tube is still in his stomach. Check the NG for placement, assess the color and amount of the return, and then place the NG to intermittent suction (see Chapter 11). Next, evaluate his urinary catheter to determine it is draining properly (see Chapter 12).

The next priority is to monitor Mr. Espinoza's pain level. If he is in acute pain, immediately consider incisional disruption. Because Mr. Espinoza is bleeding, you may need to give small increments as opposed to large amounts of morphine to prevent a further drop in his blood pressure. In addition to his physical comfort, attend to his possible anxiety about returning to the operating room. Maintain a calm voice and demeanor when caring for Mr. Espinoza.

Do not forget Mr. Espinoza's family, who are anxious to see him. It is helpful to send another staff nurse to keep them updated while you are busy in his room. When his condition stabilizes and before the family visits him, tell them about the tubes that they will see, including the reason for and function of each of the tubes. Be flexible when allowing the family to come in and visit Mr. Espinoza.

Case Study
Jason Brown, Gwen Galloway, Claudia Tran, and James White

This is your first week as an RN in a small rural hospital. You work the night shift on a medical-surgical unit. Tonight your only aide and a nurse have called in sick, which makes the unit short-staffed. You have notified the night supervisor that you need help, and she sends an aide from another floor to assist you. She tells you she can get someone on the floor to help you in about an hour, and instructs you to take care of the priority cases until that time.

You have six relatively uncomplicated patients, and you need to check their vital signs and give medications. You have four other patients about whom you are concerned:

- Jason Brown, a 64-year-old patient with a tracheostomy, has gurgling sounds coming from his trach and a frequent, nonproductive cough. His oxygen saturation level via pulse oximetry is 88%. You have orders to suction his trach prn.
- Gwen Galloway had been receiving chemotherapy and has now come back to the hospital with gastroenteritis. When you arrive on your shift, she is experiencing bouts of nausea and vomiting.

(continued)

Case Study

**Jason Brown,
Gwen Galloway,
Claudia Tran,
and James White
(Continued)**

- Claudia Tran, an 84-year-old patient from a nursing home, is post-CVA. She has a stage III pressure ulcer on her coccyx and a stage I ulcer on her left hip. She needs to be turned every 15 minutes because of rapidly developing erythema on bony prominences. She is confused and has fallen the past 2 nights when left unattended, even when restrained. Her family is visiting her now but plans to leave in 30 minutes.
- James White has COPD. The aide reports that the blood pressure from the automatic cuff is 168/100 mm Hg; his baseline is usually 130/70 mm Hg. The aide also reports that he has a severe headache but no other complaints.

Critical Thinking Questions

- Identify the order in which you would provide care to these patients. Explain your rationales as well as your interventions.

Integrated Nursing Care

Concepts

Oxygenation ➡ Perfusion ➡ Safety ➡ Wound prevention ➡ Comfort

Mr. Brown is having difficulty with airway clearance and oxygenation, so he will be your first priority. Nursing priorities always follow the "ABCs": airway, breathing, and circulation. He will require prompt tracheal suctioning and further evaluation of his respiratory status (see Chapter 14). When his oxygen saturation levels have stabilized, you can then attend to the other patients.

Next, address the dramatic change in vital signs that Mr. White is experiencing. Mr. White is at risk for a stroke if his blood pressure continues to stay elevated and is not controlled immediately. Before planning any other interventions, verify the blood pressure by taking it yourself with a manual cuff (see Chapter 1). Initial nursing assessment includes assessing the accuracy of the equipment as well as the accuracy of the information reported to you by an aide. The blood pressure you obtain is 190/110 mm Hg. Check for the physician's orders regarding possible prn blood pressure medications, such as sublingual Procardia. Call the physician right away and notify him or her of the change in Mr. White's status.

You know that Mrs. Tran is at high risk for falls if left unattended, and she may injure herself seriously if this occurs. Reducing her risk for injury is your next priority (see Chapter 3). In Mrs. Tran's case, you could ask a family member to stay the night, or at least until you get more help on the unit. Many families are willing to help if you make them aware of such situations. If the family leaves, ask the aide to remove the restraint, place the bed in a low position, and stay with Mrs. Tran until you get further help. You can delegate Mrs. Tran's positioning schedule to the aide.

Despite the obvious distress of vomiting, this is not a life-threatening situation for Mrs. Galloway; therefore, her condition is a lower priority than that of the other three patients. Mrs. Galloway requires comfort. Check if an antiemetic medication has been ordered; if not, call

Concepts

Prioritization ⬅➡ Delegation

the physician and obtain an order. Other interventions you can perform until her medication takes effect are lowering the lights, applying a cool cloth to the neck, decreasing noises, removing substances that may have a

(continued)

Case Study

Jason Brown, Gwen Galloway, Claudia Tran, and James White
(Continued)

strong odor (e.g., food and vomitus), and keeping her head elevated.

When prioritizing and delegating care, here are some questions that might help guide your decision-making process:

- Is the situation life-threatening?
- How rapidly could this patient deteriorate?
- How quickly can you remedy the problem?
- Who can provide assistance?

Whenever a patient's airway, breathing, or circulation is jeopardized, this is a life-threatening emergency. Base your priorities on the ABC criteria. Mr. Brown is your first priority because his airway and oxygenation are a problem. When a patient's condition has the potential to deteriorate rapidly, this is also a priority. In Mr. White's case, because of the spike in his blood pressure, he has the potential for a stroke. Preventing this life-threatening event requires immediate action. When two patients have problems of similar urgency such as oxygenation, respond to the problem that you can remedy the quickest. Sometimes when you have many activities to accomplish in a short period of time, it is difficult to take time to seek additional help. Many hospitals will have night supervisors to assist you with problem solving. Additionally, physicians are available by phone or in the hospital. Nonlicensed personnel such as aides are sometimes available to assist with noncritical tasks. A nursing skill to develop is prioritization of nursing care and delegation of noncritical tasks.

Case Study References

CDC (2003). MRSA (methicillin-resistant *Staphylococcus aureus*) fact sheet. Retrieved Feb. 6, 2004, from *http://www.cdc.gov/ncidod/hip/Aresist/ mrsafaq.htm*

Karch, A. M. (2004). *2004 Lippincott's nursing drug guide.* Philadelphia: Lippincott Williams & Wilkins.

Taylor, C., Lillis, C., & LeMone, P. (2005). *Fundamentals of nursing: the art and science of nursing care,* 5th ed. Philadelphia: Lippincott Williams & Wilkins

Glossary

A

abduction: movement away from the center or median line of the body

acid: substance containing a hydrogen ion that can be liberated or released

acidosis: condition characterized by a proportionate excess of hydrogen ions in the extracellular fluid; pH falls below 7.35

active transport: movement of ions or molecules across cell membranes, usually against a pressure gradient and with the expenditure of metabolic energy

acute pain: pain that is generally rapid in onset, varies in intensity from mild to severe, and may last from a brief period up to any period less than 6 months

adduction: movement toward the center or median line of the body

adventitious breath sounds: 1) abnormal breath sounds heard over the lungs; 2) sounds that are not normally heard in the lungs on auscultation

afebrile: a condition in which the body temperature is not elevated

agglutinin: antibody that causes a clumping of specific antigens

alkalosis: condition characterized by a proportionate lack of hydrogen ions in the extracellular fluid concentration; pH exceeds 7.45

Allen's test: an assessment determining the adequacy of the ulnar artery prior to accessing the radial artery for an arterial blood gas

allodynia: a characteristic feature of neuropathic pain; pain that occurs after a normally weak or nonpainful stimulus, such as a light touch or a cold drink

alopecia: baldness

alveoli: small air sacs at the end of the terminal bronchioles that are the site of gas exchange

ampule: a glass flask that contains a single dose of medication for parenteral administration

anesthetic: medication that produces such states as narcosis (loss of consciousness), analgesia, relaxation, and loss of reflexes

anion: ion that carries a negative electric charge

anorexia: lack or loss of appetite for food

antibody: immunoglobulin produced by the body in response to a specific antigen

antigen: foreign material capable of inducing a specific immune response

apnea: absence of breathing

approximated wound edges: edges of a wound that are lightly pulled together. Edges appear to be touching; wound appears closed.

arterial blood gas (ABG): a laboratory test that evaluates the oxygen, carbon dioxide, bicarbonate, and pH of an arterial blood sample, determining metabolic or respiratory alkalosis or acidosis

arteriovenous graft: a surgically created passage connecting an artery and a vein, used in hemodialysis

arthroplasty: surgical formation or reformation of a joint

atelectasis: incomplete expansion or collapse of a part of the lungs

auscultation: act of listening with a stethoscope to sounds produced within the body

autologous transfusion: a blood transfusion donated by the patient in anticipation that he or she may need the transfusion during a hospital stay

B

basal metabolism: amount of energy required to carry out involuntary activities of the body at rest

base: substance that can accept or trap a hydrogen ion; synonym for alkali

bell: (of stethoscope) hollowed, upright, curved portion used to auscultate low-pitched sounds such as murmurs

blood pressure: force of blood against arterial walls

body mass index (BMI): ratio of height to weight that more accurately reflects total body fat stores in the general population (weight in kg/height^2 in meters)

bradycardia: slow heart rate, usually below 60 beats per minute

bradypnea: abnormally slow rate of breathing

breakthrough pain: a temporary flare-up of moderate to severe pain that occurs even when the patient is taking around-the-clock medication for persistent pain

bronchial breath sounds: breath sounds heard over the trachea; high in pitch and intensity, with expiration being longer than inspiration

bronchodilator: medication that relaxes contractions of smooth muscles of the bronchioles

bronchovesicular breath sounds: normal breath sounds heard over the upper anterior chest and intercostal area

bruits: abnormal "swooshing" sounds heard on auscultation indicating turbulent blood flow

buffer: substance that prevents body fluid from becoming overly acid or alkaline

C

calorie: measure of heat, or energy; kilocalorie, commonly referred to as a calorie, is defined as the amount of heat required to raise 1 kg of water by 1°C

carbohydrate: organic compounds (commonly known as sugars and starches) that are composed of carbon, hydrogen, and oxygen; the most abundant and least expensive source of calories in the diet worldwide

cardiac arrest: sudden cessation of functional circulation of the heart (pulse), such as asystole or fibrillation, typically caused by the occlusion of one or more of the coronary arteries. Electrical activity may still be occurring and seen on the cardiac monitor as in electromechanical disassociation.

cardiac monitoring: visualization and monitoring of cardiac electrical activity

cardiopulmonary resuscitation (CPR): revival after apparent death by manually pumping the heart via the sternum and forcing oxygen into the lungs using mouth-to-mouth or rescue breathing

cardioversion: conversion of a pathological cardiac rhythm to normal sinus rhythm through low doses of an electrical device that applies synchronized countershocks to the heart

caries: cavities of the teeth

cation: ion that carries a positive electric charge

cerebral perfusion pressure (CPP): a way of calculating cerebral blood flow; formula is MAP (mean arterial pressure) minus ICP (intracranial pressure) equals CPP; normal CPP for an adult is 80 to 100 mm Hg

cerumen: ear wax; consists of a heavy oil and brown pigmentation

cholesterol: fatlike substance found only in animal tissues that is important for cell membrane structure, a precursor of steroid hormones, and a constituent of bile

chronic pain: pain that may be limited, intermittent, or persistent but that lasts for 6 months or longer and interferes with normal functioning

cilia: microscopic hairlike projections that propel mucus toward the upper airway so that it can be expectorated

colloid osmotic pressure: pressure exerted by plasma proteins on permeable membranes in the body; synonym for oncotic pressure

colostomy: artificial opening that permits feces from the colon to exit through the stoma

compartment syndrome: occurs when there is increased tissue pressure within a limited space. Leads to compromises in the circulation and the function of the involved tissue.

conscious sedation/analgesia: type of anesthesia used for short procedures; the intravenous administration of sedatives and analgesics raises the pain threshold and produces an altered mood and some degree of amnesia, but the patient maintains cardiorespiratory function and can respond to verbal commands

consciousness: the degree of wakefulness or ability to be aroused

constipation: passage of dry, hard stools

contracture: permanent shortening or tightening of a muscle due to spasm or paralysis

contusion: an injury in which the skin is not broken; a bruise

crackles: fine crackling sounds made as air moves through wet secretions in the lungs

crossmatching: determining the compatibility of two blood specimens

cutaneous pain: superficial pain usually involving the skin or subcutaneous tissue

cyanosis: bluish or grayish discoloration of the skin in response to inadequate oxygenation

D

dermis: underlying portion of the skin

diaphragm: (of stethoscope) large, flat disk on the stethoscope used to auscultate high-pitched sounds such as respiratory sounds

diastolic pressure: least amount of pressure exerted on arterial walls, which occurs when the heart is at rest between ventricular contractions

deep vein thrombosis: a blood clot in a blood vessel originating in the large veins of the legs

defecation: emptying of the large intestine; also called a bowel movement

defibrillation: stopping fibrillation of the heart by using an electrical device that applies countershocks to the heart through electrodes placed on the chest wall. It is hoped that this countershock will allow the heart's normal pacemaker to take over.

dehiscence: accidental separation of wound edges, especially a surgical wound

dehydration: decreased water volume

diabetes mellitus: a group of metabolic diseases characterized by elevated blood glucose levels resulting from defects in insulin secretion, insulin action, or both

diarrhea: passage of excessively liquid, nonformed stool

diffusion: tendency of solutes to move freely throughout a solvent from an area of higher concentration to an area of lower concentration until equilibrium is established

dynorphin: endorphin with the most potent analgesic effect

dyspnea: difficult or labored breathing

dysrhythmia: an abnormal cardiac rhythm; synonym is arrhythmia

E

ecchymosis: purplish discoloration resulting from infiltration of blood into the subcutaneous tissue

edema: accumulation of fluid in the interstitial tissues

elective surgery: surgery that is recommended but can be omitted or delayed without catastrophe

electrocardiogram (ECG/EKG): graphing of the electrical activity of the heart

electrolyte: substance capable of breaking into ions and developing an electric charge when dissolved in solution

embolus: foreign body, blood clot, or air in the circulatory system

emergency surgery: surgery that must be performed immediately to save the person's life or a body organ

endorphins: opioid neuromodulators; powerful pain-blocking chemicals that have prolonged analgesic effects and produce euphoria

endotracheal tube: polyvinylchloride airway that is inserted through the nose or mouth into the trachea using a laryngoscope

enema: introduction of a solution into the large intestine

enkephalins: opioid neuromodulators widespread throughout the brain and dorsal horn of the spinal cord; considered less potent than endorphins

enteral nutrition: alternate form of feeding that involves passing a tube into the gastrointestinal tract to allow instillation of the appropriate formula

epidermis: superficial portion of the skin

epithelialization: stage of wound healing in which epithelial cells move across the surface of a wound; tissue color ranges from "ground glass" to pink

erythema: redness or inflammation of an area as a result of dilation and congestion of capillaries

eschar: thick, leathery scab or dry crust composed of dead cells and dried plasma

eupnea: normal respirations

expiration: act of breathing out; synonym is exhalation

extension: the return movement from flexion; the joint angle is increased

extubation: removal of a tube

F

febrile: a condition in which the body temperature is elevated

fecal impaction: prolonged retention or an accumulation of fecal material that forms a hardened mass in the rectum

fenestrated: having a window-like opening

filtration: passage of a fluid through a permeable membrane whose spaces do not allow certain solutes to pass; passage is from an area of higher pressure to one of lower pressure

flatus: intestinal gas

flexion: bending of a joint so that the angle of the joint diminishes

fraction of inspired oxygen (FIO$_2$): concentration of oxygen delivered

fracture: a break in the continuity of the bone

G

gate control theory: theory that states that certain nerve fibers, those of small diameter, conduct excitatory pain stimuli toward the brain, while nerve fibers of a large diameter appear to inhibit the transmission of pain impulses from the spinal cord to the brain

gingivitis: inflammation of the gingivae (gums)

goniometer: an apparatus to measure joint movement and angles

granulation tissue: new tissue that is pink or red and composed of fibroblasts and small blood vessels that fill an open wound when it starts to heal

H

halitosis: offensive breath

hemodialysis: removal from the body, by means of blood filtration, of toxins and fluid that are normally removed by the kidneys

hemorrhage: excessive blood loss due to the escape of blood from blood vessels

hemorrhoids: abnormally distended veins in the anal area

hemothorax: blood in the pleural space

Homans' sign: pain in the calf when the toe is passively dorsiflexed; an early sign of venous thrombosis of the deep veins of the calf

hydrostatic pressure: force exerted by a fluid against the container wall

hyperextension: extreme or abnormal extension

hyperpyrexia: high fever, above 41°C

hypertension: blood pressure elevated above the upper limit of normal

hypertonic: having a greater concentration than the solution with which it is being compared

hyperventilation: condition in which there is more than the normal amount of air entering and leaving the lungs

hypervolemia: excess of blood volume

hypotension: blood pressure below the lower limit of normal

hypothermia: a body temperature below the lower limit of normal

hypotonic: having a lesser concentration than the solution with which it is being compared

hypoventilation: decreased rate or depth of air movement into the lungs

hypovolemia: deficiency of blood volume

hypovolemic shock: shock due to a decrease in blood volume

hypoxia: inadequate amount of oxygen available to the cells

I

ileal conduit: a surgical diversion formed by bringing the ureters to the ileum; urine is excreted though a stoma

ileostomy: artificial opening created to allow liquid fecal content from the ileum to be eliminated through the stoma

incident report: documentation that describes any injury or potential for injury suffered by a patient in a healthcare agency

inhalation: route used to administer medications directly into the lungs or airway passages

inspection: process of performing deliberate, purposeful observations in a systematic manner

inspiration: act of breathing in; synonym is inhalation

integument: skin

intracranial pressure (ICP): pressure within the cranial vault; normal ICP is less than 15 mm Hg

intractable pain: pain that is resistant to therapy and persists despite a variety of interventions

intradermal injection: injection placed just below the epidermis; sites commonly used are the inner surface of the forearm, the dorsal aspect of the upper arm, and the upper back

intramuscular injection: injection placed into muscular tissue; sites commonly used are the ventrogluteal, vastus lateralis, deltoid, and dorsogluteal muscles

intravenous route: route used to administer medications directly into the vein or venous system; the route of most rapid onset

ion: atom or molecule carrying an electric charge in solution

ischemia: insufficient blood supply to a body part due to obstruction of circulation

isotonic: having about the same concentration as the solution with which it is being compared

J

jaundice: condition characterized by yellowness of the skin, the whites of the eyes, mucous membranes, and body fluids as a result of deposition of bile pigment resulting from excess bilirubin in the blood; occurs in patients with liver and gallbladder diseases, some types of anemia, and hemolysis

K

ketosis: catabolism of fatty acids that occurs when an individual's carbohydrate intake is inadequate; without adequate glucose, catabolism is incomplete and ketones are formed, resulting in increased ketones

Korotkoff sounds: series of sounds that correspond to changes in blood flow through an artery as pressure is released

L

lipid: group name for fatty substances, including fats, oils, waxes, and related compounds

M

maceration: softening of tissue due to excessive moisture

medical asepsis: clean technique; involves procedures and practices that reduce the number and transfer of pathogens

metered-dose inhaler (MDI): device that delivers a controlled dose of medication with each compression of the canister

minerals: inorganic elements found in nature

N

nasal cannula: disposable plastic device with two protruding prongs for insertion into the nostrils; used to administer oxygen

nasogastric (NG) tube: a tube inserted through the nose into the stomach

nasointestinal (NI) tube: a tube inserted through the nose into the upper portion of the small intestine

nebulizer: method of delivering medication by dispersing fine particles of medication into the deeper passages of the respiratory tract

necrosis: localized tissue death

neuromodulators: endogenous opioid compounds; naturally present, morphine-like chemical regulators in the spinal cord and brain

neuropathic pain: pain that results from an injury to or abnormal functioning of peripheral nerves or the central nervous system

neurotransmitters: substances that either excite or inhibit target nerve cells

nociceptive: pain that is usually acute and transmitted after normal processing of noxious stimuli

nosocomial infection: hospital-acquired infection

NPO (nothing by mouth): nothing can be consumed by mouth, including medications, unless ordered otherwise

nutrient: specific biochemical substance used by the body for growth, development, activity, reproduction, lactation, health maintenance, and recovery from illness or injury

nutrition: study of the nutrients and how they are handled by the body, as well as the impact of human behavior and environment on the process of nourishment

O

obesity: weight greater than 20% above ideal body weight

occult blood: blood that is hidden in the stool

orthopnea: type of dyspnea in which breathing is easier when the patient sits or stands

orthostatic hypotension: temporary fall in blood pressure associated with assuming an upright position; synonym for postural hypotension

osmolarity: the concentration of particles in a solution, or a solution's pulling power

osmosis: passage of a solvent through a semipermeable membrane from an area of lesser concentration to an area of greater concentration until equilibrium is established

ostomy: an artificial opening; usually used to refer to an opening created for the excretion of body wastes

overhydration: increased water volume

P

pain threshold: the lowest intensity of a stimulus that causes the subject to recognize pain

pain tolerance: point beyond which a person is no longer willing to endure pain

pallor: paleness of the skin

palpation: an assessment technique that uses the sense of touch

partial or peripheral parenteral nutrition (PPN): nutritional therapy used for patients who have an inadequate oral intake and require supplementation of nutrients through a peripheral vein

pathogens: microorganisms that can harm humans

pediculosis: infestation with lice

pH: expression of hydrogen ion concentration and resulting acidity of a substance

percussion: the act of striking one object against another to produce sound

percutaneous endoscopic gastrostomy tube (PEG): a surgically or laparoscopically placed gastrostomy tube

perioperative nursing: wide variety of nursing activities carried out before, during, and after surgery

perioperative period: time frame consisting of the preoperative phase (starts with the decision that surgery is necessary and lasting until the patient is transferred to the operating room), the intraoperative phase (starts from arrival in the operating room until transfer to the post-anesthesia care unit), and the postoperative phase (begins with transfer to the post-anesthesia care unit and lasts until complete recovery from surgery)

peripheral neuropathy: an abnormal condition characterized by inflammation and degeneration of the peripheral nerves. Sensations reported include burning, tingling, numbness, and pins and needles.

peripheral vascular disease: pathological conditions of the vascular system characterized by reduced blood flow through the peripheral blood vessels

peritoneal dialysis: removal of toxins and fluid from the body by the principles of diffusion and osmosis; this is accomplished by introducing a solution (dialysate) into the peritoneal cavity

peritonitis: inflammation of the peritoneal membrane

petechiae: small hemorrhagic spots caused by capillary bleeding

plaque: transparent, adhesive coating on teeth consisting of mucin, carbohydrate, and bacteria

pleurae: membranes that cover the lungs

pleural effusion: fluid in the pleural space

pneumonia: inflammation or infection of the lungs

pneumothorax: air in the pleural space

podiatrist: one who treats foot disorders; synonym for chiropodist

precordium: the area on the anterior chest corresponding to the aortic, pulmonic, tricuspid, and apical areas and Erb's point

pressure ulcer: any lesion caused by unrelieved pressure that results in damage to underlying tissue

pronation: the act of lying face downward; the act of turning the hand so the palm faces downward or backward

protein: vital component of every living cell; composed of carbon, hydrogen, oxygen, and nitrogen

psychogenic pain: pain for which no physical cause can be identified

pulmonary embolism: obstruction of the pulmonary artery or one of its branches by a foreign body, air, or blood clot

pulse deficit: difference between the apical and radial pulse rates

pulse pressure: difference between systolic and diastolic pressures

pulse oximetry: noninvasive technique that measures the oxygen saturation (SpO_2) of arterial blood

pyorrhea: extensive inflammation of the gums and alveolar tissues; synonym for periodontitis

pyrexia: elevation above the upper limit of normal body temperature; synonym for fever

R

recommended dietary allowance (RDA): recommendations for average daily amounts of essential nutrients that healthy people should consume over time

referred pain: pain that is perceived in an area distant from its point of origin

residual: the amount of gastric contents in the stomach after the administration of a tube feeding

respiration: act of breathing and using oxygen in body cells

restraints: device used to limit movement or immobilize a patient

rotation: process of turning on an axis; twisting or revolving

S

sebaceous gland: gland found in the skin that secretes an oily substance called sebum

sediment: precipitate found at the bottom of a container of urine

shearing force: force created by the interplay of gravity and friction on the skin and underlying tissues; shear causes tissue layers to slide over one another and blood vessels to stretch and twist and disrupts the microcirculation of the skin and subcutaneous tissue

sinus tract: a cavity or channel underneath a wound that has the potential for infection

spirometer: instrument used to measure lung capacity and volume; one type is used to encourage deep breathing (incentive spirometry)

solute: substance dissolved in a solution

solvent: liquid holding a substance in solution

somatic pain: diffuse or scattered pain that originates in tendons, ligaments, bones, blood vessels, and nerves

Standard Precautions: precautions used in the care of all hospitalized patients regardless of their diagnosis or possible infection status; these precautions apply to blood, all body fluids, secretions, and excretions (except sweat), nonintact skin, and mucous membranes

sterile technique: surgical asepsis; being free of all microorganisms to prevent the introduction or spread of pathogens from the environment into a patient

stoma: artificial opening on the body surface

subcutaneous emphysema: small pockets of air trapped in the subcutaneous tissue; usually found around chest tube insertion sites

subcutaneous injection: injection placed between the epidermis and muscle, into the subcutaneous tissue; sites commonly used are the outer aspect of the upper arm, the abdomen, the anterior aspects of the thigh, the upper back, and the upper ventral or dorsogluteal area

sublingually: under the tongue

supination: turning of the palm or foot upward

suppository: a conical or oval solid substance shaped for easy insertion into a body cavity and designed to melt at body temperature

surfactant: lipoprotein produced by the alveolar epithelium; reduces surface tension, allowing alveolar sacs to open easily

surgical asepsis: sterile technique; involves practices used to render and keep objects and areas free from microorganisms

surgical staples: stainless-steel wire used to close a surgical wound

surgical sutures: thread or wire used to stitch parts of the body together

systolic pressure: highest point of pressure on arterial walls when the ventricles contract

T

tachycardia: abnormally rapid heart rate, usually above 100 beats per minute in an adult

tachypnea: abnormally rapid rate of breathing

tartar: hard deposit on the teeth near the gum line formed by plaque buildup and dead bacteria

thoracentesis: aspiration of fluid or air from the pleural space

thrill: palpable feeling caused by turbulent blood flow

thrombophlebitis: inflammation in a vein associated with thrombus formation

thrombosis: the formation or development of a blood clot

total parenteral nutrition (TPN): nutritional therapy that bypasses the gastrointestinal tract; used in patients who cannot take food orally; meets the patient's nutritional needs by way of nutrient-filled solutions administered through a central vein

tracheostomy: curved tube inserted into an artificial opening made into the trachea; comes in varied angles and multiple sizes

trans fat: product that results when liquid oils are partially hydrogenated; these oils then become more stable and solid; trans fats raise serum cholesterol levels

Transmission-Based Precautions: precautions used in addition to Standard Precautions for patients in hospitals who are suspected of being infected with pathogens that can be transmitted by airborne, droplet, or contact routes; these precautions encompass all the diseases or conditions previously listed in the disease-specific or category-specific classifications

triglycerides: predominant form of fat in food and the major storage form of fat in the body; composed of one glyceride molecule and three fatty acids

tunneling: a passageway or opening that may be visible at skin level, but with most of the tunnel under the skin surface

turgor: fullness or elasticity of the skin

typing: determining a person's blood type (A, B, AB, or O)

U

undermining: areas of tissue destruction underneath intact skin along the margins of a wound

V

vagal stimulus or response: stimulation of the vagus nerve that causes an increase in parasympathetic stimulation, triggering a decrease in heart rate

Valsalva maneuver: voluntary contraction of the abdominal wall muscles, fixing of the diaphragm, and closing of the glottis that increases intra-abdominal pressure and aids in expelling feces

vasoconstriction: narrowing of the lumen of a blood vessel

vasodilation: an increase in the diameter of a blood vessel

venous stasis: decreased blood flow in the venous system related to dysfunctional valves or inactivity of the muscles of the affected extremity

ventilation: exchange of gases

ventriculostomy: a catheter inserted through a hole made in the skull into the ventricular system of the brain; can be used to monitor ICP and or drain cerebrospinal fluid

vesicular breath sounds: normal sound of respiration heard on auscultation over peripheral lung areas

vial: a glass bottle with a self-sealing stopper through which medication is removed

visceral pain: poorly localized pain that originates in body organs in the thorax, cranium, and abdomen

vital signs: body temperature, pulse, respiratory rate, and blood pressure; synonym for cardinal signs

vitamins: organic substances needed by the body in small amounts to help regulate body processes; are susceptible to oxidation and destruction

W

wheezes: continuous high-pitched squeaks or musical sounds made as air moves through a narrowed or partially obstructed airway

INDEX

Page numbers followed by "f" denote figures; "t" denote tables; and "b" denote boxes

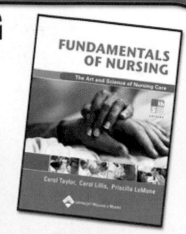
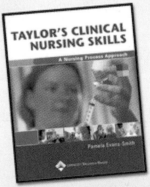
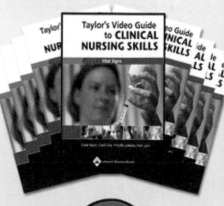